Clinical Electrocardiography

Clinical Electrocardiography
A Textbook

FIFTH EDITION

ANTONI BAYÉS DE LUNA
Autonomous University of Barcelona, Hospital de la Santa Creu i Sant Pau, Barcelona, Spain

MIQUEL FIOL-SALA
Illes Balears Health Research Institut (IdISBa), and Hospital Son Espases, Palma, Spain

ANTONI BAYÉS-GENÍS
Heart Institute, Hospital Universitari Germans Trias i Pujol, Badalona, Spain

ADRIÁN BARANCHUK
Division of Cardiology, Kingston Health Sciences Center, Kingston, Ontario, Canada

With contributions from:
ROBERTO ELOSUA
Hospital del Mar Medical Research Institute (IMIM), Barcelona, Catalonia, Spain

MANUEL MARTÍNEZ-SELLÉS
Department of Cardiology, Hospital General Universitario Gregorio Marañón, Madrid, Spain

WILEY Blackwell

This edition first published 2022
© 2022 John Wiley & Sons Ltd

Edition History
Fourth edition published 2012 by John Wiley & Sons Ltd

Registered Offices
John Wiley & Sons, Inc., 111 River Street, Hoboken, NJ 07030, USA
John Wiley & Sons Ltd, The Atrium, Southern Gate, Chichester, West Sussex, PO19 8SQ, UK

Editorial Office
9600 Garsington Road, Oxford, OX4 2DQ, UK

For details of our global editorial offices, customer services, and more information about Wiley products visit us at www.wiley.com.

Wiley also publishes its books in a variety of electronic formats and by print-on-demand. Some content that appears in standard print versions of this book may not be available in other formats.

Library of Congress Cataloging-in-Publication Data

Names: Bayés de Luna, Antoni, 1936- author. | Fiol-Sala, M. (Miquel), author. | Genis, A. Bayés, author. | Baranchuk, Adrian, author.
Title: Clinical electrocardiography : a textbook / Antoni Bayés de Luna, Miquel Fiol-Sala, Antoni Bayés-Genís, Adrián Baranchuk ; with contributions from Roberto Elosua, Manuel Martínez-Sellés.
Description: Fifth edition. | Hoboken, NJ : Wiley, 2022. | Includes bibliographical references and index.
Identifiers: LCCN 2021025949 (print) | LCCN 2021025950 (ebook) | ISBN 9781119536451 (cloth) | ISBN 9781119536468 (Adobe PDF) | ISBN 9781119536437 (epub)
Subjects: MESH: Electrocardiography–methods | Arrhythmias, Cardiac–diagnosis | Heart Diseases–diagnosis
Classification: LCC RC683.5.E5 (print) | LCC RC683.5.E5 (ebook) | NLM WG 140 | DDC 616.1/207547–dc23
LC record available at https://lccn.loc.gov/2021025949
LC ebook record available at https://lccn.loc.gov/2021025950

Cover Design: Wiley
Cover Image: © Courtesy of Antoni Bayés de Luna

Set in 9.25/12pt Palatino LT Std by Straive, Pondicherry, India

C092857_130921

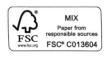

Contents

Preface

by Prof. Antoni Bayés de Luna

I am very pleased to present the 5th Edition of the book "Clinical Electrocardiography," for which in its four previous editions (1987, 1993, 1998, 2012) I was the sole author and responsible for it.

Given my age, and foreseeing the book continuity in the future, three expert cardiologists—Adrián Baranchuk, Antoni Bayés-Genís, and Miquel Fiol-Sala—accompany me in the present edition as co-authors. All three have worked for many years with me in the field of clinical electrocardiography, and together we have selected and included in the book what we considered more interesting from the work published in the last 10 years. It is therefore not a book that has four cardiologists acting as editors of the work performed by many co-authors, but a book of clinical electrocardiology in which four cardiologists become joint authors of the entire work.

I am satisfied and happy with the choice. Adrián Baranchuk has achieved success in Canada, far from his country, Argentina, and has turned his center, Queen's University, into a benchmark in arrhythmology, not only in all of America but also worldwide. Toni Bayés-Genís, my son, is a worldwide expert in heart failure who has positioned his center, Hospital Germans Trias de Badalona, as one of the best in Europe in its specialty. And finally, Miquel Fiol, the oldest of my dear collaborators for more than 40 years, is a great expert in ECG and has made original and very valuable contributions from his Hospital in Mallorca, especially in the field of ischemic heart disease.

I have been fortunate that all three have accepted this challenge. All of them have exceptional qualities that make them the best collaborators, so that this book continues to be a "work of the author" thanks to their contributions.

Nevertheless, we have had the collaboration of other experts in specific aspects. For this edition, Dr Roberto Elosua is the sole author of Chapter 8—Epidemiology, and Dr Manuel Martínez-Sellés has reviewed Chapters 22 and 23. Also I would like to thank Iwona Cygankiewicz, Wojciech Zareba, Xavier Viñolas, Ramón Brugada, Javier García-Niebla, Juan Lacalzada-Almeida, José Nunes de Alencar, Delicia Lorente Gentille, José Guerra, Gemma Vilahur, Guiomar Mendieta, Luis Alberto Escobar-Robledo, and many others, for the help they have offered me regarding specific aspects and in previous editions, and my collaborators for many years, especially Andrés Carrillo, Jaume Riba, Josep Guindo, Josep Massó, Ignasi Duran, and Diego Goldwasser. Finally, I also am very grateful to my previous secretary Montse Sauri and currently Esther Gregoris for her excellent secretarial work and help throughout the entire process of this edition.

Also, I am glad to express my gratitude to Fundación Jesús Serra-Catalana Occidente for the great support given to us in the last nearly 25 years.

Finally, our very special gratitude to Professors Hein Wellens, Paul Puech, Eugene Braunwald, and Marcelo Elizari, authors of the forewords in previous editions. I am deeply grateful to Professors Pedro Brugada and Marcelo Elizari for the excellent prologues they have written for this edition.

I want to conclude by stating that electrocardiology continues to be a key piece in cardiological diagnosis, and its contribution is irreplaceable for the benefit of the patient to correctly focus the diagnosis and treatment of our patients. We trust that this book will help to achieve this goal.

I now leave the other authors to give their opinion on it.

Antoni Bayés de Luna
December 2020

Preface

by Drs Miquel Fiol-Sala, Antoni Bayés-Genís, and Adrián Baranchuk

This 5th edition of Clinical Electrocardiography is very special. Antoni has decided to invite some of his closest collaborators as co-authors of the book.

Working with Prof. Bayés de Luna is a privilege. Each one of us that have had the opportunity to share his vision, his vast knowledge, his deep understanding of electrocardiology, and more importantly, his view about humanity, the world and the reason for our existence, has felt at some point, the immensity of his Universe.

Antoni teaches to teach, teaches how to approach any conflict, concern, or disparity, with an open mind, without prejudices, exercising tolerance to overdrive frustration and in a calm manner that calls to understanding.

He has taught generations of cardiologists around the globe, he has traveled five continents and his voice has been heard in all academic environments. In addition, his lessons, books and papers, were replicated in each corner of the planet. His books were translated to more than 10 languages, and his way to understand human electricity, has helped millions of health care providers, from students and ECG techs to professors of medicine.

What makes Antoni unique?

Maybe his capacity of "giving" without "taking." Antoni never asks for a return on what he gives. It is natural for him to keep giving and giving: knowledge, opportunities, collaborations, money. . . All these co-authors have personally experienced what is being said here. Antoni would share his grants and honorariums with his stuff and collaborators, and several times we have questioned that he is not taking his share. Money, glory, or fame is not important to Prof. Bayés' de Luna. He would not ask anything in return; however, to work with him, you have to feel the same passion.

Antoni walks at a fast pace. This is not a metaphor. Antoni literally walks at a faster pace than any of us. In order to walk at his pace and to be at his side during a conversation through the corridors of Sant Pau Hospital, you have to almost run.

This is a reflection on what it takes to collaborate with him: at the same time, we would complete a registry, write 2–3 papers, an editorial, supervise students and fellows, create slides for presentations, interact with editorial groups and much more. You want to be at his side, you have to run.

And when you think you had enough, Antoni will tell you to stop and enjoy life, family, friends, and a good glass of wine. He will not like to know that you are missing a birthday, a celebration, or an important date, because you are working too hard. If it is difficult to explain, please imagine how difficult it is to keep his pace. . .

Clinical Electrocardiography 5th edition would not be possible without the amazing collaboration and commitment from Wiley and its staff. We learnt to communicate fluently, frequently, and to design strategies that are mutually convenient. All the editors of this book are grateful to Wiley for their decision to go ahead with this new edition.

In this book, the reader will find what we call the "Bayés' spirit." We have updated some chapters and references, but we have followed the way Antoni teaches. This is the "magic" of this book. Chapter after chapter, you will immerse into the Universe of a unique man and scientist. You will understand his approach to "active" and "passive" arrhythmias, you will enjoy his definitions, repetitions, and perspective of multiple aspects of human cardiac electricity.

We welcome you to the opportunity to dig deep in the mind of this amazing colleague. Here it is, all his knowledge condensed in a book for you to enjoy.

Open the book, and enjoy this trip to knowledge, page by page, like a slow train arriving to a desired destination.

This group of co-authors is pleased to bring you the 5th edition of Clinical Electrocardiography. For all of us, a dream comes true.

Sit down, and enjoy this unique ECG book!

Adrián Baranchuk, Antoni Bayés-Genís, and Miquel Fiol-Sala
December 2020

Foreword

by Dr Marcelo V. Elizari

Again, Professor Antoni Bayés de Luna has honored me with his invitation to write the foreword to the 5th edition of "Clinical Electrocardiography: A Text Book." I believe the main reason for this invitation lies in the old and unbreakable friendship that has bonded us since our first meeting in the Symposium "Recent Advances in Ventricular Conduction," organized by Mario Cerqueira Gomes in Oporto in 1973.

While the four previous editions that preced this issue were written by Prof. Bayés de Luna as the sole author, this textbook is co-authored by renowned experts in the field of electrocardiography and arrhythmias, such as Miquel Fiol-Sala, Antonio Bayés-Genís, and Adrián Baranchuk. Prof. Bayés de Luna's strong genetic influence, for his joy, has been transmitted to his son Antoni, who has followed the path of spirituality traced by his father.

More than a hundred years ago, Wilhelm Einthoven introduced the electrocardiogram. Some years later, Thomas Lewis, his successor and Wilson's teacher, made his invaluable contribution to the understanding of the mechanisms and diagnosis of rhythm disorders, causing a profound impact in the development of electrocardiography. And afterward, the introduction of the unipolar leads by Frank Norman Wilson continued drawing the virtuous circle, marking the dawning of a new era of great progress for the interpretation of morphologic changes in intraventricular bundle branch blocks and cardiovascular diseases. In 1949, Silvio Weidmann and Edouard Coraboeuf recorded the first intracellular cardiac action potential and in the 1960s, Benjamin Scherlag developed the technique for His bundle recording.

Both advances and the advent of newer diagnostic and therapeutic tools gave rise to a new discipline: clinical cardiac electrophysiology. Besides, the deep knowledge about molecular biology has fostered the recognition and management of different familial cardiomyopathies. Thus, invasive and non invasive diagnoses have allowed the correlation of the electrocardiographic imaging with subyacent physiopathologic mechanisms. Bayés de Luna honors in this book those pioneers and researchers that

are not only part of history but also of the present and future.

The usual question is what is the reason for a new book on already so extensively discussed topics. And the answer is straightforward: there is always a place for a good book and, particularly in cardiology, a specialty that has developed in an unpredictable fashion. The publication of a medical book always marks the crystalization of a noble objective: provide medical education by mentors, whose deep knowledge and vast experience contribute to the management of patients.

Bayés de Luna and collaborators have distilled their extraordinary medical knowledge in the field of electrocardiology based on their own experience and research and always appealing to a profuse and well-selected bibliography. Since current technological advances have dramatically changed the approach to the clinical significance of any morphologic or rhythm disorder, this textbook frames the fundamental concepts covering all the possibilities for the correct interpretation of an electrocardiogram.

The 5th edition of Clinical Electrocardiography is a well-structured and well-planned medical work for advanced students, internists, trainees in cardiology, clinicians and physicians in the emergency room to find in the electrocardiogram a diagnostic resource to broadly interpret the value of images more simply and easily. However, a detailed and thoughtful history and a meticulous physical examination are essential to reach an accurate diagnosis since a normal electrocardiogram does not rule out in any way the existence of a potentially malignant cardiomyopathy. Thus, the authors alert the reader about the limitations of this diagnostic method but also, about its sensitivity and specificity as determinants of its clinical usefulness.

Every chapter deals in detail with the anatomical basis, the underlying physiopathology of the electrocardiographic and vectorcardiographic manifestations, clinical implications and differential diagnosis of every electrocardiographic pattern or rhythm disorder. A perfect logic and a rigorous plan allow the reader to easily follow the steps to diagnosis, even if unfamiliar with the diagnostic methods of electrophysiologic and clinical exploration. An asset of this edition is the systematic description of each electrocardiographic phenomenon profusely illustrated with figures, sketches, and diagrams and the bringing together of the interrelated resources for a more comprehensive analysis. In this way, the readers are presented with a remarkable teatrise that highlights the surface electrocardiogram as the "gold standard" in clinical practice and, at the same time, pays tribute and glorifies the Spanish electrocardiology and cardiology.

Antoni has always been an inspiring leader in the field of electrocardiography and arrhythmias because his intellect, clinical sagacity, and pursuit of new horizons have led him to transcendent contributions of international impact that will remain in the history of cardiology. As a prestigious scientist and mentor, he has gained the recognition of the world scientific community and has achieved top national and international positions as a cardiologist through his prestige as a scientist and teacher. The academic training in cardiology at Sant Pau Hospital, under Antoni's genuine vocation for medical education, has become the seedbed for renowned cardiologists and electrocardiologists in the world.

Lastly, I feel genuinely happy and grateful to Antoni because Pedro Brugada, another giant in the world of electrocardiology, has also been invited to write more introductory words to this book. I am sure Pedro will agree with me that this 5th edition is worth the hightest merit because the reader will learn not only clinical electrocardiography but also to interpert and apply it on a scientific basis. Certainly, this 5th edition by Bayés de Luna and his well-known collaborators will become a "must" in all medical libraries for health carers in cardiology.

Prof. Marcelo V. Elizari
February 2021

Foreword

by Dr Pedro Brugada

In November 1982, almost 40 years ago, I presented my doctoral thesis at the University of Maastricht, The Netherlands. The topic was "New Observations on the Role of the AV Junction in tachycardias in Man." The promotor was the late Hein Wellens. As co-promotors, I had no less than the Physiologist Mauritz Allessie, and the Electrophysiologists Jeronimo Farre and the late Mark E. Josephson. It was a real dream becoming true. In the eighties, I do not believe any doctoral candidate had ever had such an exquisite panel. The doctoral thesis had been written in just two years and contained no less than nine original articles already published or accepted for publication in the most outstanding cardiology journals of the time.

Four years before, I had written almost two-hundred letters to any existing organization or foundation supposed to support education and research. By the time my cardiology training at the University of Barcelona was about to finish, I had discussed with my mentor, the late Paco Navarro-Lopez, the possibility of expending some time abroad before deciding upon my future career. The idea was to learn some clinical cardiac electrophysiology at a good laboratory. Electrophysiology was a new cardiology subspecialty. Only a few centers in the world were starting to perform electrophysiological investigations in man by means of electrode catheters placed within the heart via a venous access. Scherlag had performed the first recordings of electrical activity of the His bundle in man, in vivo, and Coumel in Paris and Durrer in Amsterdam started to provoke and stop cardiac arrhythmias in the in situ human heart using the same technology. At the other side of the Atlantic, a few centers were also exploring the value and limitations of these new techniques. Among them, Kenneth Rosen in Chicago was the closest follower of the European steps. The University of Maastricht was about to open its doors in 1977 and Hein Wellens, by that time an associate of Durrer, moved from Amsterdam to Maastricht (via Liege by the way) to become the first Professor of Cardiology of the new University. Together with Durrer, he had just published the proceedings of one of the first grand meetings in electrophysiology. The book was titled: "The conduction system of the heart." I had bought that book, did my best, but

I finished by not understanding a single chapter. That was the reason I wanted to go abroad and understand that book. It could not be that I just finished my cardiology training and could not understand a word about cardiac electrophysiology.

Obtaining a position as a visitor, fellow, or whatever name you may give it, was not an easy task. I was accepted both by Rosen in Chicago and Wellens in Maastricht, but the problem was how to finance my trip—initially planned for six months. The 200 letters became 200 hours of telephonic calls, appointments at institutions and foundations. Even I visited the president of the football club Barcelona to see whether they could help finance my stay abroad. The 200 letters and answers are a genuine piece of the black history of Spain in the immediate post-Franco time. The President of the Fundacion Pablo Iglesias wrote by hand a letter to me excusing himself, not for not having a grant for me, but for the letter "because they do not even had money to pay for a secretary and a typewriter."

When all hope was almost gone, something unusual was going to happen, something that justifies explaining all of this to you in this foreword. A young but mature cardiologist of the Hospital de San Pau in Barcelona had become the new President of the Arrhythmia Section of the Spanish Society of Cardiology. The first thing this new president did was to take care of the program for trainees, residents and fellows. He wanted electrocardiography and rhythmology to become an important domain in the knowledge of the future cardiologists. As president, he created also a grant for trainees to visit other centers than the one where they were being trained. I applied for the grant and obtained it. It was presented to me by the president, who was nobody else than Antoni Bayés de Luna. The grant was 25 000 pesetas, the equivalent to €400 nowadays. When I explained the reason for me requesting the grant, Antonio put his hands on his head and said: "We must do something, with this amount you cannot expend 6 months in Maastricht." He decided to immediately double the amount of the grant.

The €800 were spent immediately with my first trip to Maastricht to introduce myself to Hein Wellens and with the second trip to move to Maastricht for the six months. Literally, I had received from Antonio the only thing that I needed: an injection of moral support. The amount of money was now irrelevant, I had accepted it, he had doubled it, and now I was committed, there was no way back. Three months after my arrival, I was offered a position as research fellow at the new university and moved rapidly the next years to present my doctoral thesis, and to become assistant, associate, and full professor in cardiology. The "primum movens" behind all this was that exceptional man Antoni Bayés de Luna.

There has been a mutual respect between us since, however, as one of the key factors in my life, I kept a respectful subordinate relation with him. As a matter of fact, he was for me the hand of the destiny that pulled me to my future and to what I appreciate as a very privileged life for my family and myself. It is with the passage of time that my respect for him started to change into something else. His support for us went beyond the explainable and then I understood that Antoni was much more than a supporting colleague, he actually had become my "oldest brother."

This is my story with Antoni Bayés de Luna. Hundreds of fellows, residents, students and thousands of colleagues could tell each a similar special relation with this very special human being.

I thought it would have been too arrogant from my side to try to explain to you how good this excellent book by Antoni and his coworkers is.

Pedro Brugada
Lede, Valentine's Day
February 2021

Recommended Reading

Baranchuk A. *Interatrial Block & Supraventricular Arrhythmias: Clinical Implications of Bayés' Syndrome.* Cardiotext, 2017.

Baranchuk A. *Brugada Phenocopy: The Art of recognizing the Brugada ECG pattern.* Elsevier, 2018.

Bayés de Luna A. The morphology of the electrocardiogram. In Camm AJ, Lüscher TF, Serruys PW (eds). *The ESC Textbook of Cardiovascular Medicine*, 3rd edn. Oxford University Press, 2019.

Bayés de Luna A, Cosín J (eds). *Cardiac Arrhythmias.* Pergamon Press, 1978.

Bayés de Luna A, Baranchuk A. *Clinical Arrhythmology*, 2nd edn. Willey-Blackwell, 2017.

Bayés de Luna A, Goldwasser D, Fiol M, Bayés-Genis A. Chapter 12: Surface electrocardiography. In Valentin Fuster, Robert A. Harrington, Jagat Narula, Zubin J. Eapen (eds). *Hurst's The Heart*, 14th edn. McGraw-Hill, 2017.

Bonow RO, Mann DL, Zipes, DP, Libby P. *Braunwald's. Heart diseases. A textbook of Cardiovascular Medicine*, 9th edn. Elsevier Saunders Pu, 2012.

Camm AJ, Lüscher TF, Serruys PW (eds). *The ESC Textbook of Cardiovascular Medicine.* Blackwell Publishing, 2006.

Cooksey JD, Dunn M, Marrie E. *Clinical Vectorcardiography and Electrocardiography.* Year Book Medical Publishers, 1977.

Fiol-Sala M, Birnbaum Y, Nikus K, Bayés de Luna A. *Electrocardiography in Ischemic Heart Disease. Clinical and Imaging Correlations and Prognostic Implications*, 2nd edn. Willey-Blackwell, 2020.

Fisch C, Knoebel S. *Electrocardiography of Clinical Arrhythmias.* Futura, 2000.

Friedman HH. *Diagnostic Electrocardiography and Vectorcardiography*, 3rd edn. McGraw-Hill, 1985.

Fuster V, Walsh RA, Harrington RA (eds). *Hurst's The Heart*, 13th edn. McGraw-Hill, 2010.

Gerstch M. *The ECG: A Two Step Approach for Diagnosis.* Springer, 2004.

Grant RP. *Clinical Electrocardiography: The Spatial Vector Approach.* McGraw-Hill, 1957.

Kligfield P, Gettes L, Wagner G, *et al. Guidelines of AHA/ACC/HRS.* Circulation 2007; 115 (10): 1306–1324. Doi:10.1161/CIRCULATIONAHA.106.180200.

Lipman BS, Marrie E., Kleiger RE. *Clinical Scalar Electrocardiography*, 6th edn. Year Book Medical Publishers, 1972.

Macfarlane PW, van Oosterom A, Pahlm O, Kligfield P, Janse M, Camm J. *Comprehensive Electrocardiology*, 2nd edn. Springer-Verlag, London, 2010.

Nadeau-Ruthier C, Baranchuk A. *Electrocardiography in Practice: What to do?* iTunes USA, 2016. https://itunes.apple.com/ca/book/electrocardiography-in-practice/id1120119530?mt=13

Piccolo E. *Elettrocardiografia e vettocardigorafia.* Piccin Editore, 1981.

Restrepo Molina G, Wyss F, Sosa Liprandi A, Barbosa M, Baranchuk A. *Texto de Cardiologia de la Sociedad Interamericana de Cardiologia.* Distribuna, 2019.

Rosenbaum M, Elizari M, Lazzari J. *Los hemibloqueos.* Editorial Paidos, 1968.

Sodi Pallares D, Bisteni A, Medrano G. *Electrocardiografía y vectorcardiografía deductiva.* La Prensa Médica Mexicana, 1967.

Surawicz B, Knilans TK. *Chou's Electrocardiography in Clinical Practice*, 6th edn. WB Saunders Company, 2009.

Tranchesi J. *Electrocardiograma normal y patológico.* La Medica, 1968.

Wagner GS. *Marriott's Practical Electrocardiography*, 10th edn. Lippincott Williams & Wilkins, 2001.

Zipes D, Jalife J. *Cardiac Electrophysiology. From Cell to Bedside.* WB Saunders, Philadelphia, 2004.

Part 1
Introductory Aspects

Chapter 1
The Electrical Activity of the Heart

Basic concepts

The heart is a pump that sends blood to every organ in the human body. This is carried out through an electrical stimulus that originates in the sinus node and is transmitted through the specific conduction system (SCS) to contractile cells.

During the rest period, myocardial cells present an equilibrium between the positive electrical charges outside and the negative charges inside. When they receive the stimulus propagated from the sinus node, the activation process of these cells starts. **The activation** of myocardial cells is an electro-ionic mechanism (as explained in detail in Chapter 5) that involves two successive processes: **depolarization**, or loss of external positive charges that are substituted by negative ones, and **repolarization**, which represents the recovery of external positive charges.

The process of depolarization in a contractile myocardial cell starts with the formation of a **depolarization dipole** comprising a pair of charges (−+) that advance through the surface cell like a wave in the sea, leaving behind a wave of negativity (Figure 1.1A). When the entire cell is depolarized (externally negative), a new dipole starting in the same place is formed. This is known as a **dipole of repolarization** (+−). **The process of repolarization**, whereby the entire cell surface is supplied with positive charges, is then initiated (Figure 1.1B).

The expression of the dipoles is a vector that has its head in the positive charge and the tail in the negative one. An electrode facing the head of the vector records positivity (+), whereas when it faces the tail, it records negativity (−) (Figures 1.1–1.3; see also Figures 5.24, 5.25, and 5.28). The deflection originating with the depolarization process is quicker because the process of depolarization is an active one (abrupt entry of Na ions, and later Ca) and the process of repolarization is much slower (exit of K) (see Chapter 5, Section "Transmembrane action potential").

If what happens in one contractile cell is extrapolated to the left ventricle as the expression of all myocardium, we will see that the **repolarization process in this case starts in the opposite place to that of depolarization**. This explains why the repolarization of a single contractile cell is represented by a negative wave, whereas the repolarization of the left ventricle expressing the human electrocardiogram (ECG) is represented by a positive wave because the repolarization process of all left ventricles starts in the zone less ischemic, the subepicardium compared with the subendocardium that is the more ischemic zone (Figure 5.28) (see Chapter 5, Section "From cellular electrogram to human ECG").

How can we record the electrical activity of the heart?

There are various methods used to record the electrical activity of the heart. The best known method, the one we examine in this book, is **electrocardiography. An alternative method**, rarely used in clinical practice today but **very useful in understanding ECG curves and therefore helpful in learning about ECGs, is vectorcardiography.**

The latter and other methods will be briefly discussed in Chapter 25. These include, among others, body mapping, late potentials, and esophageal and intracavitary electrocardiography. In addition, normal ECGs can be recorded during exercise and in long recordings (ECG monitoring, Holter technology, telemetry, etc.) (Braunwald et al. 2012, Camm et al. 2006; Fuster et al 2001) For more information about different techniques, consult our books *Clinical Arrhythmology* (Bayés de Luna and Baranchuk 2017) and *Electrocardiography in Ischemic Heart Disease* (Fiol-Sala et al. 2020), and other ECG reference books (Macfarlane and Lawrie 1989; Wagner 2001; Gertsch 2004; Surawicz et al. 2008) (see "Recommended Reading").

Clinical Electrocardiography: A Textbook, Fifth Edition. Antoni Bayés de Luna, Miquel Fiol-Sala, Antoni Bayés-Genís, and Adrián Baranchuk.
© 2022 John Wiley & Sons Ltd. Published 2022 by John Wiley & Sons Ltd.

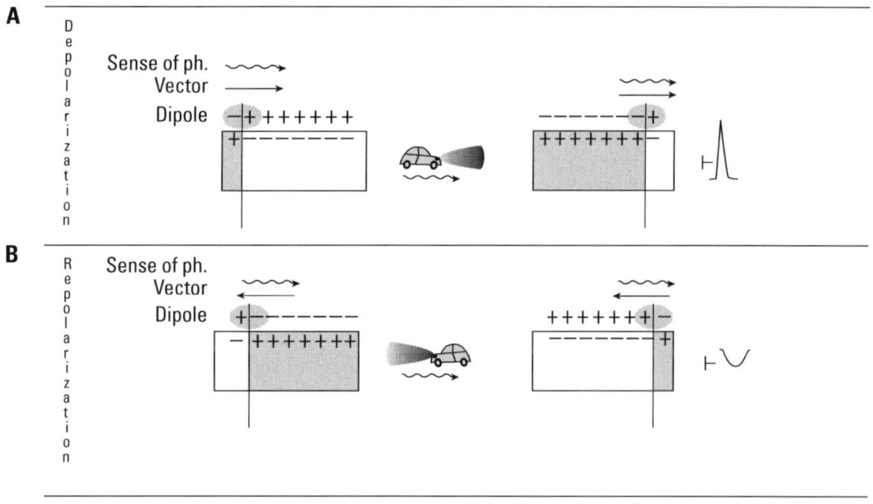

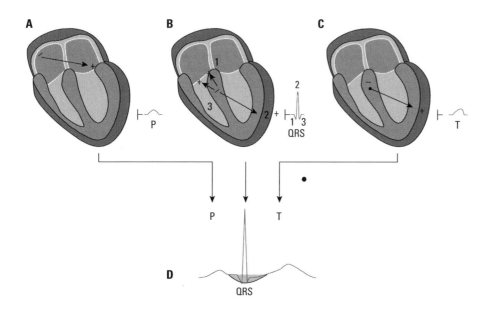

Figure 1.1 Depolarization (A) and repolarization (B) of the dipole in an isolated myocardium cell. We see the onset and end of the depolarization and repolarization processes and how this accounts for the positivity and negativity of corresponding waves (see text and Chapter 5).

Figure 1.2 The origin of P, QRS, and T deflections (A, B and C). When van electrode located in some zone of LV faces the head (+) of a vector of depolarization (P, QRS) or repolarization (T), it records positivity. When an electrode faces the tail of a vector (–), it records negativity. Atrial repolarization is hidden in the QRS (shadow area) (see text and Chapter 5).

What is the surface ECG?

The ECG is the standard technique used for recording the electrical activity of the heart. **We can record the process of depolarization and repolarization** through recording electrodes (leads) located in various places.

The depolarization process of the heart, atria, and ventricles (see Chapter 5 and Figures 5.16 and 5.18) starts with the formation of a dipole of depolarization (–+), which has a vectorial expression (——▶) that advances through the surface of the myocardium and seeds the entire surface of the myocardial cells with negative charges. A recording electrode facing the head of the vector records positivity (Figure 1.2). Later, **the repolarization process starts** with the formation of a **repolarization dipole (+–),** which also has a vectorial expression. During

this process, the positive charges of the outside surface of the cells are restored.

These two processes relate to specific characteristics of the atria and ventricles (Figure 1.2). The process of atrial depolarization, when recorded on the surface of the body in an area close to the left ventricle (Figure 1.2), presents as a small positive wave called the P wave (⌒). This is the expression of the atrial depolarization dipole (vector). **The process of ventricular depolarization,** which occurs later when the stimulus arrives at the ventricles, usually presents as three deflections (⎰), known as the QRS complex, caused by the formation of three consecutive dipoles (vectors). The first vector appears as a small and negative deflection because it represents the depolarization of a small area in the septum the first part of LV to be depolarized, and is usually directed upward and to the right and therefore, recorded from the left ventricle as a small negative deflection ("q wave"). Next, a second important and positive vector is formed, representing the R wave. This is the expression of depolarization in most of the left ventricular mass. The head of this vector faces the recording electrode. Finally, there is a third small vector of ventricular depolarization that depolarizes the upper part of the septum and right ventricle. It is directed upward and to the right and is recorded by the recording electrode in the left ventricle zone as a small negative wave ("s wave") (Figure 1.2).

After depolarization of the atria and ventricles, the **process of repolarization starts**. The repolarization of the atria is usually a smooth curve that remains hidden within the QRS complex. The ventricular repolarization curve appears after the QRS as an isoelectric ST segment and a T wave. This T wave is recorded as a positive wave from the left ventricle electrode because the process of ventricular repolarization, as already mentioned and later explained in detail (see Chapter 5, Section "From cellular electrogram to the human ECG" and Figures 5.24 and 5.25),

appears very differently from what happens in an isolated contractile cell (see Figure 5.9). Repolarization starts on the opposite side to that of depolarization, because it starts in the zone less ischemic of LV that is the subepicardium. Thus, the recording electrode faces the positive part of the dipole, or head of the vector, and will record a positive deflection, even though the dipole moves away from it (Figure 1.2C; see also Figures 5.24 and 5.25). Therefore, repolarization of the left ventricle in a human ECG (the T wave) is recorded as a positive wave, just as occurs with the depolarization complex (QRS) in leads placed close to the left ventricle surface (⌐⌐).

The successive recording of the ECG is linear and the distance from one P–QRS–T to another can be measured in time. The frequency of this sequence is related to heart rate.

The heart is a three-dimensional organ. In order to see its electrical activity on a two-dimensional piece of paper or screen, it must be projected from at least two planes, the frontal plane (FP) and the horizontal plane (HP) (Figure 1.3).

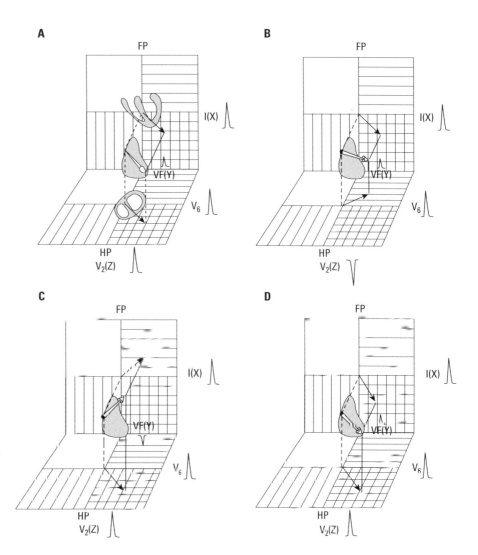

Figure 1.3 Four locations of a vector and their projection in frontal (FP) and horizontal planes (HP). **A** and **B** have the same projection in FP but not in HP. **C** and **D** have the same projection in HP but not in FP. Different positive and negative morphologies appear according to these projections. The locations of the orthogonal leads X, Y, and Z perpendicular to each other are similar to I, aVF, and V2 leads. Vertical lines correspond to the positive hemifields of aVF and V2, and horizontal lines correspond to the positive hemifields of leads I and V6. FP lead I (X) = 0°; VF (Y) = +90°; HP V2 (Z) = +90°; V6 = 0°.

The shape of the ECG varies according to the location (lead) from which the electrical activity is recorded. In general, the electrical activity of the heart is recorded using 12 different leads: six on the FP (I, II, III, aVR, aVL, aVF), located from +120° (III) to −30° (aVL). The aVR is usually recorded in the positive part of the lead that is located in −150° (see Figures 6.10 and 6.11), and six on the HP (V1–V6) located from +120° to 0° (see Chapter 6, Section "Leads" and Figures 6.10 and 6.13).

Each lead has a line that begins where the lead is placed, 0° for lead I or +90° for lead aVF in the FP and 0° for lead V6 and +90° for lead V2 in the HP, for example (see Figure 6.10), and ends at the opposite side of the body, passing through the center of the heart. **By tracing each perpendicular line that passes through the center of the heart, we may divide the electrical field of the body into two hemifields for each lead, one positive and one negative** (Figure 1.3). A vector that falls into the positive hemifield records positivity, while one that falls into the negative hemifield records negativity. When a vector falls on the line of separation between hemifields, an isodiphasic curve is recorded that is +− or −+ according to the sense of rotation of the curve (loop) (see later) (see Figures 6.14 and 6.16).

The different vectors are recorded as positive or negative depending on whether they are projected onto positive or negative hemifields of different leads (Figures 1.3 and 1.5). This is a key concept for understanding the morphology of ECG curves in different leads and is explained in Chapter 6 in more detail (Figure 6.14).

> The ECG and its different morphologies can be explained using the following sequence:
> **Dipole→Spatial vectors→Projection in frontal (FP) and horizontal (HP) planes**

What is vectorcardiography? (See Chapter 25 for more extensive information)

The vectorcardiogram (VCG) is the closed curve or loop that records the entire pathway of an electrical stimulus from the depolarization of the atria (P loop) and ventricles (QRS loop) to the repolarization of the ventricles (T loop). These loops are recorded in FP and HP, as well as in the sagittal plane. The VCG is the result of the joined heads of the multiple vectors that are formed during the consecutive processes of depolarization and repolarization of the heart (Figure 1.4). VCG loops are obtained from three orthogonal (perpendicular to each other) leads, X, Y, and Z, which are placed in positions similar to those of leads I, aVF, and V2, respectively (see Figure 1.4 and Chapter 25).

The VCG curve is a plot of voltage against voltage of the different waves generated by the heart (P, QRS, T loops), and therefore in the VCG loops, it is not possible to measure the time between the beginning of the P loop and the beginning of the QRS loop (PR interval), or the beginning of QRS and the end of the T loop (QT interval). However, we can interrupt the loops of P, QRS, and T by

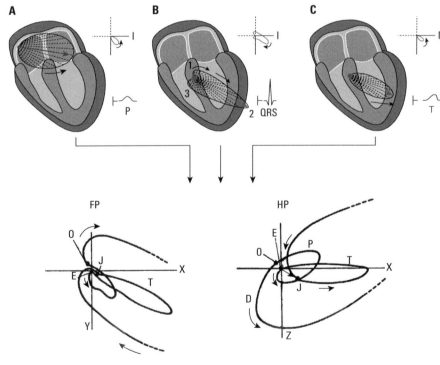

EO = P loop; OJ = QRS loop; JE = T loop; OJ = ST vector

Figure 1.4 The origin of P, QRS, and T loops (A, B and C). The vectorcardiographic curve (D) is the union of the heads of multiple vectors that form during the consecutive processes of depolarization and repolarization (see text and Figure 5.23).

cutting the tracing every 2.5 ms, which allows the duration of each loop to be measured (see Figures 10.6–10.10 and 10.22–10.25).

One advantage of the VCG is that the different rotations of the loop can be visualized. It is important to know if the stimulus follows a clockwise or counterclockwise rotation when one complex or wave is biphasic. Figure 1.5B shows how the mean vector of a loop directed to +0° that falls within the limit between the positive or negative hemifields in lead "Y" (aVF) may present a +− (↑) or a −+ (↓) deflection. The direction of the mean vector of the loop does not solve one important problem: a +− deflection is normal, but a −+ deflection may be the expression of myocardial infarction (MI). The correct morphology will be shown, however, by the direction of loop rotation (Figure 1.5). In addition, the mean vector of the QRS loop, which expresses the sum of all vectors of depolarization, does not indicate the direction of the small initial and final forces when these forces are opposed to a mean vector (Figure 1.5). However, the small part of the loop (beginning and end) that falls in the opposite hemifield of the main vector can explain the complete ECG morphology with initial (q) and final small (s) deflections (Figures 1.5 and 1.6; see also Figures 7.10 and 7.11).

> The VCG can be described using the following sequence:
> The head of multiple vectors → Spatial loops → Projection in FP and HP

ECG–VCG correlation

Bearing in mind the abovementioned information, it is clear that **to better understand the morphology of an ECG, we must consider the stimulus pathway through the heart (VCG loop) in different normal and pathological conditions and identify the projection of these loops in FP and HP**. It is important to understand how the different parts of the loop that fall into the positive or negative hemifields of each lead correspond to the different deflections of an ECG curve (Figures 1.5 and 1.6; see also Figure 5.23) (ECG–VCG correlation). **This allows the ECG curves to be drawn from the VCG loops and vice versa.**

> The key concepts around how ECG curves can be obtained from the VCG loops and vice versa (ECG–VCG correlation) are defined using the following sequence:
> Dipole → Vector → Loop → Projection in different hemifields → ECG patterns

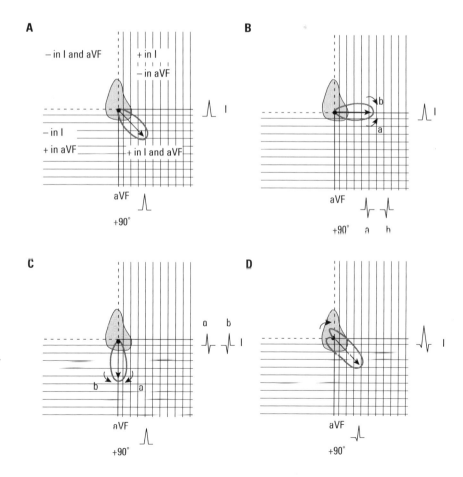

Figure 1.5 The concept of the hemifield. We see how a morphology may be +− or −+ with the same vector but a different loop rotation (B and C) (A and B). The recording of the initial and terminal deflections of qRs are well understood with the correlation of the loop and hemifields in D (see I and aVF).

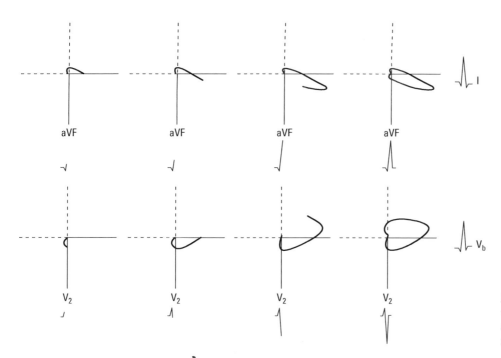

Figure 1.6 Correlation of a vectorcardiographic loop with an electrocardiographic morphology in aVF and V2.

Why do we record ECG curves and not VCG loops?

Although ECG–VCG correlation is used in this book to explain how the different ECG patterns appear, the recording of vectorcardiographic loops for diagnostic purposes is rarely used in clinical practice at present. **There are many reasons for the superiority of ECG curves over VCG loops, the main ones being as follows:**

• **The established diagnostic criteria of ECG in different pathologies are more defined and agreed-upon, compared with the VCG criteria.** They are also easier to apply. Furthermore, it has not been clearly demonstrated by experts in ECG/VCG interpretation that VCG criteria provide more diagnostic information than that taken from ECGs, even in an era when VCG criteria were most used (Simonson *et al.* 1967; Rautaharju 1988; Van Bemmel *et al.* 1992) (see later).

• **VCG loops do not show an appreciation of time (PR and QT interval)**, as previously mentioned.

• **The ECG curves–VCG loop correlation gives us all the detailed information obtainable from VCG loops.** In fact, if the origin of the ECG curve interpretation based on the projection of VCG loops in the positive and negative hemifields of different leads (ECG–VCG correlation) is understood and used, we are able to derive the same information that VCGs provide by just looking at the ECG. For example, it has been reported (Benchimol *et al.* 1972) that VCGs are essential for the diagnosis of superoanterior fascicular block (hemiblock) associated with inferior MI. However, as discussed in Chapter 13,

the same information can be obtained from the ECG if we recognize the exact pathway of the stimulus in both cases (inferior MI alone or associated with hemiblock) and we make a good ECG–VCG correlation (see Figure 13.99). Furthermore, many details provided by amplified VCG loops (the degree of ST shifts, onset of pre-excitation, characteristics of the P wave, etc.) can also be obtained from surface ECGs through amplification of the ECG waves, if necessary (see Figure 13.24) (Fiol-Sala *et al.* 2020).

• **The VCG is not useful in the diagnosis of arrhythmias.** Even information about the ectopic P wave may be correctly obtained from ECG curves. However, the recording of P loops may help to know better how is the way of stimulus in situations such as the presence of advanced interatrial block (Bayés de Luna *et al.* 2012).

• **Computerization of ECG data and not of VCG has become dominant** and, despite current limitations, it has a great future. However, as we see later on (Chapter 3, Section "Limitations"), it is necessary to improve the results of ECG computerization with better technology and the inclusion of new data (clinical setting, different scores, etc.), and we hope that in the near future become a substitute of individualized interpretations.

• **The ECG is used more than the VCG** for estimating the size of an MI (Selvester QRS scoring system) (Selvester *et al.* 1972; Wagner *et al.* 1982). However, in the era of ECG-imaging correlations, it is necessary to improve the methodology of QRS score measurement to obtain a better correlation with contrast-enhanced cardiovascular magnetic resonance measurements (see later and Chapter 3, Section "Limitations").

• **ECG and not VCG patterns have already been correlated with imaging techniques**, especially coronarography and contrast-enhanced cardiovascular magnetic resonance (CE-CMR). The correlation of ECG patterns with coronarography has allowed us to better locate the occlusion and determine the severity of ischemia in different types of acute coronary syndromes (leads with different ST shifts) (Sclarovsky 1999; Wellens *et al.* 2004; Fiol-Sala *et al.* 2020). It is also possible to obtain better classification and location of Q-wave MI (leads with abnormal Q or R waves as mirror image) using CE-CMR-ECG correlation (Bayés de Luna *et al.* 2006a, 2006b; Cino *et al.* 2006; Bayés de Luna 2007; Rovai *et al.* 2007; Van der Weg *et al.* 2009; Fiol-Sala *et al.* 2020). Similar correlations have not been done with VCG loops. Currently, a good estimation of infarction size using CE-CMR has been obtained (Kim *et al.* 1999; Moon *et al.* 2004). However, the correlation of infarct size measurement performed by surface ECG (QRS scoring system) (Selvester *et al.* 1972) with CE-CMR is not very consistent, and the CE-CMR shows larger values than the QRS score estimation (Weir *et al.* 2010). We hope that in the future it will be possible to improve these results with new equations (see Chapter 3, Section "The future"). Good results have also recently been shown by Montant *et al.* (2010) using a contrast-enhanced three-dimensional echocardiography compared with CE-CMR to identify and quantify myocardial scars (positive and negative predictive value (PV) > 90%).

• **Young physicians should realize that ECG–VCG correlation is a basis for better understanding ECG curves.** This does not mean that they need to know specific VCG criteria, such as the number of milliseconds the loop is going up and down, because these data obtained from the VCG does not add too much diagnostic information. Therefore, a recorded VCG loop is not clinically necessary. However, **it is important to remember that the ECG–VCG correlation is a key point for better understanding of how ECG curves are originated** (see below).

• Currently, **there are very few devices that still correctly record VCG curves.** At the Electrocardiology Congress held in 2009, titled with the subheading "VCG symposium," it was decided that this subheading should be suppressed (Macfarlane 2009). "Signum temporis" stated the first organizers (Sobieszczańska and Jagielski 2010). The number of VCG papers published in Medline in the 1970s and 1980s reached more than 800 per decade; today, in the first decade of this century, there are fewer than 60 and in the last decade the number is probably still lower.

• It appears that the VCG loops taken from the orthogonal leads do not give much more information of clinical interest than a conventional 12-lead surface ECG. They are also time consuming and need special devices. Although we consider that VCG is not very useful for diagnosis, we are sure that the VCG loops are very useful

for teaching and research purposes (Kors *et al.* 1990, 1998; Rautaharju *et al.* 2007; Pérez Riera 2009; Lazzara 2010). It may be that incorporating VCG loops synthesized directly from 12-lead surface ECG recordings would be an interesting option (see Chapter 3).

Why do we use ECG–VCG correlations to understand ECG patterns?

Electrocardiography and vectorcardiography are two methods for recording the electrical activity of the heart. As explained above, the **ECG is a linear curve** based on the positive and negative deflections recorded when an electrode faces the head or the tail of a depolarization and repolarization dipole, the expression of which is a vector, from leads placed in frontal and horizontal planes. The **VCG is a loop** that represents the outline of the joining of multiple dipoles (vectors) formed along the electrical stimulus pathway through the heart. The projection of these loops in frontal and horizontal planes is a closed curve that is different in morphology from the linear curves of an ECG. Both ECG curves and VCG loops, however, are completely connected so that the **ECG curve may be easily deduced from the VCG loop, and vice versa** (see ECG–VCG correlation, Figures 1.5 and 1.6). As already mentioned, this approach is considered to be the best way to understand both the normal ECG and all the morphological changes that different pathologies introduce to the ECG.

The correlation between VCG loops and projection of this on different hemifields to understand the ECG pattern (**dipole → vector → loop → hemifield sequence**) will no doubt remain a cornerstone of the teaching of the ECG (Grant and Estes 1952; Sodi-Pallares and Calder 1956; Cooksey *et al.* 1957; Cabrera 1958; Gertsch 2004).

---

1. **The deduction of the ECG from the VCG loops is crucial to better recognizing how both normal ECG curves and the many ECG changes found in different heart diseases and under special circumstances originate.**

2. Although the deductive method for teaching electrocardiography is fundamentally based on the correlation that exists between ECG curves and VCG loops, VCG criteria are not used for diagnosis.

3. **In the majority of diagrams** used to show the usefulness of **VCG** loop–ECG wave correlations, the pathway of the electrical stimulus is represented as a curve with a **continuous line** When we **record original VCG tracings**, however, dashes every 2.5 ms in the VCG loops are shown. Examples of this may be seen throughout this book (see, for example, Figures 11.25, 11.36, and 11.40).

References

Bayés de Luna A. New heart wall terminology and new electrocardiographic classification of Q-wave myocardial infarction based on correlations with magnetic resonance imaging. *Rev Esp Cardiol* 2007;60:683.

Bayés de Luna A., Baranchuk A. *Clinical Arrhythmology*, 2nd edn. Willey-Blackwell, 2017.

Bayés de Luna A, Wagner G, Birnbaum Y, *et al.* A new terminology for left ventricular walls and location of myocardial infarcts that present Q wave based on the standard of cardiac magnetic resonance imaging: a statement for healthcare professionals from a committee appointed by the International Society for Holter and Noninvasive Electrocardiography. *Circulation* 2006a;114:1755.

Bayés de Luna A, Cino JM, Pujadas S, *et al.* Concordance of electrocardiographic patterns and healed myocardial infarction location detected by cardiovascular magnetic resonance. *Am J Cardiol* 2006b;987:443.

Bayés de Luna A, Platonov P, García-Cosio F, *et al.* Interatrial blocks. A separate entity from left atrial enlargement: a consensus report. *J of Electrocardiol* 2012; 45: 445–451.

Benchimol A, Desser KB, Schumacher J. Value of the vectorcardiogram for distinguishing left anterior hemiblock from inferior infarction with left axis deviation. *Chest* 1972;61:74.

Braunwald E, Bonow RO, Mann DL, Zippes D, Libby P. *Heart Disease*, 11th edn. Elsevier Saunders, 2012.

Cabrera E. *Teoría y práctica de la Electrocardiografía*. Edic INC México, La Prensa Médica Mexicana, 1958.

Camm J, Luscher TF, Serruys PW (eds). *The ESC Textbook of Cardiovascular Medicine*. Blackwell, 2006.

Cino J, Pons-Lladó G, Bayés de Luna A, *et al.* Utility of contrast-enhanced cardiovascular magnetic resonance (CE-CMR) to assess how likely is an infarct to produce a typical ECG pattern. *J Cardiovasc Magn Reson* 2006;8:335.

Cooksey J, Dunn M, Massie E. *Clinical Vectorcardiography and Electrocardiography*, 2nd edn. YearBook MP, 1957.

Fiol-Sala M, Birnbaum Y, Nikus K, Bayés de Luna A. *Electrocardiography in Ischemic Heart Disease. Clinical and Imaging Correlations and Prognostic Implications*, 2nd edn. Willey-Blackwell, 2020.

Fuster V, Walsh RA, Harrington RA (eds). *Heart's*, 13th edn. McGraw-Hill, 2010.

Gertsch M. *The ECG: A Two Step Approach for Diagnosis*. Springer, 2004.

Grant R, Estes EH. *Spatial Vector Electrocardiography*. Blakston Co, 1952.

Kim RJ, Fieno D, Parrish T, *et al.* Relationship of CE-CMR to irreversible injury, infarct age and contractile function. *Circulation* 1999;100:1992.

Kors JA, Van Herpen G, Sitting AG, *et al.* Reconstruction of the Frank VCG from the standard ECG leads. *Eur Heart J* 1990;11:1083.

Kors JA, De Bruyne MC, Hoes AW. T axis as an independent indicator of risk of cardiac events in elderly people. *The Lancet* 1998;352:361.

Lazzara R. Spatial vectorcardiogram to predict risk for sudden arrhythmic death: Phoenix risen from the ashes. *Heart Rhythm* 2010;7:1614.

Macfarlane PW. Interview with Peter W Macfarlane by Ljuba Bacharova. *J Electrocardiol* 2009;42:223.

Macfarlane PW, Lawrie TDV (eds). *Comprehensive Electrocardiography*. Pergamon Press, 1989.

Montant P, Chenot F, Gaffinet C, *et al.* Detection and quantification of myocardial scars using CE-3D-echocardiography. *Circulation CV Imag* 2010;3:415.

Moon JC, De Arenaza DP, Elkington AG, *et al.* The pathologic basis of Q-wave and non-Q-wave myocardial infarction: a cardiovascular magnetic resonance study. *J Am Coll Cardiol* 2004;44:554.

Pérez Riera A. *Learning Easily Frank Vectorcardiogram*. Editora Mosteiro, Sao Paulo, 2009.

Rautaharju PM. A hundred years of progress in electrocardiography. 2: The rise and decline of vectorcardiography. *Can J Cardiol* 1988;4:60.

Rautaharju P, Prineas R, Zhang Z-M. A simple procedure for estimation of the spatial QRS/T angle from the standard 12-lead ECG. *J Electrocardiol* 2007;40:300.

Rovai D, Di Bella G, Rossi G, *et al.* Q-wave prediction of myocardial infarct location, size and transmural extent at magnetic resonance imaging. *Coronary Artery Dis* 2007;18:381.

Sclarovsky S. *Electrocardiography of Acute Myocardial Ischaemic Syndromes*. Martin Dunitz, 1999.

Selvester RH, Wagner JO, Rubin HB. Quantitation of myocardial infarct size and location by electrocardiogram and vectorcardiogram. In Snelin HA (ed.) *Boerhave Course in Quantitation in Cardiology*. Leyden University Press, 1972, p. 31.

Simonson E, Tune N, Okamoto N, *et al.* Vectorcardiographic criteria with high diagnostic accuracy. *Z Kreislaufforsch* 1967;56:1243.

Sodi-Pallares D, Calder R. *New Bases of Electrocardiography*. Mosby, 1956.

Sobieszczańska M, Jagielski J. The International Society of Electrocardiology: a 50 year history originated in Poland. *J Electrocardiol* 2010;43:187.

Surawicz B, Knilans TK, Te-Chuan Chou. *Chou's Electrocardiography in Clinical Practice*, 6th edn. Saunders, 2008.

Van Bemmel JH, Kors JA, van Herpen G. Combination of diagnostic classifications from ECG and VCG computer interpretations. *J Electrocardiol* 1992;25(suppl):126.

Van der Weg K, Bekkers S, Gorgels A, *et al.* The R in V1 in nonanterior wall infarction indicates lateral rather than posterior involvement. Results from ECG/MRI correlations. *Eur Heart J* 2009;30(suppl):P2981.

Wagner GS (ed.) *Marriott's Practical Electrocardiography*, 10th edn. Lippincott Williams & Wilkins, 2001.

Wagner G, Freye C, Palmer ST, *et al.* Evaluation of QRS scoring system for estimating myocardial infarction size. *Circulation* 1982;65:347.

Weir R, Martin T, Wagner G. Comparison of infarct size and LVEF by CE-CMR and ECG scoring in reperfused anterior STEMI. *J Electrocardiol* 2010;43:230.

Wellens H, Doevedans P, Gorgels A. *The ECG in Acute Myocardial Infarction and Unstable Angina*. Kluwer Academic, 2004.

Chapter 2
The History of Electrocardiography

Electrical phenomena have been observed by humans for more than 2500 years. **Thales of Miletus** in Greece (sixth century BCE) noted that amber rubbed with wool attracts light objects. In fact, the ancient Greek name for amber is *elektron*. As early as the end of the sixteenth century, the English physician William Gilbert postulated the relationship between electricity and magnetism. He was followed by Benjamin Franklin, who discovered the lightning rod in about 1750. At the end of the eighteenth century, the Italian **Luigi Galvani** discovered that electricity in animals is generated via "an electric fluid." Galvani believed that electrical stimulus preceded muscle contraction. He would become the world's first electrophysiologist (Rosen 2002; Rosen and Janse 2006).

The electrical activity of the heart was first recorded in the late nineteenth century by **Augustus D Waller** (Figure 2.1), who in 1887 recorded the curves of electrical activity of the human heart using saline-filled tube electrodes and the capillary electrometer developed by Gabriel Lippmann (Figure 2.2A,B). The first human ECG was taken to Thomas Goswell, a technician in his laboratory. Initially, he used his dog Jimmy to perform ECG recordings, but was accused of cruelty to animals because of the belts used and the practice of putting the dog's extremities in saline water. Although Waller was credited with being the first to record the electrical activity of the heart, he did not have much faith in the usefulness of electrocardiography, stating "I do not imagine the electrocardiography is likely to find any very extensive use ... just occasionally to record some rare anomaly of cardiac action" (Burch and DePasquale 1964).

In the last years of the nineteenth century, **Willem Einthoven** (1860–1927) (Figure 2.3) (Einthoven 1912; Snellen 1977; Moukabary 2007; Kligfield 2010) began to study animal action potentials using the capillary electrometer. Because he was dissatisfied with the records obtained, he made several modifications that greatly improved the tracing quality by using differential

equations to correct the poor frequency response of the original design (Figure 2.2A). With these modifications, he was able to predict the correct form of the human ECG

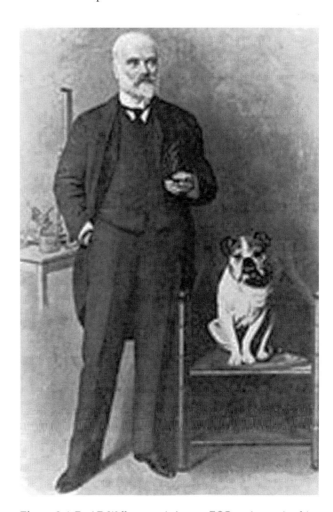

Figure 2.1 Dr AD Waller recorded many ECG tracings using his dog Jimmy, resulting in accusations of animal cruelty (Portrait of A.D. Waller Wellcome M0012782, https://commons.wikimedia.org/wiki/File:Portrait_of_A.D._Waller_Wellcome M0012782.jpg. CC-BY-4.0).

Clinical Electrocardiography: A Textbook, Fifth Edition. Antoni Bayés de Luna, Miquel Fiol-Sala, Antoni Bayés-Genís, and Adrián Baranchuk.
© 2022 John Wiley & Sons Ltd. Published 2022 by John Wiley & Sons Ltd.

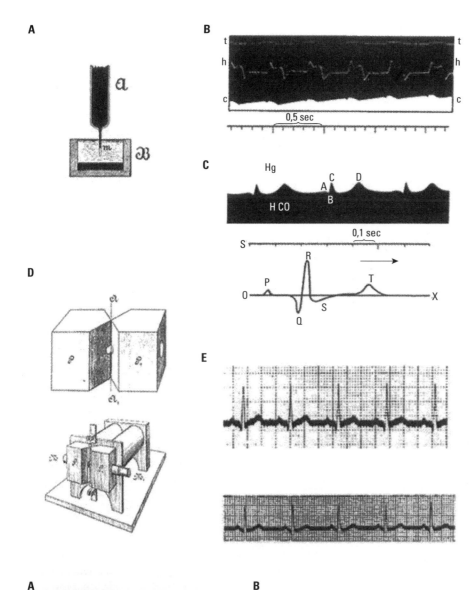

Figure 2.2 (A) Lippmann's capillary electrometer consisted of a mercury reservoir ending in a glass capillary with the upper half filled with mercury and the lower half and reservoir filled with sulfuric acid. (B) Waller's cardiogram recorded using a capillary electrometer. t = time; h = external pulsation from heart beat; c = electrical activity of heart. (C) Einthoven's recording using a capillary electrometer. Upper: A, B, C, and D waves; lower: mathematically corrected waves, now designated PQRST. (D) A string galvanometer. Upper: Poles P and P_1 of electromagnet and aperture for string. Note holes for viewing via microscopes. Lower: electromagnet with string in place and two microscopes. (E) Einthoven's ECG recordings.

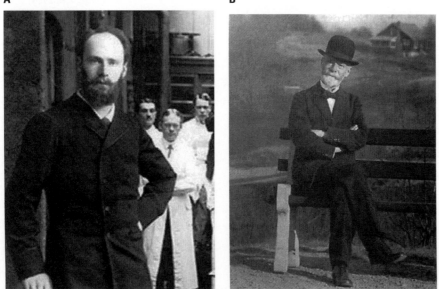

Willem Einthoven (1860–1927)

Figure 2.3 Dr Willem Einthoven in his laboratory early in his career (A) and years later (B) while visiting Frank N Wilson in Ann Arbor, Michigan.

(Figure 2.2C) and he proved his findings using a string galvanometer developed in 1902.

Einthoven's **string galvanometer** (Figure 2.2D) consisted of a silver-coated quartz filament suspended between the two poles of an electromagnet. The fixed magnetic field created by the electromagnet established a strong constant force moving from one pole to the other. Currents from the heart registered from the surface of the body were conducted through the quartz string, thereby creating a varying magnetic field of force around the long axis of the string. The interaction between the two magnetic fields, one between the poles of the electromagnet and the other depending on the magnitude of the current that flowed through the string, resulted in movements of the string that were recorded as sharp deflections.

The first electrocardiogram recorded using the string galvanometer was published in 1902. The quality of the tracings was undoubtedly very good and similar to today's tracings (Figure 2.2E). It is interesting to note that because Einthoven's laboratory was more than a mile from the academic hospital in Leyden, he developed a method for recording the ECG from a distance, which he called "Telecardiogramme."

Unlike Waller, Einthoven intuited the great potential of electrocardiography, stating that **"A new chapter has been opened in the study of heart diseases . . . by which suffering mankind is helped."** In fact, by 1906, **he had already published his first paper presenting normal and abnormal ECGs** (Einthoven 1912). With this new technique, the recording of ECG curves had a high fidelity and sensitivity and represented an undistorted, directly readable graphic record of the electrical activity of the heart. Einthoven labeled the detailed wave deflections "PQRST," instead of using the "ABCD" notations used for the waves taken with the capillary electrometer (Figure 2.2C). This avoided confusion between uncorrected and corrected records and allowed the addition of further letters if other earlier or later wave forms should be discovered. Starting with "P" to describe the first wave avoided the use of the letters "N" and "O," which were already in use for other mathematical/geometrical conventions.

The diagnostic technique introduced by Einthoven more than 110 years ago was soon manufactured by the Cambridge Scientific Instrument Company, founded by Horace Darwin, younger son of the great biologist Charles Darwin and the first to officially commercialize ECG machines. The first manufactured ECG machine was supplied to EA Schafer in Edinburgh in 1908 (Figure 2.4A). The second model, the table model, was manufactured in 1911. Figure 2.4B shows how the recording of tracings with this huge machine was performed. One of the three first complete electrocardiographs was delivered to Sir Thomas Lewis.

Today's ECG tracings no better in quality from a morphological point of view (Figure 2.2E), although now the

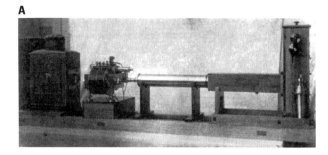

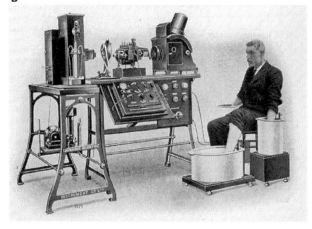

Figure 2.4 (A) The first manufactured ECG machine. (B) The second model (table model manufactured by Cambridge Scientific Instrument Company in 1911) (see text) (https://commons. wikimedia.org/wiki/File:Willem_Einthoven_ECG.jpg).

ECG is usually recorded digitally, and the devices are much smaller, and even may be recorded by a mobile phone or the ECG information may be given with the use of a watch holding the device between two hands (see Chapters 6 and 26, Figure 6.19). Even with a watch, may be recorded the ECG just pushing a bottom, what is especially useful. In any case, the ECG remains, presumably forever, the "gold standard" technique most used in everyday practice in cardiology, and possibly general medicine, throughout the world.

In hindsight, it is clear that the Nobel Prize Einthoven received in 1924 was very well deserved. He had a fascinating and creative personality added to his genius. He only looked for the truth. He once stated **"What you or I think is not important. What is important is the truth"** (Burch and De Pasquale 1964).

Prior to the discovery of the ECG, the diagnosis of heart rhythm disorders had been performed by clinical examination and polygraphic recordings of arterial and venous pulsations. The most important studies in this field were performed by the physicians Sir James Mackenzie and Karel F Wenckebach in the late nineteenth century. In the early days of electrocardiography, they were naturally suspicious of this new technique, probably because they thought that it might interfere with careful observation and the physical diagnosis of heart diseases. However, Wenckebach in particular became convinced of its importance. The ECG made the identification of many of the great concepts discovered by these pioneers much easier and more accurate. In fact, Wenckebach was able to discover with polygraphic recordings different types of second-degree atrioventricular block. The influence of both cardiologists on the evolution of the ECG, especially in the field of heart rhythm disorders, is very significant.

From a historical point of view, the two most important pioneers of clinical electrocardiography, Sir Thomas Lewis and Frank N Wilson, must be mentioned. **Sir Thomas Lewis** (1881–1945) (Figure 2.5) accomplished the daunting task of demonstrating the importance of Einthoven's discovery, especially in the field of heart rhythm disorders. He also demonstrated interesting aspects of changes in wave morphology, such as the significance of the mirror pattern in acute ischemia, and wrote the first ECG books describing the clinical usefulness of the technique (Lewis 1913, 1949). He did not, however, correctly interpret the ECG morphology in bundle branch block; this was accomplished later by other pioneer such as George Fahr (Figure 2.6). Lewis believed that there was nothing left to discover in the field of electrocardiography after 1920, and turned to peripheral circulation. **Frank N Wilson** (1890–1952)

(Figure 2.6) was the father of chest leads and the central terminal that allows us to record the so-called "unipolar leads" in the frontal plane (aVR, aVL, aVF) and the horizontal plane (precordial leads) using limb leads as a reference (Wilson *et al.* 1931, 1944). He also performed important studies on ventricular blocks and other aspects of electrocardiography.

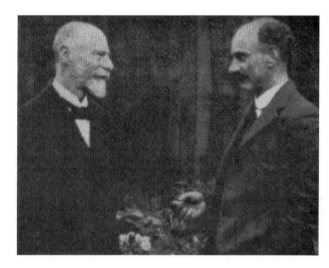

Figure 2.5 Dr Willem Einthoven, left, with Sir Thomas Lewis, right (Museum Boerhaave, Leiden).

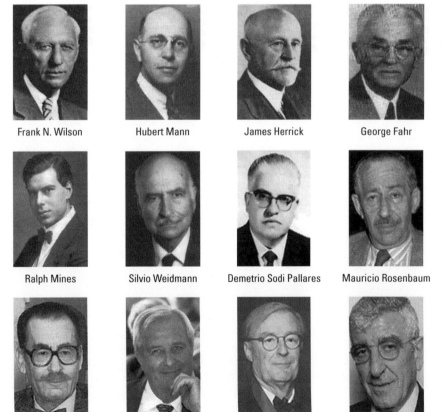

Frank N. Wilson   Hubert Mann   James Herrick   George Fahr

Ralph Mines   Silvio Weidmann   Demetrio Sodi Pallares   Mauricio Rosenbaum

Paul Puech   Philippe Coumel   Hein Wellens   Marcelo V. Elizari

Figure 2.6 Twelve pioneers of electrocardiology (see text).

Both Sir T. Lewis and F.N. Wilson became good friends with Einthoven (Figures 2.3B and 2.5) and both died at a relatively young age from acute infarction. In fact, T. Lewis was nominated several times with Einthoven as a candidate for Nobel Prize. However, finally was only awarded Einthoven, probably because in spite of the great importance of his discoveries, it was considered that the research of T. Lewis was not completely original (Bayés de Luna 2019). During the last two decades of his life, he believed that was not nothing left to discover in the field of electrocardiography and dedicated his interest to the field of peripheral circulation.

Other important researchers and pioneers before my traineeship (1960–1963) include among others (Figure 2.6) Hubert Mann (1891–1974), who recorded the first version of VCG loops (1920), and J. Herrick who published (1919) the first ECG in a patient who had a myocardial infarction (MI), and H. Pardee (1920) the first sequential ECG changes in an acute MI. As mentioned above, George Fahr (1880–1959) was the first to correctly recognize the ECG pattern of bundle branch block (Fahr and Weber 1915). In the field of basic electrophysiology, G Ralph Mines (1886–1914) first described the reentry phenomenon (Mines 1914) and S Weidmann (1921–2005), pioneer of cellular cardiac electrophysiology, recorded the transmembrane action potential (TAP) for the first time with E Coraboeuf in 1949. Also, Louis Wolff, Sir John Parkinson, and Paul Dudley White (Figure 2.7), who described the first electrocardiological syndrome, the Wolff–Parkinson–White (WPW) syndrome, in 1930, a very significant contribution to Cardiology (Wolff *et al.* 1930).

Since my training, I have had the privilege to contemplate many great advances and discoveries in the field of electrocardiography, which I consider to be not just a part of history but part of the present and the future. These include among others: (i) a better knowledge of cellular electrophysiology (Hoffman, Cranefield); (ii) a correct interpretation of intraventricular blocks from an experimental and clinical point of view (Sodi-Pallares and his group, Medrano, Bisteni, Rosenbaum and Elizari); (iii) the first studies on intracavitary electrocardiography (Alanis, Puech, Scherlag) (Figure 2.6); (iv) the discovery of total excitation of the human heart (Durrer); (v) the clinical application of new methods to the study of the electrical activity of the heart, such as exercise ECGs (Bruce, Ellestad), continuous ECG recording, especially Holter technology (Kennedy, Stern); (vi) the programmed electrophysiological studies (Wellens, Coumel, Josephson); (vii) the discovery of the critical importance of ECGs for the diagnosis of some inherited heart diseases (Moss, Schwartz, and Brugada brothers that discover the Brugada syndrome) (Figure 2.8); (viii) the importance of the diagnosis of interatrial blocks and other P wave indices and their association to atrial fibrillation, stroke, and dementia (Bayés syndrome) (Bayés de Luna, Spodick, Garcia-Cosio,

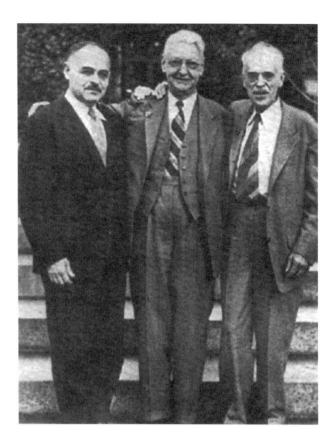

Figure 2.7 From left to right: Louis Wolff, Sir John Parkinson, and Paul Dudley White, the discoverers of the first arrhythmological syndrome (Drj).

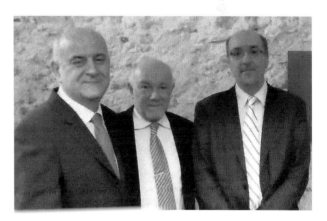

Figure 2.8 Brugada brothers. Pere in the middle with Josep and Ramon at his right and left side.

Baranchuk, Bayés-Genís, Platonov, Martínez-Sellés, Magnani, Soliman, Chen LY, etc.); (ix) advances in the knowledge of mechanisms (Moe, Antzelevitch, Jalife, Zipes) and clinical diagnosis of arrhythmias (Schamroth, Fisch); (x) the demonstration of the usefulness of ECGs in following the evolution of ischemic and other heart diseases (Sclarovsky, Birnbaum, Nikus, Fiol-Sala, Gorgels, Wagner, Bacharova, Viskin), in the diagnosis of some cardiomyopathies (Fontaine and Marcus), and of different situations such as electrolyte disturbances (Surawicz), athletes (Maron, Pelliccia, Corrado, etc.); (xi) the implementation of a scoring system to measure the size of necrotic tissue (Selvester, Wagner); (xii) the emergence of automatization and computerization of ECGs (Pipberger, Rautaharju, Willems, Macfarlane); (xiii) the importance of the ECG in many aspects related to the electrical treatment of arrhythmias and sudden death from cardioversion to pacemakers and implantable defibrillators, and, recently, resynchronization therapy (Lown, Zoll, Elmqvist, Mirowski, Moss, Cazeau, Daubert) and its drug treatment (Bigger, Breithardt, Camm, Connolly, Yusuf, Kirchhof, Kottkamp), and many others that surely deserves to be mentioned here. **All of these advances and many others will be discussed throughout the book.** Because of them, the ECG has become more useful, and more frequently used, than ever before. By sure I have forgotten many other important names. Please consult some of the books devoted to this topic ECG (see Recommended reading).

References

Bayés de Luna A. Willem Einthoven and the ECG. Antoni Bayés de Luna discusses the discovery of the ECG almost 120 years ago which has remained almost unchanged to the present day. *Eur Heart J* 2019;40: 3381.

Burch GE, DePasquale NP. *The History of Electrocardiography*. YearBook Medical, 1964.

Einthoven W. The different forms of the human electrocardiogram and their signification. *Lancet* 1912;March 30:853.

Fahr GE, Weber A. Über die ortsbestinmmung der Erregnung im menschlichen Herzen. *Deutsch Arch Klin Med* 1915;117:361.

Herrick JB. Thrombosis of the coronary artery. *JAMA* 1919;72:387.

Kligfield P. Derivation of the correct waveform of the human electrocardiogram by Willem Einthoven, 1890–1895. *Cardiol J* 2010;17:109.

Lewis T. *Clinical Electrocardiography*. Shaw-Sons, 1913.

Lewis T. *Electrocardiography and Clinical Disorders of the Heart Beat*. Shaw-Sons, 1949.

Mann H. A method of analyzing the ECG. *Arch Intern Med* 1920;25:683.

Mines GR. On circulating excitations in heart muscles and their possible relation to tachycardia and fibrillation. *Trans R Soc Can* 1914;4:43.

Moukabary T. Willem Einthoven (1860–1927): father of electrocardiography. *Cardiol J* 2007;14:316.

Pardee H. An electrocardiographic sign of coronary artery obstruction. *Arch Int. Med.* 1920;26:244.

Rosen MR. The electrocardiogram 100 years later. Electrical insights into molecular messages. *Circulation* 2002;106:2173.

Rosen MR, Janse M. Electrophysiology: from Galvani's frog to the implantable defibrillator. *Dialogues CV Med* 2006;11:123.

Snellen HA. *Selected Papers on Electrocardiography of Willem Einthoven*. Leiden University Press, 1977.

Wilson FN, McLeod AG, Barker P. The potential variations produced by the heart beat at the apices of Einthoven's triangle. *Am Heart J* 1931;7:207.

Wilson FN, Johnston FD, Rosenbaum F, *et al.* The precordial ECG. *Am Heart J* 1944;27:19.

Wolff L, Parkinson J, White PD. Bundle branch block without PR interval in healthy young people prone to paroxysmal tachycardia. *Am Heart J* 1930;5:685.

Chapter 3
Utility and Limitations of the Surface ECG: Present and Future

Introduction

More than 100 years have passed since the invention of the surface ECG and we now live in an age when new inventions and progress in medicine are seen every day, so it is astonishing that the surface ECG not only still exists but also remains as a "gold standard" technique for the study of electrical disorders of the heart. The following is an overview of the most relevant advantages and disadvantages, as well as the utility and limitations, of the surface ECG.

Utility

ECG as the best diagnostic tool (Fiol-Sala *et al.* 2020, Bayés de Luna and Baranchuk 2017)

The ECG is the best diagnostic tool for the following:
- The diagnosis and evaluation of **tachy and brady arrhythmias**, conduction disorders, at sinoatrial, at atrial, AV junction and ventricular level, and pre-excitation syndromes.
- **Differential diagnosis in cases of broad QRS tachycardia** with one strip of the surface ECG. Correct differential diagnosis (supraventricular vs. ventricular tachycardia) can be achieved in more than 90% of cases.
- **Some ECG patterns may be markers of future tachyarrhythmias, or even of global, CV, or of sudden death such as** Wolff–Parkinson–White (WPW) pattern, channelopathies and some P wave indices especially duration P wave, the advanced interatrial block (A-IAB), the P axis, and P voltage. And, also recently a score of P wave may be more useful that P wave indices alone (Alexander *et al.* 2019), and the association of P wave indices with CHA2DS2-Vasc (Maheshwari *et al.* 2019) (see Chapter 9).

The ECG also may perform, sometimes with the help of clinical history, the differential diagnosis of some types of ECG pattern such as Brugada phenocopies (Baranchuk 2018).
- Determining whether or not it is necessary **to implant a pacemaker** or cardiac resynchronization therapy (CRT) (Chapter 17).
- **The diagnosis of acute ischemic events**. In this case, it is essential to have the clinical information, but a good knowledge of ECG patterns may help to perform the diagnosis of acute coronary syndromes (ACS), and to classify them into two types: those with ST segment elevation and those with non-ST segment elevation (Bayés de Luna *et al.* 2007) (see Chapters 13 and 20).
- As said, the detection of a phenotype expression of **channelopathies** (long QT, short QT, Brugada syndrome). In other inherited heart diseases, such as hypertrophic cardiomyopathy or arrhythmogenic right ventricular dysplasia, the ECG may also help in the diagnosis, but there is no clear genotype–phenotype correlation (Bayés de Luna and Baranchuk 2017) (Chapter 21).
- The surveillance of different types of pacemakers and implanted defibrillators (ICD).

When the ECG is also important
The ECG is also important for the following:
- To presume a diagnosis of chronic ischemic heart disease (IHD), especially of chronic Q wave myocardial infarction (MI).
- The evaluation and follow-up of patients **following MI** or cardiac surgery.
- The diagnosis and study of the **evolution of other heart diseases**, such as valvular heart diseases or pericarditis (Spodick 2003), and in special circumstances, such as electrolyte imbalance (Surawicz 1967) or drug administration.

• The evaluation of **athletes and check-ups** in general, and as a pre-operative assessment for cardiac and non-cardiac surgery.

The correlation of ECG patterns with the clinical setting

The ECG is currently of great utility, not only from a diagnostic point of view, but also from a prognostic one, in addition to its use in the management of heart disease. This is clearly illustrated in the acute phase of IHD. ACS are classified into two groups to decide treatment: with ST elevation (STEMI) and without ST elevation (NSTEMI) (see above and Chapter 20).

This classification, although challenged by some authors (Phibbs 2010), is very helpful in stratifying the management of ACS and is used worldwide and accepted in all guidelines (ACC/AHA/HRS 2007, 2009).

However, it is important to note that even experts in ECG diagnosis experience problems in correctly interpreting ST changes without good clinical information (see Bayés de Luna *et al.* 2007; Jayroe *et al.* 2009; Nikus *et al.* 2010; Fiol-Sala *et al.* 2020, and Chapter 19) (see Section "Limitations").

Correlation with coronarography and imaging techniques

The correlation between ECG patterns and coronarography in cases of ACS is very valuable to better locate the occlusion site and area at risk (Sclarowsky 1999; Wellens *et al.* 2003; Fiol *et al.* 2004, 2009; Fiol-Sala *et al.* 2020).

Contrast-enhanced cardiac magnetic resonance (CE-CMR) is very useful in determining the presence and size of MI (Moon *et al.* 2004) and in demonstrating that the first area of myocardium to suffer the effects of ischemia is the subendocardium (Mahrholdt *et al.* 2005). **In patients with chronic MI** in particular, **the correlation of ECG patterns and CE-CMR** has been very useful in demonstrating and properly locating the presence of necrotic areas according to the new terminology used for heart walls (Cerqueira *et al.* 2002; Bayés de Luna *et al.* 2006a; Fiol-Sala *et al.* 2020). For example, it has been demonstrated that in post-MI patients, the R wave in V1 is caused by lateral, not posterior, MI and that "q" in aVL is caused by first diagonal occlusion (midanterior MI) rather than circumflex occlusion (high lateral MI) (Bayés de Luna *et al.* 2006b, 2008; Rovai *et al.* 2007; Van der Weg *et al.* 2009) (see Figure 13.68).

The ECG as a research tool

The ECG is used in epidemiological studies and in the safety evaluation of new drugs with recognized or potential cardiac effects (QT interval, arrhythmias, etc.).

Other benefits

ECG recording is an inexpensive, easy, and quick technique to register the electrical activity of the heart.

Limitations

• Despite the usefulness of the ECG in acute MI, many patients ($\approx$30–50%) with old MI or chronic IHD present with a **normal or non-definitively abnormal ECG** at rest and often even during exercise. If the physician is not well trained, small changes may not be correctly perceived.

• **Some severe heart diseases** such as pulmonary embolism, cardiac tamponade, acute aneurysmal dissection, or even as acute ischemic attack **may present not ECG changes at all, or only non-specific, or subtle ECG changes** that may only be interpreted correctly by those with very good ECG training, who are able to make a good correlation with the clinical setting (see Chapters 20 and 21).

• Following the emergence of **new imaging techniques** (echocardiography and especially cardiovascular magnetic resonance), the diagnosis of chamber enlargement and congenital heart disease is more precise than with electrocardiography alone. However, the usefulness of ECG recording is still important in some aspects, not only from a diagnostic point of view, but also from a prognostic one (see Chapter 10). Furthermore, although no full correlation between ECG changes and these imaging techniques has been performed, the results obtained to date have been promising (see Chapters 9 and 10).

• The ECG can be a misleading diagnostic tool if the existence or absence of underlying heart disease is identified based only on the presence of a normal or abnormal ECG pattern. Unfortunately, the **ECG does not have a talisman's power**. When faced with a patient presenting with precordial pain of unknown origin, it is a great mistake to proclaim "The ECG will settle this." While it is true that the ECG may give crucial information that may be decisive for the diagnosis, on some occasions even in the very acute phase of MI, the ECG may remain unmodified or presenting changes (f.i. positive and symmetrical T wave in right precordial leads) that may be considered normal. Therefore, it would be very dangerous to fail to integrate the ECG information with the clinical setting. On the other hand, healthy individuals sometimes present with some alterations of the ECG, which may lead to a wrong diagnosis if used alone (f.i. do not perform a new recording with deep inspiration in the presence of Q in lead III) (see Chapter 25). Therefore, **the ECG must always be interpreted in the light of the clinical context**. At present, a manual interpretation of the ECG is still advised. Automatic interpretation, which may produce a more accurate and useful computer-generated report, will likely be used more often in the future, but currently computer interpretation needs physician overreading (see later) (Kligfield *et al.* 2007).

• Clearly, a **normal ECG should not be considered a "warranty"** and in fact does not exclude the possibility of cardiac death resulting from an electrical disturbance (i.e. ventricular fibrillation or bradyarrhythmias), even on the same day that the ECG is recorded. If there is some clinical suspicion of IHD, serial ECGs should be recorded and an attempt should be made to ascertain the cause of the pain, regardless of the presence of a normal or nearly normal ECG at entrance.

• **Normal variants of the ECG may be related to body constitution, thoracic malformations**, race, or gender. **The ECG may also show transient changes** caused by metabolic or other disorders (hyperventilation, hypothermia, glucose or alcohol intake, electrolyte disorders, drug effects, etc.).

• **There are limitations inherent in the technology used.** Until recently, the recording process was based on analog techniques. These techniques present limitations because the quality of the recording decreases with time, storage become a problem, and it is impossible to transmit the recording immediately. It also has to be considered the possible presence of technical errors in the recording process (Chapter 6). Therefore, digitalized ECG is very much recommended.

• Probably the most important limitation of the ECG is not the technique itself but rather **the physician's lack of ECG expertise.** Currently, the majority of hospitals do not provide a period devoted to training by experts in ECG diagnosis. It is important that the ECG is studied with an updated mentor in a systematic and sequential way, which is what we attempt to do in this book. It is also extremely important as we have already said to interpret the ECG bearing in mind the clinical context. Once the training period is finished, periodic updated programmes are necessary. Universities, Hospitals, and Scientific Societies must organize intramural and extramural meetings, including internet courses, designed for trainees and also their mentors. This will allow the weaknesses to be identified and the knowledge to be reinforced. An adequate traineeship approach would be of great advantage for the healthcare system because it would allow for: (i) a better and quicker diagnosis, prognosis and management in many situations (acute ischemic events, patients at risk of sudden death, the need for pacemaker implant, etc.) and (ii) the avoidance of more sophisticated techniques, resulting in saved money, time, and discomfort.

• **Some limitations of the surface ECG may be overcome by other electrocardiological techniques**. It is clear that the study of the electrical activity of the heart using exercise and long-term recording (monitoring and Holter technology), intracardiac electrophysiological studies, filtering systems, body mapping, etc. (see Chapter 25), may help in some specific ways. This adds to the usefulness of the surface ECG and reduces its limitations.

Finally, the correlation with imaging techniques, especially echocardiography, cardiac multislice scanner, and cardiac magnetic resonance, complements the capacity of ECG for the diagnosis, prognosis, and management of heart diseases. We will deal with each of these aspects later along the book.

The future of electrocardiography

Undoubtedly, what is most important for the future is to try to overcome the limitations that still exist in electrocardiography. Fortunately, we are already obtaining great results in this respect. The ECG is an evolving, living science and its future is very promising, particularly if the advancements described below are achieved (Guidelines AHA/ACC/HRS 2007–2009) (see Chapter 26). Due to that, the standards for ECG interpretation require periodic review and revision (Gettes 2009).

The ECG in the digital era (see Chapter 26)

We are now immersed in the digital era, and in the field of ECG, this has given rise to the need for functional programs and devices that are portable, versatile, and interactive. Nearly all current ECG machines convert the analog ECG signal to digital form. The initial sampling rate during analog-to-digital conversion is higher than the sampling rate that is used for further processing. This oversampling was originally introduced to detect and represent pacemaker stimulus outputs which are generally <0.5 ms in duration.

Ideally, ECG machines should be small and compact, and must work in an integrated fashion in various health institutional settings, independently of the type of technology used. These systems allow us to work online and may be incorporated into telemedical services. Compression of ECGs is recommended for transmission and data storage. In an ideal world, the diagnosis could be performed by an expert in real time through the Internet and telephone, and this could then be applied to multiple scenarios (ambulance, isolated areas, ships, etc.) with poor access to assistance because of their geographic location or associated economic costs (see Figure 6.19).

Improvements in automated ECG interpretation

In spite of all, new improvements in automatic interpretation currently, all automatic recordings need to be reviewed by a physician (American College of Cardiology/

American Heart Association 2007). By entering more data about the patient (sex, age, body habitus, and clinical history) and facilitating a link to ECG-pedia—a corpus containing information taken from many ECG books and reports that can assist in the correct diagnosis—it may be possible, although it has to be proved along this century, that the need that all automatic interpretation to be reviewed will not be necessary. However, according to Surawicz (2010), a comparison between a diagnosis performed by a computer linked to an updated ECG-pedia and an ECG expert would be as interesting as a chess match between a computer and a chess master. For the moment, the ECG expert would win. Probably in the future, the match will be more equal (see Chapter 26).

New advances in correlation with imaging techniques

As previously explained, **CE-CMR is useful in detecting the presence of necrosis and the size of MI, as well as identifying, in correlation with the ECG, the location of the necrosis.** However, while the correlation between scoring ECG system and CE-CMR for estimating infarction size and measuring the left ventricular ejection fraction (LVEF) is reasonable, it is not consistent enough because the results are always larger with CE-CMR (Weir *et al.* 2010). Therefore, to obtain an accurate and reproducible estimation of infarct size and LVEF by surface ECG in survivors of acute MI using a 12-lead ECG would be a great success and something that would allow a significantly better correlation between ECG scoring and CE-CMR (Weir *et al.* 2010).

In addition, **a better definition of the diagnosis of chamber enlargement performed by ECG criteria** could be made using CMR correlation. Echocardiographic comparison underestimates the volume size of atrial chambers (Whitlock *et al.* 2010). Diagnosis would probably be more accurate if a correlation between ECG and CMR detecting chamber enlargement were performed (see Chapter 9).

Recently has been demonstrated (Lacalzada *et al.* 2018) that the presence of A-IAB in surface ECG is a surrogate of reduced LA strain measured by echo speckle-tracking, and also A-IAB is a surrogate of atrial fibrosis and LA dyssynchrony detected by CMR (Ciuffo *et al.* 2020).

The use of the ECG in new treatments of heart disease

The use of ECG in new treatments such as cardiac regeneration or the detection of cardiac rejection show promises for the future.

Rapid recording of the ECG means better treatment

Figure 20.1 shows the evolution of the ST elevation acute coronary syndrome (STE-ACS) from the 1970s to the present. Today, we can take quick decisions based on the prompt recording of the ECG and save lives, or at least reduce cardiac muscle damage, while in the past, we are not able frequently to detect the early changes and identify as abnormal or presumably abnormal some characteristics of especially ECG repolarization, such as pecked positive T wave recorded in right precordial leads (see Figure 20.4).

Improving the capacity of the ECG

Further improvements in the capacity for better diagnosis, risk stratification, prognosis, and management of heart diseases or other processes are possible (Poplack Potter 2010). This will be included in the concept of **"expanded surface ECG" or "ECG plus"** and may be accomplished by the following potential future developments:

• **Using amplification methods** in order to record the ECG (×4 amplification). This will permit the shifts of ST to be better recognized; a 0.5 mm change is sufficient for diagnosing ACS (see Figure 13.24). This will also help us to study better the P wave especially the morphology and duration so important to diagnose interatrial blocks, the initial forces of pre-excitation, intraventricular blocks, early repolarization pattern, or Brugada pattern, among others.

• **Recording the ECG at a higher speed** may be useful to detect atrioventricular (AV) dissociation.

• **Additional leads**, including Lewis leads (Bakker *et al.* 2009), esophageal leads, etc. (see Chapters 6 and 25), may be used.

• **Recording parameters such as late potentials and others to study ANS imbalance (HRV, HRT, T wave alternans, etc.).**

• **Being able in the future to record the bundle of His** deflection **externally**, which permits a better evaluation of the long PR interval and intraventricular conduction disorders. This may help in the decision-making process for pacemaker implants. This was reported to be feasible by signal averaging more than 40 years ago, but has not been implemented in commercial devices (Wajszczuk *et al.* 1978).

• **Developing the capacity** to filter some waves of the ECG to better see other waves using wavelet technology. For instance, by **filtering the T wave**, a better definition and correct identification of P wave activity may be achieved in cases of arrhythmias. While this was once reported using analog technology, it has now been demonstrated using digital technology (Goldwasser *et al.* 2011). These techniques may currently perform the correct diagnosis of different types of supraventricular tachycardias, especially in distinguishing between atrioventricular nodal reentrant tachycardia (AVNRT) and atrioventricular reentrant tachycardia (AVRT) (see Chapter 25). The next step would be to identify the presence of AV dissociation, which is crucial to the differential diagnosis of broad QRS tachycardias. Filtering the QRS to identify any hidden P-wave and to better study the characteristics of atrial fibrillation waves is another possibility (Platonov *et al.* 2012).

• **Redefining old ECG criteria with new methodology and technology**. For example, "notches and slurrings" in the QRS to diagnose some types of necrosis and many other processes, which was already published some decades ago by Horan *et al.* (1971) and now rediscovered by Das *et al.* (2006).

• **Synthesizing VCG loops from the 12-lead ECG recording**. This may be done with a conversion matrix (Edenbrandt and Pahlm 1988, Kors *et al.* 1990), or directly from a 12-lead ECG (Rautaharju *et al.* 2007). This can be useful not only for teaching, but also for some diagnostic (for instance, presence of minor pre-excitation and better study of P wave), prognostic, and research purposes. Different VCG studies have demonstrated that a widened spatial QRS–T angle is associated with subsequent CV death (Kardys *et al.* 2003) and also recently new possibilities of VCG in stratifying the risk of sudden death have been noted (Lazzara 2010). These studies have mainly been performed taking the VCG loops from the orthogonal leads x, y, and z (leads perpendicular to each other similar to leads I, aVF, and V2, see Chapter 25). As these leads are not recorded in clinical practice, the vectorcardiographic loops may be synthesized from the 12-lead ECG recording with similar results (Kors *et al.* 1990). Therefore, it may be interesting to incorporate synthesized VCG loops into the "expanded ECG" concept. In fact, although was published that the ECG frontal plane QRS-T angle should not be considered an adequate diagnostic substitute for the spatial QRS-T angle (Brown and Schlegel 2011), recent studies as yet not published seem to demonstrate that the calculation of the QRS–T angle in the frontal plane from the surface ECG will probably be equivalent to the spatial QRS–T angle taken from the VCG synthesized from an ECG.

To summarize, the new generation of cardiologists being aware of the importance of ECG. We agree with Arthur Moss that says **"We are experiencing a great renaissance of electrocardiography** (Moss 2004). With this in mind, it is important to encourage the enthusiasm of young physicians for the ECG."

References

Alexander B, Milden J, Hazim B, *et al.* New electrocardiographic score for the prediction of atrial fibrillation: the MVP ECG risk score (morphology-voltage-P wave duration). *Ann Noninvasive Electrocardiol* 2019;00:e12669.

American College of Cardiology/American Heart Association. Guidelines for the management of patients with unstable angina/non-ST-elevation myocardial infarction. *J Am Coll Cardiol* 2007;50:e1–e157.

American College of Cardiology/American Heart Association. Guidelines for the management of patients with ST elevation myocardial infarction and ACC/AHA/SCAI guidelines on percutaneous coronary intervention. *J Am Coll Cardiol* 2009;54:2205–2241.

Bakker AL, Nijkerk G, Groenemeijer BE, *et al.* The Lewis lead: making recognition of P waves easy during wide QRS complex tachycardia. *Circulation* 2009;119;e592.

Baranchuk A. *Brugada Phenocopy. The Art of Recognizing the Brugada ECG Pattern*. Academic Press 2018.

Bayés de Luna A, Cino JM, Pujadas S, *et al.* Concordance of electrocardiographic patterns and healed myocardial infarction location detected by cardiovascular magnetic resonance. *Am J Cardiol* 2006a;97:443.

Bayés de Luna A, Wagner G, Birnbaum Y, *et al.* A new terminology for left ventricular walls and location of myocardial infarcts that present Q wave based on the standard of cardiac magnetic resonance imaging: a statement for healthcare professionals from a committee appointed by the International Society for Holter and Noninvasive Electrocardiography. *Circulation* 2006b;14:1755.

Bayés de Luna A, Fiol-Sala M, Antman M. *The 12 Lead ECG in ST Elevation Myocardial Infarction. A Practical Approach for Clinicians*. Blackwell-Futura, 2007.

Bayés de Luna A, Cino J, Goldwasser D, *et al.* New electrocardiographic diagnostic criteria for the pathologic R waves in leads V1 and V2 of anatomically lateral myocardial infarction. *J Electrocardiol* 2008;41:413.

Bayés de Luna A, Baranchuk A. *Clinical Arrhythmology*, 2nd edn. Willey-Blackwell, 2017.

Brown R, Schlegel T. Diagnostic utility of the spatial versus individual planar QRS-T angles in cardiac disease detection. *J Electrocardiol* 2011;44:404.

Cerqueira MD, Weissman NJ, Dilsizian V, *et al.* Standardized myocardial segmentation and nomenclature for tomographic imaging of the heart: a statement for healthcare professionals from the Cardiac Imaging Committee of the Council on Clinical Cardiology of the American Heart Association. *Circulation* 2002;105:539.

Ciuffo L, Bruña V, Martínez-Sellés M, *et al.* Association between interatrial block, left atrial fibrosis, and mechanical dyssynchrony: electrocardiography-magnetic resonance imaging correlation. *J Cardiovasc Electrophysiol* 2020; 31:1719–1725.

Das MK, Khan B, Jacob S, *et al.* Significance of a fragmented QRS complex versus a Q wave in patients with coronary artery disease. *Circulation* 2006;113:2495.

Edenbrandt L, Pahlm O. Vectorcardiogram synthesized from a 12-lead ECG: superiority of the inverse Dower matrix. *J Electrocardiol* 1988;21:361.

Fiol M, Cygankiewicz I, Bayés Genis A, *et al.* The value of ECG algorithm based on "ups and downs" of ST in assessment of a culprit artery in evolving inferior myocardial infarction. *Am J Cardiol* 2004;94:709.

Fiol M, Carrillo A, Cygankiewicz I, *et al.* A new electrocardiographic algorithm to locate the occlusion in left anterior descending coronary artery. *Clin Cardiol* 2009;32:E1–6.

Fiol-Sala M, Birnbaum Y, Nikus K, Bayés de Luna A. *Electrocardiography in Ischemic Heart Disease. Clinical and Imaging Correlations and Prognostic Implications*, 2nd edn. Willey-Blackwell, 2020.

Gettes L. The status of the standards. *J Electrocardiol* 2009;42:213.

Goldwasser D, Bayés de Luna A, Serra G, *et al.* A new method of filtering T waves to detect hidden P waves in electrocardiogram signals. *Europace* 2011;13: 1028–1033.

Horan L, Flowers N, Johnson J. Significance of the diagnostic Q wave of myocardial infarction. *Circulation* 1971;63:428.

Jayroe JB, Spodick DH, Nikus K, *et al.* Differentiating ST elevation myocardial infarction and nonischemic cause of ST elevation by analyzing the presenting electrocardiogram. *Am J Cardiol* 2009;103:301.

Kardys I, Kors J, Kuip D, Witteman J, Hofman A. Spatial QRS-T angle predicts cardiac death in a general population. *Eur Heart J* 2003;24:1357.

Kligfield P, Gettes LS, Bailey JJ, *et al.* Recommendations for the standardization and interpretation of the electrocardiogram: Part I: The electrocardiogram and its technology: a scientific statement from the American Heart Association-Electrocardiography and Arrhythmias Committee, Council on Clinical Cardiology; the American College of Cardiology Foundation; and the Heart Rhythm Society: endorsed by the International Society for Computerized Electrocardiology. *Circulation* 2007;115:1306–1324.

Kors JA, van Herpen G, Sittig AC, van Bemmel JH. Reconstruction of the Frank vectorcardiogram from standard electrocardiographic leads: diagnostic comparison of different methods. *Eur Heart J* 1990;11:1083.

Lacalzada-Almeida J, Izquierdo-Gómez M, Belleyo-Belkasem C, *et al.* Interatrial block and atrial remodeling assessed using speckle tracking echocardiography. *BMC Cardiovascular Disorders* 2018;18:38.

Lazzara R. Spatial vectorcardiogram to predict risk for sudden arrhythmic death: Phoenix risen from the ashes. *Heart Rhythm* 2010;7:1614.

Maheshwari A, Norby FL, Roetker NS, *et al.* Refining prediction of atrial fibrillation-related stroke using the P_2-CHA_2DS_2-Vasc Score. ARIC and MESA. *Circulation* 2019;139:180.

Mahrholdt H, Wagner A, Judd RM, *et al.* Delayed enhancement cardiovascular magnetic resonance assessment of non-ischemic cardiomyopathies. *Eur Heart J* 2005;26:1461.

Moon JC, De Arenaza DP, Elkington AG, *et al.* The pathologic basis of Q-wave and non-Q-wave myocardial infarction: a cardiovascular magnetic resonance study. *J Am Coll Cardiol* 2004;44:554.

Moss AJ. A renaissance in electrocardiography. *Ann Noninvasive Electrocardiol* 2004;9:1.

Nikus K, Pahlm O, Wagner G, *et al.* Electrocardiographic classification of acute coronary syndromes: a review by a committee of the International Society for Holter and Non-Invasive Electrocardiology. *J Electrocardiol* 2010;43:91–103.

Phibbs B. Differential classification of acute myocardial infarction into ST- and non-ST segment elevation is not valid or rational. *Ann Noninvasive Electrocardiol* 2010;15(3):191.

Platonov P, Cygankiewicz I, Stridh M, *et al.* Low atrial fibrillatory rate is associated with poor outcome in patients with mild to moderate heart failure. *Circulation Arrhythmia Electrophysiol* 2012;5:77.

Poplack Potter SL. Detection of hypertrophic cardiomyopathy is improved when using advanced rather than strictly conventional 12-lead electrocardiogram. *J Electrocardiol* 2010;43:713.

Rautaharju PM, Prineas RJ, Zhang ZM. A simple procedure for estimation of the spatial QRS/T angle from the standard 12-lead ECG. *J Electrocardiol* 2007;40:300.

Rovai D, Di Bella G, Rossi G, *et al.* Q-wave prediction of myocardial infarct location, size and transmural extent at magnetic resonance imaging. *Coronary Artery Dis* 2007;18:381.

Sclarovsky S. *Electrocardiography of Acute Myocardial Ischaemic Syndromes.* Martin Dunitz, 1999.

Spodick DH. Acute pericarditis: current concepts and practice. *JAMA* 2003;289:1150.

Surawicz B. Relationship between ECG and electrolites. *J Am Heart* 1967;73:814.

Surawicz B. How to increase the accuracy of electrocardiogram's interpretation and stimulate the interest of the interpreters? *J Electrocardiol* 2010;43:191.

Van der Weg K, Bekkers S, Winkens B, *et al.* The R in V1 in non-anterior wall infarction indicates lateral rather than posterior involvement. Results from ECG/MRI correlations. *Eur Heart J* 2009;30(suppl):P2981.

Wajszczuk WJ, Stopczyk MJ, Moskowitz MS, *et al.* Noninvasive recording of His-Purkinje activity in man by QRS-triggered signal averaging. *Circulation* 1978;48:95.

Weir R, Martin T, Wagner G. Comparison of infarct size and LVEF by CE-CMR and ECG scoring in reperfused anterior STEMI. *J Electrocardiol* 2010;43:230.

Wellens HJJ, Gorgels A, Doevendans P. *The ECG in Acute Infarction and Unstable Angina.* Kluwer Academic, 2003.

Whitlock M, Garg A, Gelow J, *et al.* Comparison of left and right atrial volume by echocardiography versus cardiac magnetic resonance imaging using the area-length method. *Am J Cardiol* 2010;106:1345.

Part 2
The Normal ECG

Chapter 4
The Anatomical Basis of the ECG: From Macroscopic Anatomy to Ultrastructural Characteristics

The anatomical basis

From an anatomical point of view, the heart is made up of four cavities (Figure 4.1): two atria and two ventricles, connected by the atrioventricular (AV) valves. The pulmonary artery originates from the right ventricle and the aorta from the left ventricle. The superior and inferior vena cava are connected to the right atrium and the four pulmonary veins to the left atrium. The pacemaker of the heart is located in the sinus node close to the superior vena cava. The electrical stimulus arrives at the atrial and ventricular myocardium, where the excitation–contraction coupling is performed, through internodal tracts, the AV node, and the intraventricular conduction system (ICS) (see Figure 4.7).

The following is a description of the characteristics of the heart walls and of the specific conduction system (SCS), which are important from an electrocardiographic point of view (Figures 4.1–4.9).

The heart walls: perfusion and innervation (Cerqueira 2002; Fiol-Sala *et al*. 2020)

Our best information on the anatomical aspects of the heart walls including necrotic zones and myocardial viability has been obtained from cardiovascular magnetic resonance imaging (CMR) along with the study of the coronary tree performed by both invasive coronariography and the multislice scanner. In addition, CMR and isotopic studies are useful in studying the perfusion of the heart. Another useful technique is echocardiography, which is used to identify heart chamber volume, heart wall thickness, the presence of hypocinetic zones, and myocardial function (ejection fraction).

The left ventricle has four walls (Figure 4.1). They are currently identified as **septal, anterior, lateral, and inferior**. Historically (Perloff 1964), the term *true posterior wall* was given to the basal part of the inferior wall

that bends upward. However, using imaging techniques such as CMR, it has been demonstrated (Bayés de Luna 2006a; Fiol-Sala *et al*. 2020) that the basal part of the inferior wall bends upward in only 25–30% of cases (Figure 4.2) and that a posterior inclination of all inferior (diaphragmatic) wall is present in only 5% of cases in very lean individuals with the heart in a vertical position (Figure 4.2C). The *true posterior wall* is now known as the *inferobasal part of the inferior wall,* according to the American Societies of Imaging (Cerqueira 2002). This appears to be a suitable name given that the true posterior wall does not usually exist. From the oblique sagittal view, the anterior and inferior walls (Figure 4.3A) present one part anterior and the other posterior, and also in the horizontal axial plane, one part of the septal and lateral wall is located more anteriorly with respect to the rest of the wall (Figure 4.3B). This is completely contrary to the idea that a true and independent posterior wall exists. As previously stated, it occurs in very few cases (5%) (Figure 4.2C) and when it does occur, the orientation of the necrosis vector also is toward V3–V4, not V1–V2 (Figure 4.3A).

Despite clear findings that the true posterior wall usually does not exist (Cerqueira 2002; Bayés de Luna 2006a), correct heart wall terminology is not always used and has even been questioned (Garcia-Cosio 2008; Bayés de Luna 2008a; Gorgels and van der Web 2010; Kalinauskiene 2010; Bayés de Luna 2011). It usually takes some time to change a dogma. In their book *History of Electrocardiography* (1964), Burch and DePasquale state that:

> because of efforts by some to advance their own ideas rather than the science itself, progress in electrocardiography has, at times, been hindered. Even obviously simple problems, such as nomenclature, were made difficult because of individual prejudices. Fortunately, truth finally prevails and the best ideas supervene. However, much time and effort is required before the truth is recognized, as is well exemplified by the history of the development of the clinical use of the precordial leads.

Clinical Electrocardiography: A Textbook, Fifth Edition. Antoni Bayés de Luna, Miquel Fiol-Sala, Antoni Bayés-Genís, and Adrián Baranchuk.
© 2022 John Wiley & Sons Ltd. Published 2022 by John Wiley & Sons Ltd.

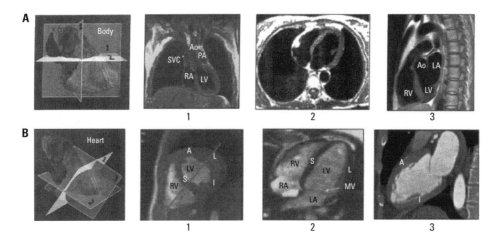

Figure 4.1 Cardiovascular magnetic resonance imaging (CMR). (A) Transections of the heart following the classical human body planes: (1) frontal plane, (2) horizontal plane, and (3) sagittal plane. (B) Transections of the heart following the heart planes that cut the body obliquely. These are the planes used by cardiac imaging experts: (1) short-axis (transverse) view, in this case at mid-level; (2) horizontal long-axis view; (3) vertical long-axis view (oblique sagittal-like). (Cerqueira 2002; Bayés de Luna *et al.* 2006a; Fiol-Sala *et al.* 2020) (Fiol-Sala *et al.* 2020).

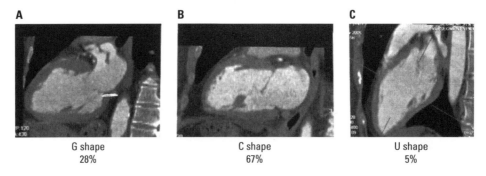

Figure 4.2 Sagittal–oblique view in a normal body build subject (A) ("G shape"), in an obese man with horizontal heart (B) ("C shape"), and a very lean subject (C) ("U shape"). We have found that the inferior wall does not bend upward in the C shape (two-thirds of cases) and is just slightly posterior in the basal part in 28% of cases (A). Only in very lean individuals with a "U shape" is the largest part of the diaphragmatic wall posterior (5% of the cases) (U shape) (5%).

This is also what happens with the concept of posterior wall/versus lateral wall. Finally, was accepted in 2015 (Bayés de Luna *et al.* 2015) the end of the dogma that posterior wall exist, and that the R wave in V1 was due to lateral not posterior MI. It was the result of several studies performed by our group and others that demonstrated (Bayés de Luna *et al.* 2006a, 2006b; Cino *et al.* 2006; Rovai *et al.* 2007; Bayés de Luna 2008a, 2008b; Bayés de Luna *et al.* 2008; Van der Weg *et al.* 2009; Fiol-Sala *et al.* 2020) that the correlation of ECG with the "in vivo" anatomy provided by CE-CMR supports this new terminology and the correlation of Q wave myocardial infarctions with these four walls: septal, anterior, lateral, and inferior (see Chapters 13 and 20).

The four walls may be projected onto the heart planes: the short axis (transverse), the vertical long axis (sagittal-like), and the horizontal long axis, both in CMR imaging (Figure 4.3) and isotopic studies (Colour Plate 1), in addition to echocardiography. These four walls are divided into 17 segments (Figure 4.4), represented in Figure 4.5 in the form of a target. Figure 4.6 shows the perfusion that the different segments receive from the coronary arteries (B–D). It is important to point out that there are some variants in coronary flow distribution as a result of anatomical variants in the coronary arteries. In 80% of cases, the left anterior descending (LAD) artery is long and wraps around the apex, and in around 80% of cases, the right coronary artery (RCA) dominates the left circumflex artery (LCX). Colour Plate 2 shows the normal coronary arteries detected with a multislice scanner.

The left ventricle may be divided into two zones (Figure 4.6): the **inferolateral zone** encompassing the inferior wall, some of the lower part of the septal wall, and nearly all of the lateral wall, which is perfused by the RCA artery and LCX, and the **anteroseptal zone** encompassing the anterior wall, an important section of the anterior part of the septal wall and a small part of the

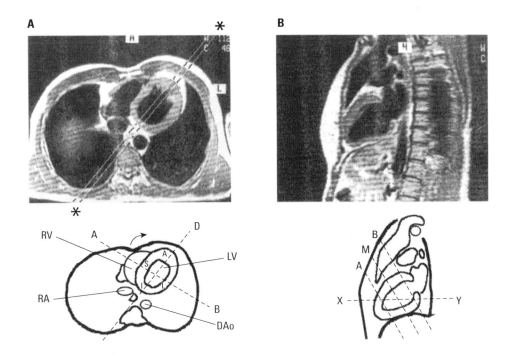

Figure 4.3 Magnetic resonance imaging. (A) Thoracic horizontal axial plane at the level of the "xy" line of the sagittal plane of right side of the figure. The four walls can be adequately observed: anterior (A), septal (S), lateral (L), and inferior (I), represented by the inferobasal portion of the wall (segment 4 of Cerqueira statement) that bends upward in this case. (B) Sagittal plane following the line seen in A (*). B, M, and A, basal, middle, and apical plane (see Figure 4.4). DAo: descending aorta; RA: right atrium; RV: right ventricle. A, S, I, L (see Figure 4.1) (Bayés de Luna *et al.* 2006a).

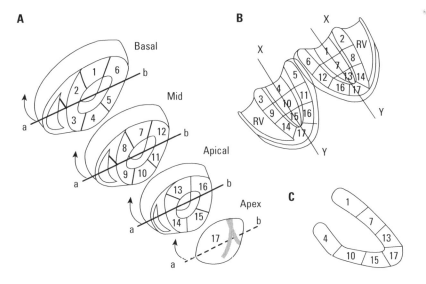

Figure 4.4 (A) Segments into which the left ventricle is divided according to the transverse (short-axis) sections performed at the basal (B), medial (M), and apical (A) levels. The basal and medial sections delineate into six segments each, while the apical section shows four segments. Together with the apex, they constitute the 17 segments into which the left ventricle can be divided, according to the classification performed by the American Imaging Societies (Cerqueira 2002). Also shown is the view of the 17 segments with the heart open in a horizontal long-axis plane (B) and vertical long-axis (sagittal-like) plane (C). RV: right ventricle (Modified from Cerqueira 2002).

mid-low lateral wall, which is perfused by the LAD artery. The lateral wall is therefore perfused mainly by the LCX and partially by the LAD and RCA. Although the anteroseptal zone is perfused by the LAD, this artery often also supplies blood to the low apical part of the inferior wall

(long LAD wrapping around the apex). The RCA perfuses the inferior wall, predominantly the mid-inferior part of the wall, the lower part of the septum and, in cases of evident RCA dominance, the entire inferior wall and part of the lateral wall. It also shares the perfusion of the right

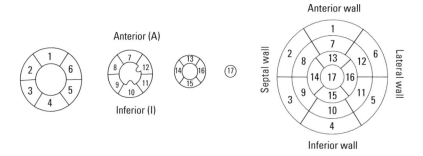

Figure 4.5 Images of the segments in which the left ventricle is divided according to the cross-sections at the basal, medial, and apical levels. Bear in mind that in this image the heart is located in the thorax strictly in a posteroanterior position. Segment 4 (inferobasal) corresponds to the classically named "posterior wall." The basal and middle sections delineate into six segments each, while the apical section shows four segments. Note in the middle section the location of the papillary muscles. On the right all 17 segments are shown in the form of a polar map ("bull's eye"), just as represented in isotopic images.

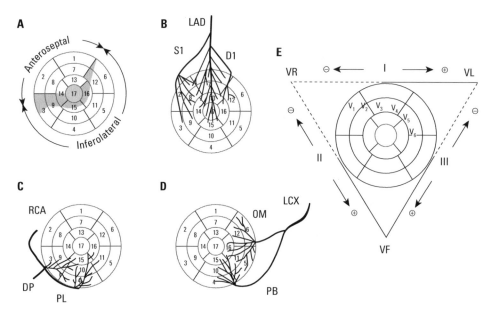

Figure 4.6 According to the anatomical variants of coronary circulation, the areas of shared variable perfusion are shown in gray (A). The perfusion of these segments by the corresponding coronary arteries (B–D) can be seen in the "bull's-eye" images. For example, the apex (segment 17) is usually perfused by the LAD but sometimes by the RCA, or even the LCX. Segments 3 and 9 are shared by LAD and RCA, and also small part of mid-low lateral wall is shared by LAD and LCX. Segments 4, 10, and 15 correspond to the RCA or the LCX, depending on which of them is dominant (the RCA in >80% of the cases). Segment 15 often receives blood from LAD. (E) Correspondence of precordial ECG. D1: first diagonal branch; LAD: left anterior descending coronary artery; LCX: left circumflex coronary artery; OM: obtuse marginal branch; PB: posterobasal branch; PD: posterior descending coronary artery; PL: posterolateral branch; RCA: right coronary artery; S1: first septal branch.

ventricle with the LAD. The LCX supplies blood to the inferolateral zone, especially the inferobasal part of the inferior wall and the lateral wall by its branch, the oblique marginal (OM) artery. The areas perfused by coronary arteries with the areas of shared perfusion are shown in Figure 4.6. The atria are perfused by a branch that usually stems from the LAD proximal part and the AV node receives perfusion mainly from the RCA (90%).

The entire atrial tissue presents a significant vagal **innervation** greater than that of the ventricles. This explains the importance of the vagus in triggering certain episodes of atrial fibrillation (see Chapter 15). In

ventricular myocardium, the sympathetic fibers run along the coronary arteries and penetrate periodically into the subepicardium. The vagal fibers are present mainly in the subendocardial zone (Zipes and Jalife 2004).

The specific conduction system: perfusion and innervation

The specific conduction system (SCS) consists of the sinus node, the internodal conduction pathways, the AV junction, and the ICS (Figure 4.7).

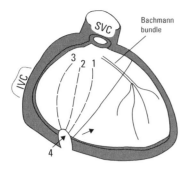

Figure 4.7 Right lateral views 1, 2 and 3 of the specific preferential conduction between two nodes in the right atrium; 4: AV node. SVC: superior cava vein and IVC: inferior cava vein.

Sinus node

The sinus node (Figure 4.7) is a small structure of the SCS located at the junction of the superior cava vein with the right atrium. Of all the SCS structures, the sinus node contains the greatest amount of automatic cells (P cells). Therefore, it is the normal site of generation of dominant pacemaker impulses: the sinus rhythm. It is traversed by the sinus node artery that perfuses it, which originates from the RCA or the CX artery (approximately 50%).

The sinus node is innervated by vagal and sympathetic fibers, which are responsible for the physiological changes of the heart rate 24 hours a day (emotions, exercise, rest).

Internodal pathways (Josephson 1978; Holmqvist *et al.* 2008)

The sinus impulse emerges to the atria at three places corresponding to the onset of three preferential internodal pathways, named Bachmann, Wenckebach, and Thorel, and is transmitted toward the AV node mainly through them. The pathways of Wenckebach and Thorel are not true bundles but rather simpler pathways that facilitate a more rapid internodal conduction. The only one that may be considered really bundle is the pathway of Bachmann. In most cases, the first activation of the left atrium (LA) takes place in the upper part of the septum, through Bachmann bundle. However, the breakthrough of the sinus impulse to the LA when the Bachmann bundle is completely blocked, may arrive though a retrograde activation of LA from zones close to coronary sinus/*fossa ovalis*.

Atrioventricular junction (Wu *et al.* 1978; Inoue and Becker 1998; Katritsis and Becker 2007)

The term atrioventricular (AV) junction should be applied to the entire area encompassing the compact AV node, the specialized tissue of the low atrium close to the AV node

and up to the coronary sinus, and the tissue from which His potentials are recorded on the atrial side of the fibrous skeleton (the proximal part of the bundle of His, the NH area). The internodal tracts come into contact with the AV node in four areas, two supero-left and two infero-right (Figure 4.8). The AV junction is followed by the bundle of His in which fibers are arranged in a parallel and linear fashion. The left branch detaches from the bundle of His, and the straight fibers give rise to the right branch (Figures 4.10 and 4.11).

The function of the AV junction is to transmit cardiac impulses from the atria toward the ventricles, with some delay in the impulse conduction. This is mainly because of the predominant presence of transitional cells in the AV junction and in the compact AV node itself.

The blood perfusion of the AV node usually (>90%) originates from a branch of the RCA, the AV nodal branch.

With regard to innervation, there is a varied network of vagal (cholinergic) fibers and sympathetic (adrenergic) fibers. This AV node network, in particular vagal innervation, is present to a greater extent than in the ventricles.

The intraventricular conduction system (Rosenbaum *et al.* 1968; Uhley 1973; Cassidy *et al.* 1984)

The bundle of His is divided into two branches: the right and the left bundle branches.

The right bundle branch

At the level of the right anterior papillary muscle, the RBB is divided in two branches that usually correspond to two selectively delimited Purkinje areas: the superoanterior region and the inferoposterior regions (Figure 4.7A).

The left bundle branch

The trunk of the left bundle branch (5–7 mm in length) is divided into two anatomically well-defined fascicles—the

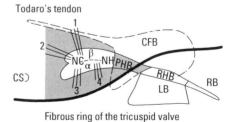

Figure 4.8 Structure of the AV junction extending further than the AV node (the compact node). The zone shaded in gray is included in the AV junction, and may be involved in the reentry circuits exclusive to the AV junction: CFB: central fibrous body; CN: compact AV node; BHP: bundle of His—penetrating portion; BHR: bundle of His ramifying portion; LB: left branch; RB: right branch. Slow conduction (α) and rapid conduction (β) pathways; 1–4: entry of fibers of internodal pathways into the AV node; NH: nodal-His transition zone; CS: coronary sinus.

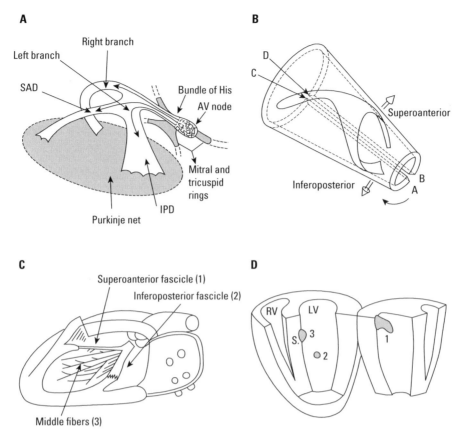

Figure 4.9 (A) Diagram of the intraventricular conduction system, starting at the AV node with its network cells, and the bundle of His with its parallel fibers moving toward the right or the left branches. The latter is divided into two fascicles: superoanterior and inferoposterior. See also the Purkinje network. (B) Left ventricle closed (trifascicular concept). (C) Left lateral view of LV: see the superoanterior (SA) division (1), the inferoposterior (IP) division (2), and the middle fibers (3) (quadrifascicular theory) or rather a quadruple input of ventricular activation theory. (D) The open left ventricle shows the three points of LV activation according to Durrer (see text). SAD and IPD: superoanterior and inferoposterior division of the LB.

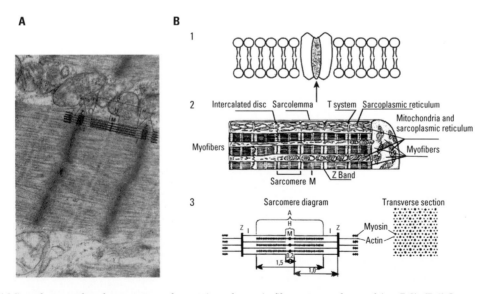

Figure 4.10 (A) Microphotography of a sarcomere where actin and myosin filaments are observed (see B-3). (B-1) Structure of the cellular membrane (or sarcolemma) showing an ionic channel. (B-2) Section of a myocardial contractile cell including all different elements. (B-3) Enlarged sarcomere scheme.

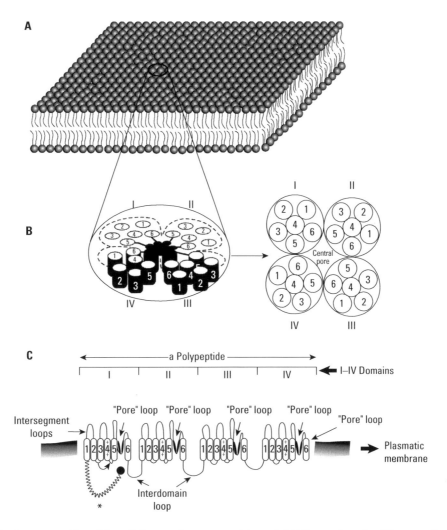

Figure 4.11 (A) Molecular composition of the cellular membrane, comprising a lipid bilayer where the different ionic channels are embedded, with pores. (B) Schematic composition of an ionic channel with its domains, each of which comprises six segments. (C) The domains are displayed. A voltage sensor is found in segment 4 of each domain. See also the ball-and-chain mechanism for channel inactivation (*).

superoanterior and the inferoposterior (Rosenbaum *et al*. 1968). This division explains why the ICS is generally considered a trifascicular system (Figure 4.9A–C). However, between these two bundles usually also exists some middle fibers (see later).

The longer and narrower superoanterior (SA) division follows the left ventricular outflow tract until the left anterior papillary muscle base is reached, whereas the shorter and wider **inferoposterior (IP) division** leads to the base of the posterior papillary muscle, an area where less hemodynamic stress exists (Figure **4.9**B). Consequently, an isolated injury in the IP division is much less frequent.

Between the two fascicles, as we have already said, **there are some middle fibers** that usually form a network, although its distribution is not uniform, configuring at times into a bundle (30% of cases) (Uhley 1973; Demoulin and Kulbertus 1972; Demoulin *et al*. 1975; Kulbertus *et al* 1976) (Figure 4.9C). The ventricular

quadrifascicular or quadruple input of ventricular activation theory is based on the existence of these fibers (right bundle branch, SA and IP divisions of the left bundle branch, and middle fibers). This theory is supported by Durrer *et al*. (1970), who demonstrated that left ventricular activation starts at three distinct points in the left ventricular endocardium (Figures 4.11D). Two are part of the papillary muscles receiving the electrical impulse through the aforementioned divisions, and the third is located in the middle anterior septal region, approximately where the middle fibers are located (Figure 4.9C).

The Purkinje network

The Purkinje network (Figure 4.9A) is formed by Purkinje fibers and occupies the entire area connecting the SCS with the ventricular subendocardium. The excitation–contraction coupling process takes place throughout this network.

Blood perfusion

Blood perfusion of the ICS takes place as follows:

1. the right bundle branch and the SA division of the left bundle branch are supplied by the LAD coronary artery;

2. the IP division of the left bundle branch receives a dual blood supply (septal branches of the LAD artery and branches of the RCA, or sometimes the CX artery; and

3. the trunk of the left bundle branch also receives a dual blood supply (LAD and RC arteries).

Ultrastructural characteristics of cardiac cells

There are two types of cells in the heart: **cardiac contractile cells**, responsible for cardiac pump function, and **specific conduction system (SCS) cells**, which are in charge of the impulse formation (automaticity) and impulse transmission to the contractile myocardium, initiating excitation–contraction coupling.

Contractile cells

Contractile myocardial cells, having no automatic capacity, are long and narrow and include three components with specific functions: activation/relaxation, contraction, and mitochondrial.

Activation/relaxation system

This is made up of the following structures:

• **The cellular membrane, or sarcolemma**, is a structure formed by two lipid layers, along which there are holes called ion channels with a radius of about 3.5Å. The flow

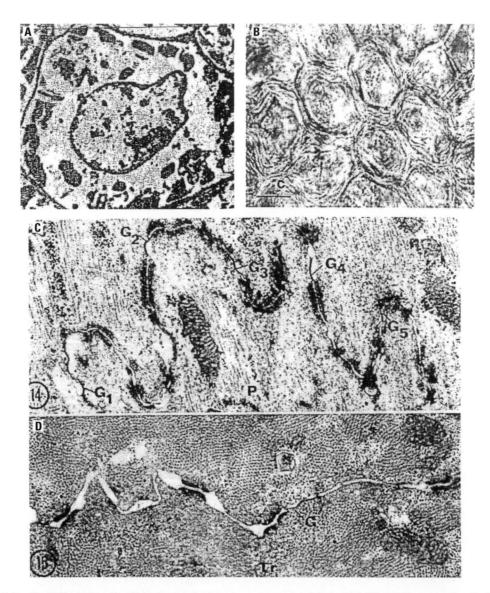

Figure 4.12 (A) P cells. (B) Purkinje cells. (C) Purkinje cells show many intercalated disks (G1–G5). (D) Transitional cells show few intercellular connections (G).

of different ions across the cell membrane takes place through these channels, which are macromolecular structures located in the bilipid layer of the cell membrane (Figure 4.10B-1). The channels through which Na^+, Ca^{2+}, and K^+ ions flow have a similar, but not identical, basic macromolecular structure. Figure 4.11 shows the Na^+ channel involving four domains of six segments each. These four domains assemble by wrapping around themselves so that the pore zones of each individual domain stay in the center, forming the central channel pore (Figure 4.11). Ca^{2+} and K^+ channels have a similar structure to Na^+ channels but with small changes in the central pore and in the connection of the four domains.

• **In the transverse tubular (T) system (Figure 4.10B-2)**, the cell membrane invaginates into the sarcomeres at the Z band level to promote electrical excitation inside the cell.

• **The sarcoplasmic reticulum (Figure 4.10B-2)** is where the calcium necessary for cell contraction is to be found. The sarcoplasmic reticulum is a specialized structure through which the T system comes into contact with the sarcomere.

The contractile system

This is organized into **sarcomeres** (Figure 4.10A,B1–3). It is the contractile unit of myocardial cells, as well as the basic component of myofibrils. Myofibrils are interconnected through intercalated disks (Figure 4.10B-2).

The mitochondrial system

The mitochondrial system (Figure 4.10B-2) provides energy to the cells.

Specific cells

There are three types of non-contractile specific cells: P cells, transitional cells, and Purkinje cells (Figure 4.12) (Martinez-Palomo *et al.* 1970; Eriksson and Thornell 1979).

• **P cells** have a polyhedric morphology with no intercalated disks (slower conduction) and are principally clustered at the center of the sinus node. They are also present in the AV node, particularly at the lower part, in the junction area with the bundle of His (nodal-His (NH) zone).

• **Transitional cells** constitute a group of heterogeneous long and narrow cells interposed among the P cells, the Purkinje cells, and the contractile cells. They have a slower conduction due to their structure (long and narrow). They are usually present in the sinus node as well as in the AV node, the bundle of His and the Purkinje–muscle junction.

• **Purkinje cells** are short and wide cells aligned linearly with many intercalated disks (faster conduction) and are frequently found in the bundle of His and bundle branches, including the divisions of these branches (Purkinje network) (see Figure 4.9). They are also found around the two nodes. They are mainly present at the NH zone of the AV node, leading to a faster conduction in this area compared to the superior and central areas of the AV node. They are also present in the internodal bundles, although less numerously.

References

Bayés de Luna A. New heart wall terminology and new electrocardiographic classification of Q-wave myocardial infarction based on correlations with magnetic resonance imaging. *Rev Esp Cardiol* 2008a;60:683.

Bayés de Luna A. Response to Garcia Cosio: "Posterior myocardial infarction is real" (Letter to Editor). *Rev Esp Cardiol* 2008b;61:431.

Bayés de Luna A. What is important is the truth (Letter to Editor). *J Electrocardiol* 2011;44:58.

Bayés de Luna A, Wagner G, Birnbaum Y, *et al.* A new terminology for left ventricular walls and location of myocardial infarcts that present Q wave based on the standard of cardiac magnetic resonance imaging: a statement for healthcare professionals from a committee appointed by the International Society for Holter and Noninvasive Electrocardiography. *Circulation* 2006a;114:1755.

Bayés de Luna A, Cino JM, Pujadas S, *et al.* Concordance of electrocardiographic patterns and healed myocardial infarction location detected by cardiovascular magnetic resonance. *Am J Cardiol* 2006b;987:443.

Bayés de Luna A, Cino J, Goldwasser D, *et al.* New electrocardiographic diagnostic criteria for the pathologic R waves in leads V1 and V2 of anatomically lateral myocardial infarction. *J Electrocardiol* 2008;41:413.

Bayés de Luna A, Rovai D, Pons LLado G, *et al.* The end of an electrocardiographic dogma: a prominent R wave in V1 is caused by a lateral not posterior myocardial infarction – new evidence based on contrast-enhanced cardiac magnetic resonance—electrocardiogram correlations. *Eur Heart J* 2015;36:959.

Burch G, DePasquale D. *History of Electrocardiography.* YearBook Medical, 1964.

Cassidy D, Vasallo J, Marchlinski F, *et al.* Endocardial mapping in humans: activation patterns. *Circulation* 1984;70:37.

Cerqueira M. Standardized myocardial segmentation and nomenclature for tomographic imaging of the heart: a statement for healthcare professionals from the Cardiac Imaging Committee of the Council on Clinical Cardiology of the American Heart Association. *Circulation* 2002;105:439.

Cino J, Pons-Lladó G, Bayés de Luna A, *et al.* Utility of contrast enhanced cardiovascular magnetic resonance (CE-CMR) to assess how likely is an infarct to produce a typical ECG pattern. *J Cardiovasc Magn Reson* 2006;8:335.

Demoulin JC, Kulbertus H. Histopathological examination of the concept of left hemiblocks. *Br Heart J* 1972;39:887.

Demoulin JC, Simar LJ, Kulbertus HE. Quantitative study of left bundle branch fibrosis in left anterior hemiblock: an histologic approach. *Am J Cardiol* 1975;36:751.

Durrer D, Van Dam R, Freud G, *et al.* Total excitation of the isolated human heart. *Circulation* 1970;80:231.

Eriksson A, Thornell LE. Intermediate myofilaments in heart Purkinje fibers. *J Cell Biol* 1979;80:231.

Fiol-Sala M, Birnbaum Y, Nikus K, Bayés de Luna A. *Electrocardiography in Ischemic Heart Disease. Clinical and Imaging*

Correlations and Prognostic Implications, 2nd edn. Willey-Blackwell, 2020.

Garcia-Cosio F. Posterior myocardial infarction is for real (Letter to the Editor). *Rev Esp Cardiol* 2008;61:430.

Gorgels AP, van der Web K. Posterior or lateral involvement in nonanterior wall infarction. What's in a name? (Letter to Editor). *J Electrocardiol* 2010;43:221.

Holmqvist F, Husser D, Tapanainus J, *et al*. Interatrial conduction can be accurately determined using standard 12 lead ECG. *Heart Rhythm* 2008;5:413.

Inoue S, Becker A. Posterior extension of human AV node. *Circulation* 1998;97:188.

Josephson ME. Paroxysmal supraventricular tachycardia: an electrophysiological approach. *Am J Cardiol* 1978;41:1123.

Kalinauskiene E. Nine times measure, 10th cut away (Letter to the Editor). *J Electrocardiol* 2010;43:220.

Katritsis D, Becker A. The AV nodal re-entrant circuit. *A proposal*. *Heart Rhythm* 2007;4:1354.

Kulbertus HE, de Laval-Rutten F, Casters P. Vectorcardiographic study of aberrant conduction anterior displacement of QRS: another form of intraventricular block. *Br Heart J* 1976;38:539.

Martinez-Palomo A, Aleanis J, Benítez D. Transitional cardiac cells of the conductive system of the dog heart. *J Cell Biol* 1970;47:1.

Perloff JK. The recognition of strictly posterior myocardial infarction by conventional scalar electrocardiography. *Circulation* 1964;30:706.

Rosenbaum M, Elizari M, Lazzari J. *Los Hemibloqueos*. Pardos, 1968.

Rovai D, Di Bella G, Rossi G, *et al*. Q-wave prediction of myocardial infarct location, size and transmural extent at magnetic resonance imaging. *Coronary Artery Dis* 2007;18:381.

Uhley H. The quadrifascicular nature of the periferal conduction system. In Dreyfus L, Kikoff W (eds) *Cardiac Arrhythmias*. Grune-Stratton, 1973.

Van der Weg K, Bekkers SCAM, Winkens B, *et al*., on behalf of MAST. The R in V1 in non-anterior wall infarction indicates lateral rather than posterior involvement. Results from ECG/MRI correlations. *Eur Heart J* 2009;30(suppl):P2981K.

Wu D, Denes P, Amat-y-Leon F, *et al*. Clinical, electrocardiographic and electrophysiologic observations in patients with paroxysmal supraventricular tachycardia. *Am J Cardiol* 1978;41:1045.

Zipes D, Jalife J. *Cardiac Electrophysiology: From Cell to Bedside*, 4th edn. WB Saunders, 2004.

Chapter 5
The Electrophysiological Basis of the ECG: From Cell Electrophysiology to the Human ECG

Types of cardiac cells: slow and fast response cells (Hoffman and Cranefield 1960)

From an electrophysiological point of view, the cardiac cells previously discussed may be grouped into two different categories (Figures 5.1 and 5.2): (i) **automatic slow response cells** (the sinus node P cells and, to a lesser extent, some of the atrioventricular (AV) junction cells) and (ii) **fast response cells** (contractile cells being the prototype of these cells). Purkinje cells are considered fast response cells, but they also have some automatic potential (Figure 5.2). Transitional cells, as the name suggests, display an intermediate transmembrane action potential (AP) between the contractile cells, the Purkinje cells, and the P cells.

The **electrophysiological characteristics during the diastole**, or resting phase (transmembrane diastolic potential (DP)), and the **systole**, or activation phase (depolarization plus repolarization–AP) **of each cell type are different**. This explains why one type of cell has an automatic behavior while the other type does not. Figures 5.1–5.3 show the different characteristics of fast and slow response cells. A distinctive characteristic of these cells is how they recover excitability; in rapid response cells, recovery is voltage-dependent, while in slow response cells, recovery is time-dependent.

Transmembrane diastolic potential (DP)

Contractile cells are polarized during the diastolic phase. This means that there is a balance between the positive charges outside the cell (Na^+, Ca^{2+}, and, to a lesser extent, K^+) and the negative charges inside the cell, mainly, the non-diffusible anion negative charges $[A^-]$, which outnumber the K^+ ion, the most important positive intracellular ion (Figure 5.4A). When two separate microelectrodes are placed on the external surface of a contractile cell in the resting phase, a horizontal line is recorded (baseline line at zero level), suggesting that there is no potential difference on the cell surface. However, if an electrode is placed inside the cell, the recording will shift downward (Figure 5.4B), showing the potential difference between the outside (+) and the inside (−) of the cell. In contractile cells, this line, called the TDP, is stable (rectilinear phase 4) at −90 mV (Figures 5.1–5.4). **Contractile cells** show an equilibrium between inward diastolic currents of Na^+Ca^{2+} (I_{bi}) and an outward K^+ current (I_{K2}). This explains why DP is not modified and remains stable. Here, DP does not reach the threshold potential (TP) ($\approx$−70 mV) by itself, but requires the impulse to be delivered by a neighboring cell (Figure 5.5).

The automatic cells of the SCS have a DP (phase 4) with an initial value of −70 mV. In this case, the inward diastolic current of Na and Ca (I_f) remains stable and rapidly inactivates the outward current of K (I_p) (Figure 5.2C). This initiates an ascending slope line, which rises to reach the TP by itself ($\approx$−55 mV). Therefore, the downward K^+ conductance (g_K) and the upward Na^+ and Ca^{2+} conductances (g_{NaCa}) cross over, initiating the automatic formation of the AP (Figures 5.1–5.3).

Transmembrane action potential

The transmembrane action potential (AP) was first recorded in 1951 by Weidman and Draper, and has four phases: phase 0, depolarization, and phases 1, 2, and 3, repolarization.

We will first discuss the concept of a dipole. **The term "dipole"** is applied to a pair of electrical charges, (+−) or (−+), that separate a positively charged zone of the cell surface from a negatively charged zone. This pair of charges exists during depolarization and repolarization, but not when these processes are completed. An electrocardiogram (ECG) records differences in potential between the positive and negative zones. These

Clinical Electrocardiography: A Textbook, Fifth Edition. Antoni Bayés de Luna, Miquel Fiol-Sala, Antoni Bayés-Genís, and Adrián Baranchuk.
© 2022 John Wiley & Sons Ltd. Published 2022 by John Wiley & Sons Ltd.

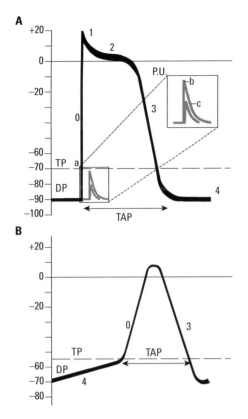

Figure 5.1 Transmembrane diastolic or resting potential (DP) and transmembrane action potential (AP) of contractile (A) and automatic (B) cells. Of particular note is the difference with regard to the DPs, which are rectilinear and far from zero in contractile cells and ascending and closer to zero in automatic cells. Only when the stimulus reaches the threshold potential (TP), after it is excited by a neighboring cell (a in A) or because it features an automatic capacity (B), is a AP generated. Note how in the rapid response cells (with no automatic capacity), a stimulus not reaching the TP (b and c in A) does not generate a AP (see box in A).

differences in potential can be expressed using a vector departing from the negative charge and heading toward the positive charge. In this way, a vector shows a magnitude calculated using the differences of potential between the head of the vector (+) and the tail (−) (Figure 5.6). The vector is recorded as a positive or negative deflection according to whether the exploratory electrode faces the head or tail of it regardless of whether the phenomenon ⌇⌇➤ is approaching or departing from the recording electrode (Figure 5.9).

Depolarization (phase 0)

The onset of phase 0 occurs both in automatic and contractile cells when the intersection of conductances (g_K, g_{NaCa}) (Figure 5.3) occurs at the TP level. This level in automatic cells is lower than in contractile cells (about −55 mV vs. −70 mV) (Figures 5.1 and 5.3).

In the fast response cells—**contractile cells**—the DP is −90 mV and is stable because during diastole there is an

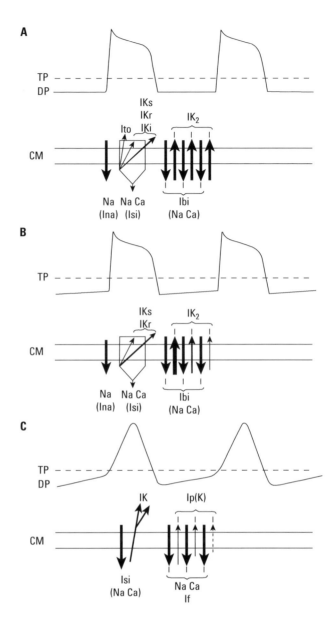

Figure 5.2 Ionic current passing through the cellular membrane (CM) in a contractile cell (fast response cell) (A), Purkinje cell (B), and automatic cell (slow response cell) (C) during systole and diastole. During diastole, the I_{K2} current is constant in contractile cells (A), but not in Purkinje cells (B) (represented by a reduction of the arrow thickness in the I_{K2} current). The outward K current (I_p) in automatic cells is even more rapidly inactivated by the inward I_f current (greater reduction or even disappearance, broken arrows representing the I_p current (C)). In a fast response cell (contractile cell) (A), the DP is stable during diastole, and the NaCa current (I_{bi}) does not predominate over the K current. This explains why in this case I_{bi} and I_{K2} arrows generally have the same size. The ionic currents of automatic and contractile cells during systole seen in more detail in Figure 5.3.

equilibrium between the inward NaCa currents (I_{bi}) and the outward K currents (I_{K2}) (Figure 5.2A). To analyze ionic changes at different levels, the voltage clamp technique is used (Coraboeuf 1971). When the DP receives

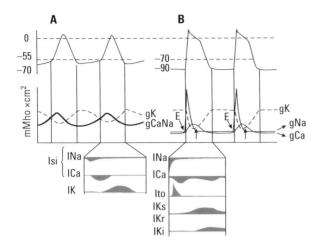

Figure 5.3 The most relevant ionic currents in automatic (A) and contractile (B) cells during systole. Contractile cells are characterized by an early and abrupt Na$^+$ inward flow and an initial and transient K$^+$ outward flow (I_{to}). These are not present in automatic cells.

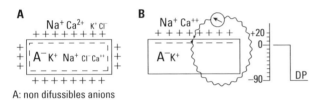

A: non difussibles anions

Figure 5.4 (A) The predominant negative charges inside the cell are due to the presence of significant non-diffusible anions which outweigh the ions with a positive charge, especially K$^+$. (B) Two microelectrodes placed at the surface of a myocardial fiber record a horizontal reference line during the resting phase (zero line), signifying no potential differences on the cellular surface. When one of the two electrodes is introduced inside the cell, the reference line shifts downward ($-90\,mV$). This line (the DP) is stable in contractile cells and has a more or less ascending slope in the specific conduction system cells.

a propagated impulse with sufficient strength to reach the TP, a AP is initiated. The AP in these cells is abrupt in the initial phase (start of phase 0) because the DP is far from zero ($-90\,mV$). According to what we already know about the membrane response curve, the AP ascending velocity is greater when the DP is far from zero (Figures 5.1 and 5.7).

This first phase of the AP, the abrupt rise of phase 0 in the fast response cells, corresponds to the QRS recording in the clinical ECG (Figure 5.8). It does not occur spontaneously because the fast response cells have a stable (contractile cells) or a slightly ascending (Purkinje cells) DP. It only initiates when the impulse delivered by the automatic cells triggers the abrupt Na$^+$ entrance of an inward Na$^+$ current, and the first part of AP is formed (Figures 5.1 and 5.3).

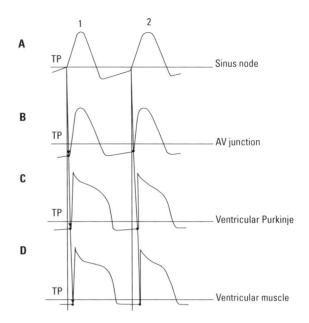

Figure 5.5 Sinus node AP (A) transmitted to the AV junction (B), the ventricular Purkinje (C) and ventricular muscle (D).

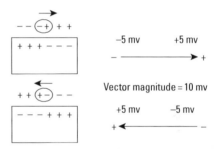

Figure 5.6 A vector is the magnitude expression of the difference in potential between the head (+) and the tail (−) of a dipole (see text).

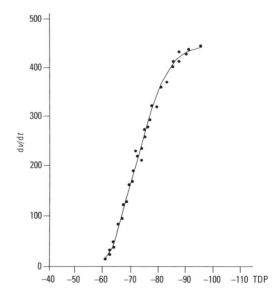

Figure 5.7 Membrane response curve. The dV/dt response depends on the transmembrane diastolic potential (DP) at each time point.

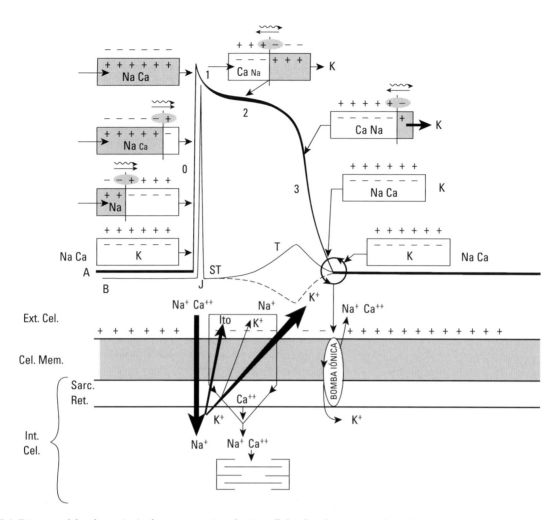

Figure 5.8 Diagram of the electro-ionic changes occurring during cellular depolarization and repolarization of contractile myocardium cells. In phase 0, when the Na inward flow occurs, the depolarization dipole (−+) is formed. In phase 2, when an important and constant K outward flow is observed, the repolarization dipole is formed (+−). Depending on whether we examine a single cell or the whole left ventricle, a negative repolarization wave (broken line) or a positive repolarization wave (continuous line) is recorded respectively (see text).

At the end of phase 0 in contractile cells (fast response cells), depolarization has already occurred as the result of the initial abrupt inward Na^+ current into the cell (rapid Na^+ channels), followed by a slow inward $Ca^{2+}Na^+$ current (slow channels). Simultaneously, a transient and brief outward K^+ current (I_{to}) occurs (Figures 5.2A, 5.3B, and 5.8).

At some moment at the beginning of phase 0, in the contractile cell, the dominant Na^+ inward and later Na^+Ca^{2+} inward currents induce the presence of negative charges outside the cell, producing in some place outside the cell a pair of charges (−+), known as the **depolarization dipole** (Figure 5.8). The depolarization dipole has a vector expression, the head of the vector being located on the positive side of the dipole.

Cell depolarization can be compared to a wave (Figure 5.6B) with positive charges at the crest and at the front and negative charges behind. As the wave advances, it leaves behind a wake of negative charges (Figures 5.8 and 5.9A). The pair of charges (−+), or dipole, may be considered the reflection of the depolarization wave. The dipole determines the recording of positive potentials at the points (electrodes) facing the dipole's positive charge, or vector head (i.e. electrode A in Figure 5.9A), and negative potentials at the points facing the negative pole of the dipole, or vector tail (Figure 5.9B).

The electrodes that face first the positive charge of the dipole and then the negative charge record a positive–negative deflection known as a **diphasic deflection**. The deflection becomes isodiphasic if the positivity equals the negativity, that is, when the electrode is confronted with the positive and negative charges of the dipole for the same span of time (Figure 5.9A-2). The complex is diphasic with

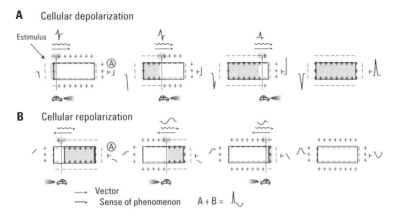

Figure 5.9 Diagram showing how the cellular electrogram curve (A + B) is produced according to the dipole vector theory. (A) Cellular depolarization; (B) cellular repolarization (see text).

positive predominance when the electrode faces the positive pole (head of the vector) longer than the negative pole (tail of the vector) (Figure 5.9A-3). Conversely, the diphasic complex is predominantly negative when the electrode faces the dipole negativity longer than the positivity (Figure 5.9A-1). The size of the deflections recorded depends on the magnitude of the dipole (vector) and the location with respect to the recording electrode (see later—Figure 6.15).

The AP originates in the automatic cells at the moment DP reaches TP and has a slow rising rate and less abrupt phase 0 rise. This is because depolarization occurs essentially through the Na and Ca slow channels (Isi) (Figures 5.2 and 5.3), because in automatic cells the initial DP is lower, or closer to zero (Figure 5.1), and the dV/dt of the response is slower, according to the membrane response curve (Figure 5.7).

The vector (→), the expression of the depolarization dipole (−+), has a magnitude and a direction (head of the vector), while the phenomenon of depolarization has a sense of movement (〜〜►). The arrow tip, the vector head, represents the positive pole of the dipole. The head of the vector during depolarization is the same as the sense of movement of the depolarization phenomenon. Conversely, the head of the vector during cellular repolarization is contrary to the sense of the cellular repolarization phenomenon (see below) (Figure 5.9B).

Repolarization (phases 1, 2, and 3)
In contractile cells
In contractile cells (Figures 5.1A and 5.8), the end of depolarization and the onset of repolarization correspond to phase 1 and the initial part of phase 2 of the AP. This phase corresponds to the J point and the onset of the ST segment in the clinical ECG.

At some point during phase 2 of the AP, the ionic permeability of the membrane for K^+ and Na^+Ca^{2+} coincides with the intersection of the Na^+Ca^{2+} and K^+ conductances (g) (conductance (g) represents an inverse value of the membrane resistance against an ion flow) (Figure 5.3—see arrows). This corresponds to the isoelectric ST segment in the ECG (Figure 5.8). When the K^+ outflow is greater than the Na^+ inflow, a **repolarization dipole** (or pair of +− charges) is formed outside the cell. Like the depolarization dipole, the vector expression of the repolarization dipole shows the vector head to be located at the positive part of the dipole (Figure 5.9).

Under normal conditions, the first area of the cell to complete repolarization is the area that was first depolarized (Figure 5.9B). The repolarization dipole is formed when the part of the cell far from the electrode (A) is already repolarized. This occurs in the second half of phase 2 (in Figure 5.9, the area opposite to electrode A). Cell repolarization can be expressed by a dipole with its negative pole facing the electrode (A).

At the end of phase 2, K^+ outflow predominates; Ca^{2+} and Na^+ inflow is progressively smaller and finally terminates at the beginning of phase 3. With this ionic movement in which the outflow of positive charges is dominant, intracellular negativity and extracellular positivity are completely restored, so that at the end of phase 3, the polarity of the cell membrane is identical to that at the onset of phase 0. During phase 3, repolarization is faster. This explains why the repolarization dipole advances more quickly toward the exploring electrode.

The repolarization dipole determines the recording of a positive potential at those points facing the positive charge of the dipole, that is, the head of the vector of repolarization, and a negative potential at the points facing the negative dipole charge, the tail of this vector. The point confronted first by negativity and then by positivity records a negative–positive reflection (Figure 5.9B-2).

Phase 3 corresponds to the downstroke of the AP curve and the T wave of the ECG (Figure 5.8). Since repolarization occurs progressively faster, the downstroke of the T wave has a steeper slope than the upstroke in the human ECG.

In the last part of phase 2, and especially in phase 3, as we already said, when the ECG T wave is recorded the K^+ outflow is quite significant and Na^+Ca^{2+} can no longer enter. Thus, at the end of phase 3, the electric polarity of the cell membrane is identical to that at the end of phase 4 (start of phase 0), with the DP at $-90\,mV$. However, the ionic conditions are not the same as those observed at the beginning of the AP: there are increased levels of Na^+ and Ca^{2+} inside the cell, while the K^+ level decreases. This ionic imbalance is corrected at the beginning of phase 4 through an active mechanism (ionic pump) (Figure 5.8).

> The repolarization dipole can also be represented by a **vector** with its head oriented toward the positive charge of the dipole. Although the sense of the repolarization phenomenon is approaching the electrode in an isolated cell (B in Figure 5.9), this electrode faces the vector tail (Figure 5.9B), resulting in the recording of a negative wave (negative T wave in the normal cell electrogram). In the human ECG, the T wave is positive (see later).

In slow response cells

In slow response cells (automatic cells), the repolarization shows an ionic mechanism similar to that of fast response cells (contractile cells), such as an ion outward K^+ current, although this ionic current is less important and less persistent. As a result, phase 1 does not occur in this case, and phases 2 and 3 are shorter (Figure 5.1B and 5.2C).

Properties of cardiac cells

Automaticity

Automaticity is the capacity of some cardiac cells to produce stimuli that may propagate to neighboring cells. As previously discussed, automatic cells with an ascending TDP (phase 4) are slow response cells. The impulse received from these cells by the neighboring contractile cells causes an abrupt Na^+ inward current through the rapid channels—rapid response cells with a stable TDP—and triggers the AP of these cells (contractile and Purkinje cells) (Figures 5.2 and 5.3).

Under normal conditions, the sinus node is the structure showing the greatest automaticity, followed by the AV node and, to a lesser degree, the ventricular Purkinje network (Figure 5.5). The increased or decreased automatism in the sinus node and other automatic cells, as well as the ventricular contractile myocardium, explains many active (tachycardias and premature complexes) and passive (sinus bradycardia and escape rhythm) rhythm disturbances (see Chapters 15–17).

Excitability

Excitability is **the capacity of all cardiac cells** (both automatic and contractile) **to respond to an effective stimulus**. Automatic cells excite themselves (spontaneous and active excitation), while contractile cells respond to a stimulus that has been propagated from an automatic cell (Figures 5.5–5.11).

Refractory period

After excitation, all myocardial cells require a certain amount of time to restore their excitability (refractory period). Recovery of excitability in rapid response cells is reached at a certain voltage level and correlates with the final part of the AP (phase 3) (voltage-dependent recovery of excitability), while in slow response cells the recovery of excitability is time-dependent. This means that excitability is not restored when phase 3 reaches a certain level, but rather when a certain period of time has elapsed, usually longer than that of the TAP (Table 5.1).

In cells with voltage-dependent recovery of excitability, four phases of refractoriness are typically observed, which correlate with different parts of the TAP (Figure 5.10):
* The phase of total inexcitability, regardless of how great the stimulus applied is, corresponds to the **absolute refractory period (ARP)** and covers great part of the systole.
* The phase of local potentials is a very short period during which potentials are initiated in the cell but are not able to propagate. The **effective refractory period (ERP)** of the cell corresponds to the sum of the ARP and the phase of local potentials (A in Figure 5.10).
* The phase of partial excitability, which corresponds to the end of AP phase 3, occurs when suprathreshold stim-

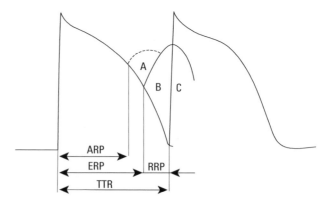

Figure 5.10 Cellular excitability phases and refractory periods in cells where excitability recovery is voltage-dependent (rapid response). During the absolute refractory period (ARP), there is no response. At the end of this period, there is a response zone with local potentials (A) called the effective refractory period (ERP). At the end of this period, a propagated response zone is initiated, but only when suprathreshold stimuli are applied (B); this is the relative refractory period (RRP), which corresponds to the zone of response to suprathreshold stimuli. The total recovery time (TRT) is equivalent to the ERP + RRP. At the end of the RRP, a normal response is initiated (C), corresponding to a AP with a morphology equal to basal morphology.

Table 5.1 Differences between rapid response and slow response cardiac cells

	Rapid (fast) response cells	Slow response cells
Location	Mainly atrial and ventricular muscle and intraventricular conduction system	Sinus node, and to a lesser degree, AV node and mitral and tricuspid rings
Level of the DTP (diastolic transmembrane potential) and types of DTP (stable or unstable)	From −80 to −95 mV. The DTP is stable in contractile cells, but in the His–Purkinje cells there is a slight diastolic depolarization and the DTP is not completely stable	About −70 mV at onset. The DTP is unstable, presenting an ascendant curve which is characteristic of the automatic structures (e.g. sinus node)
Threshold level	About −70 mV	Less than −55 mV
Phase 0 upstroke	Rapid	Slow
Height of phase 0	High, reaches +20 to +40 mV	Low, reaches 0 to +15 mV
Conduction speed	Rapid (0.5–5 m/s)	Slow (0.01–0.1 m/s)
Fast sodium channels	Present	Absent
Slow channels, mainly for Ca^{2+} (and some Na^+)	Present	Present
Inhibition of depolarization	By tetrodotoxin (puffer fish toxin), which inhibits fast Na channels	Manganese, cobalt, nickel, verapamil, etc., which inactivate slow Ca–Na channels
Duration of the effective refractory period (and consequently, recuperation of excitability) AB = Distance after depolarization, during which the cell is unexcitable	AB = Somewhat inferior to TAP duration (voltage-dependent recuperation of excitability) (TAP = transmembrane action potential)	AB = Superior to TAP duration (time-dependent recuperation of excitability)

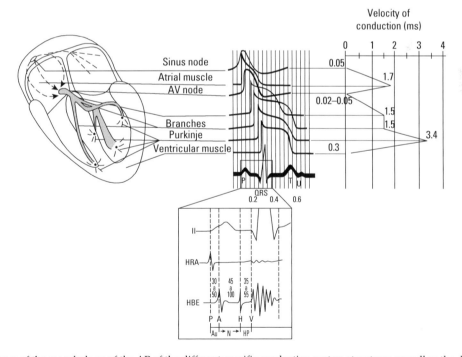

Figure 5.11 Diagram of the morphology of the AP of the different specific conduction system structures as well as the different conduction speeds (ms) through these structures. Below is an enlarged depiction of the PR interval with a hisiogram recording. HRA: High right atria; HBE: ECG of the bundle of His; PA: from start of the P wave to the low right atrium; AH: from low right atrium to the bundle of His; HV: from the bundle of His to the ventricular Purkinje.

uli are required to produce the propagated response. This phase corresponds to the **relative refractory period (RRP)** of the cell. The sum of the ERP and the RRP corresponds to the total recovery time (Figure 5.12).

• The phase of supernormal excitability (PSE) takes place at the end of the AP and at the start of diastole (phase 4). During this period, the cells respond to infrathreshold stimuli (Figure 5.13).

In an area or tissue of the SCS, the functional and effective refractory period is measured through the application of increasingly premature atrial extra stimuli (Bayés de Luna and Baranchuk 2017).

Clinically, the RRP in a conventional ECG begins when the stimulus is conducted more slowly than normal. For example, in the AV junction, a baseline PR interval of 0.20 sec is prolonged to 0.26 sec, with the shortening of the RR interval (tachycardization or premature complexes) (Figures 5.14A-2). When the stimulus falls in the AV junction ARP, it is blocked there (Figure 5.14A-3).

Conductivity

Conductivity is the **capacity of cardiac fibers to transmit the stimuli from automatic cells to neighboring cells**. The stimulus originates in the sinus node and propagates through the SCS. Conduction differs in the fast response cells (contractile and His–Purkinje system cells) (regenerative conduction) and the slow response cells, particularly in the AN and N zones of the AV junction and in the sinoatrial junction (decrementing conduction) (Figure 5.12).

The rate of conduction in the heart is essentially determined by two factors: (i) the rate of rise of TAP (dV/dt of phase 0), which is rapid in the rapid response fibers and slow in the slow response fibers and (ii) the ultrastructural characteristics. Narrow fibers (contractile and transitional cells) and those without intercalated discs (P cells) conduct stimuli slower than wide fibers with many intercalated discs (Purkinje cells). When passing from a narrow fiber zone to a wide fiber zone, the conduction increases (from the AV node to the His–Purkinje system), and vice versa (Figure 5.12).

Vulnerability

The **ventricular vulnerable period (VVP)** is a small zone located around the peak of the T wave (Figure 5.13). A stimulus falling in this zone may trigger a ventricular fibrillation (R/T phenomenon) (Figure 5.14B-4). The **atrial vulnerable period (AVP)**, located at the beginning of the ST segment (Figure 5.13), is a zone where atrial stimuli may trigger an atrial fibrillation (Figure 5.14A-4).

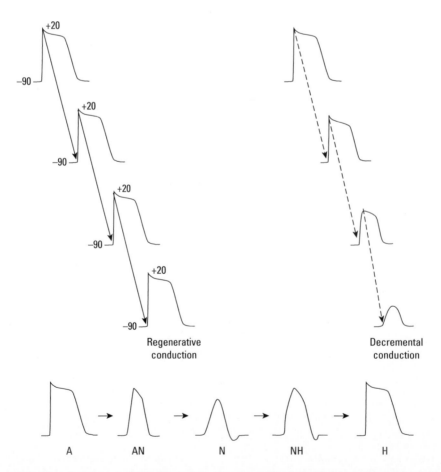

Figure 5.12 Stimulus conduction of regenerative-type (contractile cells–myocardium) and decremental-type (areas with slow response cells–AV junction and sinoatrial junction). Below: TAP of different structures from the atria to the bundle of His.

Cardiac activation

In conventional surface electrocardiography, only the activation of the muscular mass of the atria and ventricles is recorded. Sinus node activation and activation of the rest of the SCS are not recorded in surface ECG,

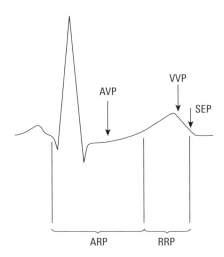

Figure 5.13 Location of refractory periods at AV level, the supernormal excitability phase or period and vulnerable periods at the atrial and ventricular level in the human ECG. ARP: absolute refractory period; AVP: atrial vulnerable period; RRP: relative refractory period; SEP: supernormal excitability period; VVP: ventricular vulnerable period.

although in Figure 5.11 the correlation between the AP of all the different parts of SCS and the surface ECG is shown. In this figure, the recording of different parts of the atria and bundle of His with intracavitary recording can be seen. This is especially important for the location of the AV block (see Chapter 17). Recording the His deflection by surface ECG through an amplifying method would greatly assist the decision-making process for pacemaker implantation (see Chapter 3, The future of electrocardiography).

Using the diagram described by Lewis, Figure 5.15 illustrates the passage of the electrical impulse through the parts of the heart responsible for surface ECG waves (A: atrial mass; V: ventricular mass), as well as the silent areas (sinus node, sinoatrial junction, and AV junction).

The normal origin of cardiac impulses: The sinus node

The normal site for the generation of pacemaker impulses in the heart is the sinus node. The sinus discharge emerges in the atria especially at three different places, corresponding to the three preferential internodal pathways (see later). In the initial sinus impulse, the whole heart is subsequently depolarized, beginning with the atria and followed, after the propagation of the impulse through the AV node and the specialized intraventricular conduction system, by the ventricles (Figure 5.11).

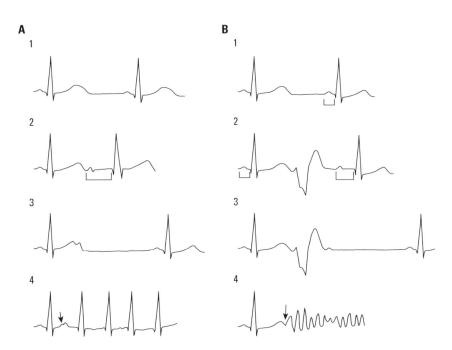

Figure 5.14 (A-1 and B-1) Normal AV conduction. (A-2) Premature atrial complex (PAC) falls in the RRP of the AV junction and the next sinus P wave shows a long PR interval. (B-2) There is an interpolated premature ventricular complex (PVC) and the next P wave shows a longer PR interval. (A-3) PAC falls in the ARP of the AV junction and is not conducted. (B-3) Due to concealed retrograde conduction in the AV junction of a PVC, the next P wave is blocked. (A-4) When a PAC falls into the atrial VP, it may trigger an atrial fibrillation. (B-4) When a PVC falls in the ventricular vulnerable period, especially in acute ischemia, a ventricular fibrillation may be triggered.

Atrial activation: The P loop

The process of atrial activation encompasses both atrial depolarization and atrial repolarization.

Atrial depolarization

Atrial depolarization follows preferential conduction pathways that do not have a uniform conduction speed through the atria. In fact, fairly concentric, isochronic lines of impulse propagation connecting the sites where activation takes place at the same time have been drawn (Figure 5.16A). Puech's studies in dogs (Puech and Grolleau 1972) and Durrer's studies in humans (Durrer *et al.* 1970) sustain the existence of radial impulse conduction in atria and ventricles. However, the conduction between the sinus node and AV node (right atrium) does not take place through the pathway first described by Wenckenbach and Thorel, that now are considered not truly bundles, rather preferential way of conduction till AV node. The conduction to the left atrium is performed preferentially through the truly bundle described by Bachmann that is located in the upper part of the atria connecting both atria. As the rest of atrial septum is of by connective tissue if the stimulus is blocked in the Bachmann bundle, the breakthrough to left atrium is performed in the lower part of atrial septum, close to AV

junction. This explains that LA is depolarized retrogradely and dues to that in leads II, III, and aVF will be recorded the P wave with a final negativity (±). Therefore, the trajectory of the atria activation is conditioned, to a large extent, by the anatomy of the septum and right atrium and, by the existence of numerous holes (superior vena cava, inferior vena cava, oval fossa, coronary sinus, etc.) (Figure 4.7).

Following these routes, the external right atrial wall is depolarized first, followed by the anterior wall and interatrial septum, with the activation wave reaching the AV junction (zone of transitional cells and the upper part of the AV node) at 0.04–0.05 sec. At the same time, the impulse reaches the left atrium, mainly through the upper and anterior part of the septum via the Bachmann bundle, and the anterior and posterior left atrial walls are subsequently depolarized. It has been demonstrated (Holmqvist *et al.* 2008) that the activation of the left atrium may take place also in a zone close to the coronary sinus. In case of Bachmann bundle block, as we have already said, the normal activation of the left atrium will take place retrogradely through this zone (Bayés de Luna *et al.* 1988).

Generally, atrial depolarization lasts 0.07–0.11 sec and is manifested in the ECG by the P wave, the first part of which corresponds approximately to right atrial depolarization and the second part to left atrial depolarization. Depolarization of the AV node is initiated approximately at the P wave midpoint.

If we consider atrial depolarization in the light of the dipole theory, we see that multiple vectors of depolarization of the right and left atria can be represented by two depolarization vectors (Figure 5.16B), the first being of the right atrium, directed forward, downward, and somewhat to the left, and the other being of the left atrium, directed to the left and somewhat backward. These two vectors reflect the sum of multiple vectors of depolarization of both atria and their respective dipoles. The morphology of the P wave is positive when the electrode faces

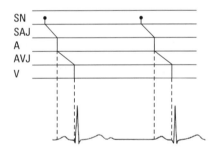

Figure 5.15 Lewis diagrams show how an impulse passes through the sinoatrial junction (SAJ), atria, AV junction (AVJ) and ventricles. (A: atria; SN: sinus node; V: ventricles).

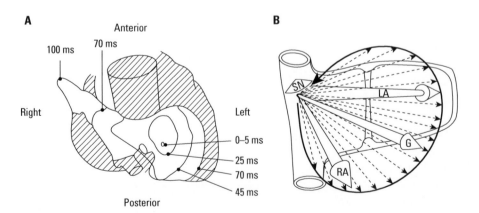

Figure 5.16 (A) Isochronic atrial activation lines (adapted from Puech and Grolleau 1972). (B) Left, right, and global (G) atrial depolarization vector and P loop. The successive multiple instantaneous vectors are also pictured.

the head of the depolarization vector and negative when it faces the tail. The mean (resultant or global) axis of atrial depolarization is the spatial sum of both vectors and is expressed as a vector directed to the left, downward, and forward (Figure 5.16B).

The entire atrial depolarization wave follows a route from right to left, back to front, and above to below, as a consequence of the right atrium activating before the left atrium. The line that delimits the route of atrial depolarization from inception to termination is conditioned in the most marked inflections by the heads of the right, left, and global vectors, but includes, as already stated, multiple sequential instantaneous vectors formed during the process of atrial depolarization. This line, which describes a counterclockwise turn because the right atrial vector is formed before the left atrial vector, is finally closed at the same starting point and **constitutes the vectorcardiographic curve of the P wave, known as the "P loop."** The projection of this loop on the positive or negative hemifield of different leads of the frontal and horizontal planes explains the morphology of the P wave in the various ECG leads (see Figure 7.4).

The atrial depolarization wave includes the entire wall from the endocardium to the epicardium because of the thinness of the atrial wall. This explains why in experimental studies the same P wave morphology is detected on both sides of the wall. The atrial depolarization vector ($\rightarrow$) has the same direction as the sense of depolarization phenomenon ($\sim\sim\rightarrow$) (see Figure 5.17).

Atrial repolarization

Atrial repolarization starts in the areas that were first depolarized and follows the same sense as atrial depolarization (Figure 5.17E). As a result, the repolarization dipole is formed with the positive charge opposite to the depolarization dipole, and the resulting repolarization vector is oriented in the opposite direction ($\leftarrow$) to the sense of repolarization phenomenon ($\sim\sim\rightarrow$). The polarity of the atrial repolarization wave (ST–Ta) is

therefore the opposite of that of the P wave. This wave is of very low voltage and longer duration than the P wave and is generally concealed by the superimposed QRS complex. Only in cases of AV block, atrial infarction, important right atrial enlargement, or sympathetic overdrive is it sometimes evident.

Transmission of the atrial impulse to the ventricle

The atrial depolarization wave reaches the proximal part of the AV node through the three internodal tracts in four areas: two supero-left areas and two infero-right areas (see Figure 4.10). The excitation wave is propagated very slowly (approximately 0.02–0.05 m/s) through the AV node, especially in its upper part, reaching the bundle of His after 65–80 ms. The electrophysiological reason for this conduction delay is related to the existence of three electrophysiologically differentiated zones in the AV node, more or less parallel to the AV fibrous ring: atrionodal (AN), nodal (N), and nodal-His (NH). The N zone has a TAP with an ascendant TDP and a slow-ascent TAP phase 0. The action potentials of the AN and NH zones are transitional with those of the atrium and bundle of His, respectively. Impulse conduction through the AV node is therefore not uniform. In the AN and especially in the N zones, there are progressively more slow response cells with lower TDP and a more slowly ascendant phase 0, which is the cause of decremental conduction of the impulse (Hoffman and Cranefield 1960). The impulse is not extinguished because on arrival at the NH zone the TAP improves in quality and conduction speed (Figure 5.12).

In the bundle of His, the propagation velocity increases greatly. Normally, this structure is the only link in the route between atria and ventricles (except when accessory pre-excitation bundles exist). This channels the impulse through a single point, thus maintaining a proper ventricular activation sequence. The bundle of His has a penetrating portion inserted in the central fibrous body

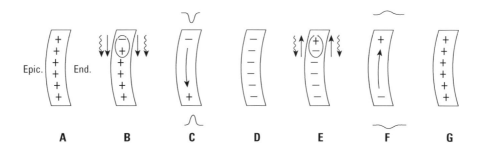

$\sim\sim\rightarrow$ = Sense of phenomenon (depolarization B and repolarization E)

$\longrightarrow$ = Vector of the phenomenon of depolarization and repolarization

Figure 5.17 (A) Atrial resting phase. (B and C) Depolarization sequence. (D) Complete depolarization. (E and F) Atrial repolarization sequence. (G) The cellular resting phase.

and a branching portion that begins at the emerging point of the fibrous body and continues to its division into two branches (Figure 4.10). The distal part of the penetrating portion and branching portion are made up of cells arranged in parallel similar to the Purkinje cells. The two branches of this bundle are mainly formed by Purkinje fibers.

The fibers of the bundle of His are destined to be included in either the right or the left branch, with longitudinal dissociation existing between them. This explains why damage to right or left side of the His bundle may produce patterns of right or left bundle branch block.

The deflections generated by depolarization of the bundle of His and bundle branches are not recorded by conventional ECGs because of the small number of fibers involved, but they correspond in time with the isoelectric space between the end of the P wave and the QRS complex (PR interval). By intracavitary recording techniques, bundle of His potentials, and even the bundle branch potentials, can be recorded as rapid bi- or triphasic deflections situated between the atrial P wave electrogram and the ventricular QRS–T complex (Figure 5.11).

Ventricular activation: QRS and T loops

This process encompasses both ventricular depolarization and repolarization.

Ventricular depolarization

Once the impulse reaches the two bundle branches, they transmit it at a conduction speed similar to that of the bundle of His. It is currently believed (see Chapter 4, The specific conduction system) that the intraventricular conduction system has three terminal divisions. This is the **trifascicular theory**, whereby the right branch represents one division and the superoanterior and inferoposterior divisions of the left branch, true anatomic fascicles,

represent the other two divisions. The importance of these two divisions has been demonstrated by Rosenbaum and Elizari (1968). However, the middle anteroseptal fibers of the left branch, which are anatomically frequently present and of variable morphological appearance, are considered another division by some authors (Uhley 1973; Kulbertus *et al.* 1976). In any case, all the respective Purkinje networks of these two divisions show abundant interconnections, especially on the left side. In fact, the experimental work of Durrer *et al.* (1970) demonstrating that the activation of the left ventricle occurs at three points favors this hypothesis (Figures 4.11C,D and 5.18A). Recently, Josephson's group (Cassidy *et al.* 1984) demonstrated that the onset of activation in the healthy human heart is very much as Durrer described it. This is the basis for the **quadrifascicular theory** of left ventricular activation. It has been suggested that some ECG changes (RS pattern in V1–V2) may be caused by the block of these middle fibers (Hoffman *et al.* 1976; Pérez-Riera 2009). However, the evidence that the block of the middle fibers of left bundle has clean ECG expression is not completely accepted. We have already commented some aspects of that in Chapter 4, and this topic will be discussed in extense in Chapter 12.

As seen in Figure 5.18A, a large part of the endocardial zone of the left septum and the free left ventricular wall is activated in the first 20 ms because of the wealth of Purkinje fibers in these zones. The subendocardial region of the free left ventricular wall has such a rapid activation that it is not recorded by peripheral or intramural electrocardiographic leads. According to the Mexican School (Sodi-Pallares *et al.* 1964), this occurs because the activation fronts originating in the subendocardium are comparable to multiple closed spheres that cancel each other transversally (Figure 5.19A,B), and do not form a single front capable of producing measurable deflections in the

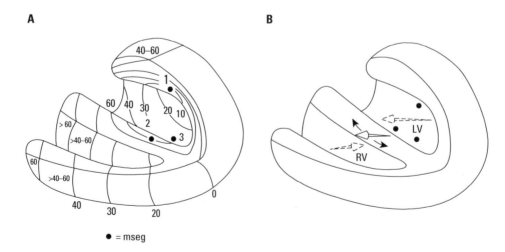

Figure 5.18 (A) The three approximate initiation points of ventricular depolarization (closed circles) (1, 2, 3) forming the isochronic lines of the depolarization sequence (Adapted from Durrer *et al.* 1970—see text). (B) See how the first vector is initiated (see text).

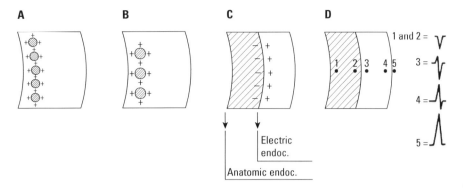

Figure 5.19 Depolarization sequence of the ventricular wall according to the Mexican School (Sodi-Pallares *et al.* 1964) (see text).

ECG leads until these spheres open and show an activation front. This only takes place well within the interior of the ventricular wall—the electrical endocardium (Figure 5.19C).

The electrodes placed in the subendocardial segment of the free left ventricular wall inscribe QS complexes like intracavitary complexes. One single left ventricular activation front mentioned earlier is formed in the subepicardial muscle lacking in Purkinje fibers (Figure 5.19C,D). This activation front, directed from endo- to epicardium, is responsible for the presence of an R wave in subepicardial intramural leads that is progressively greater as it approaches the epicardial electrode (Figure 5.19D). The limit between the rapid activation zone of the subendocardial left ventricular wall (where only QS complexes are recorded) and the slow activation subepicardial zone (QRS complexes increasingly more positive toward the epicardium) is known as the **electrical endocardium**. Its location varies according to the amount of Purkinje fibers in the different regions (from 40% to 80% of the ventricular wall thickness). This concept has been used to explain why there are often no QRS complex modifications in the presence of subendocardial necrosis. However, it has already been shown (Horan *et al.* 1971) and more recently demonstrated with contrast-enhanced cardiovascular magnetic resonance (CE-CMR) (Moon *et al.* 2004) that non-transmural necrosis with Q waves, and transmural necrosis without Q waves, may exist.

The depolarization of the initial left ventricular zones, the result of the union of the activation at the three points of Durrer (Figure 5.18A), produces a more significant vectorial force than the initial depolarization of the right ventricle. These two vector forces of opposite direction and different magnitudes produce a resultant vector directed to the right and forward (Figure 5.18A-1). The upward, downward, or intermediate direction of this vector depends especially on the position of the heart (see later) (Figures 5.20–5.22). **The resultant vector of initial ventricular depolarization is called Vector 1.** This vector accounts for the initial QRS morphology of various electrocardiographic leads (i.e. r of V1 and q of V6) and corresponds to approximately the first 10 ms of ventricular activation and the respective section of the QRS complex (Figures 5.20–5.22).

Later, part of the right ventricular wall and the midapical part of the septum and left ventricular wall depolarizes. **The sum of the two vectorial forces (right and left, from 10 to 40–50 ms) is a single vector called Vector 2**, directed to the left, slightly backward and usually downward, or occasionally slightly upward in the horizontal heart. This vector represents most of the QRS complex (i.e. S of V1 and R of V5–V6) (Figures 5.20–5.22).

Finally, the basal regions of both ventricles and the septum depolarize, producing a vector force of scant magnitude and about 20 ms in duration, shown by a vector directed upward, somewhat to the right and backward. This is due to the fact that the upper portion of the right ventricle generally depolarizes later than the upper left ventricle. This vector, known as **Vector 3**, has little electrocardiographic repercussion ("s" in the left precordial leads and terminal r in VR) (Figures 5.20–5.22).

The three vectors we have described are very useful for didactic purposes because they help explain the electrocardiographic curve. It should be remembered, however, that the route of ventricular depolarization does not consist of three vectors, but rather a succession of multiple instantaneous vectors formed during the process of ventricular depolarization, as seen in atrial depolarization. These three vectors are only a point of departure for the explanation of QRS complex morphology, which usually has two or three deflections (rS, RS, Rs, rSr', qRs). When more than three deflections exist, something that occurs in right bundle branch block (rsRs'), we may explain the corresponding morphology using other vectors. These 2–3 vectors delimit the route of ventricular depolarization approximately, and this corresponds with the normal vectorcardiographic curve of the normal heart at different positions (Figures **5.20–5.22**).

There are three basic heart positions: intermediate, vertical, and horizontal. **In the vertical heart position**, the maximum loop vector—Vector 2—is directed downward (+ 60° to + 85° or more), and the initial (first) vector is oriented upward and to the right, the loop generally rotating clockwise or moving in a figure-of-eight (Figure 5.21). **In the horizontal heart position**, the maximum loop vector—Vector 2—is directed leftward about 0 to −10°, and there is a counterclockwise loop rotation with an initial (first) vector oriented downward and to the right (Figure 5.22). **In the intermediate heart position**, the maximum vector—Vector 2—is at about +30°, but Vector 1 and the loop rotation are similar to those of the vertical heart (Figure 5.20).

Since the heart is a three-dimensional organ, the electrical forces must be projected onto two planes. The projection of the QRS loop on to the positive and negative hemifields of the different frontal and horizontal plane leads (see Chapter 6) allows the path of the impulse during depolarization of the heart to be traced and the different QRS morphologies to be deduced (see Figure 6.14).

> **Ventricular depolarization** can be divided into **three phases**, each of which can be shown as a vector.
> • **During the first phase** (10–15 ms), the initial depolarization of the ventricles and the medial septum produces a small vector (**Vector 1**) directed to the right, forward and up- or downward (more frequently upward).
> • **In the second phase** (30–40 ms), most of the free wall of both ventricles and the lower septum depolarize, initiating an important vector (**Vector 2**) directed to the left and slightly backward.
> • **In the third phase** (20–30 ms), a small vector (**Vector 3**) is generated and directed upward, somewhat backward and to the right.

Ventricular repolarization

In the human heart, the process of repolarization of the free wall of the left ventricle accounts for practically all ventricular repolarization. The route of the ventricular repolarization wave, the vectorcardiographic curve of the T wave, or **T loop**, usually has a direction and rotation similar to that of depolarization (QRS loop), although the T loop is directed somewhat less backward (Figure 5.23).

To understand why the T wave is positive in the human heart (see later), in contrast to what occurs in the normal isolated cardiac cell, we must imagine the left ventricle as an enormous cell and bear in mind that under normal conditions the subendocardium has a poorer blood supply than the subepicardium (physiological ischemia). This is because coronary circulation is terminal in the subendocardium and left ventricular intracavitary pressure also contributes to a discrete reduction in the subendocardial blood supply (physiologic underperfusion area). As a result, the subepicardial region of this enormous cell behaves like the non-ischemic zone of an isolated ischemic cardiac cell (Figure 5.24). In this case, the onset of repolarization starts where the depolarization has finalized (Figure 5.24). Consequently, an

electrode placed at A in Figure 5.24 faces the head of the depolarization dipole vector and the head of the repolarization vector in the ischemic cell (Figure 5.24). The same occurs in the human left ventricle (see later) (Figure 5.25). Therefore, the QRS complex and T wave recorded from this site will be both positive in the ischemic cell (Figure 5.24) and in the human heart (Figure 5.25). This is explained in more detail later.

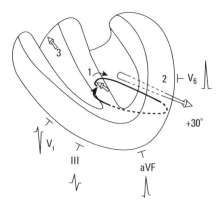

Figure 5.20 The intermediate heart: the QRS loop and the QRS morphologies in different leads (see text).

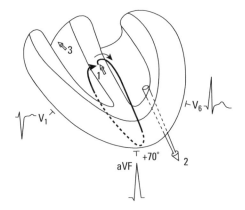

Figure 5.21 The vertical heart: the QRS loop and the QRS morphologies in different leads (see text).

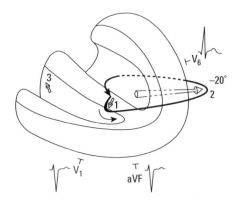

Figure 5.22 The horizontal heart: the QRS loop and the QRS morphologies in different leads (see text).

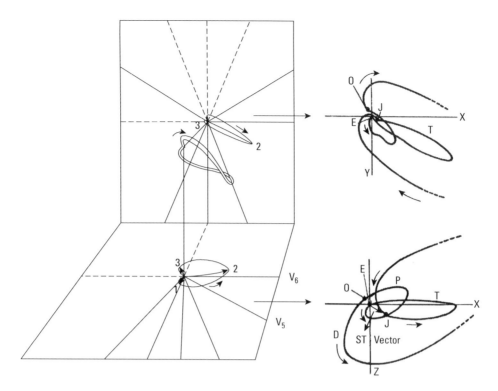

Figure 5.23 Projection of the spatial P, QRS, and T loops on the frontal and horizontal planes. Right: Onset and end of QRS loops in FP and HP.

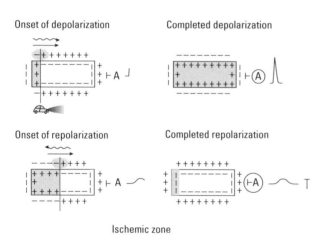

Ischemic zone

Figure 5.24 Above: Cellular depolarization in ischemic cells results in a positive complex (QRS when the recording electrode (A) faces the head of the depolarization vector). Below: Repolarization initiates first in the less ischemic zone, forming a repolarization vector with the positive charge, the vector head, directed toward exploring electrode A. For this reason, a positive deflection is recorded.

The domino model of cardiac activation

It is important to understand how the impulse originating in the sinus node, the structure with the greatest automaticity, is successively propagated to the atrial myocardium, the AV node (the next most automatic

structure after the sinus node, although this is normally not apparent because the sinus impulse depolarizes it), the specialized intraventricular conduction system, and, finally, the ventricular myocardium. When the ventricles are totally depolarized, ventricular repolarization begins. The electrical activation process (depolarization + repolarization) initiates the cardiac contraction mechanism (coupling excitation–contraction). After the electrical activation process has finished, a process of cellular rest takes place before the onset of the subsequent activation process.

This apparently complicated phenomenon of activation–rest–activation can be clearly understood by imagining a row of upright dominoes. When the first domino in the row, the sinus node, emits an impulse and moves, the next domino is pushed and falls (depolarizes), followed sequentially by the rest of the row as each domino receives the impulse (and depolarizes), propagated by the first domino. Figure 5.26 shows the correlation between each instant of this chain of falling dominoes and the conventional ECG. The black point at the end of a continuous ECG tracing indicates the exact location of the electrical impulse coinciding with different positions of the dominoes.

The white dominoes in Figure 5.26 represent nonautomatic structures. The black domino corresponds to the sinus node, the structure with the most rapid discharge cadence (or most automaticity), the cardiac

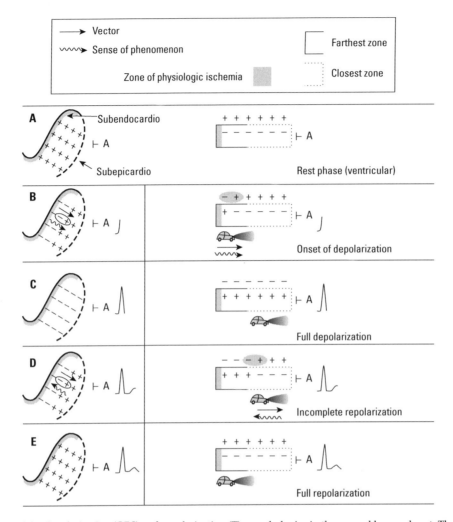

Figure 5.25 Diagram of the depolarization (QRS) and repolarization (T) morphologies in the normal human heart. The figures to the left show a view of the free left ventricular wall from above, and we see only the distribution of the charges on the external surface of this "enormous left ventricular cell." In the right column, we see a lateral view in which the changes in the electrical charges can be appreciated. With electrode A in the epicardium, a normal ECG curve is recorded.

pacemaker. The other SCS structures, which have lesser automaticity (shaded dominoes), are forced to depolarize (fall) when they receive the automatic impulse propagation from the sinus node. This process occurs in the following way: during A, the onset of the diastole, all dominoes are standing (at rest). This occurs at the beginning of the isoelectric line inscribed after the T wave. In B, the diastole is unfolding and the sinus node domino begins to move, which corresponds to the ascending phase 4 of the TAP (diastolic depolarization), while the ECG continues to record an isoelectric line. In C, the sinus node domino touches the second domino (atrial muscle), corresponding to the beginning of atrial depolarization, the correlating domino moves (D) and the recording of the P wave concludes. In E, as the SCS depolarizes the black point, it traverses the line between the P wave and QRS complex and the respective dominoes fall. In F, the onset of ventricular myocardial depolarization (the first ventricular domino falls) is accompanied by the registration of the first part of the

QRS complex. In G, the end of ventricular depolarization coincides with the termination of QRS. At this point, all the dominoes have fallen. Finally, H represents the end of ventricular repolarization, when all dominoes are again standing, as in A. This occurs at the conclusion of the T wave recording.

From cellular electrogram to the human ECG (Wilson *et al.* 1935; Cabrera 1958; Sodi-Pallares *et al.* 1964; Macfarlane and Veitch Lawrie 1989; Wagner 2001; Bayés de Luna and Baranchuk, 2017)

Why the cellular electrogram and the human ECG have different polarities of the repolarization wave

Both cellular electrograms and human ECGs represent the sum of cell or ventricular depolarization plus repolarization. In this case, the atria, which generate the P wave,

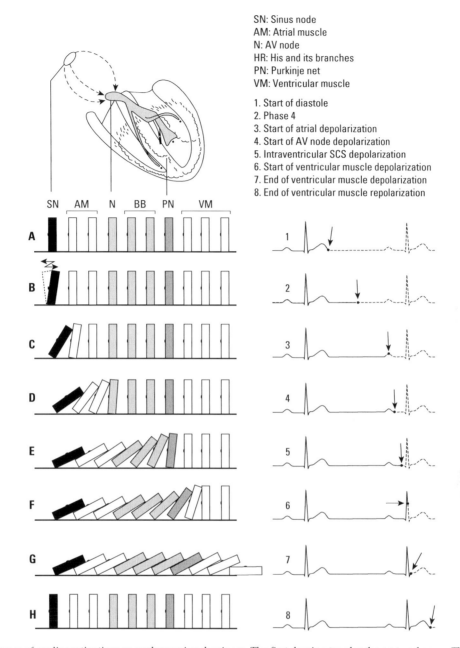

Figure 5.26 Sequence of cardiac activation: an analogy using dominoes. The first domino topples the next and so on. This occurs in the heart, when the heart structure with the most automatic capacity (the first black domino) has moved enough (C) to transmit its impulses to the neighboring cells. The black domino represents the heart pacemaker (SN: sinus node) and the gray dominoes represent cells with less automaticity, which in fact do not usually manifest, since these cells are depolarized by the propagated impulse transmitted by the black domino (SN). White dominoes usually do not feature automaticity. The point dividing the continuous line from the broken one in the ECG curve indicates the time point corresponding to these different electrophysiological situations (see inside) in the cardiac cycle.

are not taken into account and the ventricles are considered to be a large cell—left ventricle (LV)—that generates the QRS complex. In both cases, the depolarization wave (QRS) is similar $\curlywedge$, but the repolarization wave is different: negative ($\frown$) in the cellular electrogram (Figure 5.9), and positive ($\smile$) in the human ECG (Figure 5.24). Since Wilson *et al.* (1935), the discordance between cellular and human ECGs has been explained by the fact that in humans (Figure 5.24) the dipole of the repolarization wave (T wave) is initiated in the left ventricle in an area

opposite to that where the dipole of the depolarization wave starts (QRS), just as occurs in ischemic cells (see before Figure 5.24). This means that some areas of the heart that are activated earlier show a longer AP than those that are activated later.

Experimental studies on animals (Burgess *et al.* 1972; Burnes *et al.* 2001) and humans based on epicardial and endocardial AP recording during catheterism and cardiac surgery (Franz *et al.* 1987) have demonstrated that the area of shorter AP and subsequent earlier repolarization is located in the epicardium. It is well known that the epicardial zone depolarizes after the endocardial zone and also repolarizes first (Durrer *et al.* 1970; Cassidy *et al.* 1984). The Antzelevitch group (Yan and Antzelevitch 1998) has carried out studies in wedge preparations showing that the epicardium is repolarized earlier and that the end of the epicardial AP corresponds to the T wave peak. However, they found that in the middle portion of the ventricular wall (M cell area), repolarization takes longer than in the endocardium; the end of the AP in this area corresponds to the end of the T wave (Figure 5.27). There is no consensus on whether the M cell zone is the left ventricle area with the longest AP, as recently discussed (Ophof *et al.* 2007). **What is clear is that: (i) there is a myocardial area that repolarizes earlier** and, **according to most authors, is located in the epicardium; (ii) there is undoubtedly another area that repolarizes later**, and is **located in the endocardium**, or **middle portion, of the ventricular wall (M cells)** (Figure 5.27).

We can explain human ECG origins based on the fact that the **epicardium repolarizes before the endocardium** (Figure 5.25), which happens in the ischemic cell (Figure 5.24).

In a normal cellular cell, it occurs in the opposite way, as the area distal to the electrode (equivalent to the endocardium) repolarizes before the area proximal to the electrode (the epicardium) (Figure 5.9).

Theories to explain the origin of the cellular electrogram and human ECG morphologies

The origin of cellular electrograms and human ECGs may be explained by two different theories.

The first theory

This theory states that the curves of the cellular electrogram and human ECG are the result of successive recordings of cellular and human (left ventricle) depolarization and repolarization phenomenon (dipole) taken from an electrode located opposite to the initial stimulation site (depolarization), bearing in mind that when the electrode faces the head of the dipole (vector) it records positivity and when facing the tail it records negativity. As previously explained, in the human left ventricle the repolarization dipole starts in the last part that has been depolarized (the subepicardium) (see Figure 5.26), the same as in an isolated ischemic cell (see Figure 5.24). This occurs because the subendocardial area is physiologically underperfused (see before). In contrast, the first part to be repolarized in the normal cell is also the first part that has been depolarized (Figure 5.9). This explains how in the

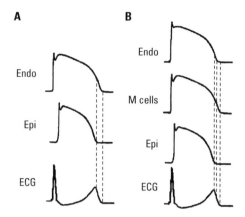

Figure 5.27 (A) The APs of endocardium and epicardium are shown. The latter, according to the theory used to explain the normal ECG, is the last to depolarize and the first to repolarize. (B) According to Yan and Antzelevitch (1998), the epicardium repolarizes first (coincides with the peak of T wave) and the endocardium later, but the area that repolarizes last is the M cell area (coinciding with the end of the T wave) (see text).

isolated electrogram, the wave of repolarization is recorded as negative ⌄ (Figure 5.9) and in the human ECG as positive (Figure 5.25) ⌄.

Figure 5.28 summarizes how the correlation between dipole, vector, and the direction (sense) of the depolarization and repolarization phenomena may account for the ECG curve, both in a normal cell (Figure 5.9) and in human beings (see Figure 5.26).

This is in fact a simplified explanation of how the ECG recording is generated. The left ventricle is considered to be responsible for the human ECG and its depolarization is represented by one vector. In practice, this is not so. The human ECG depolarization requires at least one vector, the sum of all atrial vectors that accounts for the process in which the stimulus depolarizes the atria, known as the atrial depolarization loop, or **P loop** (Figures 5.16 and 5.17), and the three vectors responsible for ventricular depolarization, or the **QRS loop** (Figures 5.20–5.22). In addition, ventricular depolarization (QRS) is followed by the ventricular repolarization wave (T wave) that is expressed by the repolarization loop, or **T loop** (Figures 5.23 and 7.18). **The projection of the P, QRS, and T loops onto the positive and negative hemifields of each lead accounts for the morphology of the ECG:**

$$\text{Dipole} \rightarrow \text{Vector} \rightarrow \text{Loop} \rightarrow \text{Hemifield} \rightarrow \text{ECG}$$

The second theory

According to this theory, **cellular and human ECGs are the sum of the subendocardial** (or cellular area most distal to the recording electrode) **and the subepicardial**

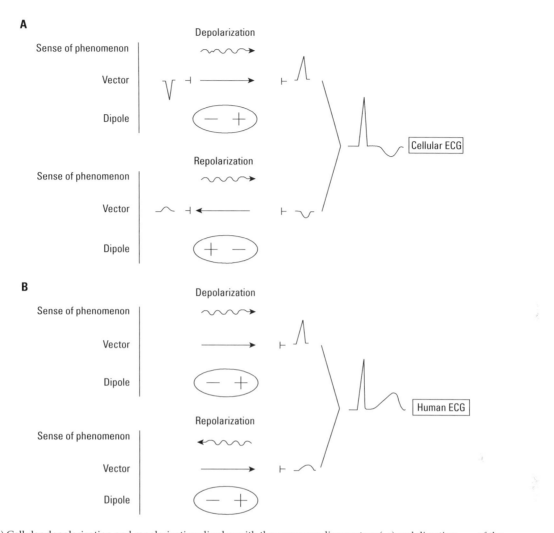

Figure 5.28 (A) Cellular depolarization and repolarization dipoles with the corresponding vectors (→) and direction ∿ of the phenomenon, which give rise to a cellular electrogram with negative repolarization wave. (B) Ventricular depolarization and repolarization dipoles, with the corresponding vectors and direction of the phenomenon and resulting human ECG curve (QRS–T curve).

(or cellular area most proximal to the recording electrode) **APs**. It should be noted that the AP phase 0 corresponds to QRS, phases 1 and 2 to the ST segment, and the end of phases 2 and 3 to the T wave (Figure 5.8). This theory is very useful in understanding the repolarization alterations observed during myocardial ischemia (changes in T wave, ST segment depression and elevation) (see Chapter 13).

Figure 5.29 shows how the sum of the APs from the area distal (A) and proximal (B) to the electrode both at the cellular (left) and ventricular (right) level accounts for the cellular and human ECG. **On the right, we can see how the human ECG is initiated**. The subendocardium ÂP corresponds to the ÂP of the left ventricular area distal to the electrode (A). At the end of depolarization (b), the electrode is facing the inner positivity of the distal area since that area is depolarized and has

negative charges on the outside and positive charges on the inside, giving rise to an ascending phase 0 of the ÂP of the subendocardium (distal area). Later on, at the end of repolarization of the distal area (c), which occurs later (2) than in the proximal area (the subepicardium) (4), the electrode is facing the inner negativity, since the outer repolarized area is already positive. Therefore, the curve returns to the isoelectric line, although, as the subendocardium repolarization ends later, its ÂP also ends later than that of the subepicardium (compare 2 with 4). The opposite is true in the case of the subepicardium ÂP. Its ÂP corresponds to the ÂP of the left ventricular area proximal to the electrode (B). When it depolarizes, it occurs later than in the subendocardial area. This zone (e) is negatively charged on the outer side and thus the electrode faces a negative charge and records phase 0 as negative (e). When this zone is repolarized (f), it occurs

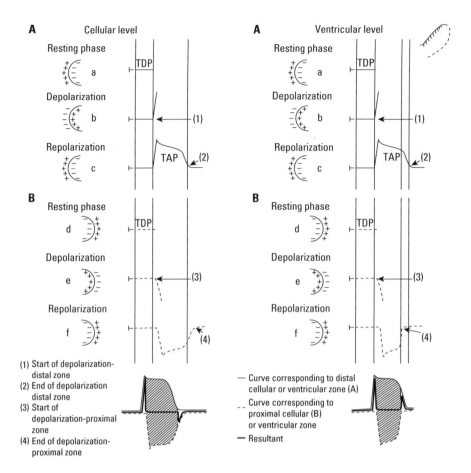

Figure 5.29 At both the cellular and the ventricular level, the sum of the AP from the area distal (A) to the electrode and the AP from the area proximal (B) to the electrode produces the cellular ECG with negative T waves and the human (ventricular) ECG with positive T waves (see text).

sooner than in the subendocardial area. The electrode faces outer positive charges because the repolarization is already complete, and the subepicardium ÂP curve returns to the isoelectric line (4) sooner than the subendocardium ÂP (2). By adding together both ÂPs (below right), it may be inferred how the human ECG is produced with positive depolarization (QRS) and repolarization (T) waves and a cancelled area in between (isoelectric ST).

On the left, the origin of a cellular electrogram is shown. It has a negative repolarization wave because the proximal zone to the electrode of the isolated cell has a longer ÂP compared with that of the distal zone (contrary to what is observed at the ventricular level). Thus, in a normal myocardial cell, the repolarization starts at the distal zone (equivalent to the subendocardium) and ends later in the proximal zone (equivalent to the epicardium). Therefore, the sum of both ÂPs explains the negativity of the T wave in a normal cellular electrogram.

1. There is considerable evidence that the **epicardium** (the most proximal area to the electrode) **is the first area of the human heart to repolarize**.

2. **Cellular electrograms and human ECGs** result from the **sum of the AP** from the distal (endocardium in the heart) and proximal (epicardium in the heart) areas to the recording electrode (Figure 5.29).

3. **According to another theory, both the cellular electrogram and the human ECG are the result of successive recordings of cellular or ventricular depolarization and repolarization (Figure 5.26).**

4. **The correlation between the contractile cell AP and the human ECG is the following (Figure 5.8):**
   - **Phase 0: QRS.**
   - **Phase 1 and start of phase 2: J point and onset of ST** segment.
   - **Phase 2 (mid-part):** ST segment isoelectric line.
   - **End of phase 2 and phase 3: T wave.**

References

Bayés de Luna A, Baranchuk A. *Clinical Arrhythmology*, 2nd edn. Willey-Blackwell, 2017.

Bayés de Luna A, Cladellas M, Oter R, *et al*. Interatrial conduction block and retrograde activation of the left atrium and paroxysmal supraventricular tachyarrhythmia. Eur Heart J 1988;9:1112.

Burgess JM, Green LS, Millar K, *et al*. The sequence of normal ventricular recovery. Am Heart J 1972;84:660.

Burnes J, Waldo A, Rudy Y. Imaging dispersion of ventricular repolarization. Circulation 2001;104:1299.

Cabrera E. *Teoría y práctica de la electrocardiografía*. La Prensa Médica Mexicana, 1958.

Cassidy DM, Vassallo JA, Klein AM, *et al*. The use of programmed electrical stimulation in patients with documented or suspected ventricular arrhythmias. Heart Lung 1984;13:602.

Coraboeuf E. Membrane ionic permeabilities and contractilephenomena in myocardium. Cardiovasc Res 1971;1(suppl 1):55.

Durrer D, Van Dam R, Freud G, Jame M, Meijler F, Arzbaecher R. Total excitation of the isolated human heart. Circulation 1970;41:899.

Franz MR, Bargheer K, Rafflenbeul W, Haverich A, Lichtlen PR. Monophasic action potential mapping in human subjects with normal electrocardiograms: direct evidence of the T wave. Circulation 1987;75:379.

Hoffman B, Cranefield P. *Electrophysiology of the Heart*. McGraw-Hill, 1960.

Hoffman I, Mehta J, Hilserath J, *et al*. Anterior conductions delay: a possible cause for prominent anterior QRS forces. J Electrocardiol 1976;9:15.

Holmqvist F, Husser D, Tapanainus J, *et al*. Interatrial conduction can be accurately determined using standard 12 lead ECG. Heart Rhythm 2008;5:413.

Horan LG, Flowers NC, Johnson JC. Significance of the diagnostic Q wave of myocardial infarction. Circulation 1971;43:428.

Kulbertus HE, de Laval-Rutten F, Casters P. Vectorcardiographic study of aberrant conduction anterior displacement of QRS: another form of intraventricular block. Br Heart J 1976;38:549.

Macfarlane PW, Veitch Lawrie TD (eds). *Comprehensive Electrocardiography*. Pergamon Press, 1989.

Moon JC, De Arenaza DP, Elkington AG, Taneja AK, John AS, Wand D. The pathologic basis of Q-wave and non-Q-wave myocardial infarction: a cardiovascular magnetic resonance study. J Am Coll Cardiol 2004;44:554.

Ophof T, Coronel R, Wilms Schopman FJ, *et al*. Dispersion of repolarization in canine ventricle and the ECG T wave: T interval does not reflect transmural dispersion. Heart Rhythm 2007;4:341.

Pérez-Riera A. *Learning Easily Frank Vectorcardiogram*. Editora e Graficas Mosteiro, 2009.

Puech P, Grolleau R. *L'activité du faisceau de His*. Sandoz, 1972.

Rosenbaum M, Elizari M. *Los hemibloqueos*. Editorial Paidos, 1968.

Sodi-Pallares D, Bisteni A, Medrano G. *Electrocardiografía y vectorcardiografía deductivas*. La Prensa Médica Mexicana, 1964.

Uhley HN. The quadrifascicular nature of the peripheral conduction system in cardiac arrhythmias. In Dreifus L, Likoff W (eds) *Cardiac Arrhythmias*. Grune-Stratton, 1973.

Wagner GS (ed.). *Marriott's Practical Electrocardiography*, 10th edn. Lippincott Williams & Wilkins, 2001.

Wilson FN, Hill I, Johnston F. The form of ECG in experimental myocardial infarction. Am Heart J 1935;10:903.

Yan GX, Antzelevitch C. Cellular basis for the normal T wave and the electrocardiographic manifestations of the long-QT syndrome. Circulation 1998;98:1928.

Chapter 6
The ECG Recording: Leads, Devices, and Techniques

Leads

The ECG waves are recorded in different forms according to the location of the explorer electrode (lead). The morphology of the ECG is determined by the location at which the lead is recorded. Because the heart is a three-dimensional organ, it is necessary to know the projection of the electrical activity at least in two planes—the frontal plane and the horizontal plane—to determine the exact direction of the different vectors that express the electrical forces of the heart. To record these forces, cables that connect the patient with the galvanometer of the ECG device are necessary, which pass through an amplifier. These cables are connected to the skin through special plaques (see Figure 6.19). **ECG devices record the electrical activity of the heart through both frontal and horizontal plane leads. There are six frontal plane leads and six horizontal plane leads (V1–V6).**

Just as it is necessary to photograph a monument or person from various angles in order to obtain comprehensive information about its size and shape (Figure 6.1), the electrical forces generated by the heart need to be recorded from different places (leads) to obtain a good electrocardiographic image of the heart. **Each lead has a lead line** which goes from the place where the lead is located to the opposite zone, passing through the center of the heart. Each of the lead lines is **divided into two segments**: the positive half, which is proximal to the positive pole and indicated by a continuous line, and the negative half, which is proximal to the negative pole and indicated by a dotted line.

Frontal plane leads
Standard limb leads: I, II, III
The three standard limb leads record the potential differences between two parts of the body. They constitute a closed circuit (Figure 6.2). Einthoven designated these leads as I, II, and III. To record these leads, electrodes are placed on the right arm, left arm, and left foot (Figure 6.2).

These bipolar leads reveal the direction and magnitude of the vectorial forces in the frontal plane (up–down, right–left). The potential differences recorded by these leads are explained in the legend of Figure 6.3.

The needle of the electrocardiograph inscribes the electrical forces as positive upward deflections (⅄) or negative, downward deflections (∨), or diphasic complexes, such as complexes consisting of both a positive–negative or negative–positive deflection (⋀∨, ∨⋀).

A positive deflection (⅄) in a certain lead represents the electrical forces pointed toward the positive electrode of this lead; a negative deflection (∨) represents electrical forces pointed toward the negative electrode of the same lead (Figure 6.3). An isodiphasic (⋀∨, ∨⋀) deflection indicates that the vectorial forces are perpendicular to the lead line (i.e. they lie on a line separating the positive and negative hemifields of the lead). The correct morphology (+− or −+ may be determined according to whether the rotation of the loop is clockwise or counterclockwise (see Figures 1.5, 1.6, 6.16, and 6.17). A deflection that has the same positive and negative height but different areas (⋀∪) is not considered isodiphasic; a deflection with some positive and negative areas but different heights (⅄∪) is considered isodiphasic.

In accordance with Kirchoff's law, Einthoven considered these three bipolar leads to be a closed circuit. Lead II = I + III is known as **Einthoven's law**. This law should always be satisfied in electrocardiography and is used as means of verifying proper lead placement and labelling.

Using the aforementioned law, **Einthoven described an imaginary equilateral triangle** superimposed on the human body as a useful visual tool, using the basic idea that electrode placement further down on the arms or legs (Figure 6.4A) is equivalent to placement on the root of the limbs (right shoulder, left shoulder, and groin) (Figure 6.4B). Although the expression of Einthoven's law as an equilateral triangle is not completely correct—it is evident that the human trunk cannot be considered a homogeneously conductive sphere with the heart at its center (Figure 6.5)—it **is the easiest way to remember the basic concepts of ECG** (hemifield, distance in angles between leads, calculation of the electrical axis, etc.). According to Einthoven's triangle, the six leads of the frontal plane form a hexagonal reference system that divides the electrical field into 12 parts separated by 30°. The scalene triangle described by Burger is probably more exact (Figure 6.6). If we follow this, the 12 parts are separated by different angles. However, on some occasions, we may explain some aspects of the ECG–VCG correlation using Burger's triangle. Figure 11.35, for example, shows that in cases of superoanterior hemiblock the last part of the frontal loop is located beyond −90° but in spite of that we do not record the "S" wave in lead I, because the positive hemifield, according Burger's triangle (dotted line around −10° in Figure 11.35), really finishes beyond −90°.

Different vectors generated in the heart (i.e. Vectors 1–6 in Figure 6.4C) result in different projections (positive, negative, and diphasic) on the three sides of the triangle (on the three standard leads of the frontal plane).

Moving the three segments of Einthoven's triangle (I, II, III) until they intersect at the triangle center, Bailey obtained a reference system (**Bailey's triaxial system**) (Figure 6.7) that does not alter the mathematical relationship between leads, I, II, and III, but facilitates the understanding of the positive and negative hemifield concepts. The frontal plane where the reference triaxial figure is situated is divided by the three leads into six spaces (**Bailey's sextants**). The positive pole of lead I corresponds to 0°, that of lead II to +60°, and that of lead III to +120°. The negative poles of these leads correspond to ±180°, −120°, and −60°, respectively. Each sextant represents a 60° arc.

Limb leads: right and left arm and left foot (aVR, aVL, aVF)

Despite the usefulness of the three bipolar standard limb leads, they reflect only the differences of potential and not the real direct potential in one specific point of the body. In order to separate the two components of standard limb leads, Wilson *et al.* (1943) joined the three vertices of the Einthoven triangle (right and left arm and left foot) with resistances of 5000 Ω to one point we refer to as the **central terminal**, obtaining at this point a potential zero (Figure 6.8A). Later, he connected the explorer electrode to the right (R) and left arm (L) and left foot (F) and obtained the absolute net potentials of these three members (right arm, left arm, and left foot): the aVR, aVL, and aVF leads. Although Wilson called these "unipolar" limb leads, really they are also bipolar because they measure differences of potential between one point and the central terminal (AHA/ACC/HRS Guidelines, Kligfield *et al.* 2007).

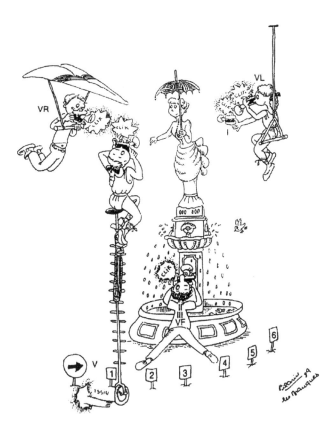

Figure 6.1 For a better understanding of a landscape, building, or statue, it is necessary to contemplate or take photographs from different angles, as shown in this case with the "Dama de la Sombrilla" (Umbrella Lady), a landmark in Barcelona. Similarly, if we want to learn about the electrical activity of the heart, it is necessary to record the activation route from different angles (leads) (drawing by Pilarín Bayés de Luna).

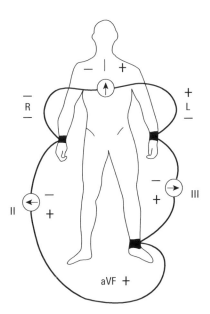

Figure 6.2 Human silhouette with the wires placed for the three classic frontal plane leads I, II, and III.

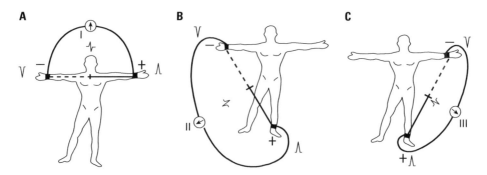

Figure 6.3 (A) Lead I records the differences in potential between the left arm (+) and right arm (−). (B) Lead II records the differences in potential between the left leg (+) and right arm (−). (C) Lead III records the differences in potential between the left leg (+) and left arm (−).

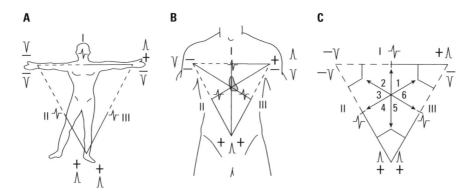

Figure 6.4 (A) Einthoven's triangle. (B) The same superimposed on a human torso. Observe the positive (continuous line) and negative (dotted line) parts of each lead. (C) Different vectors (from 1 to 6) produce different projections according to their location. For example, Vector 1 has a positive projection in I, negative projection in III, and isodiphasic projection (zero) in II.

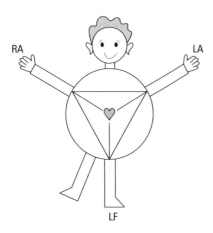

Figure 6.5 Sketch of the hypothetical human body corresponding to Einthoven's triangle: the heart in the center of a homogeneous sphere.

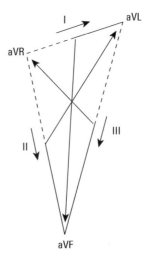

Figure 6.6 Burger's scalene triangle, which represents the electrical field of the human body more accurately than Einthoven's triangle.

To obtain better voltage complexes, Goldberger modified the Wilson system to an augmented system leads (aVR, aVL, aVF) (Figure 6.8B). These three "unipolar" leads are directed from the vertices of the three angles of Einthoven's triangle (aVR, aVL, aVF) toward the midpoint of the opposite site, intersecting the center of the triangle (Figure 6.9). Each lead has a positive pole

extending from the angle of the triangle that coincides with the respective edge to the center of the triangle, and a negative pole, extending practically from the center of the triangle to the midpoint of the opposite side of the triangle. The negative pole of each lead is situated 180°

opposite the positive pole. The direction of the lead line of aVR extends from −150° (positive pole) to +30° (negative pole); the lead line of aVL from −30° (positive pole) to +150° (negative pole); and the lead line of VF from +90° (positive pole) to −90° (negative pole).

Using the locations of the three limb leads (triaxial reference system) and combining the axes of the aVF, aVL, and aVF leads with Bailey's triaxial reference system so that the intersection of the six axes is in the center of the heart, a single figure is obtained which shows the directions, the positive and negative poles, and positive (continuous line) and negative (dotted line) parts of the six frontal plane leads (**Bailey's hexaxial system**). In this system (Figure 6.10), leads are separated by 30° angles.

There is an increased interest in revising the standard presentation of the frontal plane ECG leads by changing the lead aVR location from −150° to +30° (Case and Moss 2010). This reorients the frontal plane leads from III

to aVL into a progressive logically panoramic sequence that follows the same pattern as the horizontal precordial leads from V1 to V6 (Figure 6.11).

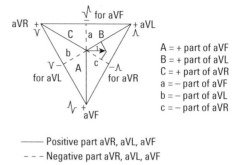

A = + part of aVF
B = + part of aVL
C = + part of aVR
a = − part of aVF
b = − part of aVL
c = − part of aVR

———— Positive part aVR, aVL, aVF
- - - - Negative part aVR, aVL, aVF

Figure 6.9 Any vector projected on aVR, aVL, or aVF produces a projection that can be positive, negative, or isodiphasic. Vector 1 has a positive projection on aVL, a negative projection on aVR, and an isodiphasic projection on aVF.

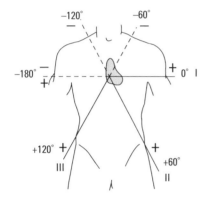

Figure 6.7 Bailey's triaxial system (see text).

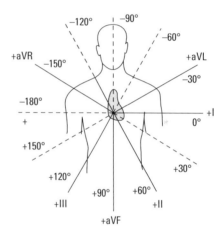

Figure 6.10 Bailey's hexaxial system (see text).

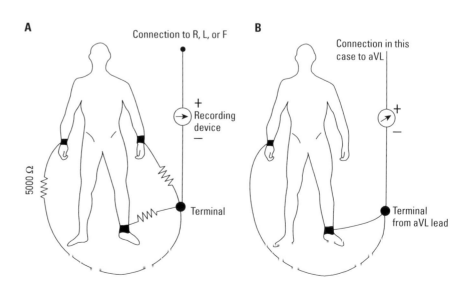

Figure 6.8 The VR, VL, and VF frontal leads. (A) Wilson's system; (B) Goldberger's system.

A

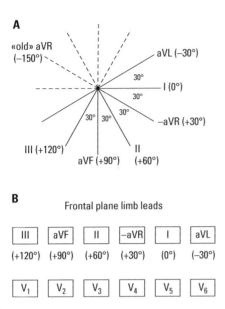

B

Frontal plane limb leads

III	aVF	II	−aVR	I	aVL
(+120°)	(+90°)	(+60°)	(+30°)	(0°)	(−30°)

| V_1 | V_2 | V_3 | V_4 | V_5 | V_6 |

Horizontal plane precordial leads

Figure 6.11 ECG lead angles and associated lead nomenclature. (A) Hexaxial lead system in the frontal plane. The change of aVR by complete electrical inversion will enter the same lead, inverted by 180° (now called—aVR in the hexaxial lead system). (B) Suggested 12-lead ECG presentation. The leads in the frontal and horizontal planes are sequentially presented in separate rows and in both cases in panoramic view from right to left from III to aVL and from V1 to V6.

Horizontal plane leads

Horizontal plane leads add necessary information about the anterior or posterior location of the electrical forces of the heart not given by the frontal plane (up–down or right–left direction of the vectors) leads. These leads are particularly useful when the cardiac vectors are perpendicular to the frontal plane because the projection of a vector in a perpendicular plane is zero. Therefore, in these cases, frontal plane leads are of little use, while the horizontal leads provide the proper information.

The horizontal plane leads used in clinical electrocardiography are based on potential differences between an exploring electrode on the chest wall and the Wilson central terminal (Figure 6.12). Therefore, although considered monopolar by Wilson, they are also effectively bipolar (AHA/ACC/HRS Guidelines, Kligfield *et al.* 2007) (see above).

The recording electrodes (+ charges) are placed at different points on the chest wall. Normally, six leads are used (V1–V6) that are located in different places on the chest (Figure 6.13A). Occasionally, additional right leads and posterior leads are added (see below). All precordial leads have a positive (continuous line) and negative (dotted line) section. In this case, despite the fact that the negative pole is in the center of the heart (central terminal), we consider for practical purposes the negative pole of

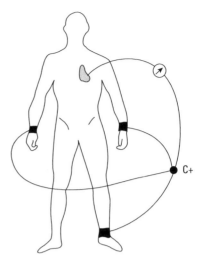

Figure 6.12 System of precordial leads (see text).

each unipolar precordial lead to be located 180° opposite from the positive pole. As we have said, these really are bipolar leads. Figure 6.13B shows the angular panoramic view of the electrodes of six usual precordial leads, and the locations of positive poles and lines of the six precordial leads.

Other additional leads or forms of presentation

The 12-lead standardized presentation of the ECG outlined by the American Heart Association more than 70 years ago has remained the "gold standard" clinical contribution and has been accepted worldwide. However, there are other leads that have been found to be useful, including the following:

• **Extreme right precordial leads (V3R and V4R) (Figure 6.13A) and extreme left precordial leads (back leads)** (V7: posterior axillary line; V8: inferior angle of the scapula; V9: left paravertebral area). These may help to diagnose right ventricle or lateral infarctions, respectively (Wellens 1999; Fiol-Sala *et al.*, 2020) (see Figures 13.48 and 13.49).

• **The use of 24 leads** (adding 12 opposed leads) (Perron *et al.* 2007).

• **The change from aVR to −aVR** with the positive pole of aVR at +30° (see above). This may create a total angular ECG system of frontal leads that may facilitate a more logically sequential study of ECG patterns (Case and Moss 2010; Bayés de Luna and Garcia-Niebla 2010) (see before) (Figure 6.11). In spite that this sequential way of presentation seems more logical has not been used in clinical practice.

• **The addition of some bipolar precordial leads (Lewis leads)** *(Baker et al. 2009) that may be useful for the* diagnosis of AV dissociation. We will discuss this in more detail later (Chapter 25).

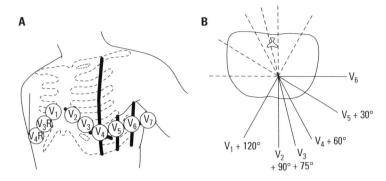

Figure 6.13 (A) Sites where the exploring electrodes are placed in precordial leads. (B) Situation of the positive pole in the six precordial leads.

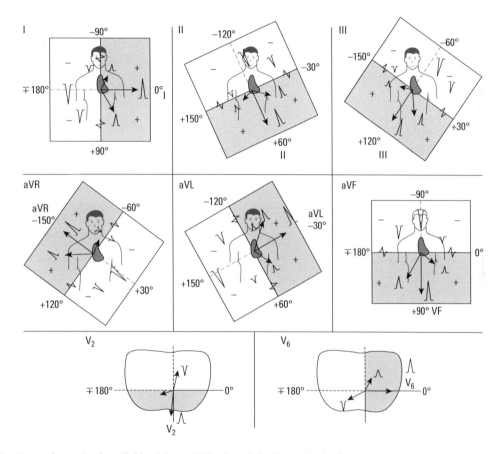

Figure 6.14 Positive and negative hemifields of the six FP leads and the V2 and V6 leads of the HP (see text).

- Esophageal leads may also be useful for some specific topics (e.g. to study atrial activation) (Rodensky and Wasserman 1962; Gallagher *et al.* 1982; Pehrson 2004) (see Figure 9.21 and Chapter 25).
- **There are also reduced and expanded lead set presentations still under study**.

Hemifield concept

In Chapter 1, we described this concept as tracing from each lead a perpendicular line that passes through the center of the heart to divide the electrical field of the body into two hemifields for each lead, one positive and one negative. In Figure 1.5, we describe the formation of the positive and negative hemifields of the frontal plane for leads I and aVF. The hemifields of the other leads of FP and HP can be depicted by drawing lines perpendicular to the frontal (I, II, III, aVR, aVL, and aVF) and horizontal leads (V1–V6) which intersect at the center of the heart (Figure 6.14) (Bayés de Luna 2012).

The positive hemifields of each lead are as follows (Figure 6.14): lead I, from −90° to +90° passing through 0°; lead II, from −30° to +150° passing through +60°; lead III, from +30° to −150° passing through +120°; lead aVR, from +120° to −60° passing through −150°; lead aVL, from −120° to +60° passing through −30°; lead aVF, from 0° to ±180° passing through +90°; and lead V6, from −90° to +90° passing through 0°. The other hemifields of horizontal plane leads are obtained in the same manner by drawing lines perpendicular to the respective leads which intersect the center of the heart.

The projection of a P, QRS, or T vectorial force on the positive and negative hemifield of any lead, or on the line separating them, initiates a positive, negative, or isodiphasic deflection, respectively in this lead. The degree of positivity or negativity depends on the magnitude and the direction of the vector (Figure 6.15). With the same magnitude, a vectorial force directed more toward the positive or negative pole of a given lead will produce a more positive or negative deflection, since the projection will have a larger amplitude; for the same

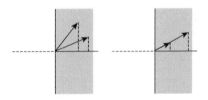

Figure 6.15 Relationship between the magnitude and direction of a vector and its positivity in a determined lead, in this case I (see text).

direction, the force with the greatest magnitude will produce the most positive or negative deflection (Figure 6.15).

Correlation between the vectorcardiographic loop and electrocardiographic morphology

Vectorcardiographic loops originate in the frontal or horizontal plane leads with different ECG morphologies, with QRS complexes more or less wide, and with positive, negative, or diphasic deflections in accordance with their projections in the respective positive and negative hemifields (Figure 6.16) (Cabrera 1958; Cooksey *et al.* 1977; Bayés de Luna 2012). (For correlation between the vectorcardiographic morphology of the loop in the frontal plane and the morphology of leads aVF and V2, see Figure 1.6.)

We believe that an understanding of the integrated dipole–vector–loop–hemifield concept, bearing in mind the correlation between the electrocardiographic curve and vectorcardiographic loop, is crucial to an understanding of clinical electrocardiography.

Up to this point, electrocardiographic deflections have been considered positive, negative, or diphasic, in order to simplify correlation with the leads' hemifields. However, under normal conditions, the QRS complex is usually triphasic when it is recorded in the leads facing the left ventricular free wall (I, aVL, V5, and V6). Using

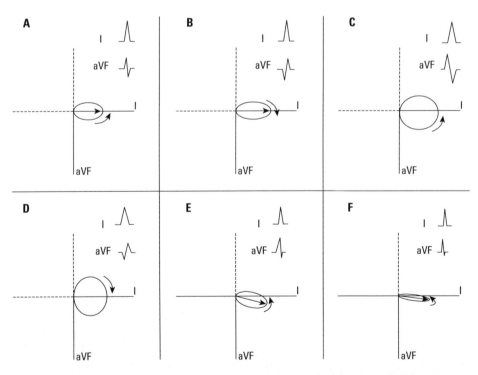

Figure 6.16 According to the direction of loop rotation, an isodiphasic deflection in a determined lead (in this case aVF) is positive–negative (A) or negative–positive (B) (see Figure 1.5). The enclosed area is larger if the loop is more open (C and D). If more of the loop lies in the positive hemifield than in the negative hemifield, the deflection is diphasic, but not isodiphasic (E, F).

leads I, II, and III in FP and V1 and V6 in HP as an example (Figure 6.17), when in FP the mean vector of QRS loop is around +60°, the morphology is qRS, and the global QRS is positive in the three leads because the main Vector 2 lies in the positive hemifield of the three leads (more positive in lead II). In leads I and II, there is an initial (q) and terminal (s) deflection because Vector 1 lies on the negative hemifield of leads I, and II (the "q" wave is less negative in I than in II), and Vector 3 falls in the negative hemifield of both leads but more in lead I than II (S wave is slightly bigger in I). Lead III usually has a small "q" in lead I but in general no "S" or only a very small "s" in lead III (see Figure 6.17A). In Figure 6.17B, the same correlation is well understood in that V6 is often recorded as qRs morphology, but in V1 the morphology is in general just rS without r′.

Recording devices

The electrocardiograph records the cardiac electrical activity conducted through wires to metal plates placed at different points, called leads. The recording device consists fundamentally of an amplifier that magnifies electrical signals, and a galvanometer which moves the inscription needle (see Chapter 2). The needle moves in accordance with the magnitude of the electrical potential generated by the patient. This electrical potential has a vectorial expression. The needle inscribes a positive or negative deflection depending on whether the explorer electrode of a given lead faces the head of the vector corresponding to the positive charge of the dipole independent of whether or not the electrical force is going toward or away from the positive pole of the lead (Figure 6.18).

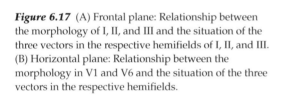
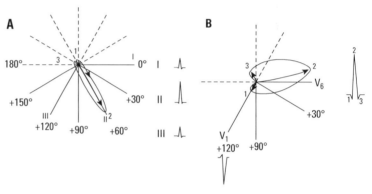

Figure 6.17 (A) Frontal plane: Relationship between the morphology of I, II, and III and the situation of the three vectors in the respective hemifields of I, II, and III. (B) Horizontal plane: Relationship between the morphology in V1 and V6 and the situation of the three vectors in the respective hemifields.

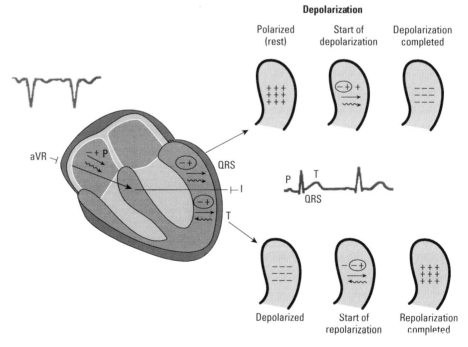

Figure 6.18 ECG recording from aVR and I. Correlation with depolarization and repolarization phenomenon.

ECG devices have to avoid oscillations and artifact distortions of ST. This can be achieved with low-frequency filtering (high-pass) with a cut-off of 0.05 Hz for routine filters or 0.67 Hz or below for linear digital filters (Garcia-Niebla *et al.* 2009). To avoid muscle tremor, high-frequency (low-pass) filtering is needed. Usually, the recommended cut-off is at least 150 Hz (or 250 Hz for children). It is recommended that the devices automatically alert if a very low high-frequency cut-off (≈40 Hz) is used (see Figure 6.24).

Until recently, the common ECG recording devices were direct-inscription analog types, that are continuous in nature, usually recording the ECG curves with ther-mosensitive paper. However, **we are now immersed in the digital era,** and in the field of ECG, this has given rise to the need for functional programs and devices that are portable, versatile, and interactive. **Nearly all current ECG machines convert the analog ECG signal to digital form**. The initial sampling rate during analog-to-digital conversion is higher than the sampling rate that is used for further processing. This oversampling was originally introduced to detect and represent pacemaker stimulus outputs which are generally <0.5 ms in duration.

Ideally, **ECG machines should be small and compact, and must work in an integrated fashion** *in the* different health institutional settings, independently of the types of technologies used. Such systems should allow us to work online and may be implemented in telemedical services. Compression of ECGs is a good idea for ease of transmission and storage. In an ideal world, the diagnosis would be performed by an expert in real time through the Internet; this could then be applied to multiple scenarios (ambulance, isolated areas, ships, etc.) with poor access to assistance because of their geographic location or associated economic costs (see Figure **6.19**B).

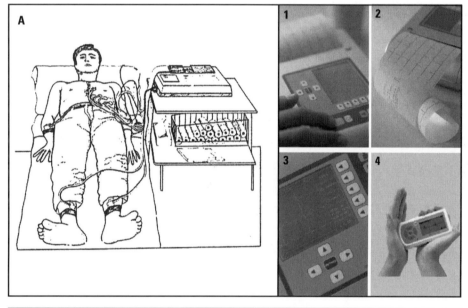

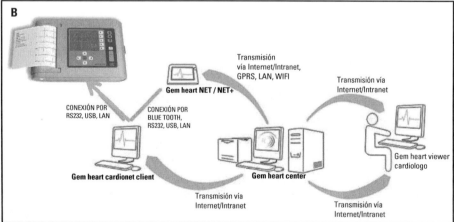

Figure 6.19 (A-1–A-3) Conventional ECG recording (see text). (A-4) Small device for self-recording an ECG strip in case of arrhythmia or precordial pain (see Figure 25.6). (B) Integrated system to visualize ECG using the Internet.

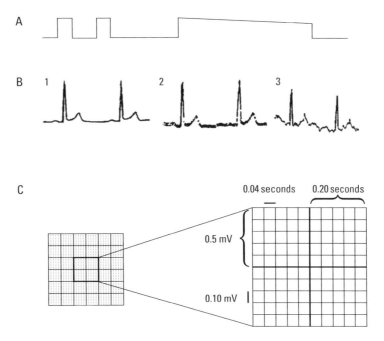

Figure 6.20 (A) Verification of proper calibration. (B) 1, Normal tracing; 2, tracing with artifacts due to alternating current; 3, tracing with artifacts due to trembling. (C) Example of a recording paper showing the distance between vertical (voltage) and horizontal (time) lines (see text).

Automatic measurement of different intervals (P, PR, QRS, QT) should be performed in different leads to detect the earliest onset and latest offset of waveforms and intervals. Particular attention should be paid to QT interval measurement (see Figure 7.9). Finally, although computer-based interpretation of the ECG is an adjunct to the ECG machine, any computerized diagnosis currently requires overview by a physician (AHA/ACC/HRS Guidelines, Kligfield *et al.* 2007) (see Chapter 3).

Recording techniques

In this section, we comment on the recording process and the technical errors that may occur during this process.

How to record an ECG

An ECG recording should be performed by trained personnel. The patient should be lying comfortably in bed or on an examination table. The room should be warm in order to minimize muscular trembling, which can produce recording artifacts. The patient's chest, wrists, and lower leg should be exposed (Figure 6.19A).

The person who records the ECG should perform the following tasks:

1 Connect the device to an electrical power source and the electrodes to the device.

2 Clean the patient's skin and place the recording electrodes at the correct sites for each lead recording. Four limb electrodes are placed (Figure 6.19): the red electrode on the right wrist; the yellow electrode on the left wrist; the green electrode, on the left leg; and the black, or indifferent electrode on the right leg. It is currently recommended that the electrodes are placed on the upper part of the arms to obtain a better recording. These electrodes are used to record the frontal plane leads. Additional electrodes are placed at different sites on the chest wall to record the precordial leads (from V1 to V6) (Figure 6.13A).

3 Adjust the baseline so that the electrocardiographic recording is centered on the paper.

4 Check the calibration of the device. Make sure that the height of the calibration deflection is 1 cm (corresponding to 1 mV) in each lead (Figure 6.20C). The morphology of the calibration deflection should also be checked. The slope of the plateau should drop down gradually as the calibration button is held down (Figure 6.20A).

5 Set the appropriate speed, normally 25 mm/s. In this case, the distance between two vertical lines of the recording paper (1 mm) corresponds to 0.04 s, and the distance between two thick lines (5 mm) is 0.20 s (Figure 6.20C). The speed of 50 mm/s is useful for better manual measurement of intervals but the quality of the recording, especially of the ST, is lower.

6 Maintain the recording line in the center.

7 Avoid artifacts such as those caused by alternating current and trembling (Figure 6.20B).

8 Record a strip of at least 20 cm for each lead. The person performing the recording should know when a long strip is needed (arrhythmias), when it is necessary to record during respiration (presence of Q in lead III), and when to

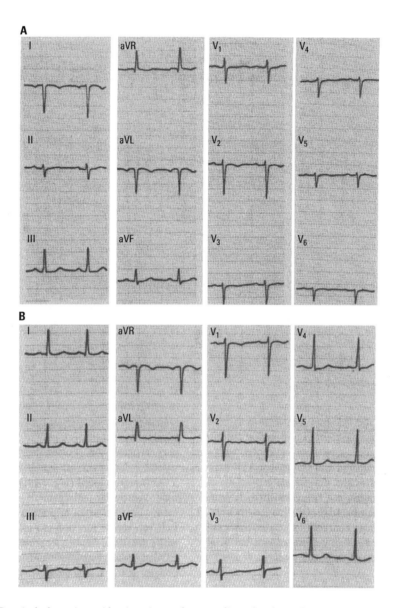

Figure 6.21 (A) An ECG typical of a patient with mirror image dextrocardia and no heart disease. (B) Normalized ECG.

record additional precordial leads (children, possible lateral or right ventricle infarct, etc.).

9 Ensure that the tracing is correctly recorded (II = I + III) and correctly label the different leads.

Technical errors in the recording process

Technical errors in the recording process may be caused by the device itself, or may be the responsibility of the recording. Errors include the following:

- **Misplacement of electrodes**, which may lead to a diagnosis of ectopic rhythm or dextrocardia (Figure 6.21) to anomalous location of the Q wave myocardial infarction (MI) (Figure 6.22) or to diagnosis false septal infarction. The latter is caused by misplacement of electrodes of V1–V2 in a high position that may record negative P wave

followed by QS instead of positive or ±P wave followed by rS pattern.

Also, a high location of V2 electrode in case of patients with superoanterior hemiblock, explain the rare ECG pattern (high R in V2 seen in these cases).

- A false diagnosis of ventricular tachycardia as a consequence of **artifacts** (Figure 6.23A).
- False diagnosis of atrial flutter in some leads (DIII) in a patient with Parkinson's disease (Figure 6.23B).
- Suppression of an otherwise visible J wave (Figure 6.24) because of the **inappropriate use of some filters** (Nuñez-Angulo 2011).

For more information, consult Lemmerz and Schmidt (1966), Drew (2006), Bayés de Luna (2019), Kligfield *et al.* (2007), and Garcia-Niebla *et al.* (2009).

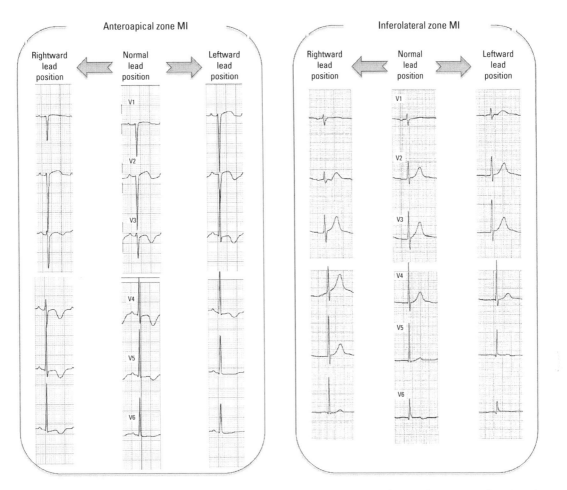

Figure 6.22 On the left, a patient with myocardial infarction of the anteroapical zone (previously named anteroseptal) in the subacute phase: normal lead position displays negative T waves up to V5. Small changes in the placement of precordial leads have significantly modified the morphology of QRS and T wave. On the right, a patient with an infarction of the inferolateral zone: moving the precordial leads a little to the right or left makes the negative T wave in V6 to disappear.

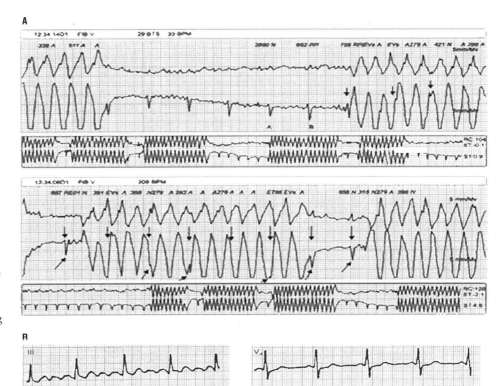

Figure 6.23 (A) Healthy 35-year-old patient, with palpitations. Holter recording shows rapid bursts with wide complexes and morphology similar to that of ventricular flutter. Detailed examination of the recording allows identification of the basal rhythm (arrows) hidden among the wide artifactual complexes. (B) Patient with Parkinson's disease whose ECG simulates atrial flutter in DIII while V4 clearly shows P waves.

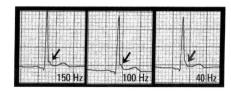

Figure 6.24 Forty-year-old patient with ECG morphology typical for early repolarization. Observe how a low-pass filter (40 Hz) can make the typical J curve disappear.

References

Baker AL, Nijkerk G, Groenemeijer BE, *et al*. The Lewis lead: making recognition of P waves easy during wide QRS complex tachycardia. *Circulation* 2009;115:1306.

Bayés de Luna A. *Clinical Electrocardiography. A Textbook*. Willey-Blackwell, 2012.

Bayés de Luna A. The morphology of the electrocardiogram. In Camm AJ, Lüscher TF, Serruys PW (eds) *The ESC Textbook of Cardiovascular Medicine*. Oxford University Press, 2019.

Bayés de Luna A, Garcia-Niebla J. To change a dogma can be very difficult. *Ann Noninvasive Electrocardiol* 2010;15:392.

Cabrera E. *Teoría y práctica de le electrocardiografía*. Instituto Nacional de Cardiología. La Prensa Médica Mexicana, 1958.

Case RB, Moss AJ. Recommendation for revision of the standard presentation of the frontal plane ECG leads including reversal of lead aVR (to aVR): it is time for a change. *Ann Noninvasive Electrocardiol* 2010;15:97.

Cooksey I, Dunn M, Massie E. *Clinical ECG and VCG*. YearBook Medical, 1977.

Drew BJ. Pitfalls and artifacts in electrocardiographty. *Cardiol Clin* 2006;24:309.

Fiol-Sala M, Birnbaum Y, Nikus K, Bayés de Luna A. *Electrocardiography in Ischemic Heart Disease. Clinical and Imaging Correlations and Prognostic Implications*, 2nd edn. Willey-Blackwell, 2020.

Gallagher JJ, Smith W, Kerr CR, *et al*. Esophageal pacing: a diagnostic and therapeutical tool. *Circulation* 1982;65:336.

Garcia-Niebla J, Llontop-García P, Valle-Racero JI, Serra-Autonell G, Batchvarov VN, Bayés de Luna A. Technical mistakes during the acquisition of the electrocardiogram. *Ann Noninvasive Electrocardiol* 2009;14:389.

Kligfield P, Gettes LS, Bailey JJ, *et al*. Recommendations for the standardization and interpretation of the electrocardiogram: Part I: The electrocardiogram and its technology: a scientific statement from the American Heart Association Electrocardiography and Arrhythmias Committee, Council on Clinical Cardiology; the American College of Cardiology Foundation; and the Heart Rhythm Society: endorsed by the International Society for Computerized Electrocardiology. *Circulation* 2007;115:1306.

Lemmerz AH, Schmidt R. *Les erreurs d'enregistrement en électrocardiographie*. Masson & Cie, 1966.

Nuñez-Angulo A. Chest pain with spurious ST elevation. *Eur Heart J* 2011;32:2349–2349.

Pehrson S. *The Oesophageal Route in Clinical Electrocardiology*. Pasquale del Bene, 2004.

Perron A, Limb T, Pahlm-Webb U, *et al*. Maximal increase in sensitivity with minimal loss of specificity for the diagnosis of ACS with the 24 leads ECG. *J Electrocardiol* 2007;40:463.

Rodensky PL, Wasserman F. Esophageal electrocardiography. Selected clinical applications. *Am Heart J* 1962;64:444.

Wellens HJ. The value of the right precordial leads of the electrocardiogram. *N Engl J Med* 1999;340:381.

Wilson F, Hill I, Johnston F. The interpretation of the galvanometric waves when one electrode is distant from the heart and the other in contact with its surface. *Am Heart J* 1943;4:807.

Chapter 7
Characteristics of the Normal Electrocardiogram: Normal ECG Waves and Intervals

A systematic and sequential approach to ECG interpretation

The interpretation of an ECG should be systematically approached in a sequential way. In this chapter, the normal value of each parameter at different ages and other ECG variants to ensure a successful ECG interpretation is discussed consecutively (Bayés de Luna, 2012; Bayés de Luna and Baranchuk, 2017). In Chapter 19, we discuss the diagnostic value of all the abnormalities of the ECG parameters. Figure 7.1A shows the temporal relationship between the different ECG waves and intervals, and Figure 7.1B shows the most frequent QRS, P, and T morphologies. In Figure 7.2, may be seen the normal activation of the atria (A), and this sequential activation according to the Lewis diagram (B). In Figure 7.2C, may be seen the infrequent alterations of P and QRS, relationship in the rare cases of sinoventricular conduction.

Heart rhythm

Heart rhythm can be sinusal or ectopic. All ectopic rhythms correspond to different types of arrhythmias (see Chapters 14–18). **Sinus rhythm** has the following characteristics:
- a positive P wave in leads I, II, aVF, and V2–V6, and negative in aVR. In leads III and V1, the P wave can be positive–negative (±); and
- the P wave is followed by a QRS complex with a fixed PR interval; in the absence of pre-excitation or AV block, its duration is between 0.12 and 0.20 s.

Under normal conditions, the discharge cadence at rest oscillates between 60 and 100 bpm and a slight variability exists between the RR intervals. Sometimes, particularly in children, this variability is more evident, most commonly related to respiration. In different pathological situations, the RR variability can be decreased, which has important clinical implications (see Chapter 25).

Under very rare pathological conditions, usually in the presence of important ionic disturbances (severe hyperkalemia) (see Chapter 23), the conduction of the sinus stimulus to the ventricles is normal through especialized fibers, but atrial activation is delayed (which explains delay of inscription of P wave and the short PR interval) or that P wave may be hidden in QRS, which explains sinus rhythm without a visible P wave (**sinoventricular conduction**) (Figure 7.2C).

Also in exceptional situations, sinus rhythm may be concealed due to extensive atrial fibrosis in the presence of large atria, particularly in valvular diseases that do not initiate measurable potentials on the surface ECG (see Figure 15.37). However, in some leads, often in V1, a small P wave may be seen.

Heart rate

Sinus rhythm is the normal rhythm of the heart. At rest, the normal sinus rate oscillates between 60 and 100 bpm. The rate will normally decrease with rest and sleep and increase with variables such as emotion, exercise, and fever. All types of normal and pathological sinus bradycardia and tachycardia will be discussed later (see Chapters 15 and 17). The heart rate can be calculated, approximately, according to the number of 0.20 s spaces (which are the spaces separated by thick lines on the ECG paper when the recording paper speed is 25 mm/s) occurring in an RR cycle (Table 7.1). Another method is to count the RR cycles occurring in 6 s and multiply this number by 10.

P wave

We will describe first the different parameters of the P wave, the wave of atrial depolarization.

To use the ECG for the study of atrial P wave in normal conditions and in pathology, we have to study the different components of the P wave, P wave parameters, named P wave indices by Magnani (Magnani *et al.*, 2010).

Clinical Electrocardiography: A Textbook, Fifth Edition, Antoni Bayés de Luna, Miquel Fiol Sala, Antoni Bayés-Genís, and Adrián Baranchuk.
© 2022 John Wiley & Sons Ltd. Published 2022 by John Wiley & Sons Ltd.

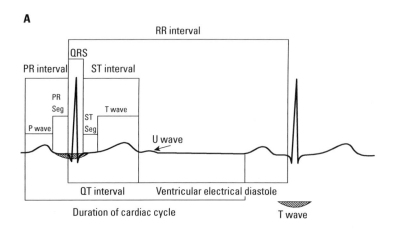

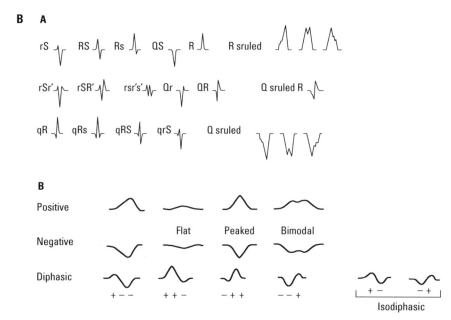

Figure 7.1 (**A**) Temporal relationship between the different ECG waves and nomenclature of the various intervals and segments. (**B**) (A) The most frequent QRS complex morphologies. (B) P and T wave morphologies.

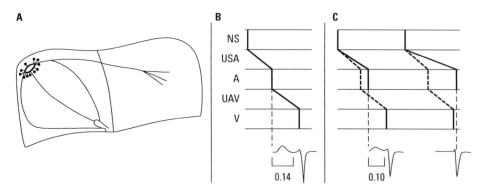

Figure 7.2 (A and B) Normal activation of the heart, with Lewis diagram. (C) One example of sinoventricular conduction with short PR interval or hidden P wave due to delay of inscription of P wave.

Table 7.1 Calculation of heart rate according to the RR interval

Number of 0.20 s spaces	Heart rate
1	300
2	150
3	100
4	75
5	60
6	50
7	43
8	37
9	33

These indices may be modified in the presence of right and left atrial enlargement and atrial blocks (see Chapter 9). The reference values are taken from studies performed in samples of healthy people (Magnani *et al.* 2010). These parameters of P are used for: (i) Diagnosis of interatrial block (IAB); (ii) Diagnosis of right and left atrial enlargement. The sensitivity for the diagnosis of right and left atrial enlargement is low; (iii) To know the risk of AF, stroke, and even dementia and death.

We will briefly describe the indices more frequently used for all these purposes (Figure 7.3) (Tables 7.2 and 7.3) (Cooksey *et al.* 1977).

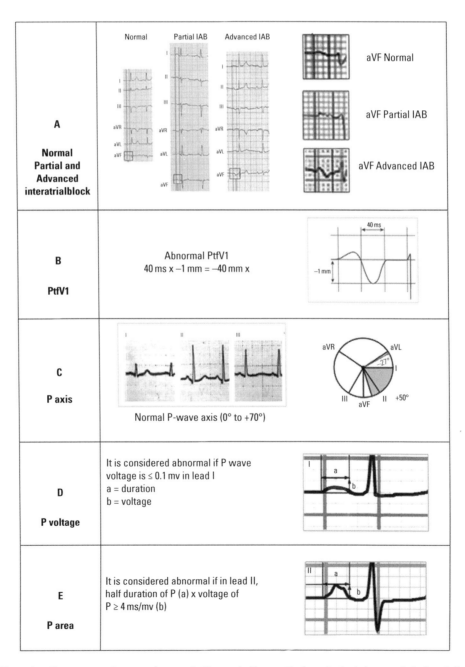

Figure 7.3 From A to E we can see the more frequently P wave índices, with the principal characteristic that define all of them.

P wave indices (Figure 7.3)

A. **P wave duration.** It is abnormal if it is ≥120 ms. It is a diagnostic criterion of partial interatrial block (P-IAB) (Bayés de Luna *et al.* 2012). In fact, to measure correctly the P wave duration, the best is to trace lines in a 6-channel device (frontal plane) and to measure the distance from the onset of P wave in the first lead that appear, to the end of P wave also in the last lead that occurs, and later measure this distance with calipers of GeoGebra method (Baranchuk 2017). The same is done to measure the PR interval.

B. **P wave morphology.** The projection of P loop is frontal and horizontal plane hemifield explains the P wave morphology in different leads (Figure 7.4). There are two important changes of the normal morphology:

• **Frontal Plane.** Biphasic (±) P wave ± in II, III, and aVF. This morphology combined with P≥120 ms, it is a diagnostic criterion of typical advanced interatrial block (A-IAB) (Bayés de Luna *et al.* 2012; O'Neal *et al.* 2016) (see later atrial blocks in Chapter 9).

• **Horizontal Plane.** P terminal force in V1 (PtfV1). It has been considered abnormal if the product of the amplitude of the negative component of P wave in V1 in mm, multiplied by the duration of this component in msec is greater than 40 ms × –1 mm (positive Morris index) (Morris *et al.* 1964; Tereshchenko *et al.*2014). However, if the electrode of V1 is not well located in 4th ICS, is two highly, there are many false positive results (Rasmussen *et al.* 2019). Also recently, some discordant results have been published regarding the value of this index as marker of AF and stroke (Inoue *et al.* 2018).

C. **Voltage.** It is considered abnormal if P wave is ≤0.1 mv in lead I (Park *et al.* 2016) (Table 7.2 and Figure 7.5).

D. **P wave axis.** It represents the location of the P wave in the frontal plane. It is normal when it is located between 0° and +75°. The P wave axis cannot be calculated in the presence of A-IAB (± in II, III, and aVF), because this represents an undetermined P wave axis, as is like the presence of S1, S2, S3 morphology that for QRS, that also does not allow to measure the QRS axis.

Table 7.2 P wave height and duration in normal adults

	Lead I	Lead II	Lead III	Lead V$_1$[a]
P height (mV)				
Mean	0.49	1.03	0.69	0.40
Range	0.2 to 1.0	0.3 to 2.0	0 to 2.0	0.05 to 0.80
P duration (s)				
Mean	0.08	0.09	0.07	0.05
Range	0.05 to 0.12	0.05 to 0.12	0.02 to 0.13	0 to 0.08
PR interval (s)				
Mean	0.16	0.16	0.16	
Range	0.12 to 0.20	0.12 to 0.20	0.12 to 0.20	

[a] Twenty-five per cent of the series had a small terminal negative deflection of the P wave in lead V1.
Adapted from Cooksey *et al.* (1977).

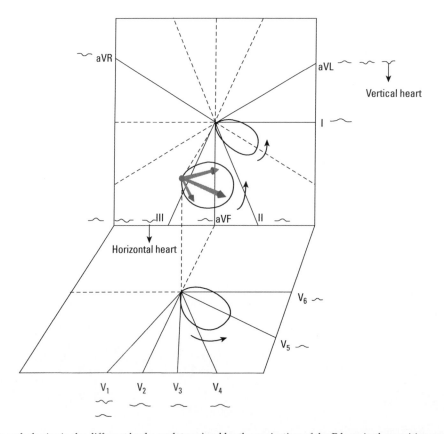

Figure 7.4 P wave morphologies in the different leads, as determined by the projection of the P loop in the positive and negative lead hemifields (see text). In a vertical heart, we have a negative P wave in aVL and in a horizontal heart, we have a negative P wave in III.

E. **P wave area**. It may be calculated in lead II by the following formula: P wave area = Half duration of P wave x voltage of P in II >4 ms/mv (Zeng *et al.* 2003).

F. **The use of scores**. It has been demonstrated that the use of an score formed by the association of duration of P wave, morphology (biphasic P wave in inferior leads) and low voltage of P wave (MVP score) (Alexander *et al.* 2019), or the association of P wave axis with 2 points to the CHA2DS2-Vasc score (Maheshwari *et al.* 2019) improves the prediction of AF and ischemic stroke.

1. **Other P wave indices**. The P wave dispersion and the PR interval are not considered now useful P wave indices, and the recording of signal averaging P wave actually seems not necessary because the amplification of the P wave obtained with a computer gives enough information on P wave morphology and duration.

How to distinguish if an atrial wave is sinusal or ectopic (Figure 7.5)

It depends on the P loop rotation as is well demonstrated in Figure 7.7. According to loop rotation (counterclockwise in the FP and HP in the case of sinus rhythm and clockwise in the case of ectopic rhythm), the P wave morphology in III and V1 varies.

Atrial repolarization (Figure 7.6)

The wave of atrial repolarization (see Chapter 5, Figure 5.17) is very flat follows the P wave and usually is hidden in the QRS complex (Figure 5.17) although in the presence of sympathetic overload may be seen (Figure 7.6). May be also recorded in cases of pericarditis and atrial infarction (Chapter 9).

The atrial rhythm may be sinusal or ectopic and depending on that the P loop rotation will be different and also the morphology of the P wave in III, V1, and aVL (Figure 7.7).

PR interval and PR segment (Table 7.2; and Figures 7.1 and 7.8)

Table 7.2 shows the mean and range of P wave height, duration, and PR interval in different leads. One recent study has demonstrated that the PR interval is longer in men and in older age (Magnani *et al.* 2010). It can be shortened due to sympathetic overdrive and prolonged in vagal predominance. The PR interval can be abnormal (shorter or longer) in different pathological situations: shorter, especially in pre-excitation syndromes (see Figure 12.2), and in some active arrhythmias (Chapter 15), and longer in different types of AV block (see Figures 17.11 and 17.12).

The PR segment is the distance between the end of P wave and QRS. It is normally isoelectric, but in sympathetic overdrive, it may be seen as downsloping (Figures 7.6

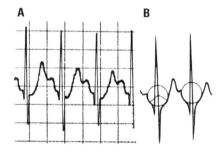

Figure 7.6 (A) A typical example of sympathetic overdrive. ECG of a 22-year-old male obtained with Holter continuous recording method during a parachute jump. (B) Drawing of the tracing that shows how the PR and ST segments form the arch of a circumference with its center located in the lower third of the R downstroke.

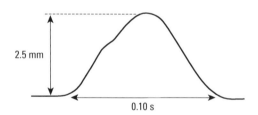

Figure 7.5 Procedure for measuring height and width of the P wave.

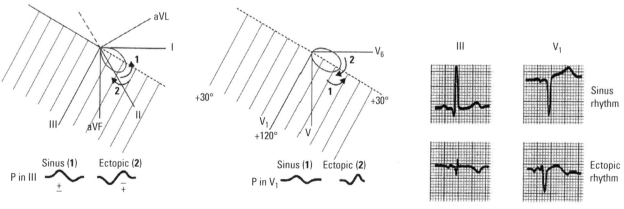

Figure 7.7 According to loop rotation (counterclockwise in the FP and HP in the case of sinus rhythm and clockwise in the case of ectopic rhythm), the P wave morphology in III and V1 varies.

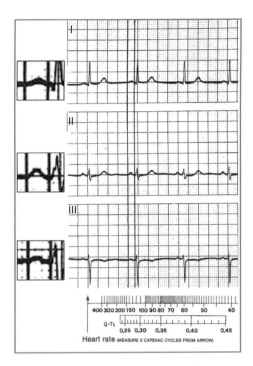

Figure 7.8 Measurement of heart rate, PR interval, and QT interval. Heart rate. The arrow is at the onset of a QRS complex. From the arrow, two cardiac cycles are measured. This distance correlates on the ruler with the heart rate, in this case 60 bpm. PR interval. The true PR interval is the distance between the first inscription of P wave and QRS complex in any lead. In this case (see solid lines), this happens in lead III but not in I and II.

and 7.8). It may also have an abnormal configuration (upsloping, or more often, downsloping) in pericarditis or atrial infarction (Figure 7.5, see also Figures 9.33, 9.35, and 19.4).

To measure the exact PR interval, it is best to utilize a device with at least three channels. The true PR interval is obtained by measuring from the onset of the P wave to the onset of the QRS complex in any of the three leads (see Figure 7.8).

QT interval (Figure 7.8) (Malik and Camm 2004; Bayés de Luna 2019; Goldenberg et al. 2008; Anttonen et al. 2009) (see also Chapters 19, 21, and 24)

The QT interval represents the sum of depolarization (QRS complex) and repolarization (ST segment and T wave). Often, particularly in the presence of a flat T wave or a U wave, it is difficult to measure the QT interval properly. It is commonly accepted that this measurement should be performed using a consistent method to ensure that equivalent measurements are taken when the QT interval is studied sequentially. The most suitable method entails considering the end of repolarization at a point

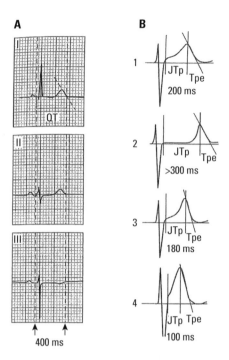

Figure 7.9 Method for measuring QT interval. The normal QT is usually less than half the RR interval. See examples of normal QT (1), long QT (2), and short QT (3 and 4). JTp = Jpoint-T peak. Tpe = T peak-end.

Table 7.3 QTc prolongation in different age groups, based on the Bazett formula: Values within the normal interval, borderline values, and altered values.

Value	1–15 years old	Adult men	Adult women
Normal	<440 ms	<430 ms	<450 ms
Borderline	440–460 ms	430–450 ms	450–470 ms
Altered (prolonged)	>460 ms	>450 ms	>470 ms

where the tangent line following the descendent slope of the T wave crosses the isoelectric line, as seen in Figure 7.9. This figure also shows how to measure the QT interval in special situations (see Figure 7.9). Table 7.3 shows the normal range of QT intervals for various ages and gender groups.

It is necessary to correct the QT interval for heart rate (QTc). The QT is clearly long when it is greater than half the RR distance. Usually, the QTc is shorter than 440 ms (99th percentile is 470 ms for men and 480 ms for women). In clinical practice, QTc may be measured with a ruler (see Figure 7.8), and it is considered that its duration should not exceed approximately 10% of the corresponding value according to heart rate.

The time of day can influence the measurement as QT is longer in the evening and at night (Bexton *et al.* 1986; Morganroth *et al.* 1991), in addition to being longer in women than in men (Molnar *et al.* 1996).

A long QT interval may be related to an inherited heart disease (congenital long QT syndrome) (Moss and Kass 2005) (see Figure 21.10) and can be acquired in diseases such as heart failure and cardiac ischemia, in some electrolyte imbalances (especially hypokalemia), and after the intake of different drugs. It is considered that a drug should not increase the QTc by >30 ms and that a change of 60 ms may result in torsades de pointes (TdP) and sudden cardiac death. Nevertheless, TdP rarely occurs unless the QTc exceeds 500 ms (Bayés de Luna and Baranchuk 2017).

A short QT interval can be found in cases of early repolarization, digitalis effect, hypermagnesemia, acidosis, among other conditions, and, rarely, in some genetic disorders associated with sudden death (short QT syndrome). Usually, in the latter case, the QT is <300 ms and the T wave is peaked and tall, especially in V2–V3.

QRS complex

The study of a normal QRS complex encompasses: (i) its FP axis (ÂQRS); (ii) polarity, morphology, and voltage.

Axis of the QRS in the FP (ÂQRS)

This is commonly between 0° and 90°, more toward 0° in the horizontal heart and toward 90° in the vertical heart. Normal hearts do not present ÂQRS beyond −30° (at −30° the differential diagnosis with partial superoanterior hemiblock must be performed), or +110° (at > 90° the possibility of right ventricular enlargement or inferoposterior hemiblock must be excluded).

Polarity, morphology, and voltage

The morphology of the QRS complex according to the loop–hemifield correlation (see Figures 1.5 and 1.6), and the projection of QRS on different hemifields in the FP and HP in a heart without rotations (intermediate heart) can be seen in Figures 7.10 and 7.11.

• Normally the QRS width should be, at most, 0.10 s and the height of the R wave should not be greater than 25 mm in leads V5–V6, 20 mm in lead I, and 15 mm in aVL, although exceptions may exist. Voltage is considered low when the sum of the QRS voltages in I, II, and III is less than 15 mm, or less than 5 mm in V1 or V6, 7 mm in V2 or V5, and 9 mm in V3 or V4.

• On the other hand, the amplitude of the Q wave should not usually be greater than 25% of the following R wave,

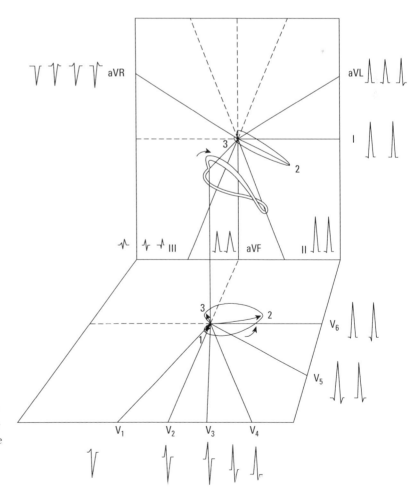

Figure 7.10 Projection of the QRS loop on the FP and HP in an intermediate heart, and morphology of the 12 ECG leads, as determined by whether the loop lies in the positive or negative hemifield of the different leads. In the case of vertical or horizontal heart, we can do the same.

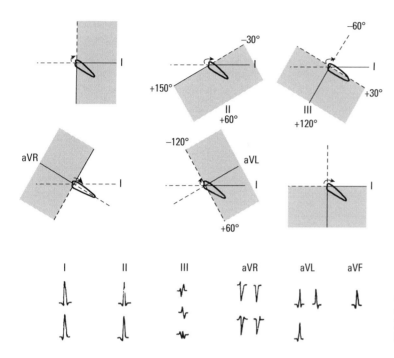

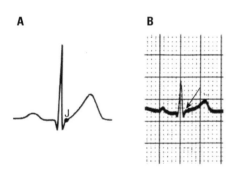

Figure 7.11 Different QRS morphologies in the six frontal plane leads, as determined by whether the QRS loop lies in the positive or negative hemifield of each lead (see text).

Figure 7.12 (A) Drawing showing the location of the J point. (B) The J point (arrow) in an ECG tracing.

although there are exceptions, particularly in III, aVL, and aVF, and it should be narrow (less than 0.04 s) and sharp.
• The normal values of intrinsic deflection time (IDT: time interval from the onset of QRS to the peak of R) in V5–V6 and in V1 are 0.045 s and 0.02–0.03 s, respectively. IDT may be somewhat higher in athletes and in the presence of vagal predominance.
• The ranges and mean values of the Q, R, and S wave voltages in 12 leads and for various ages are shown in Tables 7.4–7.6.

ST segment and T and U waves

ST segment

The ST segment is the distance between the end of the QRS (J point) and the onset of the T wave. Under normal conditions, this union is smooth and upsloping and usually short (Figure 7.12).

Normal variants:
• Sometimes, particularly in women and the elderly, the ST can be straight (see below and Figure 7.13C,D).
• The ST segment should be isoelectric, or only slightly (<0.5 mm) above or below the isoelectric line. However, the ST is often above the isoelectric line (1 or even 2 mm), especially in men and in V1–V2. Usually in these cases, the ST presents some convex inflexion with respect to the isoelectric line (Figure 7.13H).
• Especially in the presence of vagal predominance, the ST segment can present a convex elevation of, usually, 1–3 mm with respect to the isoelectric line, more commonly seen in V3–V6, and sometimes in the inferior lead. This pattern, named early repolarization (see Figure 7.14), is usually preceded by the J wave and normalizes with exercise (see Chapter 24). Recently, it has been observed that many patients with idiopathic ventricular fibrillation present this pattern with some special characteristics (Figure 7.15) (Haïssaguerre *et al.* 2008). However, from an epidemiological point of view, its presence only represents a very slight increase in the risk of sudden death (11 in 100 000 vs 4 in 100 000 in a control group) (Rosso *et al.* 2008).
• The rSr' in V1, often with a saddle-type pattern and with some ST changes, can be observed in V1 in some athletes and also in those with pectus excavatum or in a normal but more often lean individual when the V1 and V2 leads are located in a higher position (second intercostal space).

Table 7.4 Q wave voltage in millimeters in different leads and at different ages

Limb leads					Precordial leads				
Lead	Age	No. cases	Mean	Range	Lead	Age	No. cases	Mean	Range
I	24 hr	32	0.5	0.0–0.5	V_1	24 hr	41	0.0	0.0–0.0
	0–2 yr	72	0.7	0.0–2.0		0–2 yr	72	0.0	0.0–0.0
	3–5	72	0.1	0.0–1.0		3–5	72	0.0	0.0–0.0
	6–10	72	0.2	0.0–2.0		6–10	72	0.0	0.0–0.0
	12–16	68	0.1	0.0–3.0		12–16	49	0.0	0.0–0.0
	Adults	500	0.9	3.0–4.0		Adults	121	0.0	0.0–0.0
II	24 hr	32	1.5	0.0–5.0	V_2	24 hr	41	0.0	0.0–0.0
	0–2 yr	72	1.3	0.0–3.0		0–2 yr	72	0.0	0.0–0.0
	3–5	72	0.3	0.0–2.0		3–5	72	0.0	0.0–0.0
	6–10	72	0.5	0.0–3.0		6–10	72	0.0	0.0–0.0
	12–16	68	1.2	0.0–2.5		12–16	49	0.0	0.0–0.0
	Adults	500	1.1	0.0–4.0		Adults	121	0.0	0.0–0.0
III	24 hr	32	2.5	0.5–9.0	V_3	24 hr	41	0.0	0.0–0.0
	0–2 yr	72	1.6	0.0–4.0		0–2 yr	72	0.0	0.0–0.0
	3–5	72	1.4	0.0–3.0		3–5	72	0.0	0.0–0.0
	6–10	72	0.6	0.0–3.0		6–10	72	0.4	0.0–1.0
	12–16	68	1.6	0.0–5.0		12–16	49	0.0	0.0–0.7
	Adults	500	1.4	0.0–6.0		Adults	121	0.0	0.0–0.5
aVR	24 hr	32	2.4	0.0–4.0	V_4	24 hr	41	1.3	0.0–1.5
	0–2 yr	16	1.6	0.0–10.5		0–2 yr	72	0.1	0.0–1.0
	2–4	16	2.9	0.0–10.0		3–5	72	0.3	0.0–2.5
	5–10	53	1.4	0.0–10.0		6–10	72	0.2	0.0–1.5
	11–14	15	1.0	0.0–8.0		10–15	49	0.1	0.0–2.4
	Adults	151	2.0	0.0–8.0		Adults	121	0.1	0.8–1.6
aVL	24 hr	32	1.3	0.0–2.0	V_5	24 hr	41	2.2	0.0–5.5
	0–2 yr	16	0.1	0.0–0.5		0–2 yr	72	0.8	0.0–6.0
	2–4	16	0.2	0.0–1.0		3–5	72	0.8	0.0–3.0
	5–10	53	0.1	0.0–1.0		6–10	72	0.6	0.0–4.0
	11–14	15	0.1	0.0–0.5		10–15	49	0.3	0.0–2.1
	Adults	151	0.2	0.0–3.5		Adults	121	0.5	0.0–2.1
aVF	24 hr	32	1.8	0.0–6.0	V_6	24 hr	41	1.3	0.0–2.0
	0–2 yr	16	1.2	0.0–4.5		0–2 yr	72	1.1	0.0–3.0
	2–4	16	1.3	0.0–4.0		3–5	72	0.7	0.0–2.5
	5–10	53	0.5	0.0–3.0		6–10	72	0.4	0.0–3.0
	11–14	15	0.4	0.0–2.0		10–15	49	0.5	0.0–1.7
	Adults	151	0.5	0.0–3.0		Adults	121	0.4	0.8–2.7

(Adapted from Winsor 1956).

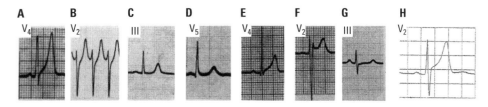

Figure 7.13 Different morphologies of atypical ST segment and T wave in the absence of heart disease. (A) Vagal overdrive and early repolarization in a 25-year-old man. (B) Sympathetic overdrive during a crisis of paroxysmal tachycardia in a 29-year-old woman. (C) Straightening of ST in a healthy 45-year-old woman. (D) Flattened ST and symmetric T in a 75-year-old man without heart disease. (E) Another illustration of early repolarization. (F) A 20-year-old man with *pectus excavatum*. Normal variant of ST segment ascent (saddle morphology). (G) Straightening of ST with prolongation of QT at the expense of the ST segment in a 22-year old male with hypocalcemia from renal insufficiency. (H) ST elevation even > 1 mm with mild convexity to isoelectric line that may be seen relatively often, especially in healthy young men.

Table 7.5 R wave amplitudes in millimeters in different leads and at different ages*

		Limb leads					Precordial leads		
Lead	Age	No. cases	Mean	Range	Lead	Age	No. cases	Mean	Range
I	24 hr	32	2.6	0.0–5.5	V₁	24 hr	41	16.7	3.0–23.0
	0–2 yr	72	4.2	0.0–10.0		0–2 yr	16	7.0	1.0–14.5
	3–5	72	5.0	2.0–10.0		2–4	16	7.5	1.0–14.0
	6–10	72	5.0	2.0–9.0		8–10	16	3.6	1.0–9.0
	10–15	49	4.8	1.3–11.4		11–14	15	5.1	0.5–15.5
	Adults	121	5.3	0.7–11.4		Adults	151	2.3	0.0–70
II	24 hr	32	5.5	1.0–2 1.0	V₂	24 hr	41	21.0	3.0–41.0
	0–2 yr	72	5.7	0.0–14.0		0–2 yr	16	13.0	4.5–22.0
	3–5	72	7.6	3.0–12.0		2–4	16	12.7	5.0–25.0
	6–10	72	7.2	3.0–13.0		8–10	16	7.8	2.0–14.0
	10–15	49	9.1	3.7–16.8		11–14	15	8.4	1.5–23.5
	Adults	121	7.1	1.8–16.8		Adults	151	5.9	0.0–16.0
III	24 hr	32	8.8	2.0–21.0	V₃	24 hr	41	20.0	14.0–26.0
	0–2 yr	72	5.6	1.0–11.0		0–2 yr	16	14.0	3.0–24.0
	3–5	72	5.6	2.0–10.0		2–4	16	13.4	6.0–25.0
	6–10	72	4.2	0.5–13.0		6–10	16	8.4	5.0–12.5
	10–15	49	6.0	0.7–15.8		11–14	15	9.2	3.0–22.0
	Adults	121	3.8	0.3–13.1		Adults	151	8.9	0.5–26.0
aVR	24 hr	32	3.7	0.0–9.0	V₄	24 hr	41	19.0	3.0–32.0
	0–2 yr	16	1.0	0.5–4.0		0–2 yr	16	20.0	3.5–35.0
	2–4	16	1.3	0.0–3.0		2–4	16	18.5	9.0–30.0
	8–10	16	1.2	0.5–6.0		8–10	16	14.9	4.0–30.0
	11–14	15	1.2	0.5–8.0		11–14	15	17.2	7.0–28.0
	Adults	151	0.8	0.0–5.0		Adults	151	14.2	4.0–27.0
aVL	24 hr	32	2.1	1.0–6.0	V₅	24 hr	41	12.0	4.5–21.0
	0–2 yr	16	4.0	0.5–8.0		0–2 yr	16	16.0	2.5–25.0
	2–4	16	3.1	0.5–7.0		2–4	16	18.4	10.0–26.0
	8–10	16	1.2	0.5–8.8		8–10	16	17.4	6.0–28.0
	11–14	15	1.6	0.5–6.0		11–14	15	16.4	6.0–29.0
	Adults	151	2.1	0.0–10.0		Adults	151	12.1	4.0–26.0
aVF	24 hr	32	6.6	2.0–20.0	V₆	24 hr	41	4.5	0.0–11.0
	0–2 yr	16	8.8	0.5–16.0		0–2 yr	16	12.0	2.0–20.0
	2–4	16	9.5	0.5–19.5		2–4	16	14.6	8.0–23.0
	8–10	16	8.5	3.5–14.0		8–10	16	12.5	6.0–19.1
	11–14	15	10.5	5.0–21.0		11–14	15	13.5	4.0–25.0
	Adults	151	1.3	0.0–20.0		Adults	151	9.2	4.0–22.0

* Adapted from American Heart Association (1956).
(Adapted from Winsor 1956).

However, this pattern should be differentiated from other ECG patterns with rSr′ in V1, especially with type II Brugada pattern (see Figure 7.16 and Figures 21.15 and 21.17) (see Chapter 21).

Measurement of the ST segment shifts

The reference points to measure ST segment elevation or depression are TP (or UP) intervals before and after the ST segment of interest (Figure 7.17A). If these intervals are not at the same level (isoelectric), the PR interval of the same cycle is used as a reference level—baseline line (Figure 7.17A). The level of the ECG tracing at the onset of the QRS complex is used if the PR interval has a downsloping morphology. ST segment elevation is measured from the upper part of the isoelectric reference line to the upper part of the ST segment and depression is measured from the lower part of the reference line to the lower part of the ST segment (Figure 7.17C).

At times, with a normal resting ECG, an exercise ECG test is required to determine the possible existence of ischemic heart disease. The test response must be compared with the clinical data to reach a diagnosis of ischemic heart disease. An ST segment that departs from a descended J point but rapidly attains the isoelectric line (depressed, rapid-ascent ST segment represents a physiologic response by the ST segment ($Q_X/Q_T < 0.5$) (Figure 7.17B).

At other times with a normal basal ECG after the exercise ECG test, the depressed ST segment slowly crosses the isoelectric line or stays depressed and pulls the T wave down, both of which are abnormal responses (Figure 7.17C,D).

Table 7.6 S wave amplitudes in millimeters in different leads and at different ages*

Limb leads					Precordial leads				
Lead	Age	No. cases	Mean	Range	Lead	Age	No. cases	Mean	Range
I	24 hr	32	6.3	0.0–15.0	V$_1$	24 hr	41	10.0	0.0–28.0
	0–2 yr	72	3.9	0.0–7.0		0–2 yr	16	4.8	0.5–14.0
	2–5	72	2.5	0.0–6.0		2–4	16	8.8	3.0–16.0
	6–10	72	1.6	0.0–3.0		8–10	16	8.6	3.0–16.0
	10–15	49	1.8	0.0–6.8		11–14	15	11.6	0.0–20.0
	Adults	121	1.0	0.0–3.6		Adults	121	8.6	2.0–25.0
II	24 hr	32	3.2	0.0–7.0	V$_2$	24 hr	41	22.0	1.0–42.0
	0–2 yr	72	2.7	0.0–5.0		0–2 yr	16	9.3	0.5–21.0
	2–5	72	1.6	0.0–4.0		2–4	16	16.0	8.5–30.0
	6–10	72	1.4	0.0–3.5		8–10	16	16.8	8.0–30.0
	10–15	49	1.6	0.0–4.9		11–14	15	20.8	7.0–36.0
	Adults	121	1.2	0.0–4.9		Adults	151	12.7	0.0–29.0
III	24 hr	32	2.3	0.0–3.0	V$_3$	24 hr	41	26.4	0.0–39.0
	0–2 yr	72	1.1	0.0–3.5		0–2 yr	16	10.2	0.5–23.0
	2–5	72	0.8	0.0–5.0		2–4	16	12.7	3.5–21.0
	6–10	72	0.7	0.0–4.0		8–10	16	16.3	8.0–27.0
	10–15	49	0.9	0.0–5.3		11–14	15	14.8	1.0–30.0
	Adults	121	1.2	0.0–5.5		Adults	151	8.8	0.0–25.0
aVR	24 hr	32	3.9	0.0–9.5	V$_4$	24 hr	41	23.0	0.0–42.0
	0–2 yr	16	6.3	0.0–14.0		0–2 yr	16	10.2	2.0–22.0
	2–4	16	5.9	0.0–14.0		2–4	16	9.0	0.0–20.0
	8–10	16	4.9	0.0–10.0		8–10	16	11.2	4.0–17.0
	11–14	15	8.3	0.0–17.0		11–14	15	8.0	1.0–16.0
	Adults	151	4.3	0.0–13.0		Adults	151	5.2	0.0–20.0
aVL	24 hr	32	6.6	0.0–16.0	V$_5$	24 hr	41	12.0	1.5–30.0
	0–2 yr	16	3.4	0.0–7.0		0–2 yr	16	6.1	1.0–13.0
	2–4	16	2.7	0.0–6.0		2–4	16	4.4	0.0–11.0
	8–10	16	3.2	0.0–7.0		8–10	16	5.7	0.5–12.0
	11–14	15	3.1	0.0–9.0		11–14	15	3.7	0.5–8.0
	Adults	151	0.4	0.0–18.0		Adults	151	1.5	0.0–6.0
aVF	24 hr	32	3.0	0.0–7.5	V$_6$	24 hr	41	4.5	0.0–13.0
	0–2 yr	16	0.7	0.0–2.5		0–2 yr	16	2.5	0.0–7.5
	2–4	16	2.1	0.0–14.0		2–4	16	1.6	0.5–5.0
	8–10	16	0.7	0.0–2.0		8–10	16	1.1	0.0–4.0
	11–14	15	0.8	0.0–2.5		11–14	15	0.9	0.0–2.0
	Adults	151	0.2	0.0–8.0		Adults	151	0.6	0.0–7.0

* Adapted from American Heart Association (1956).
(Adapted from Winsor 1956).

T wave

The study of the normal T wave encompasses: (i) its frontal plane axis, (ii) polarity and morphology, and (iii) voltage.

Axis on the frontal plane (ÂT)

Normal values range from 0° to +70°, with the limits of normality at +80° and –40°. The ÂT situated more to the left appears in sympathetic overdrive and in obese subjects with left ÂQRS. However, even in very lean normal individuals with right ÂQRS, a negative but not deep T wave can be seen in III and aVF, and a flattened T can be seen in lead II.

QRS/T spatial angle

A widened spatial QRS/T angle measured by VCG is pathological and a marker of bad outcome (Kardys et al. 2003)

(see Chapter 3). This can be synthesized from the ECG (Rautaharju et al. 2007). However, it is probable that the measurement of QRS/T angle in FP by surface ECG may have similar values (see Chapter 3).

Normal polarity: Morphology and voltage

Normal T wave morphology depends on the relationship between the ventricular repolarization loop and the positive or negative hemifields of the different leads (Figure 7.18). Figure 7.18 shows the T loop and its projection on FP and HP and Table 7.7 gives the range and mean values of the normal T wave voltage in 12 leads and for different ages.

Although typically the normal T wave has a slow ascent and more rapid descent (see Figure 7.12), this morphology is frequently absent in normal cases. Relatively often, especially in women and older persons with no

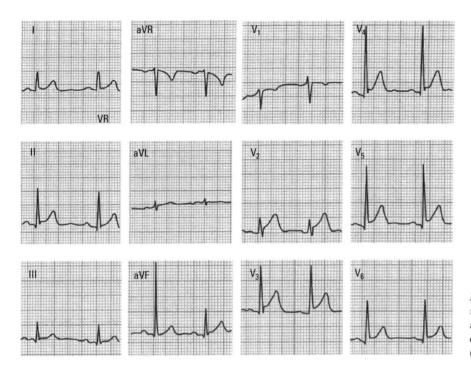

Figure 7.14 Typical ECG of early repolarization of benign type. See the ascent of the J point and ST elevation, especially in mid/left precordial leads (see text).

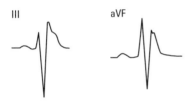

Figure 7.15 Drawing of ECG pattern of early repolarization seen especially in inferior leads with J point ≥ 2 mm. This corresponds to potentially malign pattern.

evidence of heart disease, the T wave shows a symmetric inscription (see Figure 7.13C,D). However, this pattern may also be seen in the early phase of left ventricular hypertrophy and is consistent with suspected ischemia under some specific clinical conditions (see Chapters 13 and 20).

In the frontal plane, the T wave usually follows, with some, usually small, differences, the direction of the QRS. **In I**, the T wave should be positive. In the vertical heart in aVL, the QRS is of low voltage and in this case, the T wave is usually negative. The T wave is also positive in II; sometimes is of low voltage or even flattened. **In III, aVF, and aVL**, it can be positive, flattened, or negative, according to the direction of the T loop. In aVR, it is always negative. A significant difference with ÂQRS direction is abnormal (see before).

In the horizontal plane, it is usually located more forward than the QRS (compare Figures 7.10 and 7.18).

Because of this, in V1, the T wave is flattened, slightly negative or slightly positive. However, a deep negative T wave in V1 is rarely seen in normal subjects and it is even rarer in V1–V2. It is more frequent in women and Black people. An absolutely positive and symmetric T wave in V1 is not common in normal individuals; if this appears, especially if it is peaked, and precordial pain is present, the possibility of acute ischemia must be ruled out (Figure 13.10). In V2, T is generally positive, but it can be flattened or even negative but usually asymmetrical, in some middle-aged women and Black people with no apparent heart disease. In both cases, exceptionally, without any known cause, it can be negative in other precordial leads. From V3 to V6, T should be positive.

The voltage of the T wave is lower and the duration is longer than that of the QRS complex because ventricular repolarization is slower than depolarization.

The height of the T wave does not usually exceed 6 mm in the frontal leads or 10 mm in the left precordial leads. Occasionally, the T waves are very high (up to 16–18 mm in V2–V4, especially in vagal overdrive, while in sympathetic overdrive coinciding with tachycardia, the voltage of the T wave is usually lower. In any case, T is taller in the leads that face the ÂT.

A very high T wave can be a variant of normality, but abnormalities such as hyperkalemia, subendocardial ischemia, some kinds of left ventricular enlargement, alcoholism, etc., should be excluded (Figures 13.10 and 13.15).

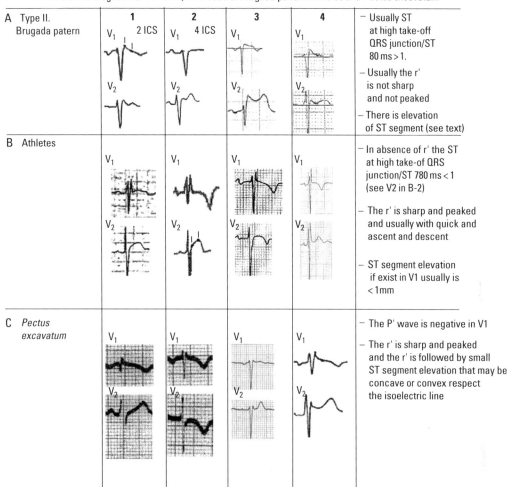

Figure 7.16 See the diagnostic differential features of ECG patterns of (A) type II Brugada, (B) athletes, and (C) *pectus excavatum* (see Table 21.9).

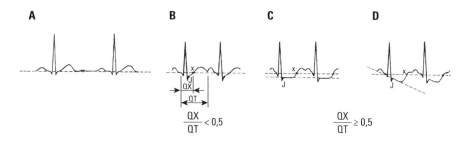

Figure 7.17 (A) Normal resting ECG. (B) A normal ECG response to exercise. Although the J point is depressed, the X point is rapidly reached so that $Q_X/Q_T < 0.5$. In (C) and (D) two types of abnormal response can be seen.

U wave

The U wave coincides with the supernormal excitation phase in the cardiac cycle. **The electrophysiological origin of the U wave is not clear**, although there are some experimental studies that suggest it is caused by repolarization of the Purkinje fibers or afterpotentials (Surawicz 1998, 2008). Recently, it has been postulated (Postema *et al.* 2009) that an increase or decrease in U wave amplitude is modulated by either an increase or decrease of the inward rectifier repolarizing current I_{k1} occurring in the terminal part of the action potential.

The U wave **is a small, low-voltage wave** that, when it is recorded, **follows the T wave** and normally has the same polarity. If not, it is always pathologic. It is best recorded in V3 and V4 and in elderly people

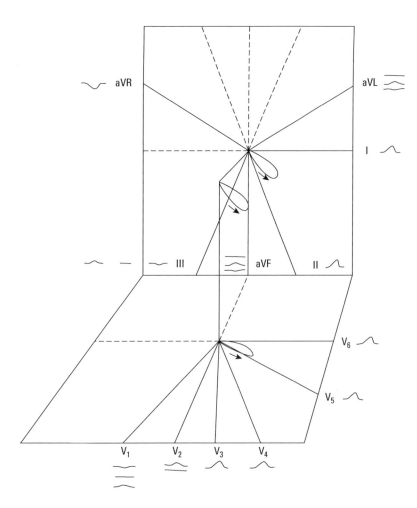

Figure 7.18 T loop and its projection on FP and HP. Observe the corresponding morphologies determined by the projection of the T loop in the positive or negative lead hemifields.

(Figure 7.19). Hypokalemia and bradycardia cause it to be more evident. Its voltage can also increase with digitalis and quinidine administration, hypercalcemia, etc.

A negative U wave in the precordial leads facing the left ventricle is a highly specific sign of heart disease, appearing especially in left ventricular hypertrophy and/or related to ischemia (see Figures 10.20, 20.15, and 20.26). Characteristically, the presence of negative U waves in right precordial leads in the presence of chest pain is highly suggestive of left anterior descending coronary artery occlusion.

Abnormalities of repolarization

The abnormalities of repolarization encompass not only the U wave alterations already mentioned, but especially the T wave disturbances and the abnormal deviations of the ST segment. These abnormalities may be of **primary origin or secondary to changes of depolarization** (Bayés de Luna 2012).

Primary T wave disturbances

These are changes of normal T wave such as T wave higher than normal or flat/negative often with prolonged QT interval. These changes are due to delayed transmembrane action potential (TAP) in some regions of the heart or some layers of the left ventricle, that appear sometimes transiently, as a result of acute subendocardial ischemia (tall and symmetric T waves) or more frequently due to transmural post-ischemic changes (deep negative T waves in V1–V4). The symmetric and positive T wave in V1–V2 in the chronic phase of lateral MI may be a mirror pattern of post-ischemic lateral involvement and not a sign of acute ischemia. Other causes, such as ischemic stroke, electrolyte imbalance, etc., may also explain changes in T wave polarity (Chapters 13 and 20).

Primary ST deviations

Primary ST deviations include the abnormal elevations and depressions of ST. They are due to changes of TAP in some regions of the heart or in some layers of the left ventricle as a consequence of acute ischemia or other causes (see changes in ST segment) (see Chapter 13).

Table 7.7 T wave amplitudes in millimeters in different leads and at different ages*

Limb leads					Precordial leads				
Lead	Age	No. cases	Mean	Range	Lead	Age	No. cases	Mean	Range
I	24 hr	41	0.3	2.0 to 3.0	V₁	24 hr	32	1,3	−4.0 to 6.0
	0–2 yr	72	2.6	0.5 to 5.0		0–2 yr	16	−2.3	−4.5 to −0.5
	3–5	72	1.7	0.0 to 4.0		2–4	16	−2.2	−5.5 to −1.0
	6–10	72	2.0	0.5 to 4.0		8–10	16	−1.7	−3.0 to 1.5
	10–15	49	2.6	1.1 to 6.8		11–14	15	−1.3	−3.5 to 0.2
	Adults	500	3.0	1.0–5.0		Adults	151	0.2	−4.0 to 4.0
II	24 hr	41	1.2	0.0 to 3.0	V₂	24 hr	32	1.3	−7.5 to 9.0
	0–2 yr	72	2.4	1.0 to 4.0		0–2 yr	16	−2.4	−6.0 to −0.4
	3–5	72	1.8	0.5 to 4.0		2–4	16	−2.6	−7.0 to −3.0
	6–10	72	2.1	0.5 to 5.0		8–10	16	0.0	−3.5 to 5.0
	10–15	49	3.0	0.9 to 6.5		11–14	15	0.7	−1.5 to 3.5
	Adults	500	3.8	1.0 to 6.5		Adults	151	5.5	3.0 to 18.0
III	24 hr	41	1.0	−1.0 to 3.0	V₃	24 hr	32	−0.4	−7.0 to 4.0
	0–2 yr	72	0.2	0.0 to 3.0		0–2 yr	16	−0.7	−5.0 to 4.5
	3–5	72	0.2	0.0 to 1.5		2–4	16	−0.7	−5.0 to −5.0
	6–10	72	0.1	0.0 to 1.0		8–10	16	1.8	−2.0 to 4.5
	10–15	49	0.4	−1.9 to 3.1		11–14	115	1.7	0.0 to 5.0
	Adults	500	0.8	−1.0 to 3.4		Adults	151	5.4	−2.0 to 16.0
aVR	24 hr	41	−0.4	−3.0 to 2.0	V₄	24 hr	32	−0.6	−7.0 to 3.0
	0–2 yr	16	−2.0	−3.0 to −0.5		0–2 yr	16	1.7	−2.5 to 5.0
	2–4	16	−2.5	−5.0 to −1.5		2–4	16	2.4	0.0 to 11.0
	8–10	16	−2.0	−3.5 to −0.2		8–10	16	3.2	0.0 to 9.0
	11–14	15	−2.2	−4.0 to −1.5		11–14	15	3.3	0.0 −7.0
	Adults	151	−2.3	−5.0 to 1.5		Adults	151	4.8	0.0 to 17.0
aVL	24 hr	41	0.1	−1.5 to 2.0	V₅	24 hr	32	1.3	−4.0 to 5.0
	0–2 yr	16	0.7	−0.5 to 2.0		0–2 yr	16	2.6	1.2 to 5.0
	2–4	16	1.4	−0.5 to 3.0		2–4	16	3.4	0.0 to 7.0
	8–10	16	0.7	−1.0 to 2.5		8–10	16	4.1	0.5 to 11.0
	11–14	15	0.8	0.5 to 2.0		11–14	15	3.1	1.0 to 5.0
	Adults	151	0.5	−4.0 to 6.0		Adults	151	3.4	0.0 to 9.0
aVF	24 hr	41	0.9	−1.0 to 3.0	V₆	24 hr	32	1.2	−3.0 to 6.0
	0–2 yr	16	0.6	0.8 to 3.5		0–2 yr	16	2.2	0.5 to 4.0
	2–4	16	1.8	−0.2 to 4.0		2–4	16	3.2	1.5 to 5.0
	8–10	16	1.4	−0.2 to 3.0		8–10	16	3.1	0.0 to 4.18
	11–14	15	1.3	0.0 to 3.5		11–14	15	2.2	1.0 to 4.0
	Adults	151	1.7	−0.5 to 5.0		Adults	151	2.4	−0.5 to 5.0

* Adapted from American Heart Association (1956).
(Adapted from Winsor 1956).

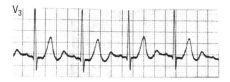

Figure 7.19 Healthy 70-year-old male (my father). Observe the prominent U wave in V3.

Secondary abnormalities of repolarization

Secondary changes encompass ST depression and/or asymmetric negative T wave and are due to changes in shape and duration of TAP of the ventricles secondary to conduction delays (bundle branch block) (see Chapter 11)

and/or ventricular hypertrophy (strain pattern) (Bacharova *et al*. 2010) (see Chapters 10 and 22).

Mixed pattern (primary and secondary)

Sometimes a mixed pattern (primary and secondary) may be seen (Figure 10.28C,D) (see Chapter 10).

All changes in the normal morphology of the T wave and the abnormal deviations of the ST segment secondary to ischemic heart disease or present in other heart diseases or situations will be discussed later in Chapters 10–13 and 20 22.

Calculation of the electrical axis

Mean electrical axis of depolarization and repolarization is the name given to the resultant vector of the forces generated by these processes. Calculation of the electrical axis of the heart is very valuable in clinical practice, as we will see throughout this book. We can measure the mean electrical axis of atrial depolarization, ÂP, and those of ventricular depolarization and repolarization, ÂQRS and ÂT. Although the direction of these three axes does not correspond exactly with the direction of the maximum vector of the P, QRS, and T loops recorded by the vectorcardiogram, in practice and for didactic purposes, we will assume that this exact correlation exists. In daily practice, we only calculate the electrical axes of P, QRS, and T in the frontal plane (I, II, III, aVR, aVL, and aVF).

Recently, measurement of the spatial QRS/T angle has been considered of interest because it may be a marker of bad prognosis (Kardys *et al.* 2003) (see Chapter 1). In clinical practice, checking the angle between ÂQRS and ÂT in FP has probably similar value.

Here, we refer exclusively to the calculation of the ÂQRS although the same procedure is used to obtain ÂP and ÂT. To calculate the ÂQRS, we must see the ECG morphologies and determine where the electrical forces are directed, as reflected by their projection on the positive or negative side of the different leads, that is, whether they lie in the positive or negative lead hemifields. We will consider first the morphology of the QRS complex with the ÂQRS at +60° and then axis deviations to the right and to the left.

ÂQRS at +60° (Figure 7.20)

If we consider a ventricular depolarization loop with the initial and terminal small vectors directed upward and to the right, and the maximum vector pointing to +60°, it is understandable that the QRS complex is fundamentally positive in I, II, and III, although with small initial and terminal negativities. In this case, ÂQRS is directed toward +60° in spite of these small negative deflections. For this reason, we will forget the small negative initial and final deflections while we calculate the mean electrical cardiac axis.

When the ÂQRS is located at +60°, which is common in many normal individuals, the QRS is mainly positive in I, II, and III with the maximum positivity in II. This is due to the fact that the projection of ÂQRS on the I, II, and III leads of Einthoven's triangle and the orientation of the axis with respect to the positive and negative hemifields of these leads are the origin of positive QRS morphologies in the three leads, but with the QRS complex having the highest voltage in lead II. This is because the vectorcardiographic loop with its corresponding main vector of ÂQRS at +60° lies mostly in the positive hemifields of I, II, and III, but has its greatest positive projection on the positive hemifield of II. This is necessarily so to satisfy Einthoven's law: II = I+III.

Considering the ECG–VCG correlation, when there are predominantly positive QRS complexes in I, II, and III, with the maximum positivity in II (ÂQRS +60°), the maximum vector of the QRS vectorcardiographic loop is directed at about +60°.

Applying the hemifield theory, when ÂQRS is at +60°, we can deduce the QRS morphology of the unipolar limb leads (aVR, aVL, and aVF). In effect, aVR has a negative morphology V because ÂQRS located at +60° falls in the negative hemifield of aVR, and is on the limit between the positive and negative hemifields of aVL. Since the loop rotates clockwise in aVL, the isodiphasism in this lead is of the V type. aVF has a positive morphology because ÂQRS at +60° remains in the positive aVF hemifield. To summarize, when ÂQRS is at +60°:

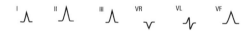

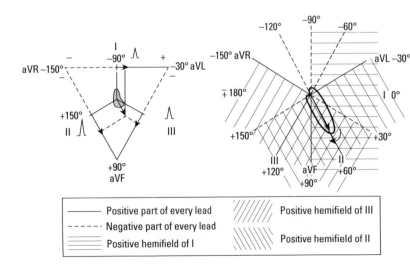

Figure 7.20 Calculation of the ÂQRS: When this is situated at +60°, the projection on I, II, and III and the situation in the positive and negative hemifields of these leads originate in I, II, and III, the morphology shown at the left of the figure.

Changes of ÂQRS to the right and to the left of +60°

As the orientation of ÂQRS on the frontal plane changes, its projection on the three sides of Einthoven's triangle and its location in the respective hemifields of the different leads varies, conditioning reciprocal changes in QRS morphology.

Applying the hemifield theory and evaluating the projection of ÂQRS on the three sides of Einthoven's triangle, I, II, and III, as was done with ÂQRS at +60°, it can be seen (Figure 7.21) how the morphology of QRS changes with the ÂQRS deviation to the right or to the left. It is recommended that the reader carry out this exercise for the entire circumference at 30° intervals, following the example of Figure 7.20 and drawing the result. As an example, we consider an ÂQRS deviated to the right and ÂQRS deviated to the left.

ÂQRS at +90°

Projection on Einthoven's triangle leads is the origin of an isodiphasic QRS complex in I and positive QRS complexes in II and III (Figure 7.22A).

The QRS loop is situated on the limit between the positive and negative hemifields of lead I and rotates clockwise; therefore, the resulting complex is isodiphasic and of the type $\wedge\!\!\!\!\vee$. The loop is projected on the positive hemifields of II and III equally, in other words, the maximum loop vector is equidistant from both directions, so the positivity is equal in II and III. This loop is situated in the positive VF hemifield and the negative aVR and aVL hemifields, resulting in

a positive complex in aVF and negative complexes in aVR and aVL. In summary, with the ÂQRS at +90°:

ÂQRS at 0°

The projection on the Einthoven triangle leads is reflected in positive QRS complexes in I and II (more in I) and negative in III, but the resulting negative complex is of low voltage because it is near the line separating the positive and negative hemifields of III (it begins at +30°) (Figure 7.23).

The loop lies in the positive aVL hemifield and the negative aVR hemifield, producing positive and negative QRS complexes in aVL and aVR, respectively. In aVF, the QRS complex is isodiphasic (maximum loop vector at 0°). If it rotates counterclockwise, as is most probable, it will be of the + type $\vee$:

In summary, with the ÂQRS at 0°:

ÂQRS calculation in clinical practice

The electrical axis of the heart is normally calculated by studying the morphologies in leads I, II, and III, as explained, but the calculation is corrected, or quality controlled, using the unipolar limb leads (see below).

As shown above, from +60°, characterized by positive QRS complexes in the three bipolar leads, deviation of the axis to the left or right produces changes in morphology that express the different situation of ÂQRS in the respective lead hemifields. These modifications are as follows: at +60°, the QRS complex is positive in I, II, and III and at −120°, it is negative in the same leads. The changes in morphology (from positive to isodiphasic or from isodiphasic to negative, or the reverse) occur at 30° intervals. They consist of progressive loss of positive area, beginning at III or I (it depends if the change goes to the left or to the right), in such a way that for every 60° a positive complex becomes negative and for every 30° a positive complex becomes isodiphasic, or one isodiphasic negative until the QRS complexes in I, II, and III are all negative at −120°. **All this can be summarized as follows.**

• **As the ÂQRS moves to the left** from +60° to +30°, until it finally reaches −120°, the QRS complexes gradually become negative beginning with III, going from positive to isodiphasic and from isodiphasic to negative with each 30° progression (Figure 7.24B).

• **When the ÂQRS moves to the right** from +60° to +90°, etc., until −120°, the complexes become negative, although commencing at I and likewise passing from positive to isodiphasic and from isodiphasic to negative with each 30° change (Figure 7.24A).

In practice, we can therefore calculate the ÂQRS (or ÂP or ÂT), based on the I, II, and III morphologies, by

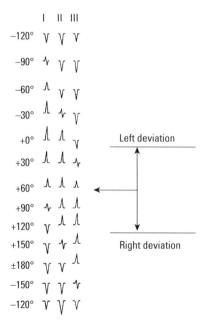

Figure 7.21 QRS morphologies at different ÂQRS situations.

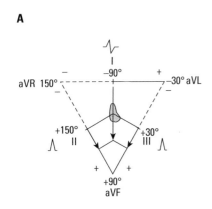

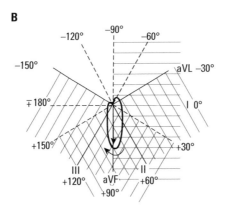

Figure 7.22 Morphologies of I, II, and III with ÂQRS at +90°.

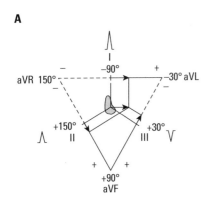

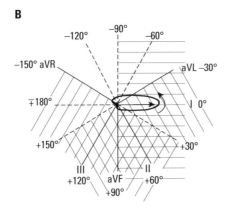

Figure 7.23 Morphologies of I, II, and III with ÂQRS at 0°.

adding or subtracting 30° in every advance from positive to isodiphasic or from isodiphasic to negative produced: adding when the change is initiated at I (in which case the morphology of I will be first altered than that of III) and subtracting when it is initiated from III (the morphology of III is then first modified than that of I).

This is how to calculate the ÂQRS at 30° intervals, but to obtain intermediate values, one proceeds as follows. If, for example, III is diphasic but more positive than negative, according to the degree of positivity, the ÂQRS value will be +50°, +40°, etc. Example:

$$\Lambda \quad \Lambda \quad \Lambda \quad + 50°$$
$$\Lambda \quad \Lambda \quad \Lambda \quad + 40°$$
$$\Lambda \quad \Lambda \quad \Lambda \quad + 30°$$

As mentioned above, the unipolar limb leads serve to calculate, adjust, or verify the calculations made of QRS in I, II, and III, For instance, if the QRS complexes in I, II, and III are positive, then ÂQRS is at +60°. However, if QRS is diphasic in aVL, with a slight preponderance of positivity, it means that ÂQRS is between +50° and +60°. Another example: if QRS is positive in I and II but negative in III,

the ÂQRS is around 0°; but if it is somewhat positive in aVF, the ÂQRS will be between 0° and +10°, whereas if it is slightly negative, the ÂQRS will be between 0° and −10°.

This is the system used in practice because it gives approximations of 5° to 10° and can be realized almost instantaneously. Figure 7.25 shows the QRS morphologies in the frontal plane leads with varying ÂQRS positions. There are more exact procedures to calculate the electrical axis of the heart on the frontal plane, but they are more complicated. As they are less useful, they will not be described here.

Figure 7.26 is an example of calculation of the ÂQRS, ÂP, and ÂT electrical axes of the heart (see legend).

Indeterminate electrical axis

The electrical axis of the heart cannot always be calculated. For instance, when there are isodiphasic complexes in various leads, as occurs in the SI, SII, and SIII morphology and in some cases of advanced right bundle branch block, the electrical forces do not have a predominant direction. Instead, the first and second parts of the complex are oriented opposing each other with respect to the center of the heart. In these cases, the global cardiac ÂQRS

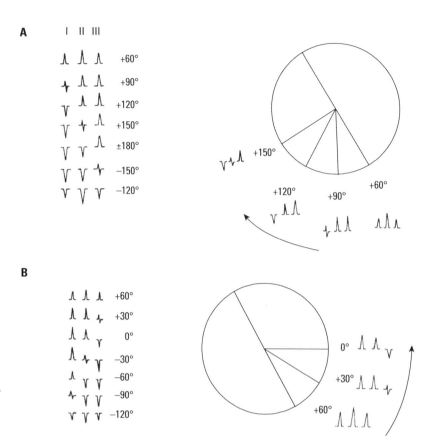

Figure 7.24 (A) When ÂQRS shifts to the right, QRS starts becoming negative from I (see text). (B) When ÂQRS deviates to the left, QRS starts becoming negative from III (see text).

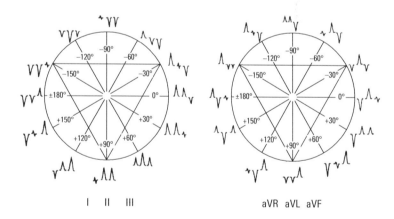

Figure 7.25 Morphology of the QRS in the six frontal plane leads for different ÂQRS positions.

cannot be calculated, although the electrical axes of the first and second parts can be, which is very useful in some cases of ventricular block (RBBB with superoanterior hemiblock) (Figure 7.27).

Rotations of the heart

The heart can rotate on three axes: Anteroposterior, longitudinal, and transversal (Figure 7.28).

Rotation on the anteroposterior axis

Rotation on this axis produces verticalization or horizontalization of the heart. The most striking changes, and the most useful for this diagnosis, are seen in aVL and aVF (frontal plane).

Vertical heart

Vertical heart is observed especially in people with very lean body habitus. The QRS loop is directed downward and rotates clockwise on the frontal plane, a large part of

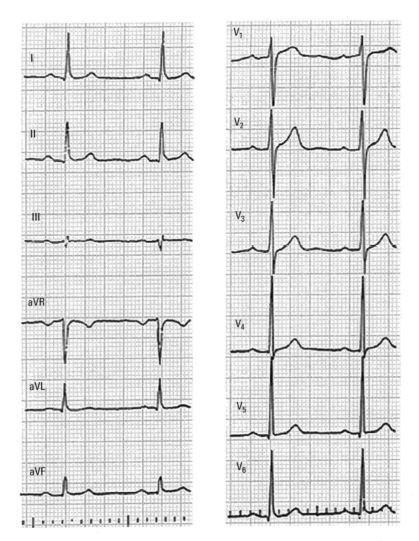

Figure 7.26 ECG of a 50-year-old male without evident heart disease and without any apparent rotation (ÂQRS = +30°, qRs in V4–V5, and qR in V6).

the loop lying on the positive aVF hemifield with its initiation generally in the negative hemifield. In aVL, the morphology is usually rS with low voltage P and T waves (Figures 7.29 and 7.30). When QS is seen in aVL, the P and T waves are usually negative or mildly positive because this morphology represents the recording of the left intraatrial potential. The morphology of HP leads may be different (Figures 7.29 and 7.30) according to the associated rotation (see later).

Horizontal heart

Horizontal heart is seen especially in obese subjects. The QRS loop is directed slightly upward until about −20°, but not more than −30°, and rotates counterclockwise on the frontal plane. It has a large part of the loop lying in the positive aVL hemifield, but with the initiation in the negative hemifield. This loop is relatively closed, in contrast to

the left superoanterior hemiblock, in which the loop is open and directed further upward. This explains the morphology of Figures 7.31 and 7.32.

Rotation on the longitudinal axis

Rotation on the longitudinal axis produces dextrorotation (clockwise) or levorotation (counterclockwise). The leads that best serve to diagnose this rotation are the precordials (horizontal plane).

Dextrorotation

In dextrorotation, the right ventricle is further forward than normal (clockwise rotation) and all the precordial leads record morphologies from this ventricle or transition morphologies between the right and left ventricles. The vectorcardiographic loop in the horizontal plane is inscribed counterclockwise, with the final part of the loop

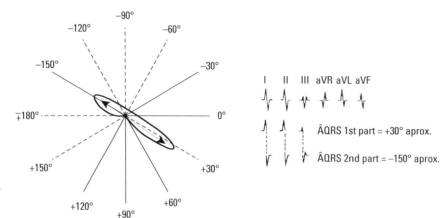

Figure 7.27 Procedure for calculating the electrical axis of the first and second parts of the QRS complex.

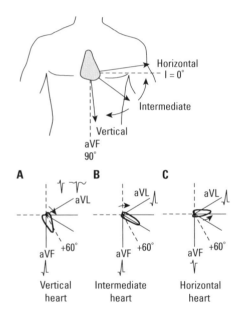

Figure 7.28 Above: ÂQRS direction in the vertical and horizontal heart. Below: QRS morphology in the vertical (A), intermediate (B), and horizontal heart (C).

directed backward and to the right (S until V6). The "q" wave in precordial leads is absent because the loop begins directly to the left (Figures 7.33 and 7.34).

Levorotation

When the heart turns counterclockwise, the left ventricle faces the intermediate precordial leads, or even the right precordial leads, explaining the Rs, qR, or solitary R morphology seen in V2 in cases of extreme levorotation. The vectorcardiographic loop in the horizontal plane rotates counterclockwise and is not as far backward as normal, and the last part of the loop is left, not right (Figures 7.33 and 7.35).

With two-dimensional echocardiography correlation, it has been demonstrated (Yanagisawa *et al.* 1981) that levorotation can be explained by aortic displacement without left ventricular enlargement necessarily being present.

The levorotation concept is useful for the explanation of the different normal variants of QRS morphology as high voltage in V2–V3. However, it is better not to use it for the interpretation of an abnormal ECG, because it is more likely that the high-voltage R morphology present

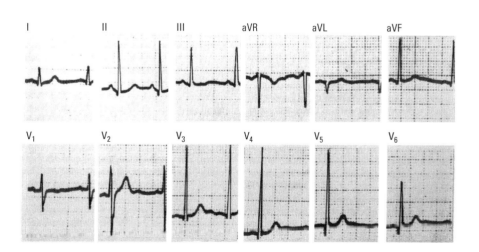

Figure 7.29 Healthy, 16-year-old, very asthenic male with vertical heart without dextrorotation.

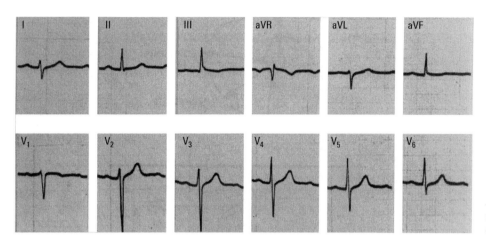

Figure 7.30 Healthy 26-year-old male with vertical and dextrorotated heart.

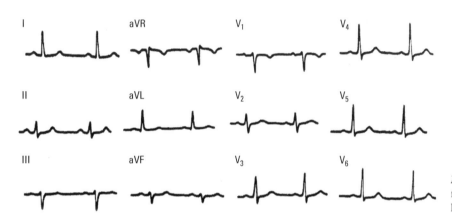

Figure 7.31 Very obese 40-year-old female with horizontal heart without levorotation.

in V2–V3 in some cases of left ventricular enlargement is due to septal hypertrophy or biventricular enlargement rather than to levorotation.

Rotation on the transversal axis

There are some doubts about the way this rotation is produced, as well as the utility and veracity of this clinical diagnosis. It is possible that in some normal or abnormal hearts the QI, QII, QIII and SI, SII, SIII morphologies described by Cabrera (1963) as caused by deviation of the cardiac apex forward or backward can be completely or partially explained by a certain degree of cardiac rotation on the transversal axis (Figure 7.36). However, these morphologies may be due to other causes. Specifically, it has been demonstrated (Bayés de Luna *et al.* 1982, 1987) that the SI, SII, SIII may be seen in normal individuals associated to conduction delay in the anterior subpulmonary area of the right ventricle, probably as a result of a variation in the right ventricular Purkinje distribution and it is also frequently seen in some cases of right ventricle enlargement (see Figure 7.27) (see Chapter 11).

Combined rotations

The normal heart is generally subject to more than one rotation. The following are the most common associations.

- Verticalization with dextrorotation, manifested by:
- VL $\bigvee$ VF $\bigwedge$ V$_6$ $\bigvee$
- With right ÂQRS (SI QIII) (see Figure 7.30).
- Horizontalization with levorotation, characterized by:
  VL $\bigwedge$ VF $\bigvee$ V$_2$–V$_4$ $\bigwedge$ or $\bigwedge$ or $\bigvee$ and V$_6$ $\bigwedge$
-
- With left ÂQRS (Figure 7.32).
- Sometimes, **horizontalization predominates over levorotation**, and in this situation the left ventricle is further above and to the left and not as far forward, the right ventricle remaining underneath and in front of the left ventricle. In these situations, the low left precordial leads can be facing the right ventricle or a transitional zone in spite of horizontalization, accounting for the persistence of S until V6. This association, horizontal heart with RS until V6, must be differentiated from hemiblock of the superoanterior division of the left bundle branch. In the latter case,

ÂQRS is beyond −30° in the frontal plane, justifying the fact that in II the R<S (compare Figure 7.31 with 11.36).

- Horizontalization with S in V6

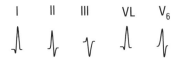

- Left superoanterior hemiblock

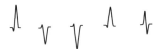

- **In vertical hearts**: (aVL, Λ
- aVL, and
- aVF) there is sometimes qR morphology in V3–V4, usually with a small S. This probably occurs because the heart is very vertical and the electrode placed at V3 is equivalent to V4–V5 (Figure 7.29).
- When there is **dextrorotation with horizontalization** (Figure 7.37), the QRS loop has a clockwise rotation on the frontal plane and a maximum vector between +10° and +30°, explaining the at times marked "q" wave in III and the S wave in I. This morphology can be confused with inferior infarction. Suggesting positional origins are: (i) a clean-cut and narrow "q" wave (less than 0.04 s), although it is relatively deep; (ii) absent or very small "q" wave in II and aVF; (iii) a negative, but asymmetric, T wave in III; (iv) minimal or non-existent initial "r" wave in aVR; (v) normality in the rest of the ECG.

Electrocardiographic variations with age

The most important characteristics of the ECG in healthy children and older persons, as compared with the adult ECG that we have been considering until now, are described below.

Infants, children, and adolescents (Figures 7.38–7.44)

The characteristics of ECGs in children and adolescents are as follows:
- Faster heart rate.
- Shorter PR interval.
- The ÂP is sometimes to the left, occasionally passing 0°, without this fact alone being abnormal.
- ÂQRS in the frontal plane moves to the right in the newborn. Over time, the QRS loop is first located to the left, and later to the back (Figure 7.38), so lead V6 acquires adult morphology before lead V1. The morphology in V6 is Λ
- when a morphology type
- still exists in V1. When the rS morphology appears in V1 in an infant, the possibility that the child is preterm should be excluded before considering left ventricular enlargement (see Figure 7.39).
- The intrinsicoid deflection time (time from the onset of QRS until the peak of R wave in V6) is normally up to 0.03 s in infants and up to 0.04 s in children.
- The heart is usually vertical or semi-vertical in early childhood, later becoming semi-vertical or intermediate.

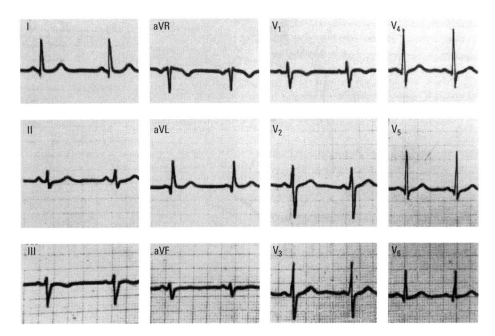

Figure 7.32 Obese 35-year old woman with horizontal and slightly levorotated heart.

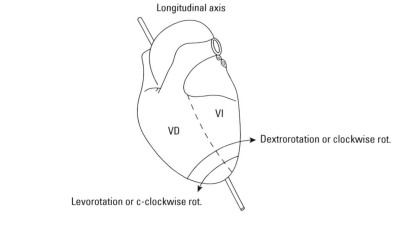

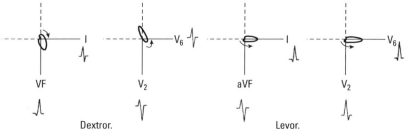

Figure 7.33 Above: Diagram to explain dextrorotation and levorotation. Below: The most common loops in the two cases and the VF, V2, and V6 morphologies.

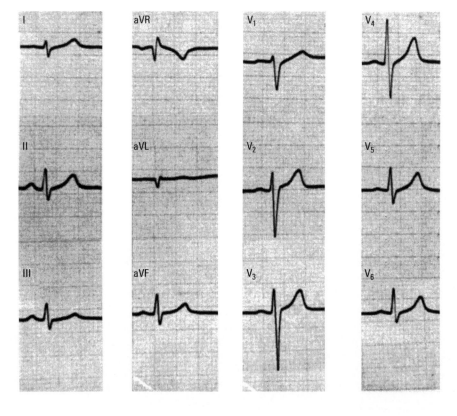

Figure 7.34 A 21-year-old asthenic male, without heart disease, with a dextrorotated heart and SI, SII, SIII morphology in the FP.

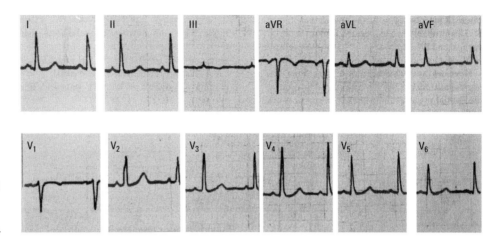

Figure 7.35 Healthy 40-year-old male with levorotated heart in horizontal plane (R in V2) but without rotations in frontal plane.

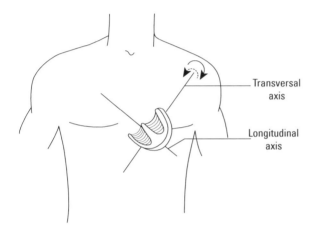

Figure 7.36 When cardiac rotation on the transversal axis exists, the apex is displaced forward or backward.

• There is rSr′ morphology in 5% of normal children (most commonly from 6 months up to 4 years). The normal r′ usually varies with respiration and is low voltage. However, the r′ seen in different heart diseases is sometimes also modified by respiration (Figure 7.40).

• The ECG in post-term newborns usually presents R in V1, even with qR (Figure 7.41). Often a dominant R wave of low amplitude remains forever. This may be a source of confusion with right ventricular enlargement and lateral myocardial infarction in adulthood.

• In contrast, the ECG in premature newborns may frequently present rS morphology in V1 (Figure 7.39). In Chapter 22, we will comment on the ECG findings that are consistent with suspected congenital heart diseases in the newborn.

• The presence of childhood repolarization morphology (Figure 7.42) manifests as an asymmetric, negative T in V1 or V1 and V2, and diphasic (−+) or humped T in the intermediate precordial leads. This morphology is caused by the T loop heading backward after the first week, and later gradually assuming a forward direction (at the end

of the first year, T is positive in V3 in 45% of the cases, and at 8 years, in 95%). At times, certain characteristics of so-called "childhood repolarization" persist until 15–20 years, especially in women. In summary, from the first day of life to the end of the first week, the T wave is positive in V1. At the end of the first week, the T loop goes backward and becomes somewhat more anterior with time (Figure 7.43).

• In some adolescents, there is a high-voltage R wave in the precordial leads (SV2+RV5 sums of up to 65mm) without echocardiographic evidence of left ventricular enlargement.

Elderly people

Several studies have found that in comparison to younger persons, the elderly present a higher incidence of the following abnormal findings:

• Arrhythmias (supraventricular and ventricular extrasystoles, atrial fibrillation, sick sinus syndrome, and AV block)

• Ventricular blocks

• Left and right ventricular enlargement morphologies

• Important repolarization alterations. In most cases, these alterations are not caused by age but by underlying heart disease.

In contrast, the following can be considered normal variants due to age:

• High prevalence of sinus bradycardia

• A somewhat longer PR interval than in the younger adult (normal upper limit: 0.22 s)

• The frontal ÂP frequently passing +60°, at least partly due to pulmonary emphysema

• The frontal ÂQRS deviated to the left (including further than 0°)

• Frequent dextrorotation ("S" wave until V6) because of the pulmonary emphysema often present in the aged

• Decrease in amplitude of all the deflections. The decrease in amplitude of initial anterior vectors accounts

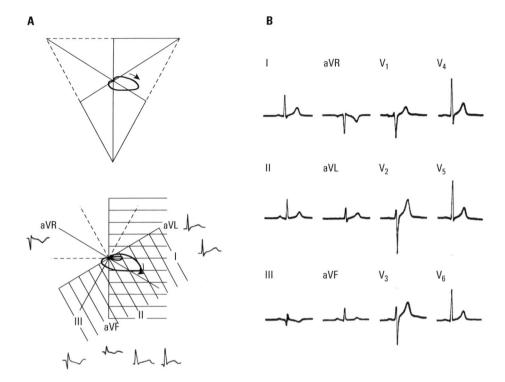

Figure 7.37 (A) QRS loop and ECG morphologies in a case with the heart dextorotated, and horizontalized. (B) An example of this type of rotation in a healthy, obese 35-year-old female.

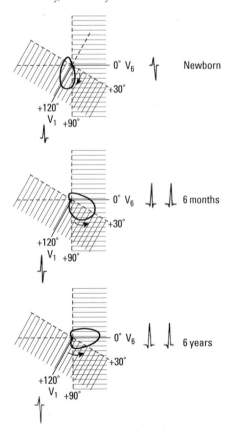

Figure 7.38 Changes in the direction of the QRS loop on the horizontal plane from birth to 6 years.

for the poor progression of "r" from V1 to V3. For this reason, diagnosis of septal infarction in the elderly is often very difficult. However, especially in some thin old women, a high-voltage R wave is seen in the left precordial leads, unaccompanied by echocardiographic evidence of left ventricular enlargement

• Reversal of the QRS–T angle in horizontal plane with respect to infants (Figure 7.44)

• Occasional depression of the ST segment greater than 0.5 mm with no evidence of heart disease.

Figure 7.45 shows the normal ECG of a man of 90 years of age (my grandfather Michel) that presents several characteristics of a normal ECG of an elderly person.

Martínez-Sellés *et al.* (2016) studied the ECG of centenarians, the final increased number of abnormal ECG patterns including P wave and QRS abnormalities and AF. The incidence of stroke and dementia was related with the presence of AF and/or A-IAB (Figure 7.46).

Other ECG variants

Gender

The presence of J point elevation > 0.1 mV (and sometimes even > 0.2 mV) in right precordial leads with ST segment of quick ascent and a little convex relative to the isoelectric line and asymmetric T wave is present more frequently in men than in women (Surawicz and Prikh 2003).

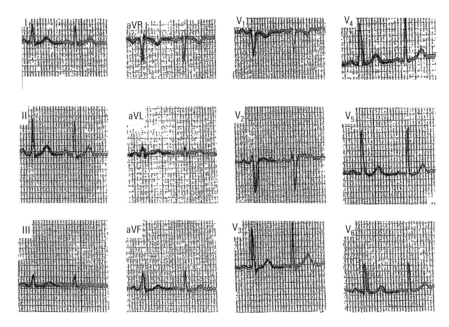

Figure 7.39 Infant preterm born. Observe the rS pattern in V1 (see text).

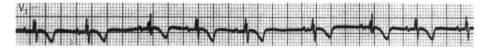

Figure 7.40 A normal 2-year-old child. Observe how the rSr′ morphology in V1 varies with respiration.

Middle-aged women often present a T wave with a symmetrical inscription in right precordials (see T wave). In fact, various sophisticated parameters of T wave morphology have gender-related differences in their prognostic predictive value for risk assessment (Porthan *et al.* 2009).

Other differences have also been found. For example, it has been shown that:

• the value of the PR interval is shorter in women than in men (Magnani *et al.* 2010);
• the duration of T wave alternans is longer in healthy women than in healthy men (Burattini *et al.* 2010); and
• women with and without left ventricular enlargement have lower QRS voltages and shorter QRS duration than men (Okin 2006).

Race

It has been demonstrated (Vitelli *et al.* 1998) that racial differences in ECG cannot be explained exclusively by variations in coronary artery disease risk factors. The healthy Black population compared to the healthy White population in the United States present QRS voltages of higher amplitude (greater Cornell voltage criteria for left ventricular enlargement), more ST/T wave changes, typically in V1–V2, and longer PR intervals. However, the QTc was shorter in African Americans.

Some other changes in comparisons between races have also been described.

Body habitus

Very lean subjects usually present ÂP and ÂQRS lifted to the right with higher voltage of QRS, especially in inferior and left lateral leads. Morbidly obese subjects usually present a low voltage of ECG (QRS and T wave), especially in precordial leads and therefore the voltage criteria for LVH are not useful (Domienk-Karlowicz *et al.* 2011). In general, the ÂQRS is shifted to the left as obesity increases (Frank *et al.* 1986). The same may be observed in anasarca (Madias *et al.* 2001).

Other factors

Transitory changes of repolarization induced by hyperventilation sometimes during exercise test, glucose and alcohol intake, etc., may be seen even in healthy young people (Figures 7.47 and 7.48).

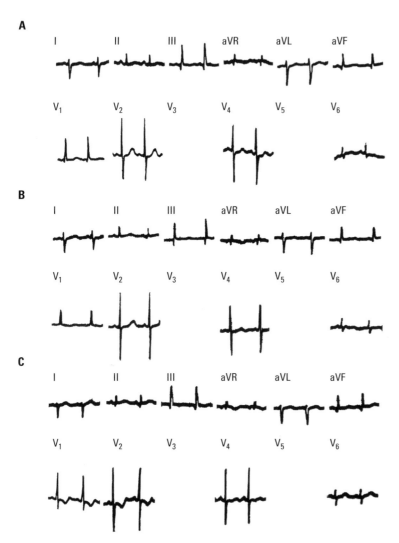

Figure 7.41 Infant, post-term born. Observe the ECG at birth (A), at one week (B) and at one month (C). The frontal plane has hardly varied, while in the horizontal plane, there was in V1 a qR morphology with positive T at birth (A), which later became at 1 month solitary R with flattened T (B) at 1 year Rs with negative T wave (C).

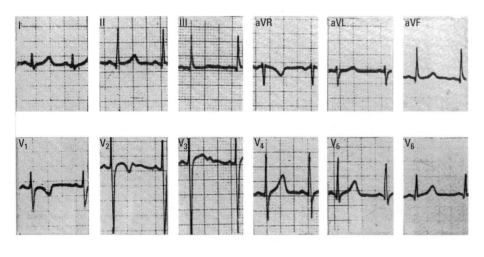

Figure 7.42 ECG typical of a healthy 2-year-old child (my daughter Miriam). Observe the infantile repolarization from V1 to V3 and how there is qRs in V5 and V6, with RS in V1. The VCG loop has moved to the left but still does not point very far backward.

Figure 7.43 Changes of T wave axis from newborn to adulthood.

Figure 7.44 Difference between ÂQRS and ÂT on the horizontal plane in infants and adults.

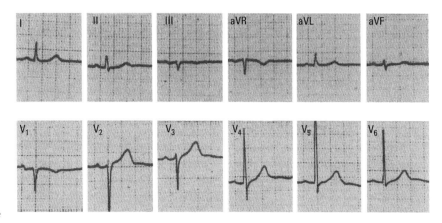

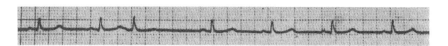

Figure 7.45 This ECG of a 90-year-old male is typical of the age with low voltage on the frontal plane and poor progression of the r from V1 to V3 and Rs in V6. In the lower strip, we can see an atrial premature beat, which is relatively common at this age.

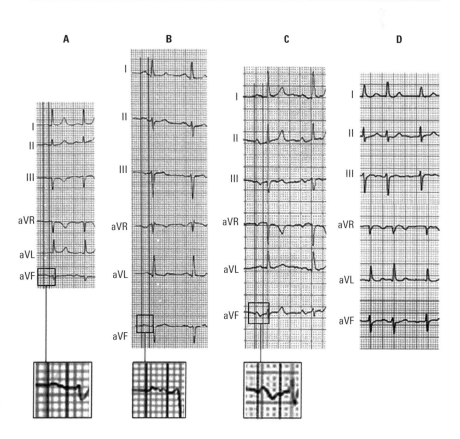

Figure 7.46 Examples of the 4 types of atrial activity: (A) normal P wave (P-wave duration <120 ms), (B) partial interatrial block (P-wave duration ≥120 ms), (C) advanced interatrial block (P-wave duration ≥120 ms plus/minus morphology in leads II, III, and aVF), and (D) atrial fibrillation.

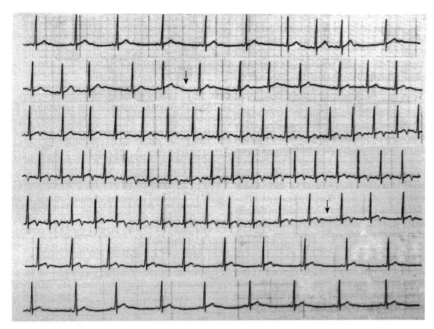

Figure 7.47 ECG of healthy 17-year-old male. Observe the modification produced during the hyperventilation test in the T wave, which goes from positive to negative, with a slight elevation in ST (arrows). It is now considered that these changes are non-specific, although connections recently established between hyperventilation and coronary spasm suggest that a review of the meaning of these changes is necessary.

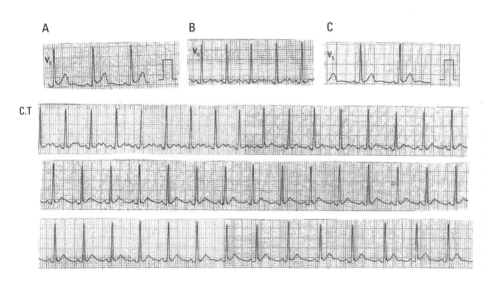

Figure 7.48 A 42-year-old man, healthy, with evident T wave changes during exercise (B). A and C correspond to ECG before and after 5 m. post exercise. Repolarization changes were suspected to be due to hyperventilation. C.T: continuous tracing during hyperventilation that induce the same changes that disappear in a few seconds.

References

Alexander B, Milden J, Hazim B, *et al.* New electrocardiographic score for the prediction of atrial fibrillation: the MVP ECG risk score (morphology-voltage-P wave duration). Ann Noninvasive Electrocardiol 2019;00:e12669.

Anttonen O, Junttila J, Maury F, *et al.* Differences in 12-lead ECG between symptomatic and asymptomatic subjects with short QT interval. Heart Rhythm 2009;6:267.

Bacharova L, Szathmany V, Mateasik A. Secondary and primary repolarization changes in left ventricular hypertrophy: a model study. J Electrocardiol 2010;43:624.

Baranchuk A. *Interatrial Block and Supraventricular Arrhythmias. Clinical Implications of Bayés' Syndrome.* Cardiotext Publishing, Minneapolis, Minnesota, USA, 2017.

Bayés de Luna A. *Clinical Electrocardiography: A Textbook.* Willey-Blackwell, 2012.

Bayés de Luna A. *The Morphology of the Electrocardiogram: The ESC Textbook of Cardiovascular Medicine.* In Camm AJ, Lüscher TF, Serruys PW (eds). 3rd edn. Oxford University Press, 2019.

Bayés de Luna A, Baranchuk A. *Clinical Arrhythmology.* 2nd edn. Willey-Blackwell, 2017.

Bayés deLuna A, Cosín J, Carrió J, *et al.* Right ventricular peripheric block: Diagnostic problems. In Alboni P (ed.) *Cardiac Electrophysiology.* Academic Press, 1982, p. 401.

Bayés de Luna A, Cosín J, Carrió I, Subirana MT, Guindo J, Torner P. Electrophysiological mechanisms of the S1,S2,S3 electrocardiographic morphology. J Electrocardiol 1987;20:38.

Bayés de Luna A, Platonov P, García-Cosío F, *et al.* Interatrial blocks: a separate entity from left atrial enlargement: a consensus paper. J Electrocardiol 2012;45:445.

Bexton R, Vellin H, Camm J. Diurnal variations of the QT interval. Br Heart J 1986;55:253.

Burattini L, Zareba W, Burattini R. Identification of gender-related normality regions for T wave alternans. Ann Noninvasive Electrocardiol 2010;15:328.

Cabrera E. *Teoría y práctica de la electrocardiografía.* La Prensa Médica Mexicana, 1963.

Cooksey I, Dunn M, Massie E. *Clinica ECG and VCG.* YearBook Medical, 1977.

Domienk-Karlowicz J, Lichodsiejewska B, Link W. ECG criteria of LVH in morbid obesity. Ann Noninvasive Electrocardiol 2011;16:258.

Frank S, Colliver JA, Frank A. The electrocardiogram in obesity: statistical analysis of 1029 patients. J Am Coll Cardiol 1986;7:295.

Goldenberg I, Zareba W, Moss AJ. Long QT syndrome. Curr Probl Cardiol 2008;33:629.

Haïssaguerre M, Derval N, Sacher F, *et al.* Sudden cardiac arrest associated with early repolarization. N Engl J Med 2008;358:2016.

Inoue YY, Ipek EG, Khurram IM, *et al.* Relation of electrocardiographic left atrial abnormalities to risk of stroke in patients with atrial fibrillation. Am J Cardiol 2018;122:242.

Kardys I, Kors J, van der Meer I, *et al.* Spatial qRS-T angle predicts cardiac death in a general population. Eur Heart J 2003;24:1357.

Madias JE, Bazaz R, Agarwal H, *et al.* Anasarca-mediated attenuation of the amplitude of electrocardiogram complexes: a description of a heretofore unrecognized phenomenon. J Am Coll Cardiol 2001;38:756.

Magnani J, Johnson W, Sullivan L, *et al.* P wave indices: Derivation of reference values from the Framingham heart study. Ann Noninvasive Electrocardiol 2010;15:344.

Maheshwari A, Norby FL, Roetker NS, *et al.* Refining prediction of atrial fibrillation-related stroke using the P_2-CHA_2DS_2-Vasc score. *Circulation* 2019;139:180. doi: 10.1161/CIRCULATIONAHA.118.035411.

Malik J, Camm AJ (eds). *Dynamic Electrocardiography.* Blackwell, 2004.

Martínez-Sellés M, Massó-van Roessel A, Álvarez-Garcia J, *et al* (The Investigators of the Cardiac and Clinical Characterization of Centenarians (4C) registry). Interatrial block and atrial arrhythmias in centenarians: prevalence, associations, and clinical implications. Heart Rhythm 2016;13:645.

Molnar J, Zhang F, Weiss J, *et al.* Diurnal pattern of QTc interval: how long is prolonged? Possible relation to circadian triggers of cardiovascular events. J Am Coll Cardiol 1996;27:76.

Morganroth J, Brozovich F, McDonald J, *et al.* Variability of the QT measurement in healthy men. Am J Cardiol 1991;67:774.

Morris JJ, Estes EH, Whalen RE, *et al.* P wave analysis in valvular heart disease. Circulation 1964;29:242.

Moss AJ, Kass RS. Long QT syndrome: from channels to cardiac arrhythmias. J Clin Invest 2005;15:2018.

Okin PM. Electrocardiography in women: taking the initiative. Circulation 2006;113:464.

O'Neal WT, Zhang ZM, Loehr LR, *et al.* Electrocardiographic advanced interatrial block and atrial fibrillation risk in the general population. Am J Cardiol 2016;117:1755.

Park JK, Park J, Uhm JS, *et al.* Low P-wave amplitude (<0,1 mV) in lead I is associated with displaced inter-atrial conduction and clinical recurrence of paroxysmal atrial fibrillation after radiofrequency catheter ablation. Europace 2016;18:348.

Porthan K, Viitasalo M, Jula A, *et al.* Predictive value of ECG QT interval and T wave morphology parameters for all-cause and cardiovascular mortality in a general population sample. Heart Rhythm 2009;6:1202.

Postema PG, Ritsema Van Eck H, Opthof T, *et al.* IK1 modulates the U-wave: insights in a 100-year-old enigma. Heart Rhythm 2009;6:393.

Rasmussen MU, Fabricius-Bjerre A, Kumarathurai P, *et al.* Common source of miscalculation and misclassification of P-wave negativity and P-wave terminal force in lead V1. J Electrocardiol 2019;53:85.

Rautaharju P, Prineas R, Zhang ZM. A simple procedure for estimation of the spatial QRS/T angle from the standard 12-lead ECG. J Electrocardiol 2007;40:300.

Rosso R, Kogan E, Belhassen B, *et al.* J-point elevation in survivors of primary ventricular fibrillation and matched control subjects: incidence and clinical significance. J Am Coll Cardiol 2008;52:1231.

Surawicz B. U wave: facts, hypotheses, misconceptions, and misnomers. J Cardiovasc Electrophysiol 1998;9:1117.

Surawicz B. U wave emerges from obscurity when the heart pumps like in a kangaroo. Heart Rhythm 2008;5:246.

Surawicz B, Parikh SR. Differences between ventricular repolarization in men and women: description, mechanism and implications. Ann Noninvasive Electrocardiol 2003;8:333.

Tereshchenko LG, Hersikson CA, Sotoodehnia N, *et al.* Electrocardiographic deep terminal negativity of the P-wave in V1 and risk of sudden cardiac death: The Atherosclerosis Risk in Communities (ARIC) study. J Am Heart Assoc 2014;3:e001387.

Vitelli LL, Crow R, Sahar R, *et al.* Electrocardiographic findings in a healthy biracial population. Am J Cardiol 1998;81:453.

Winsor T (ed). *Electrocardiographic Test Book. Volumes I and II.* American Heart Association, Inc, New York, 1956.

Yanagisawa N, Onde M, Wada T Counter clockwise rotation of the heart: a correlative study with tomographic echocardiography. J Cardiography 1981;11:981.

Zeng C, Wei T, Zhao R, *et al.* Electrocardiographic diagnosis of left atrial enlargement in patients with mitral stenosis: the value of the P-wave area. Acta Cardiologica 2003;58:139.

Chapter 8
Diagnostic Criteria: Sensitivity, Specificity, and Predictive Value

Roberto Elosua

In some situations, conventional electrocardiography is the technique with the best diagnostic accuracy. In other words, it enables us to define criteria that make it possible to determine if a certain disease process is present or absent better than any other diagnostic method (Fisch 1989; Schlant 1991).

As a whole, conventional electrocardiography is considered a reference, or "gold standard," method for the diagnosis of atrial and ventricular conduction abnormalities, ventricular pre-excitation, most cardiac arrhythmias, and acute myocardial infarction. In some situations, other electrocardiological techniques may be needed for a reliable diagnosis. For example, in some tachycardias with a wide QRS, it may be difficult to distinguish between aberrancy and ventricular rhythm with a conventional surface ECG alone. The same limitation applies when locating an accessory pathway.

In other circumstances, such as atrial and ventricular enlargement, alterations due to chronic ischemic heart disease (ECG findings of ischemia, injury, or necrosis), or other repolarization disorders, conventional electrocardiography may yield valuable information for diagnosis. However, it has less potential than other imaging techniques (for example, echocardiography for detecting atrial and ventricular enlargement, etc.).

It is important to know the true value of ECG diagnostic criteria in diseases in which electrocardiography is not the "gold standard" diagnostic tool (i.e. diagnostic criteria of atrial and ventricular enlargement, necrosis in chronic phases, tachycardia with wide QRS, etc.). The specificity and sensitivity of electrocardiological techniques in the presence or absence of disease should be known. Thus, the concepts of sensitivity, specificity, and predictive value are indispensable for such evaluations.

The validity of the diagnostic criteria of a method or technique is determined by comparing the results obtained with the method being evaluated (in this case, surface ECG or other electrocardiological technique) with the results of a "gold standard" diagnostic test, a reference test (Ransohoff and Feinstein 1979; Willems *et al.* 1985). The reference test may be another electrocardiological technique (such as endocavitary techniques in the case of wide QRS) or a different type of test (echocardiography, hemodynamic evaluations, clinical findings such as the presentation of disease, etc.). It is only in the last few years that such concepts have been applied to ECG diagnosis criteria; prior to that, electrocardiographic diagnoses were often more intuitive than rational.

The information derived from both the diagnostic test under evaluation (presence or absence of a determined ECG criterion, or positivity or negativity result of an electrocardiological technique) and the reference test considered "gold standard" for diagnosis can be represented in a table with two rows (results of the test under evaluation) and two columns (distribution of the disease according to the reference test). This is referred to as a 2 × 2 table (Table 8.1) in which four subgroups of individuals can be defined:

a. true positives (TP): those patients with the disease/abnormality properly identified by the diagnostic method under evaluation;

b. false negatives (FN): those patients with the disease but not identified as such by the diagnostic method, thus classified as healthy;

c. false positives (FP): those individuals without the disease but identified as having the disease by the diagnostic method;

d. true negatives (TN): those individuals without the disease properly identified as healthy by the diagnostic method.

Using this type of table and these four subgroups, the sensitivity, specificity, and predictive values of the diagnostic test can be estimated (Diamond and Forrester 1979; Wulff 1980; Altman and Bland 1994a, 1994b).

Clinical Electrocardiography: A Textbook, Fifth Edition. Antoni Bayés de Luna, Miguel Fiol-Sala, Adrian Bayés-Genis, and Adrian Baranchuk.
© 2022 John Wiley & Sons Ltd. Published 2022 by John Wiley & Sons Ltd.

Table 8.1 Calculation of sensitivity (SE), specificity (SP), positive and negative predictive values (PPV, NPV) of a certain electrocardiographic criterion[a]

		100 Patients with valvular heart disease			
		LAE assessed by echocardiography		Total	
		Yes	No		
100 patients with valvular heart disease	P± in II, III, VF	2	0	2	$PPV = \dfrac{TP}{TP+FP} = \dfrac{2}{2+0} \times 100 \approx 100\%$
	without P± in II, III, VF	88	10	98	$NPV = \dfrac{TN}{TN+FN} = \dfrac{10}{10+88} = 100\% = 10\%$
Total		90	10	100	

$$SE = \frac{TP}{TP+FN} = \frac{2}{2+88} \times 100 = 2\% \qquad\qquad SP = \frac{TN}{TN+FP} = \frac{10}{10+0} \times 100 = 100\%$$

[a] An example to demonstrate whether the presence of an electrocardiographic criterion (in this case, a ±P wave in II, III, and aVF in patients with valvular heart disease) does or does not predict the presence of left atrial enlargement (LAE) as detected by echocardiography.
FN: false negative; FP: false positive; NPV: negative predictive value; PPV: positive predictive value; SE: sensitivity; SP: specificity; TN: true negative; TP: true positive.

Sensitivity

The sensitivity of an ECG criterion is defined as **the percentage of individuals with a given abnormality who present that ECG criterion** (i.e. the percentage of persons with left ventricular enlargement (LVE) who present an R≥35 mm in V5). If all individuals with this abnormality (LVE) present the determined criterion, the sensitivity is 100%, in which case no false negative cases exist. Sensitivity is also defined as the probability that the result of a diagnostic test will be positive when the disease is present. Sensitivity is calculated using the following formula:

$$Sensitivity\,(\%)\,of\,a\,criterion = \frac{TP\,(true\,positives)}{TP+FN\,(false\,negatives)} \times 100$$

where TP is the number of the subjects with the disease or abnormality (in this case, LVE) who present the criterion; FN is the number of the subjects with the disease or abnormality who do not present the criterion and are classified as healthy.

Specificity

The specificity of a test (in this case, a diagnostic criterion obtained by surface ECG or another electrocardiological technique) is defined as **the percentage of individuals without the abnormality/disease who do not present the criterion. Therefore, the smaller the number of healthy individuals who present the criterion, the more specific it is**. For example, in evaluating the criterion R wave ≥35 mm in V5 for the diagnosis of LVE, the specificity is 90% if the criterion is found in only 10 out of 100 healthy individuals.

If no healthy individual presents the criterion, the specificity is 100%, no false positive cases exist. Specificity is also defined as the probability that the result of a diagnostic test will be negative when the disease is not present. Specificity is calculated using the following formula:

$$Specificity\,(\%)\,of\,a\,criterion = \frac{TN\,(true\,negatives)}{TN+FP\,(false\,positives)} \times 100$$

where TN is the number of persons without the disease or abnormality, as confirmed by a reference technique, who do not present the problem criterion (e.g. the number of subjects without LVE, confirmed by echocardiography, who do not present with the criterion R wave ≥35 mm in V5); FP is the number or persons without the disease or abnormality who present the criterion.

Specificity is determined in the control group (patients without the pathology under study) and **sensitivity in the group of subjects with the pathology** as demonstrated by reference techniques (echocardiography, angiography, clinical course, etc.), in order to define the groups with and without the disease.

Predictive values

The predictive values indicate the real clinical meaning of a diagnostic test. They represent the utility of a test result, whether positive or negative, in the clinical setting. Therefore, two predictive values can be estimated:

a. Positive predictive value (PPV): estimates the percentage of patients showing the diagnostic criteria (sign or symptom) that have the disease or abnormality. It is defined as the probability that the disease is present when the test is positive.

b. Negative predictive value (NPV): estimates the percentage of patients without the diagnostic criteria in question that do not have the disease. It is defined as the probability that the disease is not present when the test is negative.

The PPV and NPV are calculated using the following equations:

$$PPV = \frac{TP}{TP + FP}$$
$$NPV = \frac{TN}{TN + FN}$$

At this point, it is important to highlight that sensitivity and specificity are dependent on the validity of the diagnostic test. However, PPV and NPV are not only dependent on the validity of the test but also on the prevalence of the disease in the population in which the diagnostic test is being used. **Therefore, the predictive values of a diagnostic criterion depend on the frequency and burden of the disease.**

Now, using some examples, we will calculate the sensitivity, the specificity, and the predictive values of a diagnostic criterion in a specific population. If we study 100 consecutive patients with valvular heart disease (Table 8.1), we can see that the sensitivity of a +/− P wave in II, III, and aVF leads as a diagnostic criterion for the presence of left atrial enlargement (LAE) has a very low sensitivity (2%) but a very high specificity (100%). It means that very few patients with LAE present this criterion (low sensitivity), but at the same time there are no patients without LAE who would meet this criterion (high specificity). All patients with valvular heart disease accompanied by a ±P wave in II, III, and aVF (ECG criterion) will present LAE (PPV = 100%), although the absence of this ECG criterion does not exclude the previous diagnosis. Thus, 98% of the patients with valvular heart disease that have LAE do not present with P+/− in II, III, and aVF (NPV = 10%).

Table 8.2 shows an example based on a cohort of 210 post-myocardial infarction patients. In order to determine how many patients will develop malignant ventricular arrhythmias (MVA) and whether or not the presence of late potentials is useful to identify them, we need to know the predictive value for positivity and negativity of late potential techniques in this group of patients. In other words, we want to know the value of late potentials as a marker for poor prognosis in post-myocardial infarction patients. During a one-year follow-up, 10 of the 210 post-infarction patients present MVA. In Table 8.2, calculations of the sensitivity, specificity, and predictive value of the late potential technique for this group of patients are shown.

> The lower the sensitivity (SE), the greater the number of FN; the lower the specificity (SP), the greater the number of FP. The percentage (%) of FP is 100− % SP and the percentage of FN = 100− % SE.

Sensitivity and specificity are high, 90% and 80%, respectively. However, as the number of patients without MVA is very high (200 patients) in spite of the high specificity (80%), there are 40 patients without MVA who present with positive late potentials. They must be added to the group of 9 out of 10 patients with MVA who also present positive late potentials and will develop MVA during follow-up, so the PPV is very low (<20%). In contrast, the NPV will be very high (99%) because only 1 of the 161 patients without late potentials will develop MVA during follow-up. This means that if late potentials are absent in post-myocardial infarction patients, the risk of MVA during follow-up is extremely low (<1%); if they are present, it is not very useful to predict which patients will present MVA during follow-up, although the risk of MVA is somewhat higher.

Table 8.2 Calculation of sensitivity (SE), specificity (SP), positive and negative predictive values (PPV, NPV) of late potentials[a]

		\multicolumn{3}{c}{210 Post-infarction patients MVA during follow-up}	
		Yes	No	Total	
210 post-infarction patients	Late potentials (+)	9	40	49	$PPV = \dfrac{TP}{TP+FP} = \dfrac{9}{9+40} \times 100 = 18\%$
	Late potentials (−)	1	160	161	$NPV = \dfrac{TN}{TN+FN} = \dfrac{160}{160+1} \times 100 = 99\%$
Total		10	200	210	

$SE = \dfrac{TP}{TP+FN} = \dfrac{9}{9+1} \times 100 \approx 90\%$ $\qquad$ $SP = \dfrac{TN}{TN+FP} = \dfrac{160}{160+40} \times 100 \approx 80\%$

[a] An example showing the prediction of the occurrence of a clinical event (in this case, malignant ventricular arrhythmias—MVA) during follow-up in post-infarction patients using information derived from an electrocardiographic test (in this case, the presence or absence of late ventricular potentials). FN: false negative; FP: false positive; NPV: negative predictive value; PPV: positive predictive value; SE: sensitivity; SP: specificity; TN: true negative; TP: true positive.

But, what could be the impact of increasing the frequency of the disease (MVA) on the estimations of the predictive values? Let us assume that the number of post-myocardial infarction patients who had presented MVA in the course of follow-up had been higher (i.e. about 50%, or 100 out of 210). The sensitivity and specificity of the diagnostic test do not change (90% and 80%). Then, the number of patients with positive late potentials would have increased from 49 to 112 (Table 8.3). As most of these patients (90 of 112) would have presented MVA, the PPV would have been much greater (≈80%), and the NPV would have been somewhat lower (≈90% instead of 99%). This example shows that it is necessary to consider the burden of the disease (prevalence/incidence) in the evaluation of the predictive values of a diagnostic test.

We should remember that the sensitivity and specificity of ECG criteria vary inversely: highly specific criteria will be less sensitive. For example, P wave >150 ms is very specific for LAE because few persons without LAE present it, but it is also less sensitive because few persons with LAE have such a long P wave.

Because of this inverse relationship, it is difficult to find a criterion that maintains high levels of sensitivity without sacrificing specificity. However, we should remember that depending on the frequency of the disease under study, even with a relatively high specificity and sensitivity, the true utility of a sign (its PPV) may be low (Table 8.1).

Highly sensitive ECG criteria, although less specific, are useful for screening studies, while highly specific ECG signs usually confirm the existence of a disease, they often do not appear, even in the presence of it. Clinicians should know the sensitivity, specificity, and predictive values of different ECG criteria and tests to better evaluate the presence or absence of the pathology in question.

Finally, the **accuracy** of a diagnostic test or criterion represents the overall probability of a patient to be correctly classified. The accuracy is calculated as:

$$\text{Accuracy} = \text{Sensitivity} \cdot \text{Prevalence} + \text{Specificity} \cdot (1 - \text{Prevalence})$$

Bayes' theorem

To conclude, it should be remembered that the reliability of a test (in our case, an ECG criterion) increases or decreases in accordance with Bayes' theorem (Patterson *et al.* 1984). According to this theorem, when a criterion is applied to a population group that has a high prevalence of heart disease (in other words, a high a priori probability of presenting the disease), the predictive value of the criterion increases. In contrast, the predictive value decreases when applied to a population group with a low prevalence of heart disease (low a priori probability). For example, the value of ST segment depression as a sign of ischemic heart disease is much greater when observed in a population group that has a high prevalence of ischemic heart disease (i.e. middle-aged men with hypercholesterolemia, hypertension, and precordial pain) than in a population group with a low prevalence of heart disease (i.e. young adults with no risk factors).

Based on the Bayes theorem, if we know the a priori probability of having the disease, the results of the diagnostic test, and its sensitivity and specificity, we could estimate the probability of a patient having the disease according to the positive or negative result of the test (Giner *et al.* 1981; Deeks and Altman 2004). The estimation

Table 8.3 Calculation of sensitivity (SE), specificity (SP), positive and negative predictive values (PPV, NPV) of late potentials[a]

		210 Post-infarction patients MVA during follow-up			
		Yes	No	Total	
210 post-infarction patients	Late potentials (+)	90	22	112	$PPV = \dfrac{TP}{TP+FP} = \dfrac{90}{90+22} \times 100 \cong 80\%$
	Late potentials (−)	10	88	98	$NPV = \dfrac{TN}{TN+FN} = \dfrac{88}{88+10} \times 100 \cong 90\%$
Total		100	110	210	
$SE = \dfrac{TP}{TP+FN} = \dfrac{90}{90+10} \times 100 \approx 90\%$			$SP = \dfrac{TN}{TN+FP} = \dfrac{88}{88+22} \times 100 \approx 80\%$		

[a] An example showing the prediction of the occurrence of a clinical event (in this case, malignant ventricular arrhythmias—MVA) during follow-up in post-infarction patients using information derived from electrocardiographic test (in this case, the presence or absence of late ventricular potentials). In this case, the number of patients presenting ventricular malignant tachycardia during follow-up is much higher than in Table 8.2.

FN: false negative; FP: false positive; NPV: negative predictive value; PPV: positive predictive value; SE: sensitivity; SP: specificity; TN: true negative; TP: true positive.

of this probability is based on the likelihood ratios of the diagnostic test:

a. the positive likelihood ratio (LR+) informs us about how much the probability of having the disease increases given a positive result. The LR+ is calculated as the probability of a person with the disease to present a positive result in the test (True positive)/probability of a person without the disease presenting a positive result in the test (False positive).

b. The negative likelihood ratio (LR−) informs us about how much the probability of having the disease decreases given a negative result. The LR− is calculated as the probability a person with the disease presents a negative result in the test (False negative)/probability a person without the disease presents a negative result in the test (True negative). In the example shown in Table 8.3, we can estimate the LR+ and LR− of the diagnostic criterion:

- LR+ = TP/FP = 90/22 = 4.1. The probability of a patient having the disease after a positive result of the test increases by 4.1 times.
- LR− = FN/TN = 10/88 = 0.11. The probability of a patient having the disease after a negative result of the test decreases by 0.11 times.

With the estimation of the LR (+ or −) and the a priori probability, we can use the Fagan's normogram for calculating post-test probabilities of having the disease based on the Bayes theorem.

References

Altman DG, Bland JM. Statistics notes. Diagnostic tests 1: sensitivity and specificity. BMJ 1994a;308:1552.

Altman DG, Bland JM. Statistics notes. Diagnostic tests 2: predictive values. BMJ 1994b;309:6947.

Deeks JJ, Altman DG. Statistics notes. Diagnosis test 4: likelihood ratios. BMJ 2004;329:168–169.

Diamond GA, Forrester JS. Analysis of probability as an aid in the clinical diagnosis of coronary artery disease. New Engl J Med 1979;300:1350.

Fisch CH. Evolution of the clinical electrocardiogram. J Am Coll Cardiol 1989;14:1127.

Giner PF, Mayewski RJ, Mushlin AI, Greenland P. Selection and interpretation of diagnostic tests and procedures. Ann Intern Med 1981;94:555–600.

Patterson RE, Eng C, Horowitz SF. Practical diagnosis of coronary artery disease: Bayes theorem nomogram to correlate clinical data with noninvasive exercise tests. Am J Cardiol 1984;53:252.

Ransohoff DR, Feinstein AR. Problems of spectrum and bias in evaluating the efficacy of diagnosis tests. N Engl J Med 1979;299:926.

Schlant R. Guidelines for electrocardiography. Circulation 1991;85:1221.

Willems J, Robles de Medina EO, Bernard R, *et al.* Criteria for intraventricular conduction disturbances and preexcitation. J Am Coll Cardiol 1985;5:1261.

Wulff I. *Rational Diagnosis and Treatment.* Blackwell Scientific, 1980.

Part 3
Abnormal ECG Patterns

Chapter 9
Atrial Abnormalities

Introduction

This chapter examines the electrocardiographic abnormalities seen in atrial depolarization (P wave) caused by atrial enlargement and/or atrial conduction disturbances, including the rare cases of atrial dissociation. ECG changes due atrial infarction and abnormal atrial repolarization are also discussed (Zimmerman 1968; Bayés de Luna 2012).

The following issues should be taken into consideration:
- **The normal P wave** is produced by the depolarization of the right atrium, followed by the left atrium, with an interval in which both atria are depolarized (Figure 9.1A).

In fact, left atrial enlargement (LAE) and interatrial blocks (IAB) present some similar ECG criteria, especially the increase in the duration of P wave. However (see Tables 9.1 and 9.2), the sensitivity of the criteria for the diagnosis of atrial enlargement is usually very low, as has been demonstrated by correlations of the ECG with imaging techniques. Due to that, the AHA/ACC/HRA published in 2009 a consensus paper (Hancock et al. 2009) giving the recommendation, that all abnormal P waves should usually be referred as "atrial abnormalities" rather than atrial enlargement, overload, hypertrophy, or block.

However, just three years later in 2012, the International Society for Holter and Noninvasive Electrocardiology (ISHNE) published a consensus paper (Bayés de Luna et al. 2012) establishing that interatrial block was an independent and separate entity than left atrial enlargement. This was based especially on the fact that the pattern of interatrial block: (i) may be reproduced experimentally (Waldo et al. 1971; Guerra et al. 2020); (ii) may be transient (Bayés de Luna et al. 1985, 2018a); and (iii) may be recorded in the absence of atrial enlargement or necrosis (Bayés de Luna et al. 1985).

We consider that ongoing studies will probably increase in the near future the capacity of ECG to diagnose more

accurately right and left atrial enlargement. The same that has happened as we will see later with the ECG criteria for different types of interatrial block that are already well established.

Therefore, although we consider that the "umbrella" term of "atrial abnormalities" may be used to encompass globally all pathological changes of P wave that include IAB and atrial enlargement, hypertrophy or dilation, we prefer in this chapter, in spite of all limitations that exist, due to low sensitivity that currently exist, to diagnose right and left atrial enlargement using these criteria, although emphasizing his low sensitivity. We hope that we can in the future increase the accuracy of this diagnosis. Later, we will comment the well-established diagnostic criteria of all types of interatrial block (IAB).

New concepts on P wave

Along the last 10–15 years, to study the P wave has been considered very important to recognize that there are two aspects of the atria that have grant relevance for the diagnosis of P wave abnormalities. We have referring to: (i) the concept of P wave indices, that we have exposed already in Chapter 7 and (ii) the importance that has the abnormal ultrastructure of left atrium (LA) to explain the association of P wave abnormalities especially duration and morphology (A-IAB) with atrial arrhythmias, stroke and even dementia and death (Bayés de Luna et al. 2020a, b). We will comment all that along the chapter.

Atrial enlargement

As we have commented before, due to similarities of the ECG criteria for the diagnosis of LAE and IAB, the consensus paper of AHA and HR (Hancock et al. 2009) propose the term "left atrial abnormalities" to encompass all

Clinical Electrocardiography: A Textbook, Fifth Edition. Antoni Bayés de Luna, Miquel Fiol-Sala, Antoni Bayés-Genís, and Adrián Baranchuk.
© 2022 John Wiley & Sons Ltd. Published 2022 by John Wiley & Sons Ltd.

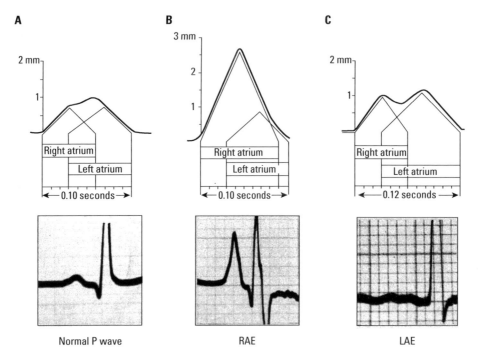

Figure 9.1 Above: diagram of atrial depolarization in a normal P wave (A), right atrial enlargement (RAE) (B), and left atrial enlargement (LAE) (C). Below: examples of the three types of P wave.

Table 9.1 Right atrial enlargement. ECG criteria with high specificity and lower sensitivity (see text)

ECG criteria	SE%	SP%
QRS criteria		
• QR or qR in V1		
Sodi-Pallares 1956; Reeves *et al.* 1981*	≈15*	>95*
QRS V1 ≤ 4 mm + QRS V2/V1 ≥ 5		
Reeves *et al.* 1981*	46*	93*
• R/S > 1 in V1		
Kaplan *et al.* 1994*	≈25*	>95*
• ÂQRS > 90°		
Kaplan *et al.* 1994*	34*	>95*
P criteria		
• P wave in inferior leads > 2.5 mm		
Kaplan *et al.* 1994*	6*	100*
Tsao *et al.* 2008**	7**	100**
• Positive part of P wave V1 > 1.5 mm		
Kaplan *et al.* 1994*	17*	100*
Tsao *et al.* 2008**	10**	96**
• Positive part of P wave V2 > 1.5 mm		
Kaplan *et al.* 1994*	33*	100*
Combined		
• Positive part of P wave in V2 > 1.5 mm + ÂQRS > +90° + R/S > 1 in V1		
Kaplan *et al.* 1994*	49*	100*

*Standards of echocardiography; **standards of cardiovascular magnetic resonance.

Table 9.2 Left atrial enlargement. ECG criteria based on P wave changes with high specificity and lower sensitivity (see text)

ECG criteria	SE%	SP%
• Morris index (Morris *et al.* 1964) (P terminal force in V1 mm/sec) (0.04 mm/sec) Munuswamy *et al.* 1984*	69*	93*
Tsao *et al.* 2008**	37**	88**
• NYAC score P ≥ 120 ms in I or II + Morris index (>0.04 mm/sec) + ÂP ≈ 0°		
Bartell *et al.* 1978	15*	98*
• P ≥ 120 ms in lead II + Terminal mode negative of P in V1 > 40 ms		
Bosch *et al.* 1981	50*	87*
• P ≥ 120 ms in lead II + Morris index (>0.04 mm/sec)		
Lee *et al.* 2007*	69%*	49%*
• Interpeaks of P wave > 40 ms		
Munuswamy *et al.* 1984*	15*	100*
Tsao *et al.* 2008**	8**	99**
• P± in II, III, VF		
Bayés de Luna *et al.* 1985*	5*	100*
• ÂP beyond +30°		
Tsao *et al.* 2008**	8**	90**
• P wave duration in II or III leads ≥ 0.12 sec		
Munuswamy *et al.* 1984*	33%*	88%*
Lee *et al.* 2007*	69%*	49%*
Tsao *et al.* 2008**	60%**	35%**

*Standards of echocardiography; **standards of cardiovascular magnetic resonance.

abnormal P wave anomalies found in both processes. However, as we have said (see before), we decided to follow in this book to comment separately on the ECG criteria of LAE and IAB although having in mind that it is necessary to follow doing the research that will allow us clearly to identify the ECG criteria that assure us the diagnosis of LAE with higher sensitivity, in the presence of P wave ≥ 120 ms and if possible even with P wave <120 ms.

Right atrial enlargement

Associated diseases and the underlying mechanism of ECG changes

The heart diseases most frequently associated with right atrial enlargement (RAE) are congenital heart disease, chronic obstructive pulmonary disease (COPD) and valvular heart disease with right ventricular involvement.

It has been observed that when the right atrium enlarges, the P wave increases in voltage and becomes peaked. The duration of the P wave does not increase because although right atrial activation may be prolonged, it never exceeds the duration of left atrial activation (Figure 9.1B).

In COPD, pulmonary hypertension, and pulmonary emphysema, the P loop often points to the right and downward (vertical), although not beyond +90°. This explains why the ÂP is generally deviated to the right (**P pulmonale**). Thus, the projection of the vertical P loop on the frontal and horizontal plane results in a low-voltage P wave in lead I and a peaked P wave of high voltage in II, III, and aVF (P ≥ 2.5 mm) (Figures 9.2B and 9.3B).

In some congenital heart diseases, such as Fallot's tetralogy, the P loop points more to the left and forward. This explains why the ÂP is displaced somewhat to the left, and consequently the P wave voltage in lead III is lower than in leads I and II (**P congenitale**) (Figures 9.2A and 9.3C). Sometimes the voltage in leads I and II is of high

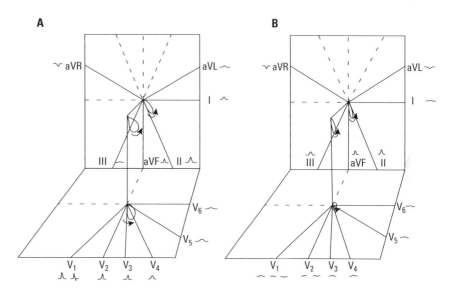

Figure 9.2 Loops of the P congenitale (A) and P pulmonale (B) waves with the morphologies in each lead. These are determined by whether the loop projection lies on the positive or negative hemisphere of each lead.

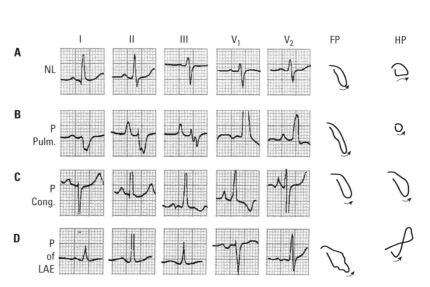

Figure 9.3 Examples of P wave morphology and loops in the following cases: (A) normal, (B) P pulmonale, (C) P congenitale, (D) left atrial enlargement.

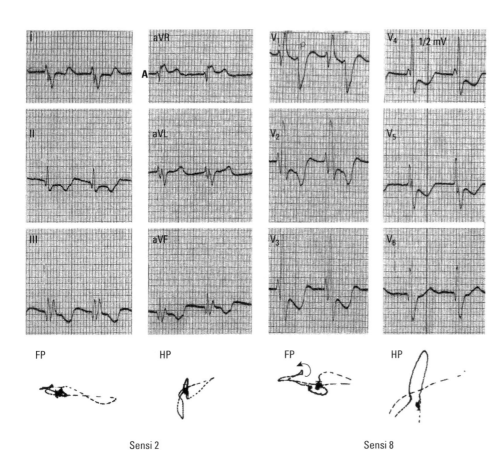

FP   HP   FP   HP

Sensi 2   Sensi 8

Figure 9.4 ECG and VCG of a one-year-old girl with Ebstein's disease. Note the long PR, the high-voltage P wave hidden in the T wave (+---mimicking rS morphology in V1), and the atypical right bundle branch block morphology.

amplitude (> 2 mm and peaked). The projection of this forward-pointing P loop on the horizontal plane produces a P wave in V1 with a voltage that may be high and positive or present with a ± morphology but with a rapid inscription diphase ⌁, the opposite to that observed in left atrial enlargement (LAE) ⌁. Exceptionally, a ⌁ pattern or even $\sqrt{}$ may appear in V1, but in V2 a predominantly positive morphology is recorded. This pattern in V1 is probably caused by the very enlarged and dilated RA, which adopts a low anterior position, and the electrode of V1 faces the negative part of the P vector. The congenital heart diseases that frequently present with these P wave characteristics in V1–V2 are **Ebstein's disease**, severe pulmonary stenosis, and tricuspid atresia. In the case of Ebstein's disease, the P wave in V1 may present with a large voltage, at times only positive and peaked, while at other times biphasic with a large negative node (P + − − −). Occasionally, the P wave voltage is similar to or even greater than the QRS voltage, with the QRS usually showing an atypical right bundle branch block (RBBB) pattern (Figure 9.4).

Electrocardiographic diagnostic criteria: imaging correlations (Table 9.1 and 9.2)

Although many diagnostic criteria were described in the past based on anatomic correlations or electrophysiological hypotheses (Sodi-Pallares 1956), the majority have been studied in the last 40 years based on echocardiography, especially with two-dimensional measurements (Reeves *et al.* 1981; Kaplan *et al.* 1994). Recently, CMR standards have been introduced for this purpose (Tsao *et al.* 2008). Table 9.1 shows the **ECG patterns** that demonstrate a very high specificity for RAE based on these studies, although the sensitivity never is ≥ 50%.

QRS criteria (indirect)

These include (Table 9.1):
• **qR (QR) morphology in lead V1** (Figure 9.5). According to Sodi-Pallares (1956), this morphology is explained by the presence of an enlarged right ventricle that is shifted forward, changing the direction of the septal vector to point forward and somewhat to the left. Consequently, lead V1 faces more toward the tail than the head of the vector and a "q" wave is recorded in V1 (Figure 9.6). **In the absence of RBBB, this criterion has a very high specificity** (> 95%) (Reeves *et al.* 1981).
• **An important difference in QRS voltage between V1 (low voltage) and V2 (high voltage)** (Figures 9.5, 9.7, and 9.8). This was attributed to a very dilated right atrium located close to V1 that acts as a barrier, thereby reducing QRS voltage in this lead. A voltage of QRS in V1 ≤ 4 mm plus a V2/V1 ratio ≥ 5 has an SP = 93% and an SE = 46% (PV = 86%) for RAE (Reeves *et al.* 1981).

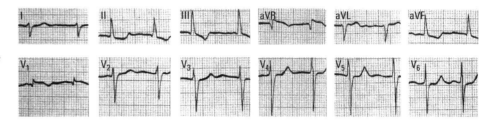

Figure 9.5 A 60-year-old woman with mitro-tricuspid valve disease who presented with QRS criteria for RAE and right ÂQRS with rS in V6 (right ventricular enlargement).

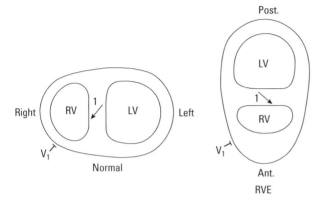

Figure 9.6 The more anterior location of the right ventricle that can be seen in right ventricular enlargement can explain how the normal first vector is seen as negative in V1.

Figure 9.7 A 52-year-old woman with double mitral and double tricuspid lesions. The difference between the very low QRS voltage in V1 and the high voltage in V2 is striking.

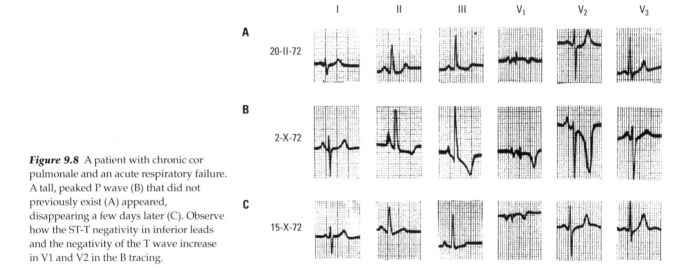

Figure 9.8 A patient with chronic cor pulmonale and an acute respiratory failure. A tall, peaked P wave (B) that did not previously exist (A) appeared, disappearing a few days later (C). Observe how the ST-T negativity in inferior leads and the negativity of the T wave increase in V1 and V2 in the B tracing.

• **R/S > 1 in V1 in the absence of other causes that may increase the R voltage in V1 (see Table 10.3). This sign has a high specificity (SP > 95 %) and low sensitivity (SE = 25 %).**
• **ÂQRS ≥ 90° (RS in lead I)** has high SP (> 95%) and a moderate SE (34%).

P wave criteria (direct)
These include (Kaplan *et al.* 1994; Tsao *et al.* 2008):
• **P voltage > 2.5 mm in inferior leads** has a low sensitivity (< 10%) but it is highly specific (100%).

• **Positive voltage of P in V1 > 1.5 mm** has a great specificity (> 95%) with low sensitivity (10%).
• **Positive voltage of P in V2 > 1.5 mm** also has a high specificity (100%) with slightly higher sensitivity (SE = 33%).

Combining QRS and P criteria
The combined criteria PV2 > 1.5 mm + ÂQRS > 90° + R/S in V1 > 1 have a correct sensitivity (≈50%) with specificity of 100% (Kaplan *et al.* 1994).

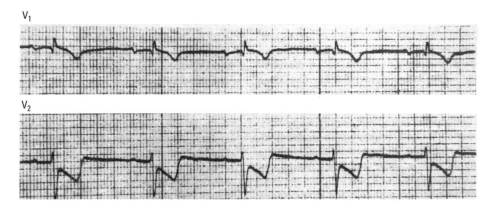

Figure 9.9 A 62-year-old woman with double mitral and double tricuspid lesions in congestive heart failure and with a history of at least 10 years of atrial fibrillation. With this rhythm, "f" waves were not seen in any lead. Unexpectedly, she changed to a sinoatrial rhythm with a PR of 0.26 sec (in atrial fibrillation and a small amount of digitalis, there was also an important AV block). The "P" wave was narrow and only visible in V1 and V2; in the other leads it appeared to be a junctional rhythm. The fact that the P wave is ± in V1 practically eliminated the possibility of ectopic rhythm.

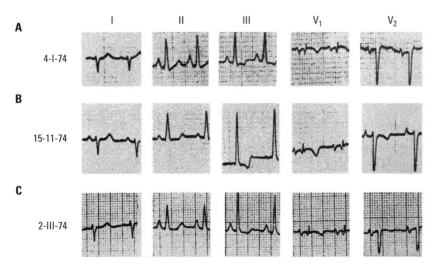

Figure 9.10 (A) A 45-year-old patient with subacute cor pulmonale. Note the right atrial enlargement (RAE) with the right ÂP. Some days later (B), the ÂP is directed to the left, returning to the right in a third ECG (C) recorded at 15 days. This example shows how atrial aberration may mask the P wave of clear RAE.

In clinical practice, the most useful criteria for RAE are those that have the highest specificity (≈ 100%) with an acceptable sensitivity (≈ 50%) (see Table 9.1).

• **The P wave criteria** are very specific but their sensitivity is very low.

• **The QRS criteria** with a QRS amplitude in V1 < 4 mm + ratio V2/V1 > 5 are highly specific (> 90%) with moderate SE (≈45%) (Reeves *et al.* 1981).

The combined P + QRS criteria with a P wave amplitude in V2 > 1.5 mm + ÂQRS > 90° + R/S ratio > 1 in V1 in the absence of RBBB have 100% specificity and 50% sensitivity (Kaplan *et al.* 1994).

False positive and false negative diagnoses of right atrial enlargement

The ECG diagnosis of RAE may be very difficult to reach for the following reasons:

• The voltage of the P wave is strongly influenced by extracardiac factors, which may result in increases (hypoxia, sympathetic overdrive, etc.) (false positive) (Figure 9.8) or decreases in voltage (emphysema, other barrier factors, atrial fibrosis, etc.), (false negative) (Bayés de Luna *et al.* 1978a) (Figure 9.9).

• The presence of associated atrial block may result in the transient or permanent disappearance of the ECG criteria for right atrial enlargement (false negative) (Figure 9.10).

• On the other hand, a high-voltage P wave may be seen in patients with exclusively left heart pathology and possible left atrial enlargement (false positive) (pseudo-P-pulmonale) (Chou and Helm 1965).

These are some of the reasons why changes in the atriogram are generally not very sensitive (many false negative) for the diagnosis of RAE. Although there are some factors that increase the incidence of false positives, they are usually fewer and therefore the specificity of ECG criteria for RAE is much higher.

Left atrial enlargement (Table 9.2)
Associated diseases and underlying mechanisms of ECG changes

In the past, the most common associated diseases were rheumatic heart diseases, particularly **mitral stenosis**.

In fact, the characteristic bimodal P wave of left atrial enlargement (LAE), seen especially in lead II, has been called "**P mitrale**." However, this type of P wave is currently seen in the presence of other causes of LAE, such as cardiomyopathies, especially dilated cardiomyopathy, arterial hypertension, and ischemic heart disease.

The P wave seen in LAE usually has a longer than normal duration due to long distance that the stimulus has to cover as a consequence of the dilated LA more than to the hypertrophy of the LA mass itself (Josephson *et al.* 1977; Velury and Spodick 1994). The enlarged left atrium first expands toward the back, so the vector of LAE points backward (Figure 9.11). Moreover, because of all that, the P loop is longer and often acquires a figure-of-eight shape in the horizontal plane (HP). All that explains that the negative component of P wave is greater than the positive, and therefore, the P wave in lead V1, in case of LA enlargement when the electrode of V1 is well located, usually has a positive–negative morphology with a **prominent negative component** that exceeds the positive component ∿ (Figure 9.12). This is not usually the case in the presence of partial IAB without LA enlargement. However, in cases of bad location of the electrode in V1, too high, a P wave, is recorded with false final negative morphology in the absence of LA enlargement. Finally, if exist associated advanced interatrial block (see later) the P wave is be positive–negative in leads II, III, and VF, and in these cases, LAE is practically always present.

An abrupt dilatation of the left atrium, which occurs in acute pulmonary edema, for example, may cause +/−P wave morphology in V1. This disappears when the clinical situation improves (Heikila and Luomanmaki 1970) (Figure 9.13).

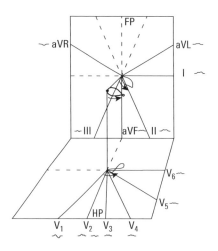

Figure 9.11 P loop of left atrial enlargement and the morphology in various leads, determined by whether the loop projection lies in the respective positive or negative hemifield of each lead (see text).

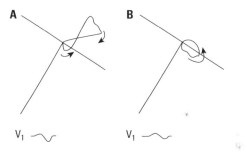

Figure 9.12 (A) P wave morphology in V1 and P loop in the case of left atrial enlargement, and (B) is a normal case or in case of isolated partial IAB.

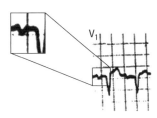
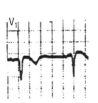
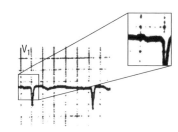

Figure 9.13 Above: An example of pulmonary edema in the acute phase of myocardial infarction (see X-ray below). Three days and 12 hours later, when the clinical improvement was evident, the ECG showed a reduction of the negative P mode in V1. This can be properly evaluated only when the V1 lead is taken at the same site. In the hospital environment, this can be ensured by marking the electrode site on the patient's skin.

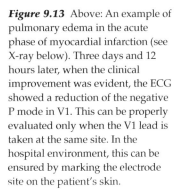
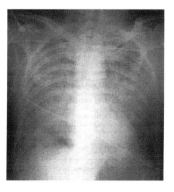

ECG diagnostic criteria: Imaging correlations (Table 9.2)

Historically, the majority of ECG criteria was based on necropsic or radiological correlations. Today, they are based on the standards of echocardiography and, more recently, CMR. (Josephson *et al.* 1977; Bartell *et al.* 1978; Bosch *et al.* 1981; Miller *et al.* 1983; Munuswamy *et al.* 1984; Bayés de Luna *et al.* 1985; Hazen *et al.* 1991; Tsao *et al.* 2008; Troung et al. 2011). Recently, it has been demonstrated by echo-speckle tracking echo, that this technique may be a surrogate of CMR (Montserrat *et al.* 2015) to demonstrate the abnormal fibrotic ultrastructure of LA wall, and even the ECG pattern of A-IAB may also be a surrogate of decrease of LA strain, and that means that the diagnosis of A-IAB by ECG is an equivalent to the presence of fibrosis in the LA wall (Lacalzada-Almeida *et al.* 2019) (Ciuffo *et al.* 2020).

As we have already commented, the P wave criteria for diagnosis of LAE have low sensitivity. Having this in mind, we will now comment on the ECG criteria of LAE.

• **Criteria based on changes of P wave** The imaging–ECG correlations have demonstrated that the best ECG criteria for LAE are the following (see Table 9.2):

• **P wave morphology in V1(P wave indices)** (see Chapter 7). A negative mode in V1 with a duration ≥ 40 ms by itself is a sign frequently seen in LAE and has a relatively good SE and high SP, according the paper of Morris (Morris *et al.* 1964). **The Morris index** has a better predictive value. This index is obtained from the product of the amplitude of the negative P wave component in V1 (in mm) and the duration of this component (in ms). A Morris index ≥ –40 mm × ms 40 ms is very specific for LAE (Figure 9.14). In practice, this means that the terminal portion of the P wave in V1 has a depth of at least one small box in the recording paper (–1.0 mm = 0.1 mV) and a duration of at least 0.04 sec. This index is very rarely seen

in normal populations (SP ≈ 90%) but the SE usually is very low. In Morris paper (1964) the SE was relatively high because all were patients with value heart disease and we are not sure about the location of electrode of V1.

In fact, recently it has been demonstrated (see before) that the morphology of Ptf V1 depends very much on the location of the electrodes of V1 (Rasmussen *et al.* 2019). If is too high (3rd of 2nd ICS), the morphology of P ± with great negative component is the rule. Also, the P in V1 may present a ± pattern or even all negative in cases of *pectus excavatum*, and other thoracic abnormalities. This may explain the discordant results obtained as a precursor of stroke. Due to that, as we are doing an observational trial to clarify this problem (Sajeev *et al.* 2019).

• **The criteria of the NYHAC score** (duration of P wave in II ≥ 120 ms + ÂP in FP close to 0° + Morris index ≥ –40 mm × ms) have a high SP (> 95%) but the SE is much lower (< 20%) (Bartell *et al.* 1978).

• The combination **of P ≥ 120 ms in lead II + negative P mode duration in V1 ≥ 40 ms** has a SE of 50% with a good SP (> 85%) (Bosch *et al.* 1981).

• **The combination of P ≥ 120 ms in lead II plus a Morris index > 0.04 mm/sec** has a high SP but a low SE (Lee *et al.* 2007).

• **The distance between two peaks of P wave** > 0.04 sec, with the second mode being taller than the first, is very specific (≈ 100%) but not sensitive (Munuswamy *et al.* 1984).

• **A positive–negative morphology of the P wave in leads II, III, and VF** (±) with a duration ≥ than 0.12 sec, **the key criteria for advanced interatrial block** with retrograde activation of the left atrium (see later), is a very specific criterion for LAE > 90% globally and 100% in valvular heart disease and cardiomyopathies, but has a very low sensitivity (< 5%) (Bayés de Luna *et al.* 1985) (Figures 9.16, 9.18 and 9.19). If present, it is a clear marker of AF in the

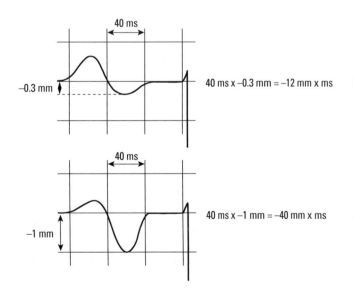

Figure 9.14 Diagram contrasting normal and abnormal negative components of the P wave in V1. When the value calculated using the width in seconds and the height in millimeters of the negative mode exceeds 40 mm × ms, it is considered abnormal.

future (Bayés de Luna *et al.* 1988) and even of stroke (Escobar-Robledo *et al.* 2018). However, as commented, its sensitivity for LAE is low (5%) (Table 9.2).

- **The P wave duration (P wave index) in leads I, II, and/ or III in LA enlargement** is ≥ 0.12 sec, and is generally bimodal. In some echocardiographic correlations, this criterion is very specific (88%) for LA enlargement, but the sensitivity is 33% (Munuswamy *et al.* 1984). In contrast, Lee *et al.* (2007) used two-dimensional echocardiography measurements to show different results (higher SE = 69%, lower SP = 49%) that were similar to those found by Tsao *et al.* (2008) using the CMR correlation (high SE = 60% and low SP = 35%). This is probably associated with the type of population used in the different studies. In the series studied by Tsao *et al.* (2008) (CMR), the patients probably present with isolated interatrial blocks more frequently, which decreases the specificity and increases the sensitivity of this criterion. The same is found in the series presented by Lee *et al.* (2007) (2D echo). The frequent presence of partial interatrial block without LA enlargement may explain this low SP (< 50%). However, since isolated partial interatrial bloc usually does not present with an important negative mode of the P wave in V1 (Figure 9.12), when we consider the association of P duration ≥ 120 ms + Morris index, or the Morris index alone, as criterion for LAE, we obtain much higher specificity (see Table 9.2). However, the value of Morris index is questionable (see other parts of this chapter).

> The duration of the P wave ≥ 120 ms alone is more a criterion for interatrial block than for LAE. It is very useful for the diagnosis of LAE, when the duration of P wave ≥ 120 ms associated with other criteria, such as bimodal and high P wave lead II, especially if P ± in II, III, and aVF and the Ptf in V1 has a positive Morris index, according to the characteristics explained before (electrode of V1 for Morris index well placed, etc. See later) (see Table 9.2, Bosch *et al.* 1981; Lee *et al.* 2007).

Other criteria

- **In the presence of atrial fibrillation (AF),** the cases of coarse f waves (≥ 1 mm) suggested the existence of LAE, especially in rheumatic heart disease patients. However, echocardiographic correlation (Morganroth *et al.* 1979) has demonstrated that the coarse "f" wave suggests especially interatrial conduction block. Moreover, AF is present in

the majority of cases (> 80%) when the left atrial diameter is > 60 mm. In a cohort of patients consecutively referred for clinical or research CMR studies, those with a history of AF had a significantly higher prevalence of LAE (47%) than patients with sinus rhythm (21%) (Tsao *et al.* 2008).

- Because of increased P wave duration, the **P/PR segment ratio > 1.8** is frequently seen in cases of LAE (Macruz *et al.* 1958).

> LAE exists if the ECG presents P wave ≥ 120 ms and presents the following characteristics:
> - **P ± in II, III, and aVF (SP > 90%)**
> - **Ptf in V1 positive (Morris index). In presence of well-located V1 electrode, and in absence of pectus excavatum and straight back syndrome or COPD**.

False positive and false negative diagnoses of left atrial enlargement

The diagnosis of LAE may often be difficult to achieve because of the following factors:

- The abnormal presence of Ptf in V1 with electrode of V1 located high (false positive) (Rasmussen *et al.* 2019).
- Many patients with thoracic abnormalities, *pectus excavatum*, and with straight back syndrome (Bayés de Luna and Baranchuk 2017) present abnormal but evident negative P waves in V1, a morphology that may be confused with LAE (false positive).
- If important atrial fibrosis exists, small and even unapparent P waves (concealed sinus rhythm) (Figures 9.9 and 15.37) may be seen, even in the presence of evident left atrial or bi-atrial enlargement. This problem increases the number of false negatives (low SE) (false negative) (Bayés de Luna *et al.* 2012).
- It is possible that young people, especially athletes, may present LAE by echo, with P wave <120 ms. It is necessary to perform an observational study to confirm that, and to be sure if this is a false negative.

Bi-atrial enlargement

Bi-atrial enlargement (BiAE) (Figure 9.15) is suspected when ECG criteria of right and left atrial enlargement coexist. Because the enlargement of two atria affects essentially different parts of the P wave, the diagnosis of bi-atrial enlargement is not as difficult as that of biventricular enlargement.

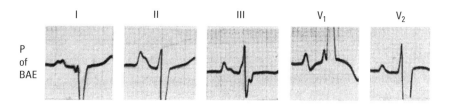

Figure 9.15 Example of P wave and loop morphology in bi-atrial enlargement (BAE).

The most important diagnostic criteria are as follows:
• **The P wave in lead II is taller (≥ 2.5 mm) and wider (≥ 0.12 sec) than normal.**
• **The first part of P wave is positive and peaked in V1–V2 (positive mode > 1.5 mm) with a slow negative node (width ≥ 1 mm)** ᐸᐳ.
• **Signs of left atrial enlargement with right ÂP. The** opposite case is not valid because the ÂP can be on the left side in isolated RAE of patients with congenital heart diseases.
• **The presence of atrial fibrillation along with QRS changes suggestive of RAE.**

Frequently, more than one criterion is found (see Figure 9.15) (P ≥ 120 ms in FP + P± in V1 with first part peaked and a slow negative mode).

Atrial blocks

Concept

The heart block may be located in different areas: at the sinoatrial and AV junction (Chapter 17), at the ventricular level (Chapter 11), and at the atrial level. This section deals with heart block at the atrial level, especially related with the concept of interatrial blocks, but we also briefly comment on blocks preferently located in RA or LA, the concept of atrial dissociation and the P wave changes due to myocardial infarction.

Various studies performed by our group (Julià *et al.* 1978; Bayés de Luna *et al.* 1985, 1988) and others, such as Spodick (Spodick and Ariyarajah 2008, 2009); Ariyarajah *et al.* (2006a), Holmqvist *et al.* (2010), and Platonov (2008), **have re-evaluated the concept that interatrial blocks and atrial enlargement are separate entities, because the ECG pattern may be considered that is due to a block if:** (i) they may appear transiently, (ii) they may exist isolated (without associated atrial enlargement), and (iii) they **may be provoked experimentally** (Waldo *et al.* 1971; Guerra *et al.* 2020) (Figure 9.16). However, in many cases, as occurs with ventricular enlargement and ventricular blocks, LA enlargement and interatrial block are both present.

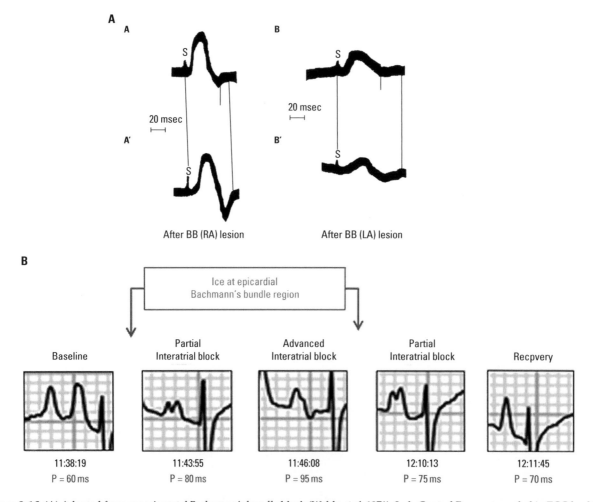

Figure 9.16 (A) Adapted from experimental Bachmann's bundle block (Waldo *et al.* 1971). Left: Control P wave recorded in ECG lead II when the atria were paced from the right atrium. Right: See the change of morphology after Bachmann's bundle lesion. P wave recorded in lead II after the creation of a lesion in the left atrial (LA) portion of Bachmann's bundle (BB). In both cases, the changes in conduction time and morphology after block are shown (adapted from Waldo *et al.* 1971). **(B)** Progressive and reversible sequence of ECG patterns of partial and advanced IAB, obtained after application of ice on the Bachmann bundle of an open chest pig.

The **evolution** from first-degree interatrial block to third-degree (advanced) interatrial block may be seen, as also happens in other types of block.

Very rarely, the atrial blocks may be located preferently in the right or left atrium, but much more often in two atria, and in the Bachmann bundle area that connects both atria. In these cases, we have an interatrial block and as the rest of atrial septum is of connective tissue in case of the block of Bachmann area, the LA has to be activated retrogradely from a zone close to AV node, and this explains that the P wave of inferior leads presents a ± morphology (see later).

Blocks located preferentially at right or left atrium (Figures 9.17 and 9.18D)

Isolated block of RA of LA are very infrequent and it is difficult to identify, only with surface ECG, the presence of a block predominantly within a single atrium. We have seen that occasionally apparently normal P waves (≤ 0.12 sec with some small notches) that presents in the VCG loop, total or near total clockwise rotation of the P loop in FP. we consider that this is due to the presence of a atrial block, preferently located in some part of the right atrium (Figures 9.17 and 9.18D) (Bayés de Luna *et al.* 1978b) because we have demonstrated by intracavitary ECG that

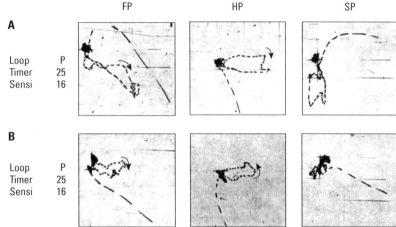

Figure 9.17 Two cases of nearly total (A) and total (B) clockwise rotation of the P loop in frontal plane (FP) that show a normal P wave (morphology and duration in the ECG). In A, the loop also rotates clockwise in the horizontal plane (HP), suggesting that the right atrial block is located in the anterior part of the right atrium.

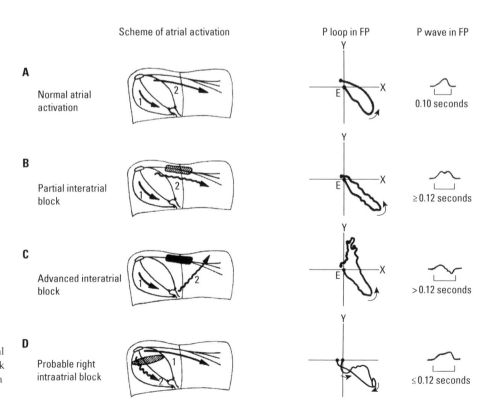

Figure 9.18 Diagram of atrial conduction under normal circumstances (A), partial interatrial block (B), advanced interatrial block with left atrial retrograde activation (AIB with LARA) (C) and probable right intra-atrial block (D).

Table 9.3 ECG classification of interatrial blocks (IAB)

1. **Typical IAB:**
   (i) Partial interatrial block (first degree*) (P-IAB)
   P wave ≥ 120 ms without negative terminal component in the inferior leads (Figure 9.18)
   (ii) Advanced interatrial block (third degree*) (A-IAB)
   P wave ≥ 120 ms with biphasic morphology in leads II, III, and aVF **(Figures 9.18–9.22)**
2. **Atypical A-IAB (Figures 9.23–9.26)**
   i) **Morphological criteria**
   - Type I: P wave ≥ 120 ms with biphasic morphology in leads III and aVF and the final component of the P wave in lead II is isodiphasic.
   - Type II: P wave ≥ 120 ms with biphasic morphology in leads III and aVF and the final component of the P wave in lead II is biphasic (±)
   - Type III: P-wave ≥ 120 ms with the first component of the P-wave isodiphasic in leads III and aVF
   ii **Duration criteria**
   - P wave < 120 ms with typical morphology (biphasic (±) P-wave in leads II, III, and aVF) **(Figure 9.26)**

* Second-degree IAB is intermittent (aberrancy) (Figure 9.27)

these cases presents a long high RA to low RA interval (Figure 9.18C).

Also, the atrial delay could be located preferently in the left atrium. This may be seen as very long and notched P waves with large slurrings present in the second part of the P wave.

Interatrial blocks

Usually, the blocks at atrial level, interatrial block, like other types of block (sinoatrial, atrioventricular, and ventricular), may be of first, second (transient block, atrial aberrancy) and third degree (see Chapter 14) (Table 9.3) (Figures 9.18A–C, and 9.19–9.21).

First-degree (partial) interatrial block (Figures 9.18B and 9.19B) (Table 9.3)

The electrical impulse is conducted normally from the right atrium to the left atrium, through Bachmann's bundle, but with a delay. Therefore, **the ECG shows a P wave of ≥ 0.12 sec**

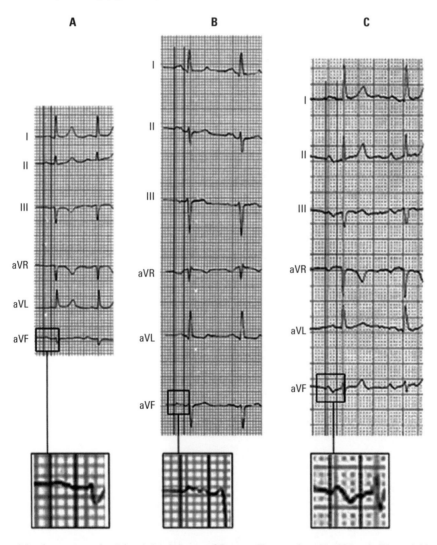

A   B   C

Figure 9.19 Examples of the three types of atrial activity: (A) normal P wave (P wave duration 120 ms), (B) partial interatrial block (P wave duration ≥ 120 ms), (C) advanced interatrial block (P wave duration ≥ 120 ms plus/minus morphology in leads II, III, and aVF).

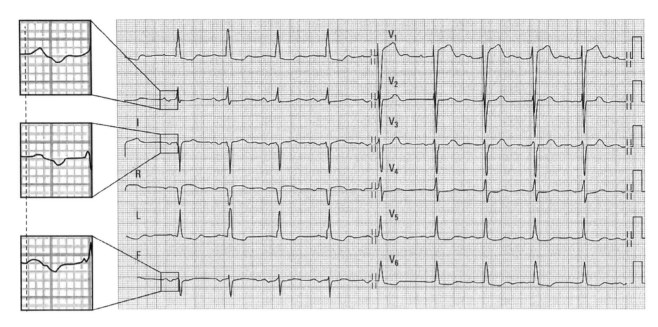

Figure 9.20 Typical ECG of advanced interatrial block (P ± in II, III, and aVF and duration > 120 ms) in a patient with ischemic cardiomyopathy. When amplified, we can see the beginning of P in the three leads.

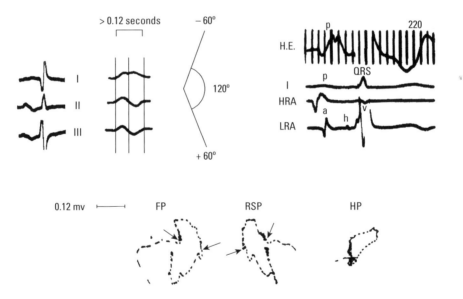

Figure 9.21 Above: P wave ± morphology in II and III typical of advanced interatrial block with retrograde conduction to the left atrium. Observe how the ÂP and the angle between the direction of the activation in the first and second parts of the P wave are measured. To the right, intra-esophageal ECG (HE) and endocavitary registrations (HRA: high right atrium; LRA: low right atrium) demonstrate that the electrical stimulus moves first downwards (HRA–LRA) and then upward (LRA–HE). Below: P loop morphology in the three planes with the inscription of the second part moving upward.

in leads I, II, or III. This ECG parameter has also been used for diagnosis of LAE (see Table 9.2). In fact, the delay in atrial conduction, rather than the increased atrial mass, explains the increase of P wave duration. As has been as previously explained, the sensitivity for LAE of this criterion in many series (Ariyarajah *et al.* 2006b; Lee *et al.* 2007; Tsao *et al.* 2008) is low because the cohort studied probably included many cases of isolated interatrial block.

The P wave morphology in V1 usually presents with a negative mode of the P wave that is less evident than in cases of LAE because the P loop is directed in a less backward direction in isolated first-degree interatrial block (Figure 9.12B) (Bayés de Luna 2012; Spodick and Ariyarajah 2008).

Finally, the prevalence of first-degree interatrial block in the general population is very high (Spodick and

Ariyarajah 2008, 2009). Recently, it has been shown to be associated with atrial fibrillation (Holmqvist *et al.* 2010), and cardiovascular and all-cause mortality (Magnani *et al.* 2011).

Third-degree (advanced) interatrial block (Figures 9.18A, 9.19B and 9.20) (see Table 9.3)

Electrical impulse is blocked in the upper part of the septum (Bachmann bundle zone), and as the rest of the septum is of connective tissue the breakthrough to LA has to be performed retrogradely from the AV junction zone (Bayés de Luna *et al.* 1985, 1988; Platonov 2008). In very rare cases, atrial dissociation may exist (see below).

Waldo *et al.* (1971) (Figure 9.16 A) demonstrated that cutting the Bachmann's bundle in dogs, and Guerra (Figure 9.16B) provoking transient A-IAB with ice in a open chest of a pig, causes a similar morphology, with P wave +– in inferior leads (Figure 9.18A, B) (Daubert 1996).

Typical ECG pattern

In typical cases, the **ECG shows** (Figures 9.19C and 9.20) **a P wave of ≥0.12 sec and ± morphology in II, III, and aVF** due to caudocranial activation of the left atrium (Puech 1956; Castillo Fenoy and Vernant 1971). Our group defined the ECG–VCG criteria (Bayés de Luna *et al.* 1985) and demonstrated that this type of block is a very specific marker for LAE (≈ 90%) but with very low sensitivity (SE). Figure 9.21 shows (A is above) the typical ECG and VCG pattern, with ± P in II, III, and aVF, and open VCG loops in FP with the final part of the loops upward. Occasionally, (B is below) the loop is closed in FT probably due to fibrosis but the second part of the loop is also upward (Figure 9.21). This figure also shows that the atrial stimulus moves first downward (HRA-LRA and after upward LRA-high esophageal). Figure 9.22 shows the endocranial

mapping in a cases of A-IAB, demonstrating the endocraneal activation of the LA.

We demonstrated (Figure 15.4) (Bayés de Luna *et al.* 1988, 1989, 1999) that this type of A-IAB is frequently accompanied by atrial fibrillation and/or atrial flutter, during follow-up especially in patients with heart diseases (see Chapter 15). Recently, this association is considered an electrocardiographic clinical syndrome (Braunwald 1998) that has been named Bayes syndrome by Baranchuk (Conde and Baranchuk. 2014a, 2014b) (Bacharova and Wagner, 2015; Baranchuk 2017).

Atypical pattern (Figures 9.23–9.26)

During the review of thousands of EG belonging to different series (Heart Failure, BAYES Register, REGICOR, Centenarians), it came to our attention that some A-IAB did not perfectly accomplish all the ECG diagnostic criteria, leading to the idea that some cases should be considered as "atypical A-IAB." A-IAB may be atypical due to two different variations of the classic definition in the 2012 Consensus: A. Changes in P-wave morphology (Figures 9.23–9.26); and B. Changes in P-wave duration (Table 9.3) (Figure 9.26).

A-IAB exist when there is evidence that left atrium is activated retrogradely. This may be assured if the last part of aVF is negative because this represents that the last part of the loops falls in the negative hemifield of aVF (beyond 0°) (Figure 9.24). This is the key point to assure that there is retrograde activation of LA. **In typical cases** of A-IAB, we have in these situations (A-IAB), a morphology ± in II, III, and aVF because the last part of atrial activation falls in the negative hemifield lead II, III, and aVF, and the duration of P waves is ≥ 120 ms. However, we found the following patterns that either present some

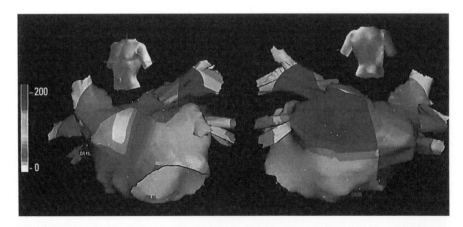

Figure 9.22 Virtual anatomic rendering of the LA in the other patient with typical biphasic (±) P wave in leads II, III, and aVF suggestive of Bachmann bundle block. Note that early left atrial activation (white) occurs at the high septal wall, as expected for Bachmann bundle conduction. Activation does not progress through the left atrial roof because of the presence of a large zone of low voltage (gray) that diverts activation toward the low septal (orange-yellow) then the low posterior (green) and finally the high posterior (violet) left atrial wall (Color Plate 6).

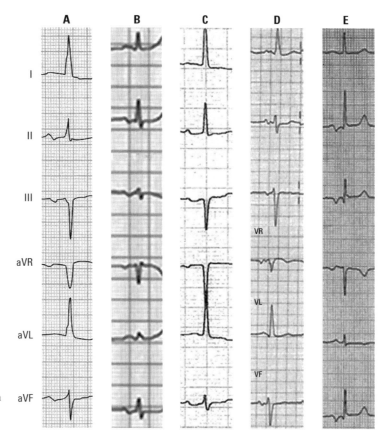

Figure 9.23 **A:** Typical A-IAB. **B:** Atypical A-IAB by duration. **C:** Type I atypical A-IAB due to morphology. The P wave is biphasic in leads III, and aVF, but the terminal component of the P wave in lead II is isodiphasic. **D:** Type II atypical A-IAB. The P wave is biphasic in leads III and aVF, but triphasic in lead II. **E:** Type III atypical A-IAB. The P wave morphology is negative in leads III and aVF, and biphasic in lead II with the initial component of the P wave in leads III and aVF isodiphasic.

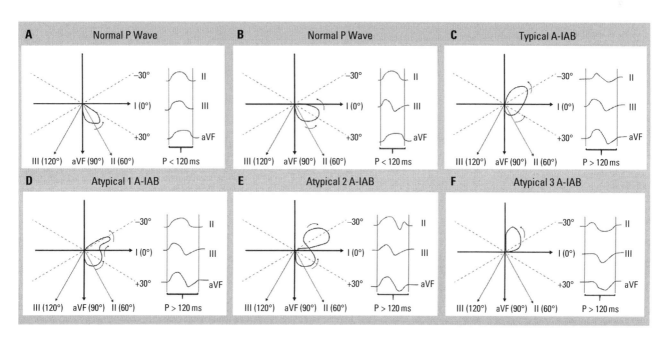

Figure 9.24 **A and B:** Normal P waves. In panel B, there is a biphasic (±) pattern in lead III. This is considered normal because the last part of the P loop falls in the negative hemifield of lead III, but it is positive in leads II and aVF, because the P loop falls in positive hemifield of these leads. **C:** Typical A-IAB. The second part of the P loop falls in the negative hemifield of leads II, III, and aVF. **D–F.** The three atypical A-IAB patterns by morphology.

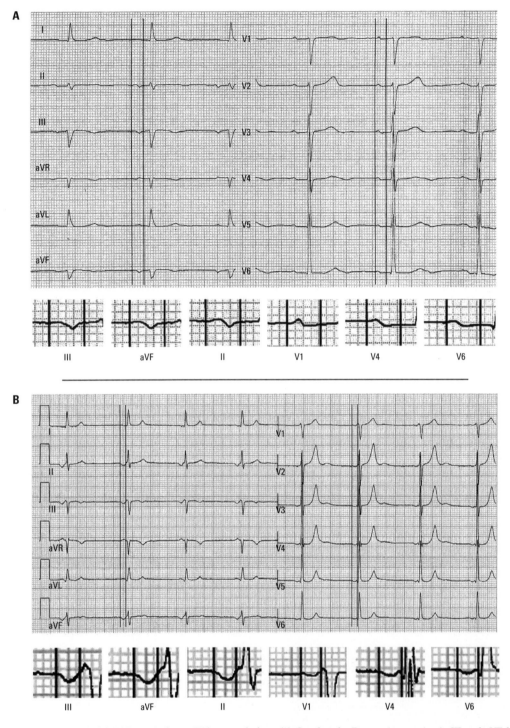

Figure 9.25 **A.** P wave in a case of A-IAB atypical type III by morphology (1). See that the P wave is negative in III and aVF, but with a
first part isodiphasic as may be seen with vertical lines. It may be confused with junctional rhythm, but in this case (see **B**), all the P wave is
negative and furthermore, the P wave is also negative in V4-V6.

morphological changes in II, III, and aVF of P wave,
but with final negativity in aVF and P duration ≥ 120 ms or a P ± in II, III, and aVF but with duration < 120 ms. Now, we explain why these patterns
may be considered atypical patterns of A-IAB.

Atypical A-IAB due to changes in P wave morphology (Figures 9.23 and 9.25)

i) **Type I:** The terminal component of the P wave in lead
II is "isodiphasic" (flat rather than negative) (Figures 9.23C
and 9.24C).

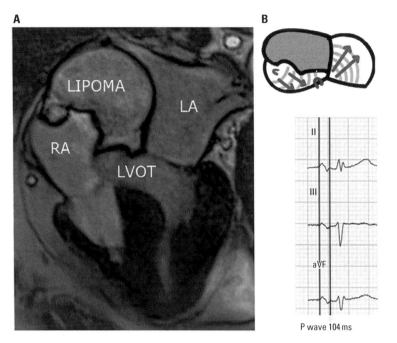

Figure 9.26 A case of 73-year-old man that has an atypical A-IAB due to duration (Figure panel B). The duration of this P wave, assessed with the use of digital calipers, is 104 ms. The patient had undergone a cardiovascular magnetic resonance (panel A) which shows a lipoma on the interatrial septum of 4×5 cm, a rare tumor that infrequently deforms both atria and compresses the superior vena cava.

ii) **Type II:** The terminal component of the P wave in lead II is "biphasic" ("negative-positive") (Figures 9.23D and 9.24E).

In these two cases, the P wave in leads III and aVF remains "biphasic" (±). The unusual morphologies of the P wave in lead II can be explained by the fact that the terminal component of the P loop falls around −30°, which corresponds to the limit between the positive and negative hemifields of lead II (**atypical pattern Type I**); or the P loop at −30° presents a final clockwise rotation moving from the negative hemifield to the positive hemifield of lead II (**atypical pattern Type II**).

iii) **Type III** (Figures 9.23E and 9.24F) is seen when the P wave morphology in leads III and aVF is completely negative, and biphasic in lead II. This pattern requires a differential diagnosis with junctional atrial ectopic rhythms (Figure 9.25). The first part of the P wave in leads III and aVF is isodiphasic. In this case, the first part of the P loop starts between 0° and −30°, and therefore, the first part of P wave is positive in lead II because it still falls in the positive hemifield of this lead that goes up to −30°, but is isodiphasic or negative in leads III and aVF, because it falls already in the negative hemifield of these leads. It requires differential diagnosis with junctional rhythm. Check the polarity of the P waves in leads V5-V6 that is positive in atypical A-IAB, and negative in junctional rhythm, and the morphology of lead II that is ± in atypical A-IAB and in junctional rhythm (Figure 9.25).

Atypical A-IAB due to changes in P wave duration (Figure 9.26)

Atypical patterns due to changes in duration occur when the morphology of A-IAB is usually typical but the duration of P wave is shorter than 120 ms, what was established in the consensus document in 2012 (Bayés de Luna *et al*). In this consensus, a cut-off for P wave duration of 120 ms was chosen due to the easy way of measurement (three grids in the ECG paper). However, several prior studies, have used 110 ms as already marker of block, a less specific but more sensitive parameter. This may be the case of young athletes that may have detected arrhythmias by echo with P wave < 120 ms.

Usually, in A-IAB there is a longer duration of P wave (≥ 120 ms) because not only the sinus impulse has to follow a longer way but also because usually, there is fibroric atrial, CM, and this provokes a delay of conduction. However, in some circumstances such as young age or in the presence of a cause of A-IAB not related with fibrosis (i.e. atrial tumor) (Figure 9.26), the presence of A-IAB may be explained by the presence of atrial block in Bachmann zone but the duration of P wave may still last less than 120 ms, because there is not fibrosis important in the rest of the atria, and consequently the degree of IAB is less.

We consider that it is important to learn these atypical patterns of A-IAB, because it will allow the proper identification of these cases as A-IAB. It also would allow differentiating Type III from junctional rhythm (Table 9.3) (Figure 9.25). Therefore, although these atypical patterns may be infrequent, it is necessary to know what the real prevalence is in different clinical setting. According our experience, we consider that don't seems that these patterns represent more danger of complications than the typical A-IAB patterns. Although it has to be proved, probably the atypical pattern that represents more advanced IAB is the atypical pattern type III by morphology.

Second-degree atrial block (Figures 9.27 and 9.28)

Second-degree interatrial block appears transiently and may be advanced (Figure 9.27) and more rarely, partial. It is also known as atrial aberrancy (Chung 1972; Julià *et al.* 1978) (Figure 9.28) because it manifests as P waves that vary in shape from one beat to another. This type of atrial block may appear in the following circumstances: (i) be induced by atrial or ventricular premature complexes (Figure 9.28); (ii) appear and disappear suddenly and transiently in one ECG; (iii) show a P wave that changes morphology in successive ECGs, progressive A-IAB (Figure 9.27).

Sometimes the interatrial block is progressive (Figure 9.29). The P wave changes from normal to P-IAB and finally A-IAB (Benito *et al.* 2017).

Changes of P wave morphology not due to atrial block (Figure 9.30)

These changes in P wave morphology, that we have discussed, are caused by variations in the atrial path of the sinus impulse through the atria. They should be differentiated from changes induced by breathing, atrial fusion beats, and artifacts, including diaphragmatic contraction (Bayés de Luna 2012).

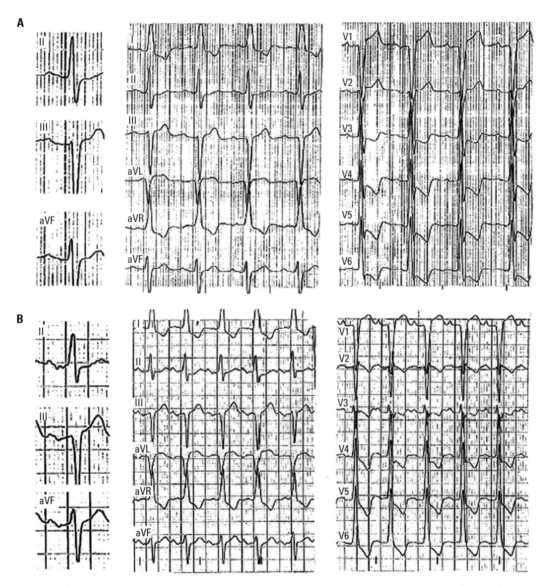

Figure 9.27 (A) Surface ECG of a 77-year-old man with hypertrophic cardiomyopathy. Heart rate of 70 bpm: P wave 160 ms (partial IAB) and QRS pattern depicting left ventricular hypertrophy with strain. (B) Same patient was hospitalized due to a febrile episode (39°). The heart rate increased to 100 bpm, the P wave depicts a typical pattern of advanced IAB (biphasic morphology in leads II, III, and aVF) and duration of 175 ms. The advanced IAB pattern is associated with a tachycardia-dependent (Phase-3) block. This ECG pattern normalized after fever was controlled and heart rate decreased.

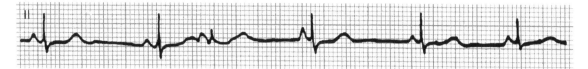

Figure 9.28 A patient with aberrant atrial conduction ectopically induced by a premature atrial complex. After this premature complex, a transitory P wave with a different morphology and a PR interval equal to previous PR intervals is observed. Other explanations to this change (atrial escape, artifact, etc.) are unlikely.

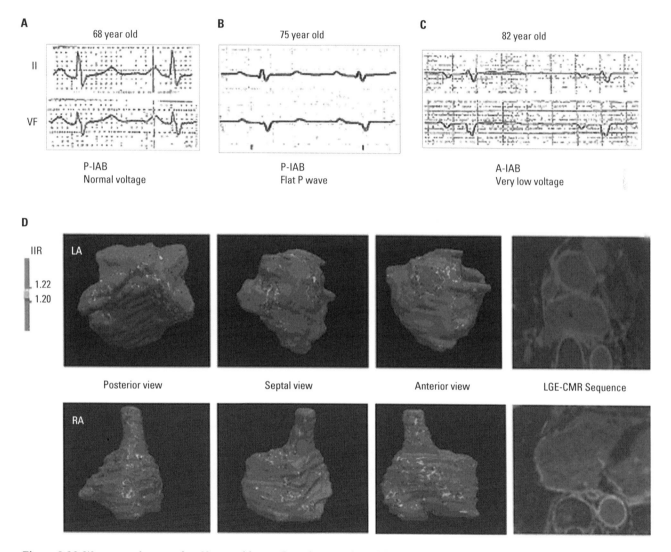

Figure 9.29 We present the case of an 82-year-old man. Over the years, his ECG pattern has developed from normal P wave to P-IAB and later A-IAB (Panel A to C) and presents short AF runs during Holter monitoring. Panel C shows that the clear A-IAB pattern with a very low voltage identifies a clear P wave with the biphasic (+) morphology. We obtained a 3D reconstruction of 3T late gadolinium enhancement cardiovascular magnetic resonance (LGE-CMR) (Panel D) showing extensive bi-atrial fibrosis with clear involvement of the upper part of the septum (Bachmann's bundle; arrows). The image intensity ratio between CMR local signal intensity of LGE and mean signal intensity of blood pool depicts the degree of fibrosis in a color scale (dense fibrosis in red) (Color Plate 7).

Atrial dissociation (Chung 1971; Zipes and De Joseph 1973; Soler Soler and Angel Ferrer 1974; Gomes *et al.* 1981)

Atrial dissociation, also known as complete interatrial block, is seen very rarely. It exists when atrial depolarization is produced by two wave fronts and the part of the atrium depolarized by one wave front remains completely separate (dissociated) from the part of the atrium depolarized by the other wave front. Only one of the two wave fronts captures the ventricles. Therefore, the electrical activation of one part of the atria is independent from that of the other part.

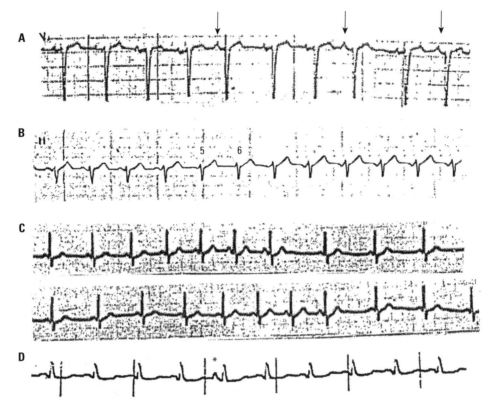

Figure 9.30 P waves with different morphologies that have to be differentiated from intermittent atrial block. (A) Late premature atrial complexes (see arrows). (B) Wandering pacemaker between the sinus node (four fast complexes) and junctional rhythm (negative P wave) (last six complexes). The fifth and sixth atrial waves are fusion beats. (C) Changes in P wave polarity and morphology in relation to inspiration. (D) Isolated change in only one P wave, probably due to an artifact.

The rhythm may be a combination of two of the following rhythms: sinus rhythm, atrial fibrillation, atrial flutter, or ectopic atrial tachycardia. The association of atrial flutter plus atrial fibrillation has been described as fibrillo flutter (Puech 1956) (see Figure 15.27).**In the presence of the combination of sinus rhythm in right atrium and atrial fibrillation in the left atrium,** sinus rhythm with regular P waves coincides with the presence of "f" waves of fibrillation (Figure 9.31). A differential diagnosis (Soler Soler and Angel Ferrer 1974) should be made with atrial aberrancy, atrial fusion beats produced by late atrial extrasystoles, diaphragmatic contractions caused by hiccups, patients with severe respiratory insufficiency, artifacts such as in Parkinson's disease (see Figure 15.42), electrical artifacts due to technical defects, pacemakers, or atrial parasystole in cases where ectopic left atrial rhythm exists. Parasystole results from a focus of unidirectional entrance block, which can capture both atria, in contrast to what occurs in atrial dissociation. Consequently, atrial fusion complexes may occur in parasystole but not in atrial dissociation. The diagnosis of atrial dissociation usually needs to be confirmed using intracavitary studies (Soler Soler and Angel Ferrer 1974). **Intravascular recording from the inferior vena cava is very useful to differentiate between false atrial dissociation**

due to diaphragmatic potential and true atrial dissociation (Figure 9.32) (Ebagosti *et al.* 1988). The electrical activity mimicking the P waves disappears completely during apnea.

Atrial dissociation is usually seen in very ill patients and, according to Chung (1971), often occurs in late stages of congestive heart failure. In fact, incidence is a rarity and misdiagnosis and confusion with the previously mentioned entities often takes place.

P wave changes in atrial infarction (Figure *9.33*)

It has been described that the **P wave may show changes in cases of atrial infarction** (see Chapter 20). The changes in the P wave appear later than the changes in STa–Ta. The following may be found: notches, slurrings, delayed ascent of the P wave or even the presence of a –+ morphology as an expression of the "Qa" wave (Zimmerman 1968). Recently, Alvarez-García *et al* (2016) has demonstrated that selective atrial coronary artery occlusion during elective percutaneous transluminal coronary angioplasty is associated with myocardial ischemic damage, atrial arrhythmias, and intra-atrial conduction delay. Our data suggest that atrial ischemic episodes might be considered as a potential cause of atrial fibrillation in patients with chronic coronary artery disease.

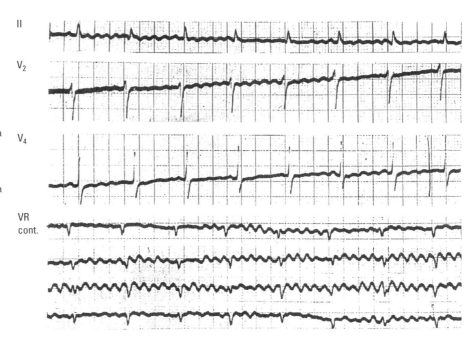

Figure 9.31 Intra-auricular dissociation: unilateral auricular fibrillation with regular ventricular rhythm at 83 bpm. In all leads, we can identify typical "f" waves of atrial fibrillation. This shows different degrees of electrical "organization," as shown in the changes in dimension and frequency of the f waves in VR (continuous trace). When the f waves are of low voltage (leads V2 and V4), we can perfectly identify P waves preceding every QRS complex with a normal PR interval. Thus, sinus rhythm coexists with auricular fibrillation that never captures the ventricles. (Figure supplied by Dr J Soler, Barcelona).

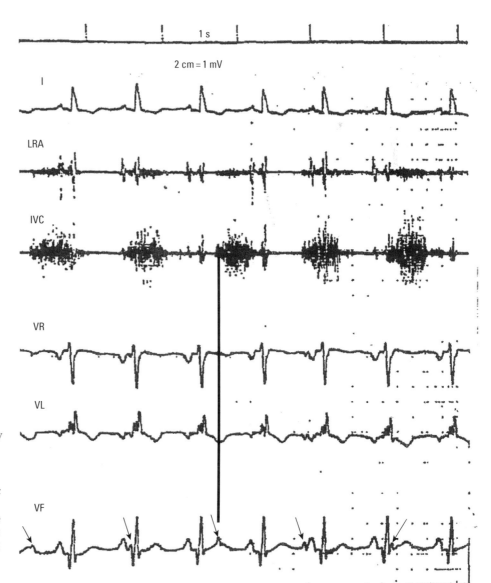

Figure 9.32 Simultaneous recording of low right atrium (LRA) and inferior vena cava (IVC) in a patient with pulmonary insufficiency. The electrical activity recorded in the surface ECG has the appearance of sinus rhythm coexisting with an ectopic atrial rhythm. After comparison with LRA and IVC recordings, we can see that the presumed ectopic atrial P waves (see VF) are caused by diaphragmatic contractions. (Reproduced with permission from Ebagosti *et al.* (1988)).

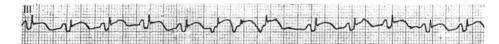

Figure 9.33 A 55-year-old patient with extensive acute anteroseptal and diaphragmatic infarction. Observe two of the most characteristic signs of atrial propagation of the infarction: (1) frequent supraventricular arrhythmias and (2) depression of the PR segment >1 mm.

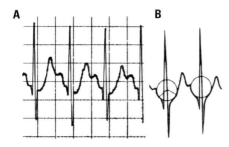

Figure 9.34 (A) Typical example of sympathetic overdrive. ECG of a 22-year-old male obtained from a Holter continuous recording device during a parachute jump. (B) Drawing of the tracing in which we see how the PR and ST segments form the arch of a circumference whose center is located in the lower third of the R downstroke.

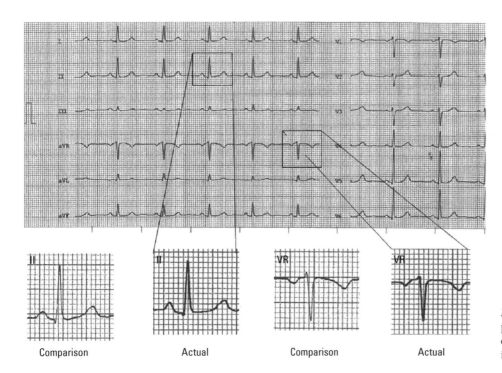

Comparison   Actual   Comparison   Actual

Figure 9.35 A case of recurrent pericarditis. Note the PR elevation in VR and a "mirror" image in lead II.

In practice, this appears very rarely, possibly because the P wave (the "Cinderella" of the ECG) is not examined carefully enough.

Atrial repolarization disturbances (Zimmerman 1968) (Figures 9.34 and 9.35)

The atrial repolarization (ST–Ta) normally has a polarity opposite to that of the P wave and is recorded between the end of P and the end of QRS (PR segment and onset of QT interval). Under normal circumstances, it is hidden by the QRS complex, although may be seen in cases of sympathetic overdrive (Figure 9.33) or first-degree AV block.

The abnormalities of atrial repolarization may be: (i) a depression of ST/Ta or (ii) an elevation of the ST/Ta.

Depressed ST/Ta: The ST/Ta depression has a polarity opposite to that of the P wave and is seen as a depression of the PR segment. Therefore, it may be seen in pericarditis and atrial infarction as an expression of atrial injury, showing a **PR segment depression in the majority of leads, except for aVR, in which a PR segment elevation in a mirror pattern is observed. When atrial infarction is suspected, a depression of at least 1 mm is required for diagnosis (Figure 9.34). PR elevation in aVR opposed to negative PR in inferior leads is sometimes seen in cases of acute pericarditis as the only change (see II and VR, Figure 9.32) (see Chapter 20).**

The depression of the PR segment can be confused with advanced interatrial block (P± in II, III, and aVF) and can mimic a false elevation of the ST segment.

Elevated ST/Ta: In this case, the P wave and ST/Ta have the same polarity. The elevation of ST/Ta recorded as an elevation of the PR segment in leads with positive P waves is occasionally seen in atrial infarction (see Chapter 13, section "Atrial infarction"). It is more specific for the diagnosis of atrial infarction than ST–Ta depression, but is rarely found (Zimmerman 1968). Elevated ST/Ta can also be seen exceptionally in other scenarios of atrial injury.

Clinical implications of P wave abnormalities: P wave indices

In recent years, it has been clearly demonstrated that the explanation of the P wave abnormalities is, especially in old people, due to the presence of LA fibrotic myocardiopathy (Kottkamp 2012; Inoue *et al.* 2018) and LA dyssynchrony (Ciuffo *et al.* 2018). Both situations may lead to the new concept of LA failure (Bisbal *et al.* 2020). The best noninvasive technique to detect both, LA fibrotic MC and LA dyssynchrony is the MR (Marrouche *et al.* 2014). However, recently (Montserrat *et al.* 2015), it has been demonstrated that echo speckle-tracking may be a surrogate for MR. Even, we can now affirm that the presence of advanced interatrial block (A-IAB) is a surrogate of decrease in LA strain detected by echo speckle-tracking, and therefore, we can affirm that the diagnosis of A-IAB in the elderly is equivalent to the presence of fibrotic LA myocardiopathy (Lacalzada-Almeida *et al.* 2017, 2018) (Bayés de Luna *et al.* 2020a). Also, recently it has been demonstrated (Ciuffo *et al.* 2020) that the presence of A-IAB is associated with atrial fibrosis and left atrial dyssynchrony detected by CMR.

Finally, some P wave indices, especially A-IAB and P wave axis, are risk markers of atrial fibrillation (Bayes syndrome) (Enriquez *et al.* 2015; Massó-van Roessel *et al.* 2017), stroke (Bayes de Luna *et al.* 2017; Enriquez *et al.* 2015) and even dementia and all types of death (Magnani *et al.* 2010, 2011; Nielsen *et al.* 2015; Martínez-Sellés *et al.* 2020a,2020b; Bayés de Luna *et al.* 2020a; Maheshwari *et al.* 2017, 2019; Martínez-Sellés *et al.* 2016; O'Neal and Zhang 2016; Park *et al.* 2016) (Figures 9.36 and 9.37).

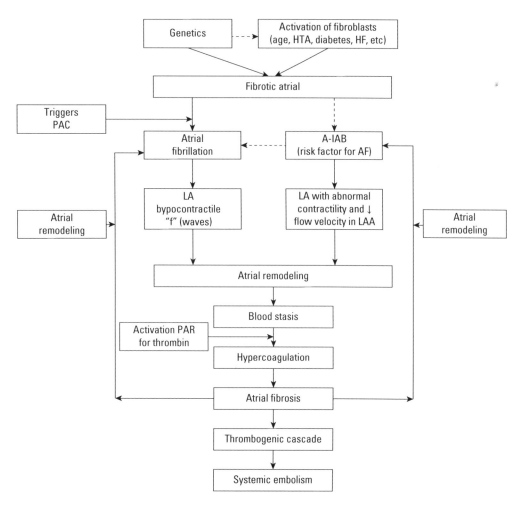

Figure 9.36 Pathophysiological events relating atrial fibrillation (AF) and advanced interatrial block (A-IAB) to systemic embolism. CM = cardiomyopathy; LA = left atrium; LAA = left atrial appendage; PAC = premature atrial contractions; PAR = protease-activated receptor.

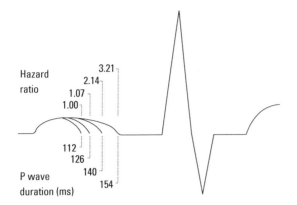

Figure 9.37 ECGs showing increasing HR for all-cause mortality in a multivariable analysis incorporating gender, age, race, heart rate, BMI, smoking habits, ratio of total to high-density lipoprotein cholesterol, hypertension, and diabetes. The figure shows the corresponding progressive increase of P wave duration by standard deviation with the respective associated HR for all-cause mortality (Adapted with permission from Magnani *et al.* 2011).

Therefore, it seems that it is already time to perform a randomized trial with two arms, NOA vs. placebo to demonstrate if anticoagulation may be useful in patients with these altered P wave indices to decrease the incidence of stroke or some other complications.

References

Alexander B, Milden J, Hazim B, *et al.* New electrocardiographic score for the prediction of atrial fibrillation: the MVP ECG risk score (morphology-voltage-P wave duration). *Ann Noninvasive Electrocardiol* 2019;24(6):e12669. doi:https://doi.org/10.1111/anec.12669.

Alvarez-García J, Vives-Borrás M, Gomis P, *et al.* Electrphysiological effects of selective atrial coronary artery occlusion in humans. *Circulation* 2016;133:2235–2242.

Ariyarajah V, Fisella ME, Spodick DH. Reevaluation of the criterion for interatrial block. *Am J Cardiol* 2006a;98:936.

Ariyarajah V, Apiyasawat S, Puri P, *et al.* Specific electrocardiographic markers of P-wave morphology in interatrial block. *J Electrocardiol* 2006b;39:380.

Bacharova L, Wagner GS. The time for naming the interatrial block syndrome: Bayes syndrome. *J Electrocardiol* 2015;48:133.

Baranchuk A. *Interatrial block and supraventricular arrhythmias: Clinical implications of Bayés' Syndrome.* Cardiotext Publishing, Minneapolis, Minnesota, USA, 2017.

Bartell H, Desser K, Benchimol A. Echocardiographic left atrial enlargement: ECG/VCG criteria for detection. *J Electrocardiol* 1978;11:355.

Bayés de Luna A. *Clinical Electrocardiography: A Textbook.* Willey-Blackwell, 2012.

Bayés de Luna A. Baranchuk A. *Clinical Arrhythmology*, 2nd edn. Wiley-Blackwell, 2017.

Bayés de Luna A, Boada FX, Casellas A, *et al.* Concealed atrial electrical activity. *J Electrocardiol* 1978a;11:301.

Bayés de Luna A, Fort de Ribot R, Coll S, *et al.* Estudio ECG/VCG del transtorno de conducción auricular derecho. Actas do VIII Congresso Luso Español de Cardiología. *Sociedad Portuguesa de cardiología*, 1978b.

Bayés de Luna A, Fort de Ribot R, Trilla E, *et al.* Electrocardiographic and vectorcardiographic study of interatrial conduction disturbances with left atrial retrograde activation. *J Electrocardiol* 1985;18:1.

Bayés de Luna A, Cladellas M, Oter R, *et al.* Interatrial conduction block and retrograde activation of the left atrium and paroxysmal supraventricular tachycarrhythmias. *Eur Heart J* 1988;9:1112.

Bayés de Luna A, Cladellas M, Oter R, *et al.* Interatrial conduction block with retrograde activation of the left atrium and paroxysmal supraventricular tachyarrhythmic treatment. *Int J Cardiol* 1989;22:147–150.

Bayés de Luna A, Guindo J, Viñolas X, *et al.* Third-degree interatrial block and supraventricular tachyarrhythmias. *EP* 1999;1:43–46.

Bayés de Luna A, Platonov P, García-Cosio F, *et al.* Interatrial blocks. A separate entity from left atrial enlargement: a consensus report. *J Electrocardiol* 2012;45:445–451.

Bayés de Luna A, Martínez-Sellés M, Bayés-Genís A, *et al.* Surface ECG interatrial block-guided treatment for stroke prevention: rationale for an attractive hypothesis. *BMC Cardiovasc Disord* 2017;17:211.

Bayés de Luna A, Baranchuk A, Niño Pulido C, *et al.* Second-Degree Interatrial block: Brief review and concept. *Ann Noninv Electrocardiol* 2018a;23(6):e12583. doi:https://doi.org/10.1111/anec.12583

Bayés de Luna A, Escobar-Robledo LA, Aristizabal D, *et al.* Atypical advanced interatrial block: Definition electrocardiographic recognition. *J Electrocardiol* 2018b;51:1091–1093.

Bayés de Luna A, Martínez-Sellés M, Elosua R, *et al.* Relation of advanced interatrial block to risk of atrial fibrillation and stroke. *Am J Cardiol* 2020a;125:1745.

Bayés de Luna A, Martínez-Sellés M, Bayés-Genís A, *et al.* Síndrome de Bayés. Lo que todo clínico debe conocer. What every clinician should know about Bayés Syndrome. *Rev Esp Cardiol (Engl Ed)* 2020b;73:758–762.

Benito EM, Bayés de Luna A, Baranchuk A, Mont L, Extensive atrial fibrosis assessed by late gadolinium enhancement cardiovascular magnetic resonance associated with advanced interatrial block electrocardiogram pattern. *EP* 2017;19:377.

Bisbal F, Baranchuk A, Braunwald E, *et al.* Atrial Failure as a Clinical Entity. *J Am Coll Cardiol* 2020;75:222–232.

Bosch X, Bayés de Luna A, Doxandabaratz R *et al.* The value of ECG and VCG in diagnosis of left atrial enlargement. In Abel H, Zamirov R (eds). *Advances in Cardiology—Electrocardiography VI.* S Karger, 1981, p. 239.

Braunwald E. Foreword. In *Bayés de Luna A Clinical Electrocardiography: A Textbook.* Futura Publishing Company, Inc, New York 1998. ISBN:0-87993-682-7

Castillo Fenoy A, Vernant P. Les troubles de la conduction interauriculaire pour bloc du faisceau du Bachmann. *Arch Mal Coeur Vaiss* 1971;64:1490.

Chou TC, Helm RA. The pseudo P pulmonale. *Circulation* 1965;32:96.

Chung E. A reappraisal of atrial dissociation. *Am J Cardiol* 1971;28:111.

Chung EK. Aberrant atrial conduction: Unrecognized electrocardiographic entity. *Br Heart J* 1972;34:341.

Ciuffo L, Inoue YY, Tao S, *et al*. Mechanical dyssynchrony of the left atrium during sinus rhythm is associated with history of stroke in patients with atrial fibrillation. *Eur H J-Cardiovasc Imaging* 2018;19:433–441.

Ciuffo L, Bruña V, Martínez-Sellés M, *et al*. Association between interatrial block, left atrial fibrosis, and mechanical dyssynchrony: Electrocardiography-magnetic resonance imaging correlation. *J Cardiovasc Electrophysiol* 2020;31:1719–1725.

Conde D, Baranchuk A. Bloqueo interauricular como sustrato anatómico-eléctrico de arritmias supraventriculares: Sindrome de Bayés. *Arch Cardiol Mex* 2014a;84(1):32–40.

Conde D, Baranchuk A. What a cardiologist must know about Bayés' Syndrome. *Rev Argent Cardiol* 2014b;82:220–222.

Daubert JC. Atrial flutter and interatrial conduction block. In Waldo A, Touboul P (eds). *Atrial Flutter*. Futura Publishing, 1996, p. 33.

Ebagosti A, Gueunoun M, Torresani J. Diaphragmatic origin of false atrial dissociation evidenced through intravascular recordings. *J Electrocardiol* 1988;21:111.

Enriquez A, Sarrias A, Villuendas R, *et al*. New-onset atrial fibrillation after cavotricuspid isthmus ablation: identification of advanced interatrial block is key. *EP* 2015;17:1289–1293.

Escobar-Robledo LA, Bayés de Luna A, Lupón J, *et al*. Advanced Interatrial Block Predicts New-onset Atrial Fibrillation and Ischemic Stroke in Patients with Heart Failure: The "Bayes Syndrome-HF" Study. *Int J Cardiol* 2018;271:174–180.

Gomes JA, Jang P, Matheson M, *et al*. Coexistence of sick sinus rhythm and atrial flutter. *Circulation* 1981;63:80.

Guerra J. Vilahur G, Bayés de Luna A, *et al*. Interatrial block can occur in the absence of left atrial enlargement: New experimental model. *Pacing Clin Electrophysiol* 2020;43:427.

Hancock EW, Deal BJ, Mirvis DM, Okin P, Kligfield P, Gettes LS. AHA/ACCF/HRS recommendations for the standardization and interpretation of the electrocardiogram part V: Electrocardiogram changes associated with Cardiac Chamber Hypertrophy a scientific statement from the American Heart Association Electrocardiography and Arrhythmias Committee, Council on Clinical Cardiology; the American College of Cardiology Foundation; and the Heart Rhythm Society. *Circulation* 2009;119:e251–e261.

Hazen MS, Marwick TH, Underwood DA. Diagnostic accuracy of the resting electrocardiogram in detection and estimation of left atrial enlargement: an echocardiographic correlation in 551 patients. *Am Heart J* 1991;122:823.

Heikila J, Luomanmaki K. Value of serial P wave changes in indication left heart failure in myocardial infarction. *Br Heart J* 1970;32:510.

Holmqvist F, Platonov P, Carlson J, *et al*. Abnormal P wave morphology is a predictor of atrial fibrillation in MADIT II patients. *Ann Noninvasive Electrocardiol* 2010;15:63.

Inoue YY, Ipek EG, Khurram IM, *et al*. Relation of Electrocardiographic Left Atrial Abnormalities to Risk of Stroke in Patients with Atrial Fibrillation. *Am J Cardiol* 2018;122:242.

Josephson ME, Kastorm JA, Morganroth J, ECG left atrial enlargement: Electrophysiologic, echocardiographic and hemodynamic correlates. *Am J Cardiol* 1977;39:967.

Julià J, Bayés de Luna A, Candell J, *et al*. Aberrancia auricular: a propósito de 21 casos. *Rev Esp Cardiol* 1978;31:207.

Kaplan J, Evans G, Foster E, *et al*. Evaluation of ECG criteria for right atrial enlargement by quantitative two-dimensional echocardiography. *J Am Coll Cardiol* 1994;23:747.

Kottkamp H. Fibrotic atrial cardiomyopathy: a specific disease/ syndrome supplying substrates for atrial fibrillation, atrial tachycardia, sinus node disease, AV node disease, and thromboembolic complications. *J Cardiovasc Electrophysiol* 2012;23:797–9.

Lacalzada-Almeida J, García-Niebla J, Bayés de Luna A, Ecocardiografía de speckle tracking y bloqueo interauricular avanzado: Speckle-Tracking echocardiography and advanced interatrial block. *Rev Esp Cardiol* 2017;70(7):591.

Lacalzada-Almeida J, Izquierdo-Gómez MM, Belleyo-Belkasem C, *et al*. Interatrial block and atrial remodeling assessed using speckle tracking echocardiography. *BMC Cardiovasc Disord* 2018;18:38.

Lacalzada-Almeida J, Izquierdo-Gómez MM, García-Niebla J, *et al*. Advanced interatrial block is a surrogate for left atrial strain reduction which predicts atrial fibrillation and stroke. *Ann Noninvasive Electrocardiol* 2019;24(4):e12632. doi:https://doi.org/10.1111/anec.12632

Lee K, Appleton C, Lester S, *et al*. Relation of ECG criteria for left atrial enlargement in two-dimensional echocardiographic left atrial measurements. *Am J Cardiol* 2007;99:113.

Macruz R, Perloff JK, Case RB. A method for the electrocardiographic recognition of atrial enlargement. *Circulation* 1958;17:882.

Maheshwari A, Norby FL, Soliman E, *et al*. Abnormal P-wave axis and ischemic stroke: the atherosclerosis risk in communities study. *Stroke* 2017;48:2060–2065.

Maheshwari A, Norby FL, Roetker NS, *et al*. Refining prediction of atrial fibrillation-related stroke using the $P_2 – CHA_2DS_2$-Vasc Score. *Circulation* 2019;139(2):180–191. doi:https://doi.org/10.1161/CIRCULATIONAHA.118.035411

Magnani JW, Johnson VM, Sullivan LM, *et al*. P-Wave Indices: Derivation of reference values from the Framingham Heart Study. *Ann Noninvasive Electrocardiol* 2010;15:344.

Magnani JW, Gorodeski EZ, Johnson VM, *et al*. P wave duration is associated with cardiovascular and all-cause mortality outcomes: the National Health and Nutrition Examination Survey. *Heart Rhythm* 2011;8:93–100.

Marrouche NF, Wilber D, Hindricks G, *et al*. Association of atrial tissue fibrosis identified by delayed enhancement MRI and atrial fibrillation catheter ablation. The DECAAF study. *JAMA* 2014;311:498.

Martínez-Sellés M, Massó-van Roessel A, Álvarez-Garcia J, *et al*. (The Investigators of the Cardiac and Clinical Characterization of Centenarians (4C) registry). Interatrial block and atrial arrhythmias in centenarians: prevalence, associations, and clinical implications. *Heart Rhythm* 2016;13:645.

Martínez-Sellés M, Elosua R, Ibarrola M, *et al*. for the BAYES Registry Investigators. Advanced interatrial block and P-wave duration are associated with atrial fibrillation and stroke in older adults with heart disease: the BAYES registry. *EP* 2020a;22:1001–1008.

Martínez-Sellés M, Martínez-Larrú E, Ibarrola M, *et al*. Interatrial block and cognitive impairment in the BAYES prospective registry. *Int J Cardiol* 2020b;321:95–98.

Massó-van Roessel A, Escobar-Robledo LA, Dégano IR, *et al*. Analysis of the association between electrocardiographic P-wave characteristics and atrial fibrillation in the REGICOR Study. *Rev Esp Card* 2017;70:841.

Miller D, Eisenbergt R, Kligfield P, *et al*. Electrocardiographic recognition of left atrial enlargement. *J Electrocardiol* 1983;16:15.

Montserrat S, Gabrielli L, Bijnens B, *et al.* Left atrial deformation predicts success of first and second percutaneous atrial fibrillation ablation. *Heart Rhythm* 2015;12:11.

Morganroth J, Horowitz J, Josephson M, *et al.* Relationship of atrial fibrillatory wave amplitude of left atrial size and etiology of heart disease. *Am Heart J* 1979;97:184.

Morris JJ, Estes EH, Whalen RE, *et al.* P wave analysis in valvular heart disease. *Circulation* 1964;29:242.

Munuswamy K, Alpert MA, Marlin RH. Sensitivity and specificity of commonly used electrocardiographic criteria for left atrial enlargement determined by M-mode echocardiography. *Am J Cardiol* 1984;53:829.

Nielsen JB, Kühl JT, Pietersen A, *et al.* P-wave duration and the risk of atrial fibrillation: Results from the Copenhagen ECG Study. *Heart Rhythm* 2015;12:1887–1895.

O'Neal WT, Zhang ZM, Loehr, *et al.* Electrocardiographic advanced interatrial block and atrial fibrillation risk in the general population. *Am J Cardiol* 2016;117:1755.

Park JK, Park J, Uhm JS, *et al.* Low P-wave amplitude (<0,1mV) in lead I is associated with displaced inter-atrial conduction and clinical recurrence of paroxysmal atrial fibrillation after radiofrequency catheter ablation. *EP* 2016;18:348.

Platonov P. Atrial conduction and atrial fibrillation. What can we learn from ECG?. *Cardiol J* 2008;15:402.

Puech P. *L'activité Lectrique Auriculaire Normale et Pathologique.* Masson Edit, 1956.

Rasmussen MU, Fabricius-Bjerre A, Kumarathurai P, *et al.* Common source of miscalculation and misclassification of P-wave negativity and P-wave terminal force in lead V1. *J Electrocardiol* 2019;53:85–88.

Reeves WC, Hallahn W, Schwitter EEJ, *et al.* Two-dimensional echocardiographic assessment of ECG criteria for right atrial enlargement. *Circulation* 1981;64:387.

Sajeev JK, Koshy AN, Dewey H, *et al.* Poor reliability of P-wave terminal force V1 in ischemic stroke. *J Electrocardiol* 2019;52:47.

Sodi-Pallares D. *New Basis of Electrocardiography.* Mosby Co. Medical, 1956.

Soler Soler J, Angel Ferrer J. Complete atrial dissociation versus diaphragmatic action potentials. *Br Heart J* 1974;36:452.

Spodick DH, Ariyarajah V. Interatrial block: a prevalent, widely neglected and portentous abnormality. *J Electrocardiol* 2008;41:61.

Spodick DH, Ariyarajah V. Interatrial block. The pandemic remains poorly perceived. *Pacing Clin Electrophysiol* 2009;32:662.

Troung QA, Charipar EM, Ptaszed LM, *et al.* Usefulness of electrocardiographic parameters as compared to comuted tomography measures of left atrial volume enlargement: from the ROMICAT trial. *J Electrocardiol* 2011;44:257–264.

Tsao CW, Josephson ME, Hauser TH. Accuracy of electrocardiographic criteria for atrial enlargement: validation with cardiovascular magnetic resonance. *J Cardiovasc Magn Reson* 2008;10:7.

Velury V, Spodick D. Atrial correlates of PV1 of left atrial enlargement and relation to intraatrial block. *Am J Cardiol* 1994;73:998.

Waldo A, Harry L, Bush H Jr, *et al.* Effects on the canine P wave of discrete lesions in the specialized atrial tracts. *Circulation Res* 1971;29;452

Zimmerman HA. *The Auricular Electrocardiogram.* Charles C. Thomas Publishers, 1968.

Zipes DP, De Joseph R. Dissimilar atrial rhythm in man and dog. *Am J Cardiol* 1973;32:618.

Chapter 10
Ventricular Enlargement

Concept: preliminary considerations

The electrocardiographic concept of chamber enlargement includes wall hypertrophy, chamber dilation, and a combination of the two. Anatomically, the term "ventricular hypertrophy" refers to an increment in myocardial mass and fiber size, while "dilation" is an increase in the volume of the internal cavity.

The electrogenesis of the morphologies that appear with **ventricular enlargement** are conditioned **more by wall hypertrophy than cavity dilation**, the opposite of what occurs in atrial enlargement. On the other hand, for years it has been affirmed (Sodi-Pallares 1956) that ventricular block homolateral to the cavity involved influences the morphology. In any case, it is clear that the modifications undergone in the P, QRS, and T loops account for the morphological alterations found in the 12 ECG leads.

Mild or even moderate degrees of ventricular enlargement may **not affect ECG results**. When heart disease involving the ventricles is not very important, such as the right ventricle with mild pulmonary stenosis, or of the left ventricle with mild aortic stenosis, it can progress for some time without ECG signs of ventricular enlargement, despite the fact that the chamber enlargement has already produced some hemodynamic overload. On the other hand, with the passing of time, often the same severity of the disease responsible for the enlargement will more or less alter the ECG, signaling the stage of the disease (see below).

Echocardiography is a sensitive, innocuous, and reproducible method for determining left ventricular dilation and left ventricular mass. Its reliability is comparable to that of anatomic and angiological studies (Reichek and Deveraux 1981), and it provides more exact information than isotopic studies (Subirana *et al.* 1981). The dimensions of the right ventricle can be even better measured using two-dimensional echocardiography (Bommer *et al.* 1980).

Cardiovascular magnetic resonance imaging (CMR) is a reproducible standard of reference technique for the assessment of ventricular mass and volumes (Sheridan 1998). The correlation between CMR left ventricular mass measurements and post-mortem left ventricular weights in humans has a correlation coefficient with a range of 0.95–0.99 (Allison *et al.* 1993). CMR results correlate closely with those of echocardiography with possibly even greater accuracy in the measurement of ventricular mass (Reiter *et al.* 1986). Diagnostic and prognostic utility of the ECG for left ventricular enlargement (LVE) defined using CMR imaging in relation to ethnicity has been studied (Jain *et al.* 2010). It has been demonstrated that the ECG has a low sensitivity but high specificity with some race-related differences, if the echocardiography is the standard reference technique. However, we are not aware that any systematic comparison of the two techniques (echocardiography and CMR) exists in order to better determine the accuracy of ECG criteria for ventricular enlargement.

Critical review of the electrocardiographic concepts of systolic and diastolic overload

The ventricles are subject to two types of hemodynamic overload: systolic and diastolic. They suffer **systolic overload** when ventricular emptying is impaired. In the left ventricle, this occurs with aortic stenosis, aortic coarctation, and arterial hypertension, as well as in some cases of ischemic heart disease. In the right ventricle, systolic overload occurs with pulmonary stenosis and pulmonary hypertension. The ventricles suffer **diastolic overload** when there is excessive diastolic filling, phenomenon that occurs in the left ventricle with aortic regurgitation and in the right ventricle with atrial septal defect (ASD).

Cabrera and Monroy (1952) coined the electrocardiographic terms "systolic overload" and "diastolic overload"

Clinical Electrocardiography: A Textbook, Fifth Edition. Antoni Bayés de Luna, Miquel Fiol-Sala, Antoni Bayés-Genís, and Adrián Baranchuk.
© 2022 John Wiley & Sons Ltd. Published 2022 by John Wiley & Sons Ltd.

based on this hemodynamic concept. They report that there are ECG morphologies characteristic of these two types of ventricular overload. According to this study, systolic overload is manifested in the right ventricle by a high-voltage R morphology in V1 with a negative asymmetric T wave, while in the left ventricle, it is manifested by a high-voltage R wave in V5–V6, again with a negative asymmetric T wave. Diastolic overload in the right ventricle, in contrast, is manifested by the rSR' pattern in V1 with a negative asymmetric T wave and by a high-voltage qR morphology with a positive, tall, symmetric, and peaked T wave in the left ventricle. Our opinion is that while Cabrera's terminology is applicable in some cases, its indiscriminate use is not correct. It may be considered that, regardless of the underlying heart disease, **the ECG morphology of Cabrera's diastolic overload usually corresponds to mild or moderate stages of right or left ventricular enlargement, while the systolic overload morphology usually reflects advanced stages of ventricular enlargement ("strain pattern")** (Bayés de Luna 2012).

New concepts

Probably, correlation exists between the changes in myocardial fibers that produce myocardial "strain," detected with imaging techniques, with the electrophysiological changes that exist when LVH develops the ECG pattern of "LVH with strain" (electrical remodeling). A new conceptual model has recently been developed in which the structural, bioelectrical, and biochemical changes are interconnected and may explain ECG changes and have prognostic implications (Bacharova *et al.* 2010, 2011).

Right ventricular enlargement: hypertrophy and dilation

Concept and associated diseases

Right ventricular enlargement (RVE) is manifested in patients with systolic overload (pulmonary stenosis, pulmonary hypertension usually due to mitral valve disease) by wall hypertrophy **(right ventricular hypertrophy),** which in advanced cases is associated with some degree of dilation **(right ventricular dilation).** Dilation appears earlier in heart diseases with hemodynamic diastolic overload, such as ASD. However, in some processes (pulmonary embolism or acute decompensation in a patient with chronic obstructive pulmonary disease (COPD)), acute right ventricular dilation can appear without evident wall hypertrophy, which occurs rarely in the left ventricle.

RVE is observed mainly in infants and children with diverse types of **congenital heart disease** (pulmonary stenosis, ASD, pulmonary hypertension, Ebstein's disease,

etc.) and in adults with **valvular heart disease** (historically, mitral stenosis with right heart repercussion in particular) or some type of **cor pulmonale.**

Mechanisms of ECG changes

The existence of any type of RVE counteracts more or less the normally dominant left ventricular forces, directing the dominant forces (QRS loop and vector) to the right and forward or backward (Figure 10.1). Associated right ventricular conduction delay influences the presentation of RVE morphology. Consequently, it is not necessary that the right ventricular mass exceed the left in order for the ECG morphology of RVE to appear. The resultant depolarization vector is directed to the right because of the following association: increase in mass plus conduction delay. In global and significant RVE, the direction of repolarization is usually altered due to the fact that the right ventricular subendocardium begins to repolarize when subepicardial wall depolarization has not yet concluded, and due to the presence of some degree of right ventricular block. As a result, the T loop and corresponding T vector often follow the opposite direction to the QRS loop, which is analogous to what occurs in the left side in advanced left ventricular hypertrophy (LVH).

It should be remembered that it is difficult, if not impossible, to make an ECG diagnosis of mild RVE because the powerful left vector forces overwhelm mild, and even moderate, degrees of RVE. Therefore, the specificity and especially the sensitivity of the ECG criteria for the diagnosis of mild and moderate RVE are lower than those for diagnosing LVE.

The QRS loop in RVE has different morphologies, but mainly it is directed **to the right and forward or backward** (Figure 10.2) (see later). Projection of these loops on the frontal and horizontal planes (on the positive and negative hemifields of the different leads) illustrates the ECG modifications seen in RVE (Figures 10.2 and 10.3).

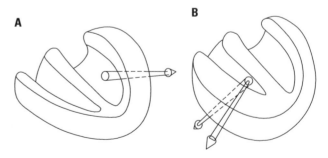

Figure 10.1 Right ventricular enlargement (RVE) counteracts the usually dominant forces of the left ventricle (A), shifting the dominant forces to the right (B), sometimes forward and other times backward (B).

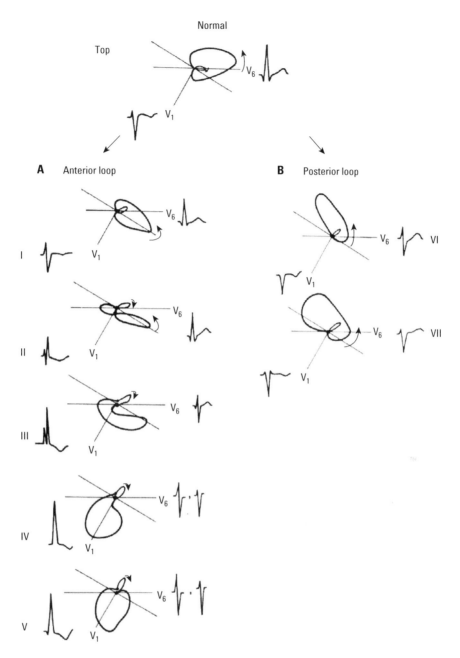

Figure 10.2 Top. Parting from a normal loop in the horizontal plane. Progressive degrees of right ventricular enlargement (RVE) always produces a rightward shift in direction, sometimes forward (A) and other times backward. (B) If the loop moves forward, (A) it produces different QRS morphologies in V1 as it becomes progressively more anterior, with R gradually becoming taller and T more negative (from I to V). Often, the loop begins rotating counterclockwise and ends up rotating clockwise, producing an rSr' morphology in V1 identical to that seen in partial right ventricular block. (B) If the RVE directs the loop to the right and backward, a normal morphology (rS) or QS or rSr' can be seen in V1, always with a marked S in V6 (VI and VII).

Changes of QRS–T in cases of progressive anterior and right QRS loop displacement (Figures 10.2 and 10.3)

This type of loop is seen in global RVE in particular, in cases of left valvular heart disease with pulmonary hypertension and in congenital heart diseases with evident RVE. With time, RVE increases in intensity and **the QRS loop becomes progressively more anterior, with its final portion directed more to the right.** In the first phase, it conserves the counterclockwise rotation in the horizontal plane (Figure 10.2I). Later, when the whole loop becomes anterior and more to the right, it rotates in a figure-of-eight or clockwise pattern (Figure 10.2II–V).

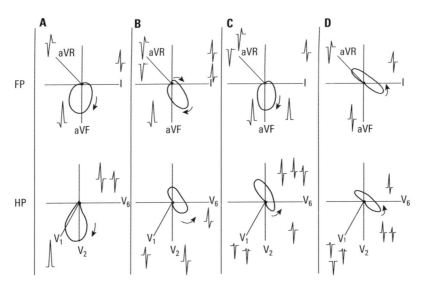

Figure 10.3 Diagram of the QRS loops in the frontal plane (FP) and horizontal plane (HP) in patients with right ventricular enlargement (RVE). B corresponds to the type of moderate RVE seen in mitral stenosis, while A corresponds to severe RVE as seen in severe pulmonary stenosis. C and D correspond to the RVE frequently seen in cor pulmonale, with right ÂQRS (C) or SI, SIII, SIII (D). The SI, SII, SIII morphology is also encountered in some cases of zonal right ventricular block, and in normal individuals. In cor pulmonale, the SI, SII, SIII morphology is probably due to late depolarization of the anterosuperior subpulmonary zone of the right ventricle, which is caused by RVE.

Type I QRS loop (Figures 10.2 and 10.3A)

This loop shows a clockwise rotation in the frontal plane and all the loop located more anteriorly (Figure 10.2A1). This loop is frequently observed in mitral stenosis with mild pulmonary hypertension, although it can be seen in almost all heart disease with mild global RVE.

The ECG **changes** (Figures 10.2–10.4) seen are as follows:
• **Frontal plane: ÂQRS somewhat to the right,** often with Rs or RS pattern in lead I, and sometimes with a small "q" (qR) in aVF and with Qr or rSr' in aVR. This is the result of the frequent clockwise rotation of the loop in the frontal plane, with some last portion lying in the negative hemifield of lead I (Figure 10.3A).
• **Horizontal plane: (i) V1:** The VCG loop maintains usually the counter clockwise rotation, but as a consequence of the more anterior position of the loop, there is an increase of "r" in V1, with R/S near 1, often with prominent R but with R < S; **(ii) V5–V6:** An Rs or RS pattern sometimes with a small "q" morphology is frequently seen in V5–V6. The **T wave** is frequently flat or mildly negative in V1 (and occasionally in V2–V3).

Type II, III, IV, or V QRS loop (Figure 10.2)

The QRS loop has a figure-of-eight rotation **in the horizontal plane** in type II, a predominantly clockwise rotation in types III and IV, and an exclusively clockwise rotation in type V. **In the frontal plane,** a progressively larger part of the final portion of the loop is observed in the negative hemifield of lead I (Figure 10.3B). The type IV and V loops of Figure 10.2 are seen in severe global RVE (severe pulmonary stenosis or severe pulmonary hypertension). The loop rotates clockwise and a large part

of the loop is directed to the right (Figures 10.2 and 10.3B). In the types II and III of Figure 10.2, a lesser part of the loop is directed to the right and the frontal plane loop morphology falls between types A and B of Figure 10.3.

The ECG changes in the frontal plane are as follows (Figures 10.2, 10.3–10.5):
• **S wave in lead I:** the greater the S wave is, the larger the loop portion directed to the right (larger in types IV and V compared to types II and III).
• **Dominant R wave in III and VF and terminal R in VR.**
• **ÂQRS right-deviated,** with the exception of the ÂQRS being left-deviated in an ostium primum-type ASD (see Figure 10.6).

The ECG changes in the horizontal plane are as follows:
• **V1 and V2: Different morphologies with a dominant R wave and a mostly negative and asymmetric T wave, according to the degree of RVE,** are seen in Figures 10.2 and 10.4–10.9. These include the range from a rsR' pattern to a unique R wave with an asymmetric and negative T wave (diastolic and systolic patterns of Cabrera) (see before). In all types (II, III, IV, and V, Figure 10.2), the T wave is usually negative in V1 and its negativity in other precordial leads reflects the increment in the degree of hypertrophy. The ST segment is commonly depressed. However, in some children with moderate and not longstanding RVE, the T wave in V1 can be positive (Figures 10.4C-10 and 10.10).

The rsR' morphology in V1 with a negative, asymmetric T is most often seen in ASD, which evolves more with right ventricular dilation than with hypertrophy (Figures 10.2II and 10.7). However, it can also be seen in

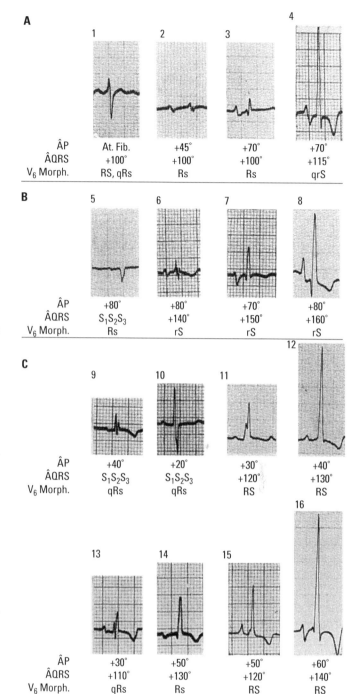

Figure 10.4 Right ventricular enlargement (RVE) is fundamentally seen in three types of processes: (A) valvular diseases with right repercussion, especially mitral stenosis; (B) lung diseases with right repercussion (cor pulmonale); and (C) certain congenital heart diseases. In (A), we can see different V1 morphologies, as well as ÂP, ÂQRS, and V6 morphologies, in different cases of mitral stenosis with associated RVE: (1 and 2) Mitral stenosis with mild pulmonary hypertension. (3) Mitral stenosis with moderate pulmonary hypertension and functional tricuspid regurgitation. (4) Mitral stenosis with severe pulmonary hypertension. The same characteristics can be seen in (B) in different types of cor pulmonale. Cases (5) and (6) correspond to chronic cor pulmonale secondary to chronic obstructive pulmonary disease (COPD) in elderly patients. Cases (7) and (8) are two cases of subacute cor pulmonale in young patients with severe pulmonary hypertension. (C) Several cases of congenital heart diseases: (9) A 9-year-old girl with mild pulmonary stenosis. (10) A case of mild pulmonary stenosis in a young boy. (11) Moderate pulmonary stenosis in a 10-year-old girl. (12) Severe pulmonary stenosis in a 16-year-old female. (13) Ostium secundum-type atrial septal defect (ASD) with mild pulmonary hypertension in an 8-year-old girl. (14) Ostium secundum-type ASD with important pulmonary hypertension in a 29-year-old woman. (15) A 10-year-old girl with typical Fallot's tetralogy. (16) A 15-year-old boy with a typical Eisenmenger syndrome. Observe how in the three situations (A, B, and C), morphologies are seen in V1 from rS or rSr' to R alone (with high voltage), according to the severity of the disease and the degree of evolution.

other heart diseases with mild RVE, such as mild pulmonary stenosis (Figure 10.4C-9).

The solitary R morphology in V1 and usually V2 with negative, asymmetric T recorded in V1–V3 and even V4 is seen in cases of important RVE and closed interventricular septum as isolated severe pulmonary stenosis, or idiopathic pulmonary hypertension (**the "barrier-type"** of the Mexican School) (Figure 10.7). In Fallot's tetralogy (pulmonary stenosis with overriding aorta and ventricular septal defect), the morphology

changes from solitary R with negative T in V1 to RS with positive T in V2, because the last part of the loop is located backward (compare Figures 10.8 and 10.9) (**the "adaptation type"** morphology of the Mexican School) (Sodi-Pallares 1956). In addition, an RS morphology with a positive T wave in V1 can be seen in moderate, not long-standing cases of Fallot's tetralogy (Figure 10.10).

• **Left precordial leads:** Usually RS or even rS morphology are recorded.

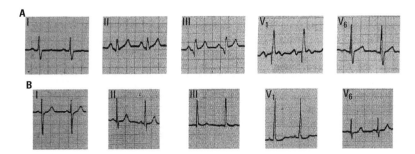

Figure 10.5 Two cases of severe right ventricular enlargement (RVE), one with great dilation of right ventricle and the other with great right ventricular hypertrophy. (A) Atrial septal defect with marked right ventricular dilation (arrow). (B) Typical ECG of RVE in a 12-year-old patient with severe pulmonary stenosis.

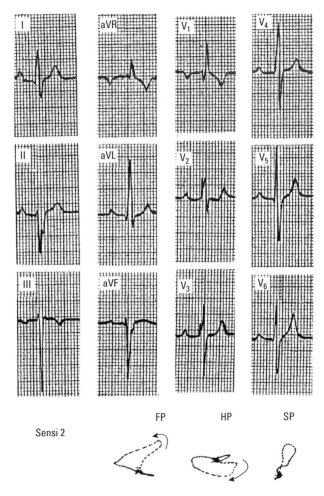

Figure 10.6 Typical morphology of ostium primum-type atrial septal defect (ASD). Observe the rSr' morphology in V1 with the ÂQRS in the frontal plane extremely deviated to the left and the ECG–VCG correlation.

Other electrocardiographic features of the anterior QRS loop

Other ECG features include:
• **increase in intrinsicoid deflection time in V1** (>0.03 sec);
• **the QRS lasting less than 0.12 sec,** unless there is associated advanced right bundle branch block (RBBB). However,

the RVE morphology is partly due to a degree of associated right peripheral block, as previously discussed.

A similar pattern in V1 may be seen in the evolutive process of RVE in different diseases (Figure 10.4)

Throughout **the evolution of right-sided heart diseases,** the QRS loop often suffers modifications, gradually **passing from the type I loop to the type V loop,** seen in Figure 10.2, over the years. **The reverse can happen after corrective surgery** in these cases (see later) (Figure 10.11).

The different ECG patterns of Figure 10.4 may be seen in congenital heart disease (Figure 10.4C), mitral stenosis (Figure 10.4A), or cor pulmonale (Figure 10.4B). The patterns with solitary R in V1 are more frequently seen in congenital heart disease with concentric RVE as pulmonary stenosis or severe pulmonary hypertension (Eisenmenger syndrome, Figure 10.4C-12 and C-16) than in mitral stenosis or ASD because these latter heart diseases usually present with milder RVE. However, if associated severe pulmonary hypertension is present, the same morphologies with solitary or predominant R can also be seen in V1 in patients with mitral stenosis (Figure 10.4A-4). Even young patients with subacute cor pulmonale and severe pulmonary hypertension may present occasionally this ECG pattern (Figure 10.4B-8). However, old patients with severe COPD usually present with the type VI or VII QRS loops (Figure 10.2) (QS or rSr' in V1 with rS or RS in V6), but with a rightward-directed ÂQRS in the FP or an SI SII SIII pattern (types C and D, Figure 10.3) during the course of the disease.

Changes of QRS–T in cases of progressive posterior and right QRS loop (Figures 10.2, 10.3, 10.12, and 10.13)

These types of loops (VI and VII of Figures 10.2, 10.3, 10.12, and 10.13), presenting significant posterior and right final forces, are especially seen in **COPD and, more rarely, in some cases of mitral stenosis.** In these cases, the RVE is located in basal posterior zones in particular, and the heart presents with a verticalized and descended position because of the low diaphragmatic

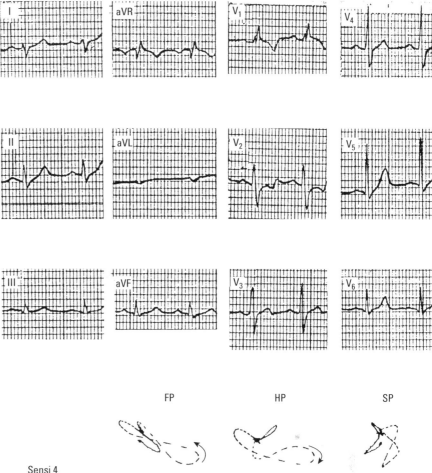

Figure 10.7 Typical morphology of ostium secundum-type atrial septal defect (ASD). Observe the rSr' morphology in V1, the right-deviated ÂQRS, and the ECG–VCG correlation.

Sensi 4

FP   HP   SP

situation frequently found in COPD. All these factors explain the predominance of the posterior forces in COPD (Figure 10.2VI–VII).

In typical cases, the QRS loop has a clockwise rotation with an open loop in the frontal plane (Figures 10.3C and 10.10), but often a folded frontal loop with a maximum axis situated at +30° to –150°, similar to the loops seen in patients with anterosuperior segmental right ventricular block and certain normal individuals (SI, SII, SIII morphology), is observed (Figures 10.3D and 10.13).

The ECG changes are as follows:
- **Frontal plane:** Two different morphologies, according to loop type: **(i) SI, SII, SIII-type ECG,** with SII≥SIII (Figure 10.2 types VI–VII and Figure 10.3D); **(ii) lead I with an S wave** (Rs or rS), **unique R in III and VF,** terminal R in aVR and right ÂQRS (Figures 10.3C and 10.12).
- **Horizontal plane: (i) V1–V2:** An **rS morphology,** sometimes with slurred S or rSr', or even QS, with rS in V2 occasionally of a much higher voltage than S in V1. The T wave is generally negative in V1 and sometimes negative in V2–V3. The P wave may also be negative, although of low voltage, in V1. **(ii) In V5–V6:** marked S or R<S (rS pattern) (Figure 10.12).

Diagnostic ECG criteria: anatomic and imaging correlations (Tables 10.1 and 10.2)

Because of the difficulties in finding diagnostic criteria for RVE that are both specific and sensitive, many have been described (Walker *et al.* 1955; Reeves 1970). Their utility largely depends on the population studied and the technique used to detect RVE. We must remember that: (i) the higher sensitivity of one criterion, the lower the specificity and (ii) criteria based on left precordial lead alterations are more sensitive but less specific, and those based on V1–V2 modifications are more specific but less sensitive.

Sensitivity increases when a population with a higher incidence of congenital heart disease or advanced right ventricular involvement is studied. Likewise, the use of autopsy material for ECG correlations can distort the results because only patients with an advanced stage of the disease are studied. Therefore, an improved evaluation of the ECG criteria for RVE can be carried out when non-invasive imaging techniques such as **echocardiography and cardiovascular CMR** are used to compare diagnostic results. **Echocardiography** has been useful in detecting right ventricular mass and volume (Bommer *et al.* 1980), showing a good correlation with autopsy

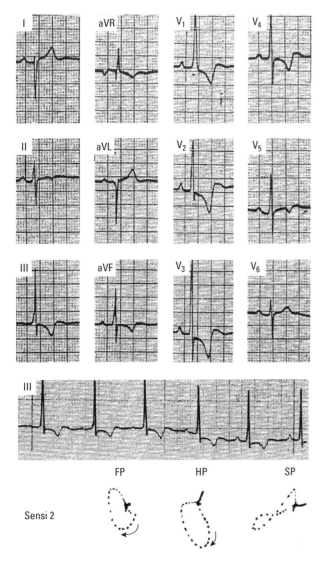

Figure 10.8 An 8-year-old patient with important pulmonary valve stenosis with a gradient over 100 mm Hg. The patient presents with a typical RVE morphology with a barrier-type systolic overload (R in V1–V2 with negative T wave). The ÂP in the ECG seems deviated leftward. In fact, the patient presents with wandering pacemaker between sinus and junctional rhythm (see strip of lead III). Note the ECG–VCG correlation.

Horan and Flowers (1980) conceived a score point system (Table 10.2) based on combinations of different criteria for RVE. This score is not useful in the presence of ventricular block or lateral infarction.

In daily practice, we must try to use very specific criteria (about 90% or more) (Table 10.1), despite the lower sensitivity, which will reduce the number of false-positive diagnoses.

In contrast, when making epidemiological studies or in cases of computerized or semi-computerized ECG interpretations (Minnesota Code) (see Chapter 25), it is necessary to use more sensitive criteria for preliminary screening.

To summarize, what can be affirmed is that in the presence of heart diseases with right involvement, and in the absence of RBBB, lateral infarction or Wolff–Parkinson–White (WPW) pattern, the ECG criteria shown in Table 10.1 are very specific for RVE.

Value of other electrocardiological techniques

Macfarlane *et al.* (1981) postulated that hybrid criteria derived from a 12-lead ECG plus three orthogonal leads would produce a sensitivity ranging from 55% to 65%. However, this scoring system has not been popularized. Pipberger *et al.* (1982) used a new classification system for epidemiological studies that increased sensitivity at the expense of specificity. It may be useful to carry out the preliminary screening.

Diagnosis of right ventricular enlargement in clinical practice (Figures 10.6–10.13)
The following are the most commonly used criteria:

• ÂQRS ≥ 110° (R < S in lead I)

• V1 = R/S > 1 and/or S in V1 < 2 mm and/or R ≥ 7 mm and/or qR

• V6 = R/S ≤ 1 and/or S V5–V6 > 7 mm.

Sensitivity will increase if there is more than one criterion (see score, Table 10.2), and in the presence of P wave abnormalities suggestive of right atrial enlargement (see Chapter 9).

Special characteristics of some types of right ventricular enlargement
Acute right ventricular dilation

We will now examine the ECG changes found when abrupt right ventricular overload accompanied by pulmonary hypertension induce right ventricular dilation. This includes cases of decompensated cor pulmonale and pulmonary embolism.

Decompensated cor pulmonale

Patients with cor pulmonale often present with acute hypoxemic episodes accompanied by pulmonary hypertension

(Prakash 1981). In the past, isotopic techniques have also been used (Subirana *et al.* 1981) (Figure 10.5), but echocardiography and CMR give better results because they are more reproducible and accurate. From a practical point of view, the use of CMR is at large scale now difficult in 2020 (see also LVE: Diagnostic ECG criteria).

We can assume that the diagnosis of RVE using the QRS criteria of right atrial enlargement (see Table 9.1; Figure 9.5) is usually certain because these criteria are usually a consequence of RVE.

In Table 10.1, ECG criteria with a specificity better than 85–90% and a corresponding low sensitivity are listed (Walker *et al.* 1955; Prakash 1981). To enhance sensitivity,

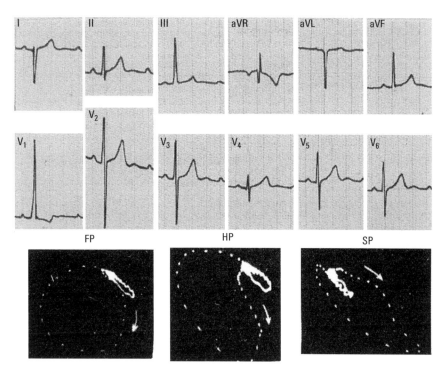

Figure 10.9 A 3-year-old patient with typical tetralogy of Fallot. The ECG corresponds to the Mexican School-named "RVE with adaptation-type systolic overload" (R in V1 with negative T and rS in V2 with positive T). Note the ECG–VCG correlation.

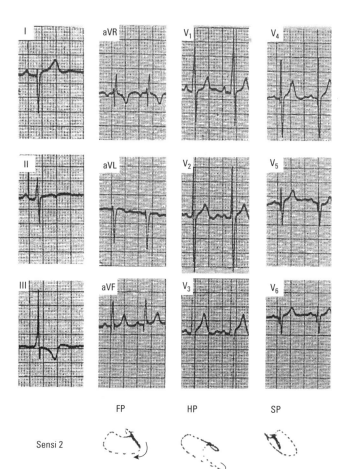

Figure 10.10 A 7-year-old patient with moderate Fallot's tetralogy and RS with positive T wave morphology in V1. Note the ECG–VCG correlation.

Sensi 2

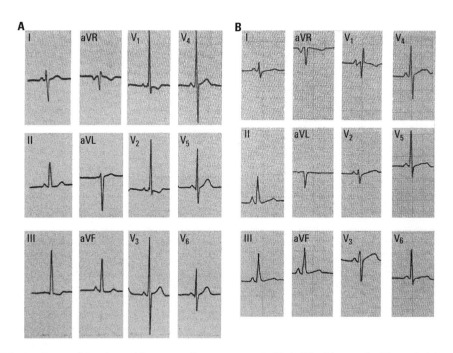

Figure 10.11 (A) ECG of an 8-year-old patient with severe pulmonary stenosis (Rs in V1 with negative T wave). After surgery (B), the morphology regressed considerably (rSR′ in V1).

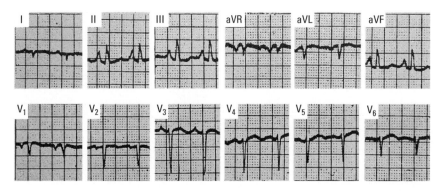

Figure 10.12 A 65-year-old patient with important chronic obstructive pulmonary disease (COPD) and no left heart disease. There is a typical P pulmonale as well as other signs of right ventricular enlargement (RVE), with the QRS loop posterior and to the right (P negative in V1, absence of the first vector in the HP, rS in V6, ÂQRS ≥110°, etc.).

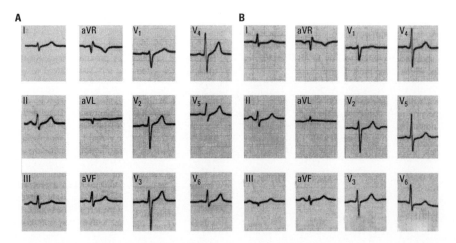

Figure 10.13 SI, SII, SIII morphology in a normal case (A) and in chronic obstructive pulmonary disease with right ventricular enlargement (RVE) (B). The ECG morphologies often do not differ. In some cases, the P and T wave pattern can help distinguish them.

Table 10.1 ECG criteria for right ventricular enlargement.

Criterion		Sensitivity (%)	Specificity (%)
V_1	$R/S\,V_1 \geq 1$	6	98
	$R\,V_1 \geq 7\,mm$	2	99
	qR in V_1	5	99
	S in $V_1 < 2\,mm$	6	98
	IDT in $V_1 \geq 0.35\,sec$	8	98
$V_5 - V_6$	$R/S\,V_5 - V_6 \geq 1$	16	93
	$R\,V_5 - V_6 < 5\,mm$	13	87
	$S\,V_5 - V_6 > 7\,mm$	26	90
$V_1 + V_6$	$R\,V_1 + S\,V_5 - V_6 > 10.5\,mm$	18	94
ÂQRS	$ÂQRS \geq 110°$	12–19	96
	$S_I\,S_{II}\,S_{III}$	24	87

that are generally reversible but accompanied by alterations in the right ventricular structure or function. In these cases, right ventricular dilation can appear without ventricular wall hypertrophy, at least in the initial stages. Dilation of the right ventricle may therefore be the initial, and sometimes the only, sign of cor pulmonale (Kilcoyne *et al.* 1970).

There are certain ECG changes that lead us to suspect that the degree of pulmonary hypertension varies abruptly as a consequence of decompensation in patients with cor pulmonale. These include:

• **ÂQRS changes,** oriented more than 30° to the right of its usual position, with RS or rS persisting until V6.

• **Presentation of a flattened or negative T wave in the right precordial leads** due to associated pulmonary affection that disappears when the affection is over (Figure 10.14). A negative T wave in the right precordial leads can also be seen in ischemic heart disease (see Chapter 13), in which case it is usually not so transient and is sometimes accompanied by a QS morphology that may also be found in right ventricular dilation (usually only in V1). The marked differences in clinical setting help to establish the diagnosis.

Table 10.2 Electrocardiographic criteria for right ventricular enlargement in adults without conduction detects known not to have infraction.

Sign	Points
1. Ratio reversal (R/S V_5: R/S $V_1 \leq 0.4$)	5
2. qR in V_1	5
3. R/S ratio in $V_1 > 1$	4
4. S in $V_1 < 2\,mm$	4
5. R in V_1 + S in V_5 or $V_6 > 10.5\,mm$	4
6. Right axis deviation $>110°$	4
7. S in V_5 or $V_6 \geq 7\,mm$ and each $\geq 2\,mm$	3
8. R/S in V_5 or $V_6 \leq 1$	3
9. R in $V_1 \geq 7\,mm$	3
10. S_1, S_{II} and S_{III} each $\geq 1\,mm$	2
11. S_I and Q_{III} each $\geq 1\,mm$	2
12. R' in V_1 earlier than 0.08 and $\geq 2\,mm$	2
13. R peak in V_1 or V_2 between 0.04 and 0.07	1
14. S in V_5 or $V_6 \geq 2\,mm$ but $<7\,mm$	1
15. Reduction in V lead R/S ratio between V_1 and V_4	1
16. R in V_5 or $V_6 < 5\,mm$	1

Interpretation of point score:

10 points: Right ventricular enlargement

7–9 points: Probable right ventricular enlargement or hemodynamic overload

5–6 points: Possible right ventricular enlargement or hemodynamic overload.

These criteria do not take into account serial electrocardiographic comparisons. Such additional data may be the interpreter's impression of the likelihood of fixed enlargement or dynamic overload.(Adapted with permission from Horan and Flowers (1980)).

• **Deviations of the ST segment** in frontal and/or horizontal plane leads.

• **Appearance of RBBB morphology.** A depressed or even elevated ST with a new RBBB pattern may be found in patients with important pulmonary hypertension. With adequate treatment, clinical outlook and ECG alterations may improve.

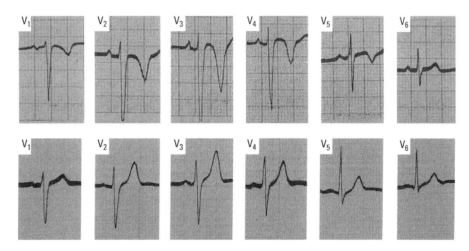

Figure 10.14 A 60-year-old patient with chronic cor pulmonale. Because of respiratory infection, the patient presented with an ECG morphology of acute right ventricular overload (above) that ceased in a few days (below).

Pulmonary embolism

The most common ECG signs found in pulmonary embolism may be similar to those commonly found in acute decompensated cor pulmonale, including the following:

• **ST segment deviations and negative T wave in right precordial leads that may be transient (Figure 10.15).**

• **ÂQRS deviation to the right** with a McGinn–White pattern (SI QIII with negative TIII morphology) that often coincides with negative T waves in V1–V3 (Figure 10.15).

This pattern is very characteristic of pulmonary embolism (high specificity) but does not appear frequently (low sensitivity). When it does appear, it usually corresponds to a major embolism. A differential diagnosis must be made, especially for inferior myocardial infarction (see Chapter 13).

• **New appearance of RBBB.** This usually represents massive embolism, often with evident ST deviation (Figure 10.16).

• **The presence of sinus tachycardia,** which is very frequent. However, it is not sometimes found in elderly people with some type of sick sinus syndrome (see Chapter 17).

• **A normal ECG.** We have to remember that this occurs **relatively often,** especially in mild/moderate pulmonary embolism (Chapter 21).

Right ventricular enlargement in children

In the neonatal period, it is difficult to diagnose RVE because there is already a physiological RVE. Nonetheless, any of the following criteria suggest the existence of abnormal RVE in the newborn (Burch and

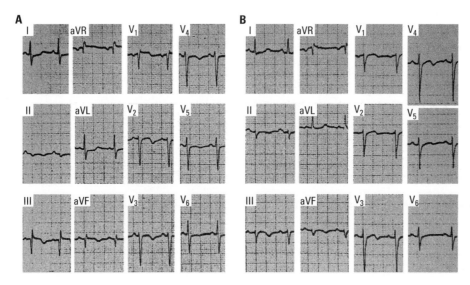

Figure 10.15 (A) A 59-year-old patient with pulmonary embolism and typical McGinn–White morphology: SI, QIII, negative TIII. (B) The ECG after the patient recovered.

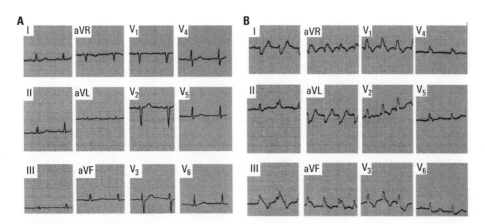

Figure 10.16 (A) Pre-operative ECG of a 58-year-old female with no heart disease. (B) During the post-operative period, the patient presented with a massive pulmonary embolism with an ECG that showed a sharply right-deviated ÂQRS, advanced RBBB, and sinus tachycardia. The patient died a few minutes later.

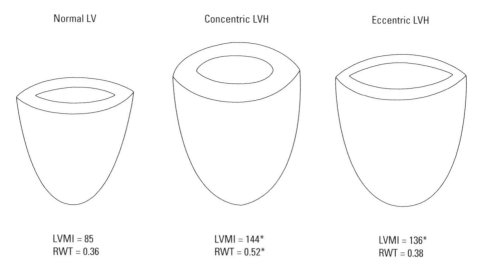

| Normal LV | Concentric LVH | Eccentric LVH |

LVMI = 85   LVMI = 144*   LVMI = 136*
RWT = 0.36   RWT = 0.52*   RWT = 0.38

Figure 10.17 Patterns of left ventricular geometry in hypertensive patients. LVMI: left ventricular mass index; RWT: relative wall thickness (Reproduced from Ganau *et al.* 1992).

DePasquale 1967; Moss and Adams 1968; Rowe and Mehrizi 1968; Fretz *et al.* 1992):
- **qR in V1,**
- **solitary R in V1 over 20 mm,**
- **S in V6 greater than 11 mm** after the 2nd day of life, **positive T in V1** after the 4th day, as long as T is also positive in the left precordials, and
- **P wave taller than 4 mm.**

Later on and until adulthood, some of these signs undergo modifications. RVE is then suggested by:
- **R/S ratio over 1 in V1** at 2 or 3 years of age, with intrinsicoid deflection time (IDT) ≥0.03 sec (except for post-term infants) or
- an **rSr′ morphology in V1** may be a normal variant, frequently due to bad location (V1 too high) of V1 electrode. May also be seen in *pectus excavatum* and other thoracic abnormalities. It is especially more indicative of RVE when: (i) R′ has a high voltage, (ii) the morphology does not vary with respiration (see Figure 7.40), (iii) it is accompanied by a marked S in V6, and (iv) ÂQRS is right-deviated beyond +120°.

Indirect signs of right ventricular enlargement

We consider the following to be indirect signs of RVE:
- **clear signs of right atrial enlargement in the absence of tricuspid atresia;**
- **signs of left atrial enlargement in the presence of mitral stenosis; or**
- **atrial fibrillation accompanying mitral stenosis.**

Regression of ECG signs

Regression of RVE signs is frequently seen post-surgery in patients with congenital heart diseases such as ASD or pulmonary stenosis (Figure 10.11). After correction of Fallot's tetralogy, post-operative ECG often shows advanced RBBB (see Chapter 11) (Figure 11.12), masking the regressive changes of the RVE.

Differential diagnosis (Table 10.3)

Differential diagnosis of right ventricular enlargement with dominant R or rSr′ morphology in V1

A differential diagnosis should be made with all cases that present with prominent R in V1, as a result of an anterior and mainly right-oriented loop (Table 10.3).
- **Normal variant.** Prominent R (RS) or rSr′ in V1 is seen with some frequency in 2.5% of normal adults, particularly in those with extreme counterclockwise rotation (RS) or thoracic abnormalities (rSr′), such as pectus excavatum or straight back syndrome. A low-voltage RS morphology in V1 may be seen in post-term newborns, even into adulthood (see Chapter 7). As we have already commented, the location of V1 lead too high, usually originates a QRS pattern with final r′ in V1. Therefore, the valve of PtfV1 as abnormal P wave indices is controversial (see Chapter 9).
- **Sometimes prominent R, especially in V2, can result from positional changes** (extreme counterclockwise rotation, massive pleural effusion, etc.). In these cases, the T wave is usually positive in V1 if there is no coexistent heart disease.
- **Right bundle branch block.** Regardless of whether the RBBB is partial or advanced, a dominant R morphology can be seen in V1, V2. The rsR′ morphology with QRS <0.12 sec, corresponding to classic, isolated partial RBBB, may be identical to the morphology observed in RVE. This morphology typically appears in ASD, but it can also be seen in mitral stenosis and early-stage congenital heart diseases with systolic overload, such as pulmonary stenosis.

Table 10.3 Presence of prominent R or r′ in V1: differential diagnosis.

Clinical setting	R or R^N(r′) morphology in V1	QRS width	P wave morphology in V1
1. No heart disease • Electrode misplacement • Hypermature • Normal variant: Fewer Purkinje fibers in anteroseptal zone or extreme counter clockwise rotation • Thorax abnormalities (pectus excavatum) (see Figure 7.16)	2nd RIS 4th RIS <10 mm	<0.12 sec <0.12 sec <0.12 sec	P– in 2° IS P$_+$ or ± In 4° IS Normal Final negativity
2. Classical RBBB		From <0.12 to >0.12 sec	Normal
3. Atypical RBBB • Ebstein's disease • Arrhythmogenic RVD/C Low voltage in V1 or Σ wave • Brugada syndrome (see Table 21.9)		Usually ≥0.12 sec May be 0.12 sec Sometimes ≥0.12 sec	Usually peaked and/or ± Usually pathologic Normal
4. Right or biventricular enlargement (athletes) or even LVH (Hypertrophic or others CM)		<0.12 sec	Usually tall and peaked. Sometimes ±
5. Wolff–Parkinson–White syndrome		From <0.12 to >0.12 sec	Normal P wave with short PR
6. Lateral MI	rs in V$_1$ RS in V$_2$	<0.12 sec	Usually normal
7. Block of middle fibers (especially if the pattern is transient (see Chapter 11)?	Prominent R in V$_1$ or more frequently V$_2$	<0.12 sec	Usually normal

This rsR′ morphology usually represents a less important degree of RVE than the presence of solitary R morphology (Figure 10.2). Therefore, the same patient can show first, one morphology and then the other in the course of the disease (see Figure 10.4).

• **Atypical RBBB.** These include the ECG pattern seen in some congenital (Ebstein's disease) and inherited heart diseases (arrhythmogenic right ventricular dysplasia, some Brugada pattern).

• Cases of LV or biventricular enlargement including athletes. Also in some cases of **hypertrophic cardiomyopathy** (HCM), or other types of cardiomyopathy with isolated LVE involving the septum, a tall R wave in V1 (>7 mm), usually with a deep S in the same lead, may be seen. An increase in the first vector due to septal hypertrophy is probably responsible, although there is not always a deep Q wave in V5–V6 because the enlarged first vector is directed more forward than to the right.

• **Type II and III WPW pre-excitation.** There is no problem if initial slurrings are visible (δ wave) and the PR interval is short. When there is an important degree of pre-excitation, an exclusive R morphology in V1 may be seen (see Figure 12.2).

• **Lateral infarction** (see Figures 13.72 and 13.76). The QRS pattern in V1 may present with prominent R (rR, RS) with a usually positive T wave (Bayés de Luna *et al.* 2006). It has been very well demonstrated with ECG-MR correlations that prominent R in V1 in patients with ischemic heart disease, is due to lateral MI, not to posterior MI that now we know, does not exist (Bayés de Luna *et al.* 2015). The QRS is consistently less than 0.12 sec. The differential diagnosis between RVE and lateral infarction can be difficult with conventional electrocardiography alone. Lateral myocardial infarction is supported by the presence of positive and an especially tall and symmetric T wave in V1–V2 and often abnormal Q waves in II, III, and aVF of associated inferior myocardial infarction. RVE is favored by a negative T wave in V1–V2, a right ÂQRS, and atrial signs of right atrial enlargement.

- **Block of middle fibers.** In the absence of lateral infarction or RVE, the presence of transient prominent R in V1–V2 may be explained by a **block of left bundle middle fibers** (see Chapter 11, Anteroseptal middle fiber block. Myth or reality? Figures 11.44–11.47).

Differential diagnosis of right ventricular enlargement with rS or Qs morphology in V1

The presence of a QRS complex without final anterior forces and consequently with rS morphology in V1 or even QS (see Figure 10.2VI), or, at most, rSr' with a low-voltage r' (Figure 10.2VII), sometimes with a much deeper S wave in V2, can cause confusion between this type of RVE and left ventricular or biventricular hypertrophy, septal infarction, or zonal right ventricular block, a frequently associated pathology. We will discuss the most important ECG characteristics in these cases.

In this type of RVE, the S waves are prominent until V6, there is dominant R in V3 R–V4R and in aVR there is a terminal R because often the final vector is oriented backward, but also upward and to the right (see Figure 10.3C and D). Sometimes there is a shallow S in V1 with greater voltage of S in V2, with an RS pattern until V6. In biventricular hypertrophy, a deep S in V2 with small S in V1 (shallow S in V1) may also exist, but in left precordials, there is a R or Rs pattern.

In LVH, the forces are directed backward and to the left, originating a tall R wave in V5–V6 and usually a deep S in right precordials, V3R and V4R. Moreover, in the frontal plane, ÂQRS is deviated to the left and in aVR, the terminal r is minimal or not found.

Biventricular enlargement diagnosis is possible when there is a much larger S wave in V2 than in V1, with R or Rs morphology in V6, and SI, SII, SIII morphology, or right ÂQRS in the frontal plane.

In chronic septal infarction a negative post-ischemic T wave is seen from V1 to V2, V3, frequently with QS or qrS in the same leads, and with an R/S ratio in V6>1 and a generally normal P wave.

The C loop of Figure 10.3 ("SI, RII, RIII"-type) (Figure 10.12) should be distinguished from inferoposterior hemiblock (IPH) of the left bundle branch (see Chapter 11). In IPH, the q of III and aVF is more marked, the R/S ratio in V6>I, and the atriogram is not suggestive of right atrial enlargement.

The D loop of Figure 10.3 ("SI, SII, SIII"-type) (Figure 10.13) is explained by the existence of zonal right ventricular block and/or RVE (see Chapter 11). In patients with COPD, this type of loop is usually due to associated RVE with a certain degree of zonal conduction delay in the right ventricle (Bayés de Luna *et al.* 1987). However, the presence of the SI, SII, SIII pattern in normal individuals is likely to be caused more by a variation in the distribution of the right ventricular Purkinje fibers with some physiological delay of conduction than by a true right peripheral block (see Figure 11.19). In addition, the differential diagnosis between the SI, SII, SIII pattern and hemiblock of the superoanterior division of the left bundle branch must be made. The morphology is that of SI, SII, SIII in RVE and/or peripheral right ventricular block, with SII ≥ SIII and a low-voltage R in I (Figure **10.3**D), while in left superoanterior hemiblock (SAH), there is an exclusive R wave in lead I with high voltage and SII < SIII.

Differential diagnosis of right ventricular enlargement in the presence of ST/T changes

These changes may be seen as the most evident findings in cases of RVE, especially in acute dilation of the right ventricle. The clinical setting may be very useful to rule out other etiologies, especially ischemic heart disease.

Diagnosis of RVE in the presence of ventricular blocks
Advanced RBBB

In the presence of advanced RBBB (QRS ≥ 0.12 sec) (Figure 11.13A), RVE is suggested when the following are found:

- **rsR' morphology is extended beyond V2**. This is seen especially in right ventricular dilation (ASD, etc.).
- **High-voltage R'**. The taller the R', the greater the likelihood of associated RVE. However, there are instances of RBBB with tall R' without RVE, and vice versa.
- **Solitary R in V1**. This results from the anterior orientation of the whole loop. Sometimes there is a solitary R of low voltage in emphysematous subjects (Figure 11.13A). It is frequently associated with the absence of "q" in V6.
- **'rS' morphology in I and 'qR' in III**. In this case, the possibility of inferoposterior division hemiblock added to the advanced RBBB must be ruled out.
- **P wave criteria of right atrial enlargement.**

Advanced LBBB

In the presence of advanced LBBB (QRS ≥ 0.12 sec), RVE is suggested (Figure 11.13B) when the following are found:

- **ÂQRS is to the right**, with an RS morphology in lead I that may not be explained by other causes (see Figure 11.27).
- There is **evident "r" in V1** in the absence of myocardial infarction.
- In precordial leads, the **transition to an Rs pattern goes beyond V4**.

Clinical implications

The ECG diagnosis of RVE is difficult, but when achieved, it generally indicates that significant enlargement is present. The prognosis of important global RVE (tall R in V1) with narrow QRS is worse than isolated advanced RBBB (tall R in V1 with wide QRS).

The differential diagnosis in patients presenting with a prominent R wave or rSr' in V1 has been discussed previously (see Table 10.3).

The sensitivity of ECG criteria for RVE is relatively low. Therefore, a normal ECG may be found in many cases of mild/moderate RVE or even acute right ventricular dilation (pulmonary embolism). However, its specificity is very high (see Tables 10.1 and 10.2).

The echocardiography measurement of RV wall is more sensitive for the diagnosis of RV hypertrophy than ECG criteria (Prakash 1981).

Left ventricular enlargement: hypertrophy and dilation

Concept and associated diseases

Electrocardiographic signs are fundamentally caused by hypertrophy of the ventricular wall (LVH) and are frequently associated with partial left bundle branch block (LBBB). It is sometimes possible to infer the diagnosis of ventricular dilation accompanying the hypertrophy (see later).

In heart diseases with diastolic volume overload (e.g. aortic regurgitation), dilation of the cavity is associated with hypertrophy (eccentric hypertrophy) earlier than in heart diseases with systolic pressure overload, such as aortic stenosis and hypertension (concentric hypertrophy) (Ganau *et al.* 1992) (Figure 10.17).

The acquired heart diseases that most frequently produce LVE are valvular diseases, especially aortic valve disease, systemic hypertension, and cardiomyopathies, including coronary cardiomyopathy. The congenital heart diseases that most often produce isolated LVE are aortic stenosis, aortic coarctation, and fibroelastosis. Depending on the severity and evolutive stage of the heart disease, different ECG morphologies may appear (see later).

Mechanism of ECG changes

The increment in left ventricular mass enhances the already dominant vectorial depolarization forces of the left ventricle, which shift backward and often somewhat

more upward, in cases of predominance of enlargement of the left ventricular free wall (Figure 10.18B). If important enlargement of the septum predominates, the vectorial forces are directed to about 0° in the horizontal plane or even somewhat forward (Figure 10.18C). In advanced LVH (the term LVH is more frequently used than left ventricular enlargement—LVE), ventricular repolarization direction changes because the subendocardium begins to repolarize when subepicardial depolarization is still incomplete. Associated left ventricular block also plays a role in this process (Piccolo *et al.* 1979; Bayés de Luna *et al.* 1983). This explains why the T loop and vector are directed opposite to the QRS in advanced LVH. It also accounts for the abnormal ST vector opposed to QRS at the conclusion of ventricular depolarization (J point). These circumstances determine that in advanced LVH, the QRS and T loops are abnormal and assume opposing directions (Figure 10.19B–E).

Different types of QRS and T loops are seen in LVE. In Figure 10.19, five of the most common configurations are shown. The type A loop corresponds to mild or moderate LVH, while B- and C-type loops correspond to more severe cases. Type D corresponds to the LVH sometimes observed in HCM and type E to LVH with a predominance of apical septal hypertrophy over free wall hypertrophy. This figure summarizes the morphological features of these loops. Loop projection on the frontal and horizontal planes (on the positive and negative hemifields of the different leads) accounts for the ECG alterations found in LVH, which will be described later.

However, it is important to remember that mild or even some moderate degrees of LVH may not change the ECG.

Changes in the QRS complex (Figures 10.19–10.25)

• The maximum loop vector increased in voltage is directed to the left, generally farther to the back than normal and more upward. When we discuss the diagnostic criteria of LVH, we will comment on the voltage limits of QRS for this diagnosis. In any case, the LVH explains the taller R wave in the left precordial leads and in leads I and aVL, and the deep S wave in the right precordials leads V1, V2, or V3. In V4, there is a deep S wave, a transitional morphology, or a tall R wave.

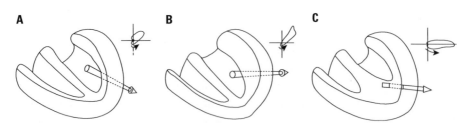

Figure 10.18 (A) Under normal conditions, the dominant forces of ventricular depolarization are directed downward, backward, and to the left. In cases of predominantly enlarged free left ventricular wall (B), the forces are generally directed more to the back and frequently upward, and in cases of predominantly enlarged septum (C), the forces can be directed to 0° or even somewhat forward.

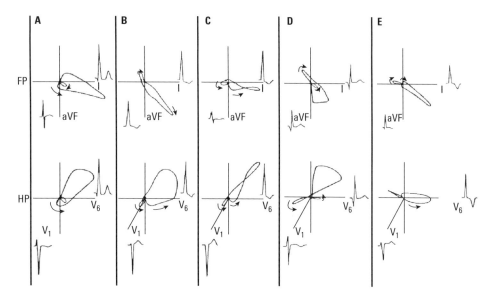

Figure 10.19 Diagram of the QRS and T loops in the frontal plane (FP) and horizontal plane (HP) in mild or moderate left ventricular enlargement (A) and severe enlargement (B and C). The D loop (or similar) is seen in some cases of hypertrophic cardiomyopathy, and the E loop is seen in cases of apical hypertrophic cardiomyopathy. Note in the five cases the typical morphology that appears in aVF, I, V1, and V6 according to the loop–hemifield correlation.

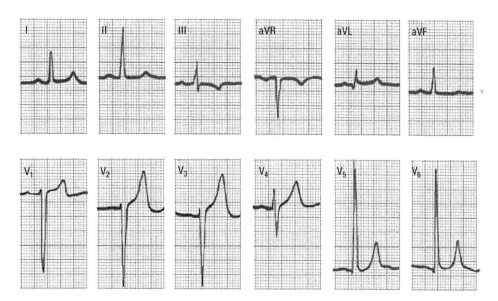

Figure 10.20 Typical ECG of a 22-year-old male with important, although not very long-standing, aortic regurgitation. It corresponds to moderate left ventricular hypertrophy but satisfies the diagnostic criteria for LVE (Romhilt–Estes score). In effect, R in V5–V6 > 30 mm (3 points); intrinsicoid deflection time (IDT) = 0.07 sec (1 point); duration of QRS = 0.10 sec (1 point). Total: 5 points. Left ventricular dilation is suggested by IDT > 0.07 sec and the R wave height in V6 greater than that in V5.

When septal hypertrophy (especially in the apical zone) predominates over that of the left ventricular free wall (asymmetric septal HCM), or when there is biventricular enlargement, the maximum loop vector can be fairly anterior (at about 0°), and the QRS may even show an RS pattern in lead V2 or even V1 (Figures 10.19E and 10.25). This morphology can be confused with isolated levorotation, or all causes of high R in V1 and/or V2 in the absence of RVE (see Table 10.3).

• **A delay in recording the maximum loop vector**, accounting for increased IDT (time till the take-off of QRS) in the left precordial leads and usually in aVL. The IDT is not of value in classical bipolar leads (I, II, III). The IDT is considered to be increased when it exceeds 0.045 sec. Occasionally, slightly higher values are seen in athletes or vagal overdrive, for example. In LVE with the loop onset to the left and forward (left ventricular strain pattern), IDT measurement is useless because the right

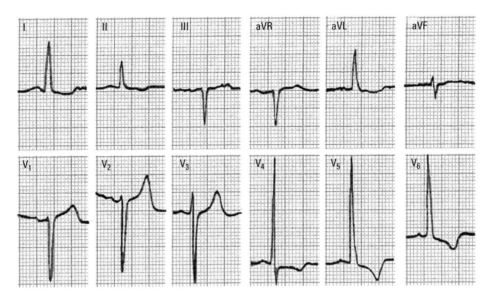

Figure 10.21 ECG of a 47-year-old male, typical of severe, long-standing aortic stenosis. The left ventricular hypertrophy pattern is typical. R in V4–V5 > 30 mm (3 points); ST–T opposite to R in V4–V6 (3 points); IDT = 0.055 sec (1 point). Total: 7 points (Romhilt–Estes score).

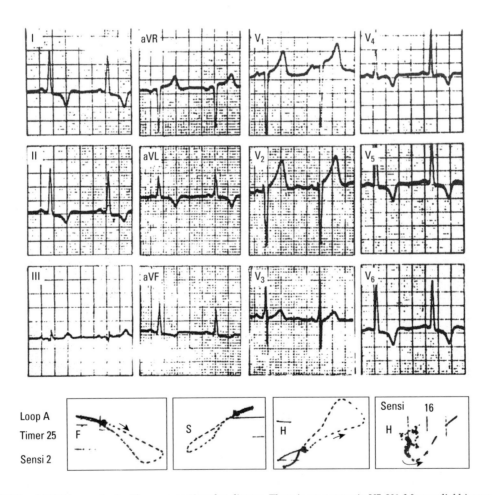

Figure 10.22 ECG and VCG in a patient with severe aortic valve disease. There is no q wave in V5–V6. Myocardial biopsy showed more than 10% of septal fibrosis.

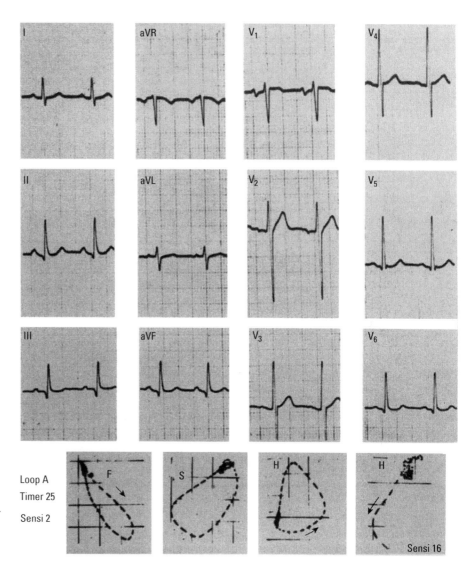

Figure 10.23 ECG and VCG in a patient with severe aortic valve disease. There is q wave in V5–V6>1 mm. Myocardial biopsy showed less than 10% of septal fibrosis.

Loop A
Timer 25
Sensi 2

initial forces are reduced. Classically, it was thought that cases with severe but not long-standing aortic regurgitation that frequently present with a normal onset of ventricular activation to the right (q in I and V6) have a larger IDT (Figure 10.20) than those with aortic stenosis of similar severity and characteristics (Figure 10.21). This is explained because loops with the initial forces to the left are seen less frequently in patients with not long-standing aortic regurgitation (Figure 10.19A) (see below).

• **Slightly longer QRS loop.** The duration of the QRS complex, which is normally around 0.10 sec, is extended to 0.11 sec. The presence of QRS≥0.12 sec is explained by associated advanced LBBB.

• **Direction of the initial forces.** The initial forces, especially in patients with long-standing aortic valve disease and severe and long-standing LVE, are frequently directed forward and to the left because of **associated partial LBBB** (Piccolo *et al.* 1979) **and/or septal fibrosis** (Bayés de Luna *et al.* 1983). The latter has been demonstrated in patients with aortic valve disease with septal biopsy performed during open heart surgery. The results of septal biopsy show that the q wave in V5–V6 is related more to the degree of septal fibrosis than to the type of hemodynamic overload (systolic or diastolic) (Cabrera and Monroy 1952). The greater the septal fibrosis, the smaller the q wave. Every case with a "q" wave <1 mm or absent presented with more than 10% septal fibrosis, and vice versa (Figures 10.22 and 10.23). Since aortic stenosis presents with more septal fibrosis than aortic regurgitation, a conspicuous q wave is more often seen in the latter. However, in the long follow-up of cases of aortic regurgitation, the "q" wave in V5–V6 is not usually recorded or is seen to have decreased markedly (Figure 10.20). The initial forces to the right ("q" wave) frequently seen in cases of ventricular enlargement of severe but not long-standing aortic regurgitation are frequently more marked than normal and are followed by a high-voltage R wave. This is due to septal hypertrophy in the absence of septal fibrosis and/or a delay in impulse conduction in the peripheral portions of the left intraventricular conduction

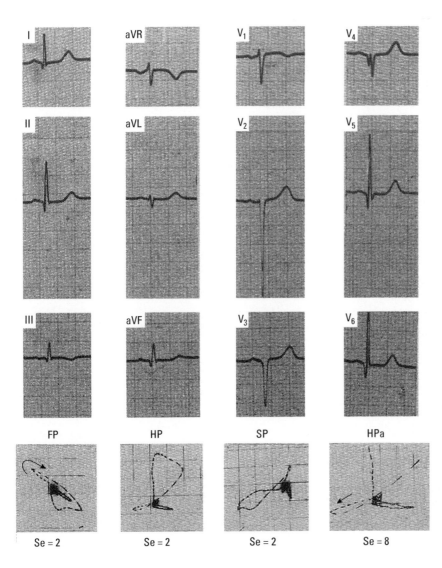

Figure 10.24 Typical but infrequent ECG of obstructive hypertrophic cardiomyopathy in a 25-year-old patient. There are no voltage criteria for left ventricular enlargement, but the deep, clean Q wave in V5–V6 and QS in the middle precordials, together with the "q" wave of the frontal plane (FP) and the absence of repolarization alterations in the leads with abnormal Q wave, suggested the diagnosis, which was confirmed by echocardiography.

system that is greater than by the proximal portion. The septal forces are more evident because the left ventricular wall vector takes longer to form.

Very conspicuous "q" waves are observed in 10–35% of cases of HCM, with the "q" wave sometimes more prominent than the "R" wave, with QS or QR patterns appearing (Figures 10.19D and 10.24). However, the presence of a prominent Q wave attributed to septal hypertrophy is a poor predictor of septal thickness (Moro *et al.* 1995). It is essential to rule out the "Q" wave of necrosis. The Q waves of HCM are thinner and, although they may be deep, they are usually followed by positive T waves (Figure 10.24) (see Chapter 13).

• **QRS loop in the frontal plane** (Figure 10.19). Because the heart frequently assumes a horizontal position in

LVH, the QRS loop usually rotates counterclockwise in the frontal plane, deviating a little more to the left than normal. This may explain an rS morphology in III and an aVF and the slightly left ÂQRS deviation that may be seen, especially in long-standing aortic stenosis (Figure 10.21). However, if the loop rotates clockwise, as is often the case in congenital aortic stenosis with vertical heart, a dominant R may appear in the QRS complex in II, III, and aVF (Figure 10.19B).

• **The terminal portion of the loop remains on the left** (Figure 10.19). Due to the final predominance of left ventricular depolarization over right (opposite to normal), the terminal portion of the loop remains in the positive hemifield of I, V6, and at times V5. As a result, no S waves are found in these leads.

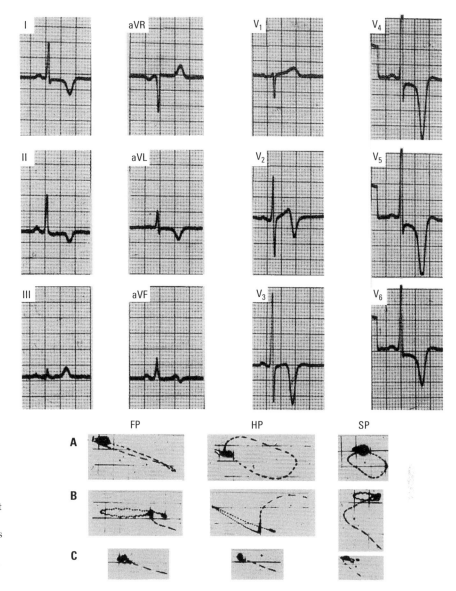

Figure 10.25 ECG and VCG of an asymptomatic patient who had been diagnosed with coronary artery disease because of deep negative T waves. The ECG shows a morphology characteristic of hypertrophic cardiomyopathy, with mainly apical involvement (tall R without "q" in V5–V6 and very deep negative T waves in different leads). The VCG shows the typical T loop morphology ("arrow point") directed to the back and right. (A: global loop, B: T loop, C: initial vectors).

Changes in ST and T (Figures 10.19, 10.25, 10.26, and 10.27B)

Two factors contribute to the appearance of repolarization alterations: the severity of the lesion and the duration of its evolution (Figures 10.19, 10.25, 10.26, and 10.27B). In valvular disease, as well as in hypertension or cardiomyopathies, the ST–T changes are determined especially by the duration of evolution.

• **In heart diseases with more or less important LVH but not long-standing**, there is usually no clear ST segment depression and the T loop conserves its normal orientation (it is sometimes more anterior), although it is generally more symmetric. The T wave is still positive, but it is more symmetric and has a straight ST segment, even in moderate or severe but not long-standing LVH. Its morphology differs somewhat according to the type of hemodynamic overload and is typically taller in diastolic overload (aortic regurgitation). The latter case usually shows a more evident q wave (Figure 10.26B,C). This relatively unaltered ECG does not mean that the valvular heart disease is mild, but that it is not very long-standing if it is severe (Figures 10.20 and 10.26B,C). These morphologies are sometimes similar to those seen in healthy lean adolescents and adults. However, in the latter, the junction of ST and the T wave is smooth, and the T wave is asymmetrical with a slow upward slope (Figure 10.27A).

• **As LVH increases, in part conditioned by the elapsed years of evolution but also because of the severity of the heart disease** (especially the severity of aortic stenosis that increases with time), whether or not the LVH is secondary to systolic or diastolic hemodynamic overload, the T wave evolves from the positive morphology to the typical pattern of ST segment depression convex with respect to the baseline, with a final negative T wave with

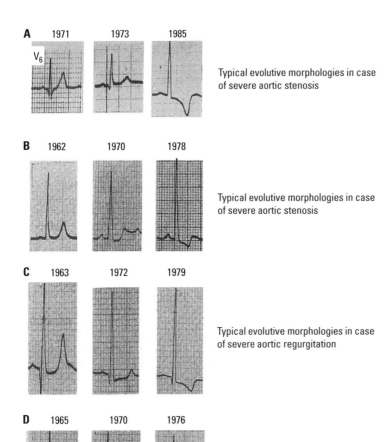

A 1971   1973   1985

Typical evolutive morphologies in case of severe aortic stenosis

B 1962   1970   1978

Typical evolutive morphologies in case of severe aortic stenosis

C 1963   1972   1979

Typical evolutive morphologies in case of severe aortic regurgitation

D 1965   1970   1976

Evolutive morphologies in case of severe coronary hypertensive patient

Figure 10.26 Four typical examples of morphology evolution. (A and B) are two cases of important aortic stenoses, the second lacking the q wave from the first ECG, and the first case with a progressive reduction in q depth coinciding with the repolarization "strain pattern." (C) shows advanced aortic regurgitation with a progressive decrease in the q wave with the appearance of "strain pattern," while in (D), we see a patient with ischemic and hypertensive heart disease. As the ECG evolves, we can observe the changes in the ECG patterns (see text).

asymmetric branches (Figure 10.26A–C). This so-called "**strain pattern**" occurs because the repolarization of the free wall starts in the subendocardium. The ST vector and T loop are therefore opposite to QRS and the initial part of the T loop is recorded more slowly (Figures 10.19A,B and 10.26A–C). The presence or not of a small "q" wave is more related to the degree of septal fibrosis and/or partial LBBB than to the type of hemodynamic overload (Figures 10.22, 10.23, and 10.26A–C). The partial LBBB may also help to explain the appearance of repolarization abnormalities (Bisteni 1977).

• The T wave and ST segment changes secondary to depolarization abnormalities, in this case LVH (secondary changes), are also associated to primary changes (prolonged AP duration) that may be related to ischemia or the effects of digitalis or other drugs, originating a **mixed morphology** with a more homogeneously recorded T wave and/or a more important ST depression, especially in long-standing cases. The T wave is thus deeper and/or more symmetric and the deviation of ST from the baseline is more conspicuous and less convex (Figure 10.28). The contribution of both primary (QT prolongation–AP

prolongation) and secondary (reduced conduction velocity) changes to the ECG pattern of LVH has been recently studied using an analytical computer model (Bacharova *et al*. 2010).

• It has been suggested (De Piccoli *et al*. 1987) in an ECG–echocardiographic study that patients with systolic overload of the left ventricle and negative ST–T have normal ventricular geometry, while patients with diastolic overload of the left ventricle and negative ST–T have an abnormal geometry of the left ventricle.

• The presence of a very deep negative and symmetric T wave in leads with an exclusively tall R wave is very suggestive of an apical type of **HCM**. In this case, the abnormal repolarization may appear early on in the evolution of the disease.

Diagnostic ECG criteria: anatomic and imaging correlations (Tables 10.4 and 10.5)

In the last 60 years, many ECG criteria for LVE have been proposed (Sheridan 1998; Van der Wall *et al*. 1999). In the beginning, most were based on radiological and necropsic studies, followed by echocardiographic correlations. It

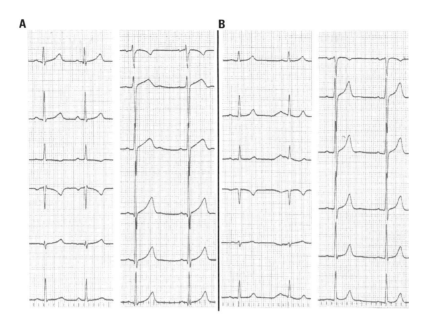

Figure 10.27 (A) ECG if a healthy, lean, adolescent and (B) if a patient with hypertension. Observe the mild differences in the ST segment/T wave. In (A), there is from the beginning an upsloping of the ST segment (V4–V6, I, and II). In contrast, in (B), there is a rectified ST with symmetric T wave (V5, V6, I, II, VF).

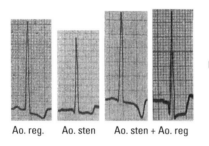

Four cases with atypical morphologies

Ao. reg.   Ao. sten   Ao. sten + Ao. reg

Figure 10.28 Four examples of atypical morphology of ST/T according to the concept of systolic and diastolic overload. The second is an aortic stenosis that looks like aortic regurgitation (there is "q"), while the first is an aortic regurgitation that mimics stenosis (exclusive R wave without "q"). The last two cases correspond to double aortic valve disease (stenosis + regurgitation), one without q and the other with very conspicuous q. The first case with evident septal fibrosis and the second with mild septal fibrosis (see text). These last two cases show very altered repolarization because a primary repolarization disorder appeared during the course of the secondary disorder, due to ventricular enlargement.

has been demonstrated (Reichek and Deveraux 1981) that left ventricular mass measured by echocardiography correlates with anatomic post-mortem weight, showing a high sensitivity (93%) and specificity (95%).

Using echocardiographic validations, the ECG criteria may obtain, at least in some subsets of patients, a sensitivity of about 50% while maintaining a 90% specificity. M-mode echocardiography is very useful in assessing left ventricular mass in patients with normal cardiac shape, as is the case in most hypertensive patients. Using two-dimensional echocardiography, left ventricular mass can be accurately assessed, even in patients with distorted left ventricular geometry due to myocardial infarction or RVE.

CMR is the ideal imaging technique for the assessment of left ventricular mass and volume, with good reproduc-

ibility and probably even greater measuring accuracy than echocardiography. In ventricles of normal shape, including those found in athletes, both echocardiography and CMR are the "gold standard" technique for accurately assessing cardiac dimensions, mass, and volume with a correlation close to 100%. However, CMR is more precise, accurate, and reproducible, especially in patients with distorted left ventricular (IHD patients with myocardial infarction scars). The echocardiography is cheaper and has better time resolution, but it is more expertise-dependent than CMR. Currently, the definitive correlation of the two techniques to certify the ECG criteria for the diagnosis of LVE is lacking. For all that, CMR is unrealistic for large-scale use in clinical practice.

The ECG has a high specificity (SP ≈ 90%) comparable to echocardiography (few false positives), **but the**

Table 10.4　ECG criteria for left ventricular hypertrophy according to ECG and echocardiography (*) and cardiovascular magnetic resonance imaging (**) correlations: sensitivity, specificity, and cardiovascular risk of death (see text).

Criteria	Sensitivity (%)	Specificity (%)	CV risk of death (adjusted hazard ratio and 95% CI) according to Hsieh *et al.* (2005)
(A) Voltage and duration of QRS			
1) Sokolow and Lyon (1949)	21* 26**	89* 92.6**	1.9 (1.6–2.2)
2) Cornell voltage (Devereux *et al.* 1984)	16* 15.1**	97* 97.3**	3.1 (2.5–3.8)
3) Framingham adjusted Cornell voltage (Norman and Levy 1993)	17 (men)* 22 (women)* 15.1**	98* 97.2**	1.4 (1.2–1.6)
4) Cornell duration product (Mulloy *et al.* 1992; Okin *et al.* 1995)	50* 14.8**	96* 97.3**	2 (1.5–2.6)
5) 12 leads sum (Siegel and Roberts 1982)	6	91.7	2.6 (2.1–3.2)
6) 12 leads sum voltage and QRS duration (Siegel and Roberts 1982)	7.5	96.7	2.7 (2.3–3.1)
7) Talbot *et al.* (1976) (see text)	Low	High	—
(B) Scores systems			
1) Romhilt and Estes ≥4 (1966)	18* 15.9**	99* 97**	2.9 (2.5–3.4)
2) Romhilt and Estes ≥5 (1966)	15* 5.7**	100* 99.1**	3.7 (3.0–4.4)
3) Framingham (Levy *et al.* 1990)	6.9* 7**	98.8* 99.2**	3.4 (2.4–4.9)
4) Perugia (Schillaci *et al.* 1994)	34* 24.7**	93* 93.2**	2.9 (2.5–3.3)
5) Glasgow R.I. (Morrison *et al.* 2007)	23.9*	95*	—
(C) Regression models			
1) Rautaharju *et al.* LV mass index equation (1988)	38.8*	70*	2.6 (2–3)
2) Wolf *et al.* logistic regression (1991)	53.7 (men)*	94.9 (men)*	3.7 (2.7–5)
3) Casale *et al.* logistic regression (1987)	63.4 (women)* 62 (necropsis)	92.9 (women)* 92 (necropsis)	3.3 (2.8–3.9)

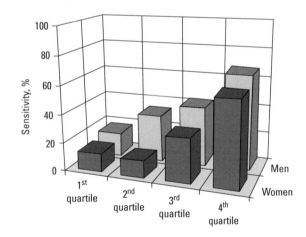

Figure 10.29　Three-dimensional bar graph showing sensitivity of the ECG criteria (Cornell voltage, Romhilt–Estes score, left ventricular strain) according to quartiles of severity of LVH (left ventricular mass assessed by echocardiography). (Reproduced with permission from Schillaci *et al.* 1994).

sensitivity (SE) of the ECG is much lower (more false negatives), **especially in early stages of LVH**. The SE increases very much according to the severity of LVH in the population studied (Schillaci *et al.* 1994) (Figure 10.29). However, it is important to remember that the ECG is a superior predictor to echocardiography for cardiovascular complications.

There are various ECG methods to detect LVH, which may be categorized as follows: (i) voltage criteria, including the product of QRS voltage and duration; (ii) point score systems; and (iii) the regression equation models (Hsieh *et al.* 2005) (Table 10.4).

ECG criteria based on QRS voltage

The ECG diagnosis of LVH is based mainly on the increase of the QRS voltage generated by the increase of left ventricular mass. The voltage criteria correlates better with ventricular wall thickness than with left ventricular mass, and the sensitivity of the ECG criteria declines with cavity dilation. As with many diagnostic techniques, specificity of these criteria is better than sensitivity. **Table 10.4 shows many of the voltage criteria with its sensitivity, specificity, and accuracy.** We will now comment on the most used criteria.

The best-known QRS voltage criteria and voltage × duration products are as follows:

• **The Sokolow–Lyon criteria (Sokolow and Lyon 1949)** in which there is a LVE when SV1 + RV5–6 ≥ 35 mm. Nonetheless, although it is very specific (≈90–95%) (very few false positives), as happens with other voltage criteria, it has a low sensitivity (≈20–25%).

• The **ECG criterion RVL + SV3 > 24 mm for men and > 20 mm for women (Cornell voltage criteria)** (Devereux *et al.* 1984; Casale *et al.* 1985, 1987). This is no more sensitive than the Sokolow–Lyon criterion, with mild higher specificity (>95%). With the **Cornell product, a modified Cornell voltage criterion,** a higher sensitivity without compromising specificity is obtained (Mulloy *et al.* 1992; Okin *et al.* 1995). The calculations, however, are tedious. Furthermore, in other series, the sensitivity is found to be lower. Even in those studies that **corrected the Cornell voltage** with the inclusion of body mass index (Norman and Levy 1993), sensitivity does not increase to above 50%.

- The **sum of 12-lead voltage** has been used in aortic valve disease patients with necropsic and hemodynamic correlations (Siegel and Roberts 1982) and in hypertension patients with echocardiographic correlations (Koito and Spodick 1989; Rodriguez Padial 1991) (see Chapter 21).

- **Talbot *et al.* (1976)** studied the utility of diverse scalar and orthogonal ECG criteria for diagnosis of LVE, and the repercussions of associated diseases (myocardial infarction and ventricular block) on the usefulness of these criteria. **The criterion R in aVL ≥ 11 mm** in the absence of left axis deviation **was found to be the most specific one in every group** (92% in isolated LVE with a sensitivity of 10%), while in the presence of SAH, the voltage of R ≥ 16 mm in aVL had similar specificity for LVE (see later). Almost the same results were obtained when myocardial infarction was found to be associated.

- **Murphy *et al.* (1983)** studied the sensitivity of 30 ECG criteria for LVH alone or combined with RVE in four scenarios (ischemic heart disease, systemic hypertension, valvular heart disease, and cardiomyopathy). Some ECG criteria frequently showed a high sensitivity for one disease but not for others. Precordial voltage criteria were more sensitive for those with hypertension and valvular disease.

- **High QRS voltage is determined by the relationship between ventricular wall thickness and cavity radius.** If the product of the two exceeds 300 mm, the Sokolow index is always ≥ 35 mm. This explains how a **large dilation with thin walls and a small radius with thick walls both produce large QRS voltage.**

- **The importance of the degree of LVH.** The sensitivity of ECG for diagnosing LVH (Van der Wall *et al.* 1999) varies from 21% to 54%, with **sensitivity increasing as the degree of hypertrophy increases**, although this is not apparent in all ECG–LVH criteria. According to Devereux *et al.* (1984), the sensitivity of the ECG when using the Cornell voltage criteria for ECG–LVH increased from 27% for mild LVH to 57% for severe cases, with a specificity of 97% that indicated a low risk of false-positive readings. These data are fairly consistent with other studies, such as the Perugia score (Figure 10.29). On the other hand, methods using combinations of various criteria also demonstrated improved sensitivity. **Each of the results shown in Table 10.4 has to be contemplated in light of this.** The sensibility, especially of different criteria, varies widely

according to population, the grade of hypertrophy, and the methodology used. We have shown the different sensitivity values of **Cornell voltage criteria and Perugia score** according to the severity of LVH. In addition, the Romhilt–Estes score ≥4 has an SE of 54% in the original paper (necropsic study) (Romhilt and Estes 1966); in a recent paper using CMR as a standard and in other types of population, it was only 15.9% (Jain *et al.* 2010).

Point score systems
Romhilt–Estes score
Romhilt and Estes (1966) devised a score (Table 10.5) that attained a global specificity of 97% and a sensitivity of ≈55% in a post-mortem series of mostly hypertensive and coronary patients. Compared with the voltage criteria, this system is somewhat more accurate (see Table 10.4). In this series, 58% of hypertrophic patients scored 5 points and 62% at least 4 points, while only 2 patients (3%) without hypertrophy scored 5 points. In patients with hypertension, sensitivity was 45% and in coronary patients it was 55%. When hypertension and coronary disease coexisted, sensitivity was 88%.

Although an objective demonstration has yet to be carried out, the Romhilt–Estes point system would probably improve in sensitivity with little loss of specificity if the following additions or modifications would be performed: (i) ST–T vector opposite to QRS with digitalis = 2 points instead of 1; (ii) other repolarization alterations (flattened or negative T, straightened ST, negative U) = 1 point; and (iii) atrial flutter or fibrillation = 2 points. As mentioned above, however, in other group of populations that are based on standards of echocardiography or CMR

Table 10.5 Romhilt–Estes score. There is left ventricular enlargement if 5 or more points are obtained. Left ventricular enlargement is probable if the sum is 4 points.

A. Criteria based on QRS modifications

1. Voltage criteria	3 points
One of the following should be present:	
– R or S in the FP ≥ 20 mm	
– S in V_1–V_2 ≥ 30 mm	
– R in V_5–V_6 ≥ 30 mm	
2. ÂQRS at −30° or more to the left	2 points
3. Intrinsicoid deflection in V_5–V_6 ≥ 0.05	1 point
4. QRS duration ≥ 0.09 sec	1 point

B. Criteria based on ST-T changes

1. ST–T vector opposite to QRS (∿) without digitalis	3 points
2. ST–T vector opposite to QRS (∿) with digitalis	1 point

C. Criteria based on P wave abnormalities

1. Negative terminal P mode in V_1 ≥ 1 mm in depth and 0.04 sec in duration	3 points

for validating LVH, the sensitivity of this score is much lower while maintaining a very high specificity (≈100%).

Framingham score (Levy et al. 1990)

This is based on the presence of a strain pattern and at least one of the following voltage criteria: (i) R I+S III≥2.5 mV; (ii) S V1/V2+R V5/V6≥3.5 mV; (iii) the S wave in V1/V2/V3>2.5 mV+R wave in V4/V5/V6≥2.5 mm.

The Perugia score

This involves positivity in one of the following three criteria: (i) Cornell voltage: S V3+R aVL>24 mm (men) or 20 mm (women); (ii) left ventricular strain pattern; (iii) Romhilt–Estes score≥5 (Schillaci *et al.* 1994).

The Glasgow Royal Infirmary score

This shows similar results and confirms that the point score systems are the best criteria for assessing LVH (Morrison *et al.* 2007).

Regression models

Regression equations for estimating left ventricular mass were used to identify LVH. Table 10.4 shows the most common models. However, they are not used in clinical practice, although they may be implemented in automatic interpretation. The accuracy in detecting LVH and evaluating risk of cardiovascular death is similar to the best voltage or score systems (see Table 10.4).

Diagnosis of left ventricular hypertrophy in clinical practice (Figures 10.20 and 10.21)

It is evident that very specific criteria are required for clinical use, even at the cost of sensitivity (Figures 10.20 and 10.21). The ideal situation would be a specificity as close as possible to 100% with the highest possible sensitivity (see Table 10.4). Of all the criteria described in Table 10.4, the ideal is a criterion that identifies LVE well and may furthermore predict risk of cardiovascular events in a multivariate analysis (see Table 10.8). The following may be used for this purpose:

• A Romhilt–Estes score ≥5 points

• The Cornell voltage (R aVL+S V3>24 mm in men and 20 mm in women)

• R aVL≥11 mm or ≥16 mm in the presence of SAH, which is easy to remember and highly specific but not highly sensitive.

Limitations of the diagnostic criteria

Having already commented on some of the limitations of the diagnostic criteria due to methodology used, type of patient cohort, etc., we will now expand on some of these aspects (Levy *et al.* 1990; Hsieh *et al.* 2005; Jain *et al.* 2010).

Methodological considerations

Statistical studies have demonstrated that the diagnostic value of the ECG criteria for LVE largely depends on the real incidence of the disease in the population studied in accordance with Bayes' theorem (Selzer 1981). In effect (Table 10.6), in a group of severely hypertensive patients, 90% had anatomic LVE. Within this context, the possibility that a positive ECG for LVE actually corresponds to anatomic LVE is quite high (720 of 740 subjects, or 97%). In contrast, in a group of asymptomatic adults, the possibility that a LVE ECG corresponds to anatomic LVE is much smaller (8 of 206 subjects, 4%).

In a study performed with pathologic correlation, the heart disease was in an advanced stage of development. As already discussed, the sensitivity of different criteria varies according to the degree of LVH. Moreover, the correlation between the anatomy of the heart and the ECG is poor (Silverman and Silverman 1979), among other reasons, because differentiating a normal heart from a hypertrophied heart is not always easy; heart weight measurement depends on the dissection technique employed, and the thickness of the muscular wall is difficult to measure correctly due to loss of muscle tone and controversy over the most appropriate procedure for taking these measurements.

All these inconveniences have spurred correlation with imaging techniques, such as ventriculography, echocardiography, and, more recently, CMR, which allows *in vivo* correlations with different evolutive periods of the disease. The latter two have the enormous advantage of being innocuous and therefore reproducible (see before).

CMR as a standard for the diagnosis of LVH has been used recently (Jain *et al.* 2010). The authors found similar results regarding specificity for the majority of ECG criteria. However, the sensitivity was much lower in some parameters than in the original papers published on different criteria. Furthermore, some ethnicity differences exist (Table 10.7). The authors admit that, having defined LVH at the 95 percentile of the left ventricular indexed mass, the sensitivity of the ECG–LVH criteria would have increased if the cut-off had been placed at a lower percentile level. This is just another example of how the **results on specificity are fairly high and constant, but the results on sensitivity, that are lower, may have many differences according to the methodology used.**

Limitations conditioned by constitutional factors

The diagnostic capability of the ECG varies with different constitutional factors (age, gender, physical habitus, etc.), to the extent that the same criterion can be positive or negative depending on the existence of one factor or other. If these factors are kept in mind, the diagnostic capability of the ECG can be increased in an important percentage of cases. We will examine some of these factors.

Table 10.6 Diagnostic value of ECG criteria of left ventricular enlargement in accordance with Bayes' theorem.

		ECG criteria for LVE		
		Positive	Negative	Total
Severe hypertension group (1000 cases)				
90% has anatomical LVE:				
900 cases with anatomical LVE		720	180	900
100 cases without anatomic LVE		20	80	100
	Total	740	260	1000
Predictive accuracy		720/740 = 97%		
Asymptomatic adults group (1000 cases)				
1% has anatomical LVE:				
990 cases without anatomic LVE		198	792	990
10 cases with anatomic LVE		8	2	10
Predictive accuracy	Total	206	794	1000
		8/206 = 4%		

Table 10.7 Diagnostic characteristics of traditional ECG criteria for detecting MRI-defined left ventricular enlargement in the overall MESA cohort (N = 4967 participants).

ECG criterion	Sensitivity (95% CI)	Specificity (95% CI)		ROC area (95% CI)
Sokolow–Lyon voltage	26.0 (21.7–30.7)	92.6	(91.8–93.3)	0.59 (0.57–0.62)
Romhilt–Estes ≥ 4	15.9 (12.4–19.9)	97.0	(96.5–97.5)	0.56 (0.55–0.58)
Romhilt–Estes ≥ 5	5.7 (3.6–8.6)	99.1	(98.8–99.4)	0.52 (0.51–0.54)
Cornell voltage	15.1 (11.7–19.1)	97.3	(96.7–97.7)	0.56 (0.54–0.58)
Perugia score	24.7 (20.5–29.4)	93.2	(92.4–93.9)	0.59 (0.56–0.61)
Minnesola code 3.1	16.9 (13.3–21.1)	95.5	(94.9–96.1)	0.56 (0.54–0.58)
Framingham score	7.0 (4.7–10.1)	99.2	(98.9–99.4)	0.53 (0.52–0.54)
Lewis index	23.2 (19.0–27.7)	88.7	(87.8–89.6)	0.56 (0.54–0.58)
Adjusted Cornell voltage*	15.1 (11.7–19.1)	97.2	(96.7–97.7)	0.56 (0.54–0.58)
LV strain pattern	10.7 (7.8–14.2)	97.0	(96.5–97.5)	0.54 (0.52–0.55)
Cornell duration product	14.8 (11.4–18.8)	97.3	(96.8–97.7)	0.56 (0.54–0.58)
Sokolow–Lyon duration product	12.5 (9.4–16.2)	98.4	(98.0–98.8)	0.56 (0.54–0.57)
Gubner and Ungerleider	13.8 (10.5–17.7)	94.5	(93.8–95.2)	0.54 (0.52–0.56)

* Framingham adjusted.

- **Changes with age**. The voltage criteria are of dubious value in subjects under 25–30 years of age because isolated voltage criteria are frequently present without LVE. For this reason, the use of different voltage criteria for children, adolescents, and young adults has been proposed. In adolescents between 11 and 16 years of age, SV2 + RV5–6 can attain ≥65 mm without LVE taking place. In some series, R exceeds 35 mm in 30% of healthy males between 20 and 40 years of age. Therefore, the SV1 + RV5–6 criterion for LVE should be raised to above 40 mm or even higher for some authors. In contrast, QRS voltage in the elderly usually declines due to myocardial fibrosis or other causes. Repolarization alterations should therefore be considered more important in the diagnosis of LVE, even in the absence of voltage criteria. It is thought that the voltage of the maximum spatial QRS vector decreases 6% per decade from the age of 20 to 80.
- **Changes in body habitus**. Very lean individuals and women with a left mastectomy have a higher QRS voltage, which can lead to a false diagnosis of LVE if this criterion is used alone for the diagnosis. Characteristically, some older persons, especially women who have suffered significant weight loss, display an ECG typical of LVE, but LVH is not found in the autopsy ("little old lady ECG"). Obese individuals or persons with any other type of intracardiac (e.g. myxedema) or extracardiac barrier effect (pleural or pericardial effusion, emphysema, etc.) can have LVE without meeting the usual voltage criteria. (Chapter 7. ECG changes with body habitus).
- **Changes according to gender or race**. Men show a greater QRS voltage in the frontal and horizontal plane leads, especially in the latter. In women, if the electrode is placed over the left breast, a lower voltage may be recorded. Furthermore, voltage is higher in Black people than in White people (Velury and Spodick 1994). The differences in SE and SP in different races have been reported (Table 10.7) (Jain *et al.* 2010).
- **Changes of voltage and heart volume**. There is no unanimous agreement as to whether increased left

ventricular blood volume that produces left ventricular dilation increase or decrease the surface ECG voltage; both direct and inverse relations have been described. Different factors contribute to this discrepancy (Brody effect, state of the myocardial fibers, etc.) (Amoore 1985). These facts illustrate the difficulties of interpreting R wave changes produced during the exercise test (see Chapter 25). For some authors (Clemency *et al.* 1982), the sensibility of the ECG criteria diminishes with ventricular dilation.

• **Day-to-day variations in voltage.** Willens *et al.* (1972) demonstrated that ECG and VCG voltage can vary on a daily basis. This is another factor that can modify the sensitivity and specificity of the voltage criteria for diagnosing LVE.

Value of other electrocardiological techniques

Using orthogonal leads, Macfarlane *et al.* (1981) found a score designed from a hybrid system (12-lead ECG+3 orthogonal leads) with a sensitivity of 65–75% and a specificity of 90–95%. Pipberger *et al.* (1982) obtained a lower specificity at the expense of increasing sensitivity with a coding system for patients with severe hypertension or aortic valve disease. This method may be useful for performing a preliminary screening. In order to improve the diagnostic accuracy of LVE, sophisticated electrocardiological procedures may be used. For instance, a better correlation with the ventricular mass is obtained with a multiple dipole technique (126 leads) (Pipberger 1979) compared to that with three orthogonal leads or a standard ECG. Considering the ease of calculating ventricular mass by echocardiography, however, the effort required to carry out this complicated technique is not worthwhile.

Special characteristics of some types of left ventricular hypertrophy

Left ventricular hypertrophy in children (Moss and Adams 1968; Rowe and Mehrizi 1968)

Because of the predominance of the right ventricle in the newborn, the diagnosis of LVH at this age presents certain peculiarities. **The following criteria suggest LVE in the neonatal period:**

• **S in V1 larger than 20 mm** in the full-term newborn and larger than 25 mm in the pre-term newborn. In the latter case, the right physiological overload is of a shorter duration than that of the full-term infant.

• **R wave in V6 greater than 16 mm.**

• **R/S ratio in V1 less than 1** in the full-term newborn.

• **T wave in V1 positive after the 4th day of life**, as long as T is negative in the left precordial leads.

• **Q in V6 over 3 mm.**

• **Left-deviated ÂQRS** (beyond 30°).

As the years pass, the QRS loop, anterior and to the right in the infant after the first few weeks of life,

becomes posterior and to the left, as in the adult (see Figure 7.44). However, the posterior position of the loop, manifested by rS in V1 with "r" similar in size to "q" in V6, is a sign suggestive of LVH in children under 2 years of age who are not pre-term. In contrast, very high voltage in V5 and V6 with R superior to 30 mm and unaccompanied by S, if the "r" in V1 is notably larger than "q" in V6, is frequently observed in children without heart disease.

A normal QRS complex for age with a P wave characteristic of left atrial enlargement also suggests LVH.

Tables have been published (Moss and Adams 1968) that show the normal values for the different ECG parameters from birth to adulthood. Values which are out of the normal range according to these tables suggest an abnormality.

Left ventricular dilation vs. left ventricular hypertrophy

When ECG criteria for LVE are found, the most constant echocardiographic sign is the increase of left ventricular mass. This is seen in practically 100% of patients, while left ventricular dilation is detected in less than 50%.

In contrast, the presence of a clear dilation of left ventricle is especially seen in cases of dilated cardiomyopathy. This generally occurs earlier in heart disease with diastolic overload (e.g. aortic regurgitation) than in heart disease with systolic overload (e.g. aortic stenosis).

When an R wave satisfies the voltage criteria for LVH, the following signs suggest associated left ventricular dilation:

• R voltage in V6 exceeding that of R in V5.

• Abrupt transition from a complex with a deep S in a chest lead to one with a tall R in the next lead to the left (Figures 10.30 and 10.31).

• In successive ECGs, the reduction in R wave height in the left precordial leads as other hypertrophy signs become more severe.

• QRS complexes with IDT ≥ 0.07 sec.

• Low voltage in the frontal plane.

• It has been reported that patients with isolated left ventricular dilation and normal thickness of the left ventricular wall may present with an increase of the QRS voltage (Toshima *et al.* 1977). However, Reichek and Deveraux (1981) found that in patients with severe chronic aortic regurgitation and massive cardiomegaly, the usual criteria for LVH were often absent.

Indirect signs of left ventricular hypertrophy

The following may be considered indirect signs of LVH:

• Clear signs of left atrial enlargement in the absence of mitral stenosis.

• Atrial fibrillation in the elderly.

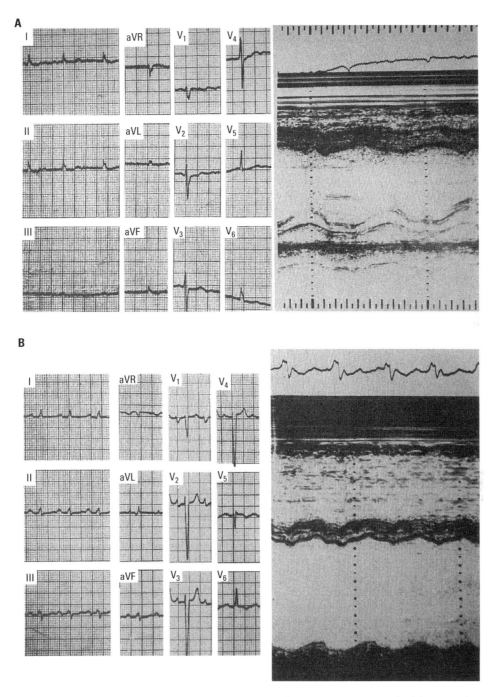

Figure 10.30 (A) Patient with mitral and aortic valve disease with atrial fibrillation. No ECG criteria for left ventricular enlargement are met but it is very apparent the presence of very low voltage in FP (see text). The echocardiography demonstrates an evident increase in ventricular mass and dilated left ventricular. (B) Patient with heart failure and evident left ventricular dilation in the echocardiography. Both ECGs showed many of the features of dilated cardiomyopathy.

• A negative U wave in leads facing the left ventricle in the absence of ischemic heart disease.
• The presence of advanced LBBB. In this case, it is recommended to always perform an echocardiogram.
• Poor progression of the R wave from V1 to V3. This morphology can also be seen in older persons with no apparent heart disease and patients with septal infarction.

LVH in cardiomyopathies and heart failure

Patients with hypertrophic CM usually present with voltage criteria and also repolarization alterations (strain pattern) of LVH (see Figure 21.3). However, it may occasionally present abnormal Q waves (Figure 21.1), and in cases of apical HCM, the negative T wave is often very deep and peaked (see Figure 21.2). Finally, patients with

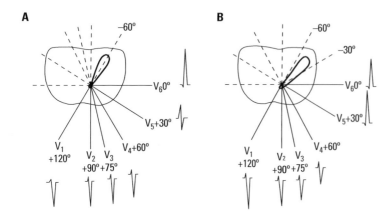

Figure 10.31 In cases with left ventricular dilation, a narrow, very posterior QRS loop is often seen (A), which explains why there is sometimes a progression from an rS complex in a lead to qR on the next to the left, with the intermediate RS morphology absent (B) (see Figure 10.30B).

HCM and low voltage of QRS have been shown to present with more frequently dilated cardiomyopathy in a long follow-up (Figure 21.4) (see Chapter 21).

Different types of restrictive CM may present striking ECG signs of LVH, including "strain pattern," but also "Q" waves of pseudo-necrosis and prominent R waves in V1 as described in Chapter 22. In this chapter, the most characteristic ECG signs found in patients with heart failure, including the changes of voltage of QRS related to the presence of anasarca, are described (Figure 22.5).

Regression of ECG signs of left ventricular hypertrophy
This may be seen in hypertensive patients in particular. With treatment, the left ventricular mass is reduced and, frequently, a clear improvement in the ECG may also be

observed (Figure 10.32). Furthermore, a regression of left ventricular strain pattern after valve replacement in case of severe aortic stenosis, usually not long-lasting evolution, may be seen.

Differential diagnosis
LVE should be distinguished from LBBB, some cases of WPW pre-excitation and ischemic heart disease, especially anteroseptal infarction.

• **LVE versus LBBB.** The QRS complex never measures 0.12 sec in isolated LVE, whereas this is the rule in advanced LBBB. Therefore, when QRS is 0.12 sec or more, there is associated advanced LBBB or SAH with an important degree of left ventricular parietal block. Partial LBBB or septal fibrosis accounts for the lack of

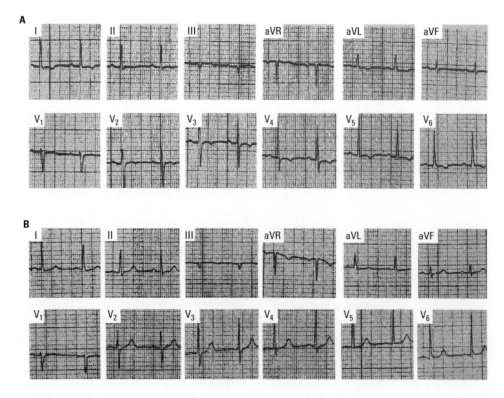

Figure 10.32 A 56-year-old male with hypertensive heart disease. ECGs before treatment (A) and 7 months later (B). Observe the reduction in the left ventricular enlargement morphology.

"q" wave in V6 in patients with LVE (Piccolo *et al.* 1979; Bayés de Luna *et al.* 1983) (see above). The negative T wave seen in advanced LVE is likely due, at least partially, to some degree of LBBB accompanied by hypertrophy (Bisteni 1977) (see before).

• **Type I and II WPW pre-excitation.** WPW pre-excitation, especially types I and II, can generate tall R waves in V5–V6 and small or even absent "r" in V1 that may be confused with LVH or LBBB, especially since there is no initial "q" and there is an abnormal repolarization. Careful measurement of the PR interval and the identification of the δ wave clarify this confusion (Chapter 12).

• **Ischemic heart disease.** The following differential diagnosis has to be performed:

  – **Lateral ischemia vs. LVH.** In cases of normal QRS and negative T wave in lateral leads (V5–6, I, VL), the following criteria suggest isolated LVE (Beach *et al.* 1981): (a) depression of the J point, (b) an asymmetric T wave with a more rapid upslope, (c) positivity in the final part of T wave, and (d) a T wave that is more negative in V6 than in V4.

  – **The presence of QS in right precordial leads in patients with LVE.** The presence of QS in V1–V2 in patients with LVE is a challenge because the presence of associated myocardial infarction has to be ruled out. The following data may suggest the presence of associated myocardial infarction in cases of QS pattern in V1: (a) a notch or slurrings at the beginning of QRS, (b) the presence of fragmented QRS, or (c) the presence of a negative symmetric T wave in V1–V2. If needed, contrast-enhanced CMR can accurately identify whether myocardial necrosis is present in cases of dubious Q waves in V1–V2 (see Chapter 13) (Bayés de Luna *et al.* 2006).

Diagnosis of left ventricular hypertrophy in the presence of ventricular blocks

In the presence of advanced right bundle branch block

The sensitivity of the criteria is lower but the specificity remains high. According to Vanderberg *et al.* (1985), **LVH is suggested with a sensitivity of about 30% and a specificity >90% when:**

• the terminal negative P wave in V1 ≥1 mm in depth and ≥0.04 sec in duration;
• the Romhilt–Estes score ≥5;
• RV5 ≥20 mm;
• RI ≥10 mm.

The Sokolow–Lyon index in the presence of RBBB has a high specificity (100%) but a low sensitivity (4%) because of the presence of a small S wave in V1.

In the presence of advanced left bundle branch block

Scott in 1973 found with **anatomic correlation** studies that all patients with advanced LBBB studied post-mortem presented with LVH and that the sensitivity of ECG criteria for LVH was only a little lower than in cases with no

LBBB. Also, studies performed with **echocardiographic correlations** showed that the diagnosis of LVH in the presence of LBBB is feasible. We will now look at the most important criteria.

A sensitivity of 75% for four cumulative criteria (RVL ≥11 mm, QRS axis −40°, or beyond, SII > SIII, SV1 + RV5 or RV6 ≥40 mm and SV2 ≥25 mm) with a specificity of 90% were found by Kulka *et al.* (1985) using an echocardiographic correlation. The author claims that LVE can be reliably diagnosed both in the presence of LBBB and under normal conditions.

A higher Sokolow–Lyon score in 80% of patients with LBBB and an augmented ventricular mass confirmed by echocardiography were reported by Lopes *et al.* (1978).

In intermittent LBBB, SV1 increases and RV5–6 decreases without modifying the Sokolow–Lyon criteria (Cokkinos *et al.* 1978).

The diagnosis of LVE in patients with LBBB can be made using the echocardiogram as a control when the sum of SV1 + RV6 ≥45 mm with a sensitivity of 86% and a specificity of 100% (Klein *et al.* 1984). However, the sensitivity of this criterion is lower than that in other studies (Gertsch 2004).

Sometimes the vertex of R wave is more peaked because Vector 4 has a greater magnitude.

There are criteria for clear left atrial enlargement.

In the presence of superoanterior hemiblock

The following criteria suggest LVE:

• The index SIII + (R+S of greatest voltage in precordials >30 mm for males and >28 mm for females) with echocardiography correlations has a high specificity and sensitivity (Gertsch *et al.* 1988).

• The R wave voltage in VL ≥16 mm strongly suggests LVE (Talbot *et al.* 1976), but the sensitivity of this criterion is low (Figure 11.40).

Clinical implications

ECG diagnosis of LVE is not easy and should always be carried out after careful observation of the QRS complex changes (above all, voltage criteria) and ST–T variations (ST segment and T loop opposite to QRS). Despite these precautions, false-positive and false-negative diagnoses are made. However, **an apparently normal ECG is more often seen in LVE than an ECG characteristic of LVE is seen in a normal individual.**

In aortic valve disease, the presence of the signs of LVE (tall R and "strain pattern" of repolarization) suggests significant and long-lasting heart disease and a poor prognosis (Greve *et al.* 2012).

Epidemiologic studies have shown that in patients with **arterial hypertension,** the presence of ECG signs of LVE is a marker for poor long-term prognosis, leading to an increase in overall cardiac mortality and sudden cardiac death (see Chapter 22, The ECG in arterial hypertension).

It should be kept in mind (see before), however, that **ECG criteria have important limitations** due to methodological problems (ECG criteria, for example, yield very different results in a group of severe hypertensive patients than in a group of healthy young people, in accordance with the Bayes' theorem), constitutional factors (i.e. variations with age, body habitus, etc.), and timing and recording technique (i.e. daily variations in QRS voltage). In fact, false-positive and false-negative diagnoses of LVE are common.

When confronted with an ECG tracing suggestive of advanced (long-standing) LVE (tall R and "strain pattern"), it is important that LBBB, type I and II WPW, and ischemic heart disease are ruled out.

From a prognostic point of view, LVH is a strong independent predictor of future cardiovascular events (Haider *et al.* 1998; Gardin *et al.* 2001; Bluemke *et al.* 2008) and the ECG is widely used to detect LVH. Although the SE of the ECG is low in predicting LVH, its SP is very high. Thus, the prognostic value of the ECG when the diagnosis of LVH is made is even greater than that of echocardiography.

The Framingham study (Kannel *et al.* 1969) indicated that one-third of men and a quarter of women with LVH who met ECG criteria that included evident repolarization disturbances in the ECG died within 5 years of diagnosis. Currently, with the new treatment of hypertension and ischemic heart disease, surely the prognosis will be much better. The multi-ethnic study of atherosclerosis (Jain *et al.* 2010) has shown **the association of different ECG criteria for LVH defined by CMR with the incidence of cardiovascular events** (Table 10.8). The ECG–LVH criteria that predicted an increased risk of cardiovascular events in this multivariate study were: a Romhilt–Estes score >5, Cornell voltage, and the Framingham score in particular. Based on this study, we use the Romhilt–Estes score >5 and Cornell voltage criteria in our clinical practice (see before).

Recently, it has been demonstrated (Subirana *et al.* 2011) that the associated LVH in a population of sudden death victims studied by necropsy in Mediterranean countries is higher when compared to Anglosaxon countries.

In patients with STEMI, the presence of LVH is associated with more adverse clinical outcome (Stiermaier *et al.* 2018).

The presence of LVH appears to be associated with more severe disease in patients with acute ischemic stroke (Tziomalos *et al.* 2018).

In patients with hypertension, the presence of ECG markers of LVH is a risk factor of future CV events (Tanaka *et al.* 2018).

The presence of ECG criteria of LVH predicts recurrences of AF after ablation of paroxysmal AF (Li *et al.* 2018).

In patients with LVH presents an increase risk predictor of sudden cardiac death (Porthan *et al.* 2019).

Table 10.8 Association of ECG correlates of LVH with incident total CVD events (n = 307 among 4938 participants followed for a median of 4.8 years).

ECG criterion	CV event rate[||]		Unadjusted HR (95% CI)	Adjusted HR (95% CI)
	No LVH	LVH		
$SV_1 + SV_2 + RV_5 (\geq 4.2\,mV)$	3.34	5.92*	1.74 (1.32–2.31)[†]	**1.64 (1.21–2.21)**[†]
Sokolow–Lyon voltage	3.45	5.83*	1.77 (1.28–2.44)[†]	1.26 (0.90–1.76)
Romhilt–Estes ≥4	3.50	7.51*	2.21 (1.47–3.32)[†]	1.05 (0.69–1.61)
Romhilt–Estes ≥5	3.54	13.59*	4.07 (2.38–6.95)[†]	**2.02 (1.15–3.54)**[‡]
Cornell voltage	3.55	6.55[†]	2.01 (1.28–3.16)[†]	**1.65 (1.03–2.63)**[§]
Perguia score	3.36	7.14*	2.32 (1.71–3.16)[†]	1.36 (0.99–1.88)
Minnesota code 3.1	3.54	5.42*	1.62 (1.35–1.94)[†]	1.15 (0.76–1.74)
Framingham score	3.53	14.08*	3.95 (2.35–6.64)[†]	**2.04 (1.20–3.49)**[‡]
Lewis index	3.43	5.34*	1.67 (1.24–2.24)[†]	1.19 (0.87–1.60)
Adjusted Cornell voltage[¶]	3.55	6.51[†]	1.98 (1.26–3.13)[†]	**1.65 (1.03–2.63)**[§]
LV strain pattern	3.51	7.89*	2.34 (1.53–3.58)[†]	1.14 (0.73–1.76)
Cornell duration product	3.48	8.57*	2.84 (1.89–4.24)[†]	**1.67 (1.09–2.54)**[§]
Sokolow–Lyon duration product	3.59	6.41[§]	1.78 (1.02–3.09)[§]	1.26 (0.71–2.23)
Gubner and Ungerleider	3.55	5.32[§]	1.52 (1.02–2.26)[§]	1.01 (0.67–1.51)

Hazard rate is adjusted for age, BMI, gender, hypertension, diabetes, total and HDL cholesterol, pack-years of smoking, ethnicity, lipid and hypertensive medication, number of alcohol drinks per week, and physical activity.

* $P \leq 0.0005$.
[†] $P < 0.005$.
[‡] $P \leq 0.01$.
[§] $P < 0.05$.
[||] Measured per 10 000 person-days.
[¶] Framingham adjusted.

Biventricular hypertrophy

Concept and associated diseases

Biventricular hypertrophy is found especially in valvular and congenital heart disease with biventricular involvement. The diagnosis of biventricular enlargement can often pose serious difficulties, especially when the enlargement of one of the ventricles is very prominent and masks the forces generated by the other enlarged ventricle, or when both ventricles are similarly enlarged. This can result in a "balanced" normal QRS complex. The presence of atrial and repolarization abnormalities can be useful for diagnosing biventricular enlargement.

ECG diagnosis of biventricular enlargement is even more difficult than the diagnosis of isolated ventricular enlargement. In adults with advanced heart disease, dilation of the ventricles usually is associated with wall hypertrophy.

On some occasions, the ECG, or at least the QRS complex, is normal due to equilibrium between the forces of the left and right ventricles, both of which are hypertrophied. **Other times, the ECG manifestations of LVH completely dominate the picture**, obscuring the presence of right ventricular hypertrophy. This situation is partly responsible for the low sensitivity (generally 25%) of many of the ECG criteria for diagnosis of right ventricular hypertrophy. Finally, **sometimes LVH** is hidden and not diagnosed by ECG, especially in cor pulmonale.

At other times, biventricular enlargement is diagnosed by ECG, but during autopsy, it is revealed that only the left ventricle was enlarged. This has occurred in almost 50% of some series (Chou 1979). The ECG criteria most commonly responsible for the false-positive diagnosis of associated RVE were an R larger than 7 mm in V1 and R V1 + SV6 > 10.5 mm.

Electrocardiographic diagnosis: ECG criteria

The specificity of ECG criteria is low, generally ≈50%, and the sensitivity is even lower (usually under 20%). However, correlation studies between bi-dimensional echocardiography and CMR will probably improve specificity at the very least.

The most useful ECG criteria for the diagnosis of biventricular hypertrophy are the following:
- **Tall R in V5–V6 with right ÂQRS** in not very lean individuals (≥+90°, Figure 10.33). The possibility of IPH coexisting with LVE should be ruled out.
- **Tall R in V5–V6 with tall R in V1–V2.** WPW-type pre-excitation must be ruled out.
- **QRS complex within normal limits accompanied by important repolarization disturbances** (negative T and ST depression), especially if the patient has **atrial fibrillation.** This type of ECG is seen in the elderly with advanced heart disease and biventricular enlargement.

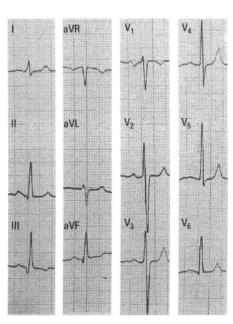

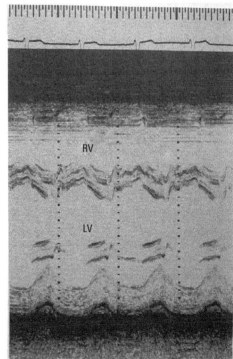

Figure 10.33 Patient with mitral–aortic–tricuspid valve disease and ECG signs of right and left ventricular and left atrial enlargement. The echocardiogram confirmed this.

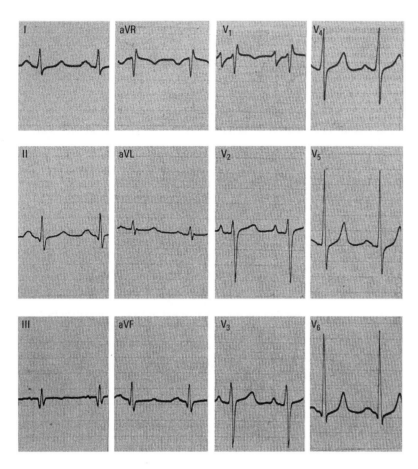

Figure 10.34 Example of bi-atrial and biventricular enlargement. A 35-year-old patient with mitral stenosis and regurgitation, aortic regurgitation, and significant pulmonary hypertension with sinus rhythm (see text).

• **Small (shallow) S in V1, deep S in V2, and a dominant R in V5–V6, with right deviated ÂQRS in the frontal plane, or SI, SII, SIII-type morphology (Figure 10.34).**
• High voltages in the intermediate precordials with a tall R in left precordials (frequent in large ventricular septal defect) (**Katz–Watchell sign**) (Figure 10.35).

Diagnosis in the neonatal period

In the neonatal period, biventricular enlargement is suggested by:

• direct signs of RVH and LVH;
• direct RVH signs plus one of the following: (i) "q" wave of 2 mm or more in the left precordial leads, (ii) conspicuous R in V6, or (iii) negative T in the left precordials;
• the criteria of LVH plus R>S waves in V1;
• an apparently normal ECG in the presence of cardiomegaly not caused by pericardial effusion.

The presence of RVE signs and an ÂQRS deviated beyond −30°, however, do not suggest biventricular enlargement, but rather RVE and SAH. This type of ECG suggests in children the existence of common atrioventricular canal or double outlet right ventricle.

Other electrocardiological methods

Macfarlane *et al.* (1981) has applied a point system based on the orthogonal leads that allow quantified criteria to be used to diagnose biventricular hypertrophy. According to this author, the sensitivity when using these criteria ranges from 42% to 64% and the specificity exceeds 90%.

Diagnosis of biventricular hypertrophy in the presence of ventricular block

In the presence of right bundle branch block

Biventricular hypertrophy is suggested in the presence of: rsR′ morphology in V1, V2 and sometimes V3, with a high R′ voltage or exclusive R in V1–V2, and qRs morphology in V5–V6, as well as, occasionally, V4 with a good voltage R (>20 mm) (see Figure 11.13C).

In the presence of left bundle branch block

Biventricular hypertrophy is suggested when there are signs of LVH plus right ÂQRS, and/or evident "r" in V1 in the absence of myocardial infarction.

Enlargement of the four cavities

This diagnosis is suggested by the association of ECG signs typical of isolated enlargement of the four cavities. This rarely occurs. However, the diagnosis is possible in certain situations, such as the coexistence of biventricular enlargement with atrial fibrillation or other ECG signs of left atrial enlargement plus indirect criteria of right atrial enlargement (QRS ratio of voltage V2/V1 ≥ 5), or a P wave of clearly bi-atrial enlargement (see Figure 10.35).

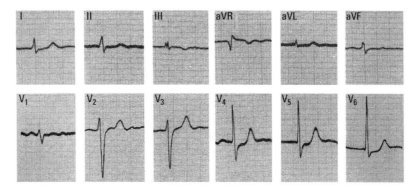

Figure 10.35 An example of biventricular enlargement (see text). Patient aged 42 years with mitral stenosis and regurgitation as well as tricuspid stenosis and regurgitation in atrial fibrillation. See the SI, SII, SIII pattern in the frontal plane, big voltage difference in V1–V2, and high R-voltage in V6 (see text).

References

Allison J, Flickinger F, Wright J, *et al*. Measurement of LV mass in hypertrophic cardiomyopathy using CMR: comparison with echocardiography. *Magn Reson Imaging* 1993;11:329.

Amoore JH. The Brady effect and change of volume of the heart. *J Electrocardiol* 1985;18:71.

Bacharova L, Szathmany V, Mateasik A. Secondary and primary repolarization changes in LVH: a model study. *J Electrocardiol* 2010;43:624.

Bacharova L, Estes E, Bang I, *et al*. Second statement of the working group of ECG diganosis of LVH. *J Electrocardiol* 2011;44:568.

Bayés de Luna A. *Clinical Electrocardiography: A Textbook*. Willey-Blackwell, 2012.

Bayés de Luna A, Serra Genís C, Guix X, *et al*. Septal fibrosis as determinant of Q waves in patients with aortic valve disease. *Eur Heart J* 1983;4(suppl E):86.

Bayés de Luna A, Carrio I, Subirana M, *et al*. Electrophysiological mechanism of SISIISIII morphology. *J Electrocardiol* 1987;20: 38–44.

Bayés de Luna A, Wagner G, Birnbaum Y, *et al*. A new terminology for left ventricular walls and location of myocardial infarcts that present Q wave based on the standard of cardiac magnetic resonance imaging: a statement for healthcare professionals from a committee appointed by the International Society for Holter and Noninvasive Electrocardiography. *Circulation* 2006;114:1755–1760.

Bayés de Luna A, Rovai D, Pons LLado G, *et al*. The end of an electrocardiographic dogma: a prominent R wave in V1 is caused by a lateral not posterior myocardial infarction-new evidence based on contrast-enhanced cardiac magnetic resonane-electrocardiogram correlations. *Eur Heart J* 2015;36:959.

Beach C, Kensure ACF, Shrot D. Electrocardiogram of pure left ventricular hypertrophy ad its differentiation from lateral ischaemia. *Br Heart J* 1981;46:285.

Bisteni A. El proceso de repolarización ventricular en las hipertrofias y sobrecargas ventriculares. *Arch Inst nac Card Mexico* 1977;47:385.

Bluemke D, Kronmal R, Lima J, *et al*. The relationship of left ventricular mass and cardiovascular events: the MESA study. *J Am Coll Cardiol* 2008;52:2148.

Bommer K, Weinert L, Neumann A, *et al*. Determinations of right atrial and right ventricular size by two-dimensional echocardiography. *Circulation* 1980;60:91.

Burch GE, DePasquale NP. *Electrocardiography in the Diagnosis of Congenital Heart Disease*. Lea-Febiger, 1967.

Cabrera E, Monroy JR. Systolic and diastolic loading of the heart. II ECG data. *Am Heart J* 1952;43:669.

Casale PN, Devereaux R, Alonso D, *et al*. Autopsy validation of improved ECG criteria of left ventricular hypertrophy. *J Am Coll Cardiol* 1985;5:511.

Casale PN, Devereux R, Alonso D, *et al*. Improved sex-specific criteria for left ventricular hypertrophy for clinical and computer interpretation of ECG: validation with autopsy findings. *Circulation* 1987;75:565.

Chou TCh. *Electrocardiography in Clinical Practice*. Grune and Stratton, 1979.

Clemency J, Bergere P, Bricand H ECG and VCG in the evaluation of LVH due to pressure overload. *Eur Heart J* 1982;3(suppl A):37.

Cokkinos D, Demopoulos JN, Heimonas ET, *et al*. Electrocardiographic criteria of left ventricular hypertrophy in left bundle-branch block. *Br Heart J* 1978;40:320.

De Piccoli B, Nicolosi GL, Franceschi M, *et al*. Correlazioni elettro-ecocardiografiche nei sovraccarichi del ventricolo sinistro. *Rev Latina Cardiol* 1987;2:25.

Devereux R, Casale P, Eisenberg R, *et al*. ECG detection of left ventricular hypertrophy using echocardiographic detection of LV mass as the reference standard. *J Am Coll Cardiol* 1984;3:1982.

Fretz E, Rosenberg H, Kennedy W, *et al*. Diagnostic value of ECG patterns of right ventricular hypertrophy in children. *J Am Coll Cardiol* 1992;19:126A.

Ganau A, Devereux R, Romen M, *et al*. Patterns of left ventricular hypertrophy and geometric remodeling in essential hypertension. *J Am Coll Cardiol* 1992;19:1550.

Gardin J, McClelland R, Kritzman D, *et al*. M mode echocardiography predictors of cardiovascular mortality in an elderly cohort. *Am J Cardiol* 2001;87:1051.

Gertsch M. *The ECG. A Two-Step Approach to Diagnosis*. Springer-Verlag, 2004.

Gertsch M, Theler A, Fogloia E. ECG detection of LVE in the presence of left anterior fascicular block. *Am J Cardiol* 1988;61:1098.

Greve A, Boman K, Gohke-Baerwolf C, *et al*. The impact of ECG in asymptomatic aortic stenosis. *Circulation* 2012;125:346–353 Doi:https://doi.org/10.1161/CIRCULATIONAHA.111.049759.

Haider AW, Larson MG, Benjamin EJ, *et al*. Increased left ventricular mass and hypertrophy are associated with increased risk for sudden death. *J Am Coll Cardiol* 1998;32:1454.

Horan LG, Flowers NC. Electrocardiography and vectorcardiography. In Braunwald E (ed.) *Heart Disease*. Saunders, 1980, p. 198.

Hsieh B, Pham M, Froelicher V. Prognostic value of ECG criteria for left ventricular hypertrophy. *Am Heart J* 2005;150:161.

Jain A, Tandis H, Dalal D, *et al*. Diagnostic and prognostic utility of ECG for left ventricular hypertrophy defined by CMR in relation to ethnicity: the MESA study. *Am Heart J* 2010;159:652.

Kannel WB, Gordon T, Offutt D. Left ventricular hypertrophy by electrocardiogram. Prevalence, incidence, and mortality in the Framingham study. *Ann Intern Med* 1969;71:89.

Kilcoyne M, Davis AL, Ferrer JA. Dynamic ECG concept useful in the diagnosis of cor pulmonale. *Circulation* 1970;42:903.

Klein RC, Vera Z, DeMaria AN, *et al*. Electrocardiographic diagnosis of left ventricular hypertrophy in the presence of left bundle branch block. *Am Heart J* 1984;8:502.

Koito H, Spodick DH. Electrocardiographic RV6:RV5 voltage ratio for diagnosis of left ventricular hypertrophy. *Am J Cardiol* 1989;63:252.

Kulka E, Burggraf GV, Milliken JA. Electrocardiographic diagnosis of left ventricular hypertrophy in the presence of left bundle branch block: an echocardiographic study. *Am J Cardiol* 1985;55:103.

Levy D, Labib S, Anderson K, *et al*. Determinants of sensitivity and specificity of ECG criteria for left ventricular hypertrophy. *Circulation* 1990;81:815.

Li SN, Wang L, Dong JZ, *et al*. Electrocardiographic left ventricular hypertrophy predicts recurrence of atrial arrhythmias after catheter ablation of paroxysmal atrial fibrillation. *Clinical Cardiology* 2018;41:797.

Lopes MG, Pereirinha A, De Padua F. The diagnosis ventricular hypertrophy in the presence of bundle branch block: an ECG/VCG and echocardiographic correlation. In Antaloczy Z (ed.) *Modern Electrocardiology*. Excerpta Medica, 1978, p. 423.

Macfarlane PW, Chen CY, Boyee D, *et al*. Scoring technique for diagnosis of ventricular hypertrophy from three orthogonal lead electrocardiogram. *Br Heart J* 1981;45:402.

Moro E, D'Angelo G, Nicolosi GL *et al*. Long term evaluation of patients with apical hypertrophic cardiomyopathy. Correlation between quantitative echocardiographic assessment of apical hypertrophy and clinical-electrocardiographic findings. Correlation between quantitative echocardiographic assessment of apical hypertrophy and clinical-electrocardiographic findings. *Eur Heart J* 1995;16:210.

Morrison I, Clark E, Macfarlane P. Evaluation of electrocardiographic criteria for left ventricular hypertrophy. *Anadolu Kardiyol Derg* 2007;7(suppl 1):159.

Moss AJ, Adams FH. *Heart Disease in Infants, Children and Adolescents*. Williams and Wilkins, 1968.

Mulloy T, Okin P, Dovereux R, *et al*. ECG detection of LVE by the simple QRS voltage-duration product. *J Am Coll Cardiol* 1992;20:1180.

Murphy ML, Thenabadu PN, Blue LR, *et al*. Descriptive characteristics of the electrocardiogram from autopsied men free of cardiopulmonary diseases—a basis for evaluating criteria for ventricular hypertrophy. *Am J Cardiol* 1983;52:1275.

Norman J, Levy D. Improved ECG detection of echocardiographic LVE. *J Am Coll Cardiol* 1993;21:1680.

Okin P, Roman M, Devereux R, *et al*. Electrocardiographic identification of increased left ventricular mass by simple voltage-duration products. *J Am Coll Cardiol* 1995;25:417.

Piccolo E, Raviele A, Delise P, *et al*. The role of left ventricular conduction in the electrogenesis of left ventricular enlargement. *Circulation* 1979;59:1944.

Pipberger HP. Performance of conventional orthogonal and multiple-dipole electrocardiograms in estimating LV muscle mass. *Circulation* 1979;60:1350.

Pipberger H, Simonsen E, Lopes ET, *et al*. The ECG in epidemiological investigations. A new classification system. *Circulation* 1982;65:1456.

Porthan K, Kentta T, Niiranen TJ, *et al*. ECG left ventricular hypertrophy as a risk predictor of sudden cardiac death. *Int J Cardiol* 2019;276:125.

Prakash R. Echocardiographic diagnosis of right ventricular hypertrophy: correlation with ECG and necropsy findings in 248 patients. *Cathet Cardiovasc Diagn* 1981;7:179.

Rautaharju PM, La Croix A, Savage D, *et al*. ECG estimates of LV mass versus radiographic cardiac size and the risk of CV disease. *Am J Cardiol* 1988;62:59.

Reeves TJ. *Year Book of Medicine*. Year Book Medical Publishers, 1970, p. 385.

Reichek N, Deveraux RB. Left ventricular hypertrophy: relationship of anatomic, echocardiographic and electrocardiographic findings. *Circulation* 1981;63:1391.

Reiter S, Rumberger J, Feiring A, *et al*. Precision of measurements of right and left ventricular volumes by cine computed tomography. *Circulation* 1986;74:890.

Rodriguez Padial L. Usefulness of total 12-lead QRS voltage for determining the presence of left ventricular hypertrophy in systemic hypertension. *Am J Cardiol* 1991;68:261.

Romhilt D, Estes E. A point score system for the ECG diagnosis of left ventricular hypertrophy. *Am Heart J* 1966;75:752.

Rowe RD, Mehrizi A. *The Neonate with Congenital Heart Disease*. WB Saunders Co, 1968.

Schillaci G, Verdechia PP, Borgioni C, *et al*. Improved ECG diagnosis of left ventricular hypertrophy. *Am J Cardiol* 1994;74:714.

Selzer A. The Bayés theorem and clinical electrocardiography. *Am Heart J* 1981;101:363.

Sheridan D. *Left Ventricular Hypertrophy*. Churchill Livingstone, 1998.

Siegel R, Roberts WC. Electrocardiographic observations in severe aortic valve stenosis: correlative necropsy study to clinical, hemodynamic and ECG variables demonstrating relation of 12-lead QRS amplitude to peak systolic transaortic pressure gradient. *Am Heart J* 1982;103:210.

Silverman M, Silverman B. The diagnostic capabilities and limitations of the ECG. In Hurst JW (ed.) *Update, I: The Heart*. McGraw-Hill, 1979, p. 13.

Sodi-Pallares D. *Bew Basis of Electrocardiography*. CB Mosby Co., 1956.

Sokolow M, Lyon T. The ventricular complex in left ventricular hypertrophy obtained by unipolar precordials and limb leads. *Am Heart J* 1949;27:161.

Stiermaier T, Pöss J, Eitel C, *et al*. Impact of left ventricular hypertrophy on myocardial injury in patients with ST-segment elevation myocardial infarction. *Clin Res Cardiol* 2018;107:1013.

Subirana MT, Carrió I, Bayés de Luna A *et al*. Valor de la escintigrafía con 201-talio (RT) en el diagnóstico de crecimiento ventricular derecho (CVD): correlación con la electrovector cardiografía. *Rev Esp Cardiol* 1981;34:1.

Subirana MT, JuanBabot JO, Puig T, *et al.* Specific characteristics of sudden death in a Mediterranean Spanish population. *Am J Cardiol* 2011;107:622.

Talbot S, Dreifus L, Watanabe Y, *et al.* Diagnostic criteria for computer-aided electrocardiographic 15-lead system. Evaluation using 12 leads and Frank orthogonal leads with vector display. *Br Heart J* 1976;38:1247.

Tanaka K, Tanaka F, Onoda T, *et al.* Prognostic value of electrocardiographic left ventricular hypertrophy on cardiovascular risk in a non-hypertensive community-based population. *Am J Hypertens* 2018;31:895.

Toshima P, Koga J, Kimura N. Correlations between ECG, VCG and echocardiographic findings in patients with LV overload. *Am Heart J* 1977;94:547.

Tziomalos K, Sofogianni A, Angelopoulou SM, *et al.* Left ventricular hypertrophy assessed by electrocardiogram is associated with more severe stroke and with higher in-hospital mortality in patients with acute ischemic stroke. *Atherosclerosis* 2018;274:206.

Van der Wall E, Van der Laarse A, Plum B, Bruschke A (eds). *Left Ventricular Hypertrophy.* Kluwer Academic, 1999.

Vanderberg B, Sagar K, Romhilt D. ECG criteria for the diagnosis of left ventricular hypertrophy in the presence of complete right bundle branch block. *J Am Coll Cardiol* 1985;5:511.

Velury V, Spodick DH. Axial correlates of PV1 in left atrial enlargement and relation to intraatrial block. *Am J Cardiol* 1994;73:998.

Walker I, Helm R, Scott R. Right ventricular hypertrophy at autopsy: correlation with electrocardiographic findings. *Circulation* 1955;11:215.

Willens J, Poblete P, Pipberger H. Day-to-day variation of the normal ECG and VCG. *Circulation* 1972;45:1057.

Wolf HK, Burgraaf G, Cuddy E, *et al.* Prediction of LV mass from the ECG. *J Electrocardiol* 1991;234:121.

Chapter 11
Ventricular Blocks

Definition of terms

Historically (Sodi *et al.* 1964; Cooksey *et al.* 1977; Laham 1980; Alboni 1981; Macfarlane and Veitch Lawrie 1989), it was thought that an electrical impulse was usually blocked in the trunk of the right or the left bundle branch, respectively, producing ECG patterns of right bundle branch block (RBBB) or left bundle branch block (LBBB). However, it was also known that ECG morphologies similar to right or left bundle branch block patterns may be produced not only by trunk injuries, but also by injuries located more proximal to the bundle of His of right or left branches, or distal to the trunk in the periphery (parietal) (Narula 1977; Sung *et al.* 1976; Horowitz *et al.* 1980).

While the concepts of superoanterior division block and inferoposterior division block of the left bundle branch (hemiblocks) have already been defined (Rosenbaum *et al.* 1968), it is currently under debate whether a pattern expressing surely blockage of the middle fibers of the left bundle branch exists (Bayés de Luna *et al.* 2012). An additional ECG pattern for the diagnosis of right zonal blocks has also been described (Bayés de Luna *et al.* 1982).

Finally, there are cases with mild increase of QRS duration (≥110 ms) due to non-specific diffuse conduction delay but without any typical pattern of right or left bundle branch block.

Anatomic considerations (see also Chapter 4)

The ventricular conduction system is formed by the right and left bundle branches, their respective divisions and their interconnected Purkinje networks (Figure 11.1).

There are three distinct terminal fascicles within the ventricular conduction system: the right bundle branch, the superoanterior division of the left bundle branch, and the inferoposterior division of the left bundle branch.

They form the basis of the **three-fascicular concept of the intraventricular** conduction system (Rosenbaum *et al.* 1968). The middle fibers of the left bundle might be considered another terminal area, although very often they are not fascicles but instead show a fan-shaped morphology, potentially forming the fourth input of ventricular activation (Uhley and Rivkin 1964; Durrer *et al.* 1970).

The right bundle branch is at first subendocardial; later, it penetrates the septal myocardium before reaching the moderator band. Anatomically speaking, the divisions are not well-defined, but are considered to consist of approximately two that encompass a unique Purkinje network. From an electrophysiological point of view, the network may act as two separate areas and produce zonal blocks.

The left bundle branch has two anatomically well-defined divisions: the superoanterior division, which is longer and narrower, and the inferoposterior division. The midseptal fibers are distributed between them with an inconsistent presentation and variable morphology (Figure 11.2). The electrophysiological significance of these fibers is still not completely understood, but as previously mentioned, it appears that a block in this area may induce a particular ECG pattern (see later).

Electrophysiological considerations

From an electrophysiological point of view, blocks at a ventricular level, as with the other types of heart block (see Chapter 11), may be **first degree or partial ventricular.** In this case, the stimulus may always cross the fascicle, or area in question, but it is delayed. In **third-degree block or advanced ventricular,** the stimulus cannot activate the blocked area through the normal pathway. In **second-degree ventricular block,** the presence of the block is intermittent.

Impulse conduction may be delayed on either the right or left side at a proximal or peripheral level.

Clinical Electrocardiography: A Textbook, Fifth Edition. Antoni Bayés de Luna, Miquel Fiol-Sala, Antoni Bayés-Genís, and Adrián Baranchuk.
© 2022 John Wiley & Sons Ltd. Published 2022 by John Wiley & Sons Ltd.

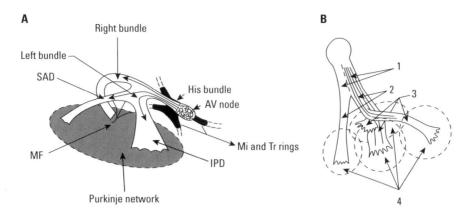

Figure 11.1 Anatomic distribution of the intraventricular conduction system from the left side (A) and from front to back (B): (1) a lesion at the hisian level; (2) a lesion at the truncal level; (3) the left bundle branch divisions; (4) the peripheral level. IPD: inferoposterior division; MF: middle fibers; Mi and Tr rings: mitral and tricuspid rings; SAD: superoanterior division.

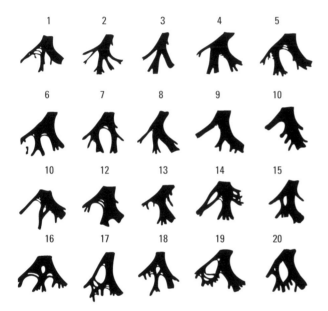

Figure 11.2 Different pathologic aspects of the middle fibers of the left branch in 20 normal cases, according to Demoulin and Kulbertus (1972) (Reproduced from Demoulin and Kulbertus (1972), with permission from BMJ Publishing Group Ltd.).

Table 11.1 Right bundle branch block (delayed right ventricular activation).

	The conduction delay zone can be situated at different points in the His–Purkinje system (see text). More frequently, it is in the proximal part, especially in the trunk of the right bundle (see text).
Global	• The ECG morphology depends especially on the grade of the block, not on its location (see leads aVR, V1, and V6 in Figure 11.17). Some types of peripheral block present ECG differences: Third-degree (advanced) morphologies correspond to type III of the Mexican School (1964) First-degree (not advanced) morphologies correspond to types I and II of the Mexican School (Sodi *et al.* 1964) Second-degree corresponds to a special type of ventricular aberration.
Zonal	• With no conspicuous r′ in V1 (superoanterior or inferoposterior zonal block) and QRS <0.12 sec (see text)

Proximal blocks are the most frequent, with the zone involved usually located in the proximal part of the left or right bundle branch trunks, or in the proximal portion of the superoanterior or inferoposterior divisions. Proximal blocks include the infrequent cases in which a block is the result of the involvement of the corresponding His fibers (see Figure **11.1**). In right peripheral block, the lesion is located in the distal part of the branch or in the corresponding Purkinje network. Left peripheral block, if global, involves the entire left Purkinje network; if partial (superoanterior or inferoposterior division), only the corresponding Purkinje network is involved.

From an **electrocardiographic point of view**, the **pattern of RBBB** and **LBBB,** including the **patterns of**

superoanterior and inferoposterior hemiblocks, are well-defined (Tables 11.1–11.6). We will look at them first individually, then as a simultaneous block of two or three of these structures. In each case, we will briefly mention the clinical and prognostic implications of these types of blocks. We will refer to the combined blocks as "bifascicular" or "trifascicular" because it is helpful to think of these four structures (right bundle branch, left bundle branch trunk and superoanterior and inferoposterior divisions of the left bundle branch) as being equivalent to fascicles (Figure 11.2). We will also describe the possible ECG expression of the middle block fibers (Chapter 5) (Figure 11.3) (see later anteroseptal middle fibers block).

The ECG morphologies of different degrees of right or left bundle branch block are the result of abnormal activation of right and left ventricle due to the presence of the block (Wilson 1941; Grant and Dodge 1956; Sodi *et al.* 1964; Strauss and Selvester 2009; Strauss *et al.* 2011) (Tables 11.1–11.4).

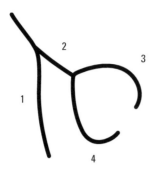

Figure 11.3 To classify bifascicular and trifascicular block, we assume that four intraventricular fascicles exist: (1) right bundle branch; (2) trunk of the left bundle branch; (3) the superoanterior division of the left bundle branch; (4) the inferoposterior division of the left bundle branch. For these purposes, the middle fibers are not considered to be a fascicle.

The ECG morphology on the RBBB is similar irrespective of the origin of the block, whether it is located in the trunk (e.g. bundle branch block) in the hisian fibers (Aguilar *et al.* 1977; Narula 1977; Sobrino *et al.* 1978; Castellanos *et al.* 1981) or is caused by an extensive peripheral block. However, some cases of peripheral block present with special morphological characteristics (i.e. Ebstein's disease, arrhythmogenic right ventricular dysplasia). In all of these cases, there is an abnormal and delayed right ventricular depolarization with the different degrees of conduction delay.

The ECG morphology of the LBBB is also similar at all levels, except in some cases of LBBB at a peripheral level that may have more slurrings and wider QRS than when the block is in the proximal part of the left bundle. **In the case of hemiblocks,** the morphology when the block is peripheral and predominantly affects the area of the Purkinje network dependent on the corresponding fascicle may be similar to the typical ECG pattern seen in cases of superoanterior or inferoposterior block at a proximal level of the fascicle.

Abnormal and delayed activation (the activation phenomenon encompasses depolarization + repolarization) **of part of a ventricle** (divisional or zonal block) **or the entire ventricle** (right or left bundle branch block) **produces vectors directed toward the blocked zone that are more important in a third-degree block than in a first-degree block.** For example, the right ventricle in third-degree RBBB is the last part of the heart to depolarize and it produces vectors directed from left to right and from the posterior to the anterior. This aspect is very important for understanding how changes in depolarization produced by ventricular blocks modify the vectorcardiographic loop and consequently the electrocardiographic morphology of different types of block in the corresponding leads.

ECG diagnosis of advanced (third-degree) RBBB and LBBB patterns offers the following features:
• **The diagnosis is performed mainly in the horizontal plane leads** (V1 and V6).

• **The QRS should measure 0.12 sec or more (see Table 11.5 for LBBB) and the slurrings** should be in the direction opposite to the T wave.
• **Depolarization of the ventricle corresponding to the blocked area** is effected transseptally from the contralateral ventricle (Sodi *et al.* 1964; Van Dam and Janse 1974; Windham *et al.* 1978), which modifies and delays the sequence of ventricular activation. The variations in the activation sequence and cardiac contraction occasioned by this anomalous activation can be confirmed by echocardiography or other imaging techniques (Frais *et al.* 1982; Strasberg 1982).
• **Septal repolarization** dominates over that of the free left ventricular wall and is responsible for the ST–T changes seen in advanced bundle branch block.

Third-degree right and left bundle branch blocks are better termed "advanced" than "complete." This is because if there were no transseptal depolarization from the opposite ventricle to the blocked zone, the right ventricle could theoretically still be depolarized by the impulse that slowly advances through the normal route.

Patients **with advanced bundle branch block, especially on the left side, often present with an enlarged homolateral ventricle.** It seems clear that a certain degree of conduction block in the area of the homolateral ventricle plays an important role in the electrogenesis of ventricular enlargement morphologies (Piccolo *et al.* 1979) (see Chapter 10). In addition, the partial bundle branch block patterns (right and left) have ECG patterns that are often similar to patterns found in the respective ventricular enlargements. In fact, atrial blocks also have ECG patterns that are often similar to atrial enlargement (see Chapter 9).

In general, **the anatomic substrate is more diffuse than its ECG expression** (Lenegre 1964). Frequently, when the ECG morphology reflects isolated advanced right or left bundle branch block, the entire ventricular conduction system is involved to some degree.

Right bundle branch block (Table 11.1)

This type of block produces a somewhat important global delay in right ventricular activation. We will first examine the different aspects of RBBB according to whether the resulting morphology corresponds to third-degree, or advanced, RBBB (QRS ≥0.12 sec and rsR' in V1); second-degree, or intermittent, RBBB; or first-degree, or partial, RBBB (QRS < 0.12 sec and rsr' or rsR' in V1). We will then discuss **zonal right ventricular block (RVB).**

Third-degree (advanced) right bundle branch block

The blockade site of advanced RBBB can be proximal or peripheral. Proximal block includes those cases caused by involvement of the His fibers corresponding to the right bundle branch, but this block is more often located in the proximal part of the right bundle. In peripheral block, the conduction delay is located either in the distal part of the right bundle branch (moderator band) or in the terminal ramifications of the branch (Purkinje network). The most frequent blocks are located in the proximal part of the right bundle. In both cases, proximal or peripheral origin, we use the same terminology because all have the same ECG pattern (RBBB).

Activation (Figures 11.4, 11.5, and 11.7)

Advanced RBBB of proximal origin
In proximal RBBB
In **proximal RBBB**, the impulse is blocked in most cases in the proximal area of the right bundle, and consequently the **ventricular depolarization** starts normally, with the impulse descending by the left bundle branch, but it does not descend by the right branch, or it does so with a delay of 60 ms or more. This is sufficient time for transseptal depolarization of the entire septum, originating from the left ventricle. Recently, studies performed with three-dimensional endocardial mapping (Auricchio *et al.* 2004) have demonstrated that all patients with RBBB pattern have a single right ventricular septal break with a mean transseptal activation time of ≈60 ms. The QRS loop is modified by the left–right direction of transseptal depolarization and predominates over that of the free left ventricular wall, generated important vectors directed forward, to the right and somewhat upward

(Sodi *et al.* 1964). The projection of this loop on the frontal and horizontal planes accounts for the different lead morphologies according to the loop–hemifield concept (see Chapters 1 and 6).

The horizontal loop, which shows the most important changes for the diagnosis of this type of block, rotates counterclockwise and is directed somewhat more forward than normal. Afterward, it moves forward and to the right with a delay (slurrings). The changes of the loop configuration in this plane are the key to understanding V1 and V6 morphologies in advanced RBBB. In the frontal plane, the last part of the loop also presents with slurrings with an upward and unusually rightward direction (Figures 11.4–11.6). Peñaloza *et al.* (1961) reproduced each of these changes in humans through progressive RBBB induction by pressuring the right bundle during heart catheterization (Figure 11.6).

To comprehend these variations, **we can imagine ventricular depolarization in advanced RBBB to be represented by four vectors** (Figures 11.4 and 11.5). Since depolarization initiates normally, Vector 1 does not vary due to RBBB. Vector 2 is somewhat diminished in voltage and slightly anterior, influenced by the anterior and right forces of powerful Vector 3, which begins at this moment and moves in the opposite direction. Vector 3 represents transseptal depolarization and is very important. Although the depolarization is of a relatively small ventricular mass, this process is slow due to the scarce number of Purkinje fibers in the septum. In the field of electrocardiography, the vectors that take longer to form are the most prominent. Vector 4, which is directed for-

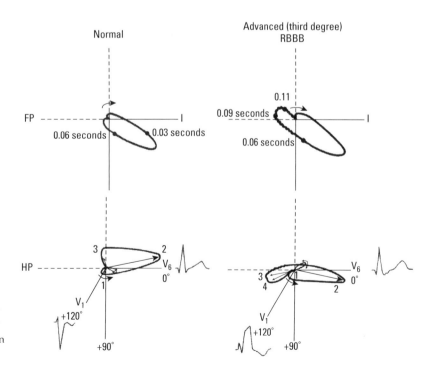

Figure 11.4 Frontal (FP) and horizontal (HP) plane loops in a normal patient and in a patient with advanced RBBB. Observe how this type of block does not modify the general loop direction in the FP, but it is a somewhat more anterior in the HP.

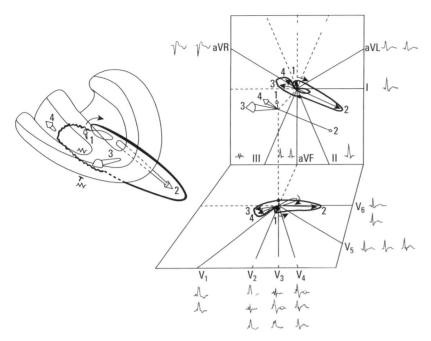

Figure 11.5 Left: QRS and T vectors and loops in advanced (third-degree) RBBB. The thinner area of the right wall corresponds to the so-called trabecular zone. The intracavitary and epicardial QRS morphologies in this zone are the same (rsr's') because of the thinness of the wall. Right: projection of the four vectors on the two planes and the resultant morphologies most often encountered in clinical practice (see text).

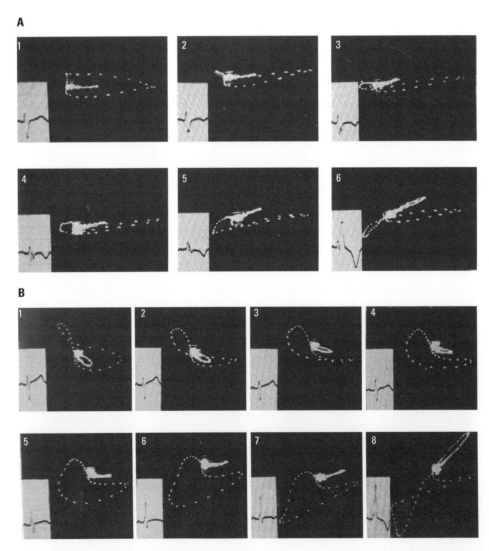

Figure 11.6 The sequential appearance of progressive ECG–VCG patterns of experimental RBBB in humans after touching the zone of the right bundle with catheter in a patient with a healthy heart (A) and in a patient with right ventricular hypertrophy (B). In both cases, progressive changes in V1 and horizontal loop may be seen. The progressive changes of the horizontal loop shows that the ECG patterns are similar in both cases (rs, RS, and rsR' (rR')), but the morphology of the loop is very different (Source: Reproduced with permission from Peñaloza *et al.* 1961).

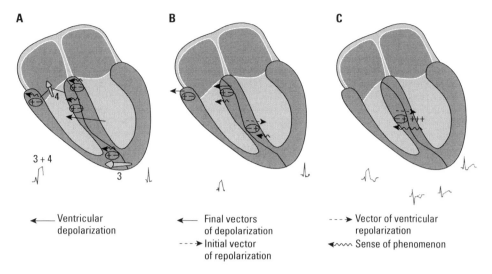

Figure 11.7 Diagrams of the formation of the dipole and vector of depolarization and repolarization in advanced RBBB (see text).

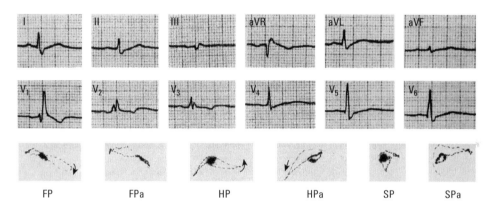

Figure 11.8 ECG of a healthy 75-year-old woman with no heart disease. For more than 15 years, the ECG was unchanged. This is a case of advanced RBBB in a normal heart with no apparent rotations (ÂQRS in the first half of QRS = +30° and there is a qRs in V5). FPa: frontal plane amplified; HPa: horizontal amplified. See the final part of QRS depolarization that produces R in aVR and V1.

ward, to the right and upward, accounts for the late depolarization of the superior portion of the septum and part of the right ventricular wall.

The ventricular repolarization does not depend on the free left ventricular wall as is the norm, but rather on the septum. Septal depolarization predominates over that of the free left ventricular wall. Consequently, repolarization begins on the left side of the septum, where depolarization starts (Figure 11.7B), before depolarization of the right side of the septum is complete. For this reason, from its onset, repolarization (ST) is opposed to depolarization (end of R) and usually draws the final part of the R wave in V1 somewhat below the isoelectric line (Figure 11.7B,C). In the surface ECG, this is not visible in the leads that face the left ventricle, where the ST segment is normally isoelectric. Finally, when depolarization is complete, a single repolarization vector is formed, directed from right to left, a little downward and backward (Figure 11.7C). The T loop is therefore situated to the left and somewhat

downward and backward, opposite to the slurrings formed by Vectors 3 and 4.

These alterations in the QRS and T loops are responsible for the changes observed in ECG patterns and loops in advanced RBBB described below (Figure 11.8).

In peripheral RBBB

In peripheral RBBB, right ventricular activation is also delayed, but the activation sequence is different because the transseptal component is missing.

It has been demonstrated (Horowitz *et al.* 1980) that the activation time in the right ventricular apex, the area where right ventricular depolarization commences, is normal or almost normal when the block results from a lesion of the moderator band or Purkinje network. This is the key to distinguishing between proximal and peripheral RBBB (Figure 11.9).

The impulse in peripheral RBBB is detained at the peripheral level, and there is no transseptal activation of

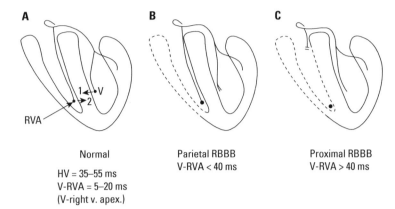

Figure 11.9 (A) Normal HV and V-right ventricular apex (RVA). (B) In peripheral right ventricular block (parietal RBBB), the V–RVA interval is normal, or in any case with a delay, less than 40 ms. (C) If the rsR′ morphology is caused by proximal RBBB, the V–RVA interval will be greater than 40 ms.

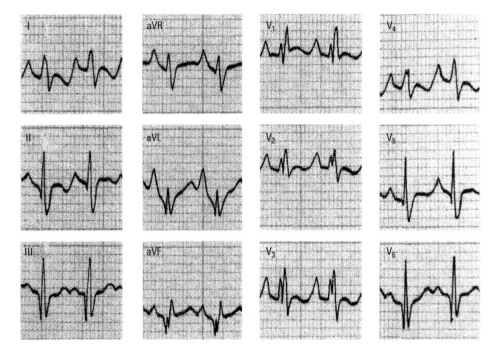

Figure 11.10 ECG of a 6-year-old girl with Ebstein's disease. Observe the high P wave, the rsr's' morphology from V1 to V3 and the prominent "q" in III and aVF.

the right ventricle, as in the case of proximal RBBB, but it represents the same delay of activation of this ventricle. This explains why the ECG pattern is similar to that of proximal RBBB.

In Ebstein's disease (Figure 11.10), activation is delayed in the atrialized zone of the right ventricle (Bialostosky *et al.* 1972).

Epicardial mapping of patients with arrhythmogenic right ventricular dysplasia has shown that right activation delay is caused by a peripheral block (Fontaine *et al.* 1987) (Figure 11.11).

There are also frequent RBBBs of peripheral origin after certain types of surgery for congenital heart diseases (Fallot's tetralogy) (Figure 11.12).

A delay of conduction in the basal part of RV related to RV dilation may explain the presence of final wide R in

aVR in cases of patients with heart failure and LBBB more than an associated partial true RBBB (see Figure 11.30) (Van Bommel *et al.* 2011).

ECG changes (Figures 11.8, 11.10–11.12)

QRS duration
In a proximal block due to the transseptal activation of the right ventricle described above, the duration of the QRS complex is longer than normal, 0.12 sec or more. **In a peripheral block,** it is ≥0.12 sec, often ≥0.14 sec, and even ≥0.16 sec, particularly when right ventricular enlargement coexists.

ÂQRS in the frontal plane
In a proximal block, the axis is not usually deviated with respect to its anterior direction, except for terminal slurrings

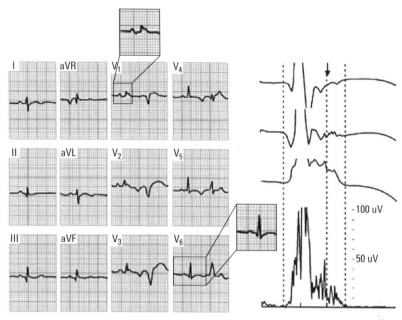

Figure 11.11 Typical ECG pattern of a patient with arrhythmogenic right ventricular cardiomyopathy. Note the atypical RBBB, premature ventricular complexes (PVC) from the right ventricle and negative T wave in V1–V4. We can also see how QRS duration is clearly longer in V1–V2 than in V6. The patient showed very positive late potentials (right). Below: a typical echocardiographic pattern showing the distortion of the right ventricular contraction (arrow).

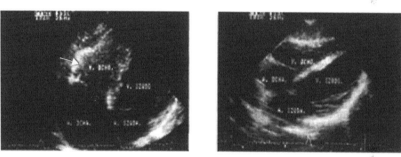

Figure 11.12 (A) Preoperative ECG in an 8-year-old with Fallot's tetralogy. Observe the rsR′ morphology in V1 with QRS<0.12 sec and right-deviated ÂQRS. (B) Postoperatory ECG. Advanced RBBB morphology (rsR′ in V1, QRS>0.12 sec), with no changes in ÂQRS, is observed. The QRS morphology, however, does not help to determine the proximal or peripheral origin of the block (see text).

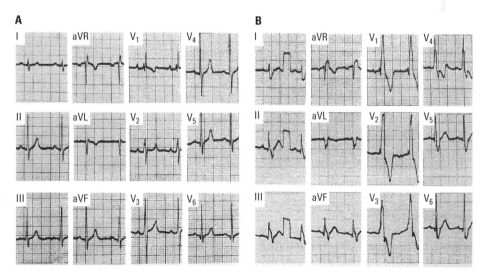

directed upward and to the right (see Figures 11.4 and 11.5). Extreme deviation to the left or right is observed in bifascicular block, advanced RBBB + superoanterior hemiblock-left deviation or inferoposterior hemiblock-right deviation (see later).

The association of RBBB with right ventricular enlargement produces a right-deviated ÂQRS that has to be differentiated from advanced RBBB with inferoposterior hemiblock. Aside from the clinical manifestations, the following suggests advanced RBBB with right ventricular enlargement: (i) ECG signs of right atrial enlargement and (ii) a shallow Q in II, III, and aVF (see Chapter 10).

In a peripheral block, if right ventricular enlargement coexists, the axis is also usually deviated to the right (see

Figures 11.10–11.12). In the post-operative RBBB that occurs after surgery for congenital heart disease, an ÂQRS hyperdeviated to the left practically ensures the proximal origin of the block (Sung *et al.* **1976**).

ECG diagnostic criteria (Table 11.2)
Proximal block (Figure 11.8)
- **QRS complex in the frontal plane**: The delayed final forces directed upward and to the right (Vectors 3 and 4) produce the following constant alterations in I, aVL, and aVR: wide "S" in I and aVL and terminal wide "R" in aVR. In the other leads, the morphology is more variable and is affected by the orientation and magnitude of the slurred forces. In an intermediate-positioned heart, S is slurred in II and aVF and the final forces are isodiphasic or slightly positive in III.
- **QRS complex in the horizontal plane**: The initial loop forces are deviated slightly forward and the final forces are directed forward and to the right, generating the typical rsR' morphology in V1, with a negative asymmetric T in V1 and V2 (r = Vector 1, s = Vector 2, R" = Vectors 3 + 4). V5 and V6 have a qRs morphology with a wide "s" (q = Vector 1, R = Vector 2, s = Vectors 3 + 4). In V3–V4 intermediate leads, we find variable morphologies, most of which are the type shown in Figure 11.5.
- **ST segment and T wave**: As mentioned above, the T wave moves in the direction opposite to the slurrings and therefore is negative in V1, V2, and aVR, and positive in I, aVL, V5, and V6. In the intermediate precordial leads, the T wave varies, although it is more often positive or flat than negative (see Figure 11.5). The ST segment is slightly depressed in V1–V2 and isoelectric in the rest of the leads.

Peripheral block
- In general, the ECG morphologies of global advanced peripheral RBBB are indistinguishable from those of proximal RBBB. However, in some situations (such as Ebstein's disease), a peculiar rsr's' morphology can be seen in V1–V2, with final slurrings (see Figure 11.10) that are different from those of classic RBBB. An atypical RBBB pattern may also be seen in arrhythmogenic right ventricular dysplasia (see Figure 11.11).

Association with other processes (Figure 11.13)

Diagnosis of associated right ventricular enlargement
The following criteria can suggest right ventricular enlargement (RVE) (see also Chapter 10):

Table 11.2 ECG features of advanced proximal RBBB.

- QRS ≥0.12 sec
- V1 rsR' with slurring in R'
- V6 qRs with slurring in S
- VR qRs with slurring in R

- A qR morphology in V1 in the absence of septal infarction. This morphology (Chapter 9) is very suggestive of right atrial enlargement, which is often associated with RVE.
- A rsR' morphology extended beyond V2. This is especially seen in cases of right ventricular dilation (i.e. atrial septal defect).
- A high-voltage R'. As R' increases in height, so does the likelihood of associated RVE. However, there are instances of tall R' without RVE, and vice versa.
- A solitary R in V1 with QRS ≥0.12 sec. This results from the anterior orientation of the whole loop. This solitary R can be low-voltage in emphysematous subjects (Figure 11.13A). It is frequently attended by the absence of "q" in V6.
- An "rS" morphology in lead I and "qR" in lead III. In this case, the possibility of inferoposterior division hemiblock in addition to advanced RBBB must be considered.

Diagnosis of associated left ventricular enlargement (Figure 11.13B)
In an echocardiographic correlation study (Vanderburg *et al.* **1985**), the most sensitive and specific criteria for diagnosing left ventricular enlargement in the presence of advanced RBBB were described. They are:
Tall R in V6 >20 mm.
Deep S in V1, and
qR in lead I and rS in lead III.

Biventricular enlargement
Biventricular enlargement may be diagnosed when in the presence of ECG criteria of RBBB, we see a tall R' in V1 and V2 and sometimes V3–V4 with a qRs morphology in V5–V6 with high R voltage. (>20 mm) (see Figure 11.13C).

Ischemic heart disease
The association of RBBB with chronic Q wave myocardial infarction and also the ECG changes in this pattern due to acute ischemia are described extensively in Chapter 13.

Pre-excitation
This association is infrequent and the diagnosis difficult. We briefly discuss it in Chapter 12.

Differential diagnosis
The differential diagnosis of all ECG patterns with dominant R morphology in V1 or rSr' is described in Chapter 10 (see Table 10.3).

Clinical implications
Advanced RBBB morphology appears in 0.3–0.4% of the normal population (Barret *et al.* 1981). If heart disease is present, the prognosis will be determined by the type of associated disease. In isolated advanced RBBB, the prognosis is good (Rotman and Frietwaser 1975) with no

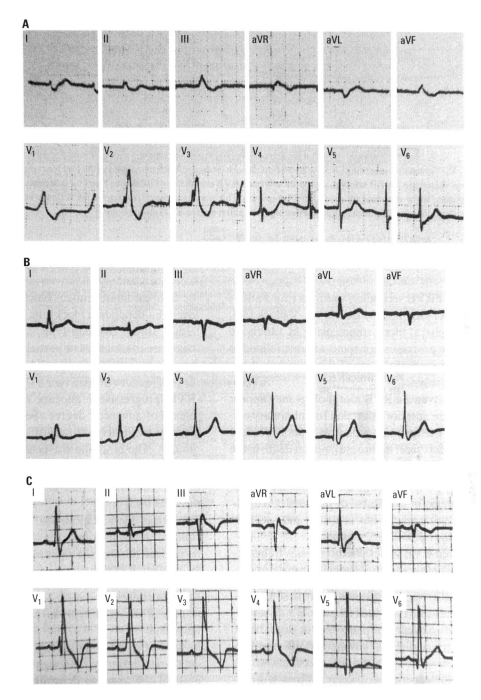

Figure 11.13 (A) Both the frontal plane and the horizontal plane are typical of advanced RBBB with right ventricular enlargement in an elderly patient with chronic obstructive pulmonary disease (COPD). In this case, it is common to see solitary R in V1–V3 and RS in V4–V6 (see text). (B) ECG of an elderly patient with arterial hypertension. The ÂQRS and the morphology and voltage of QRS in the precordial leads suggest left ventricular enlargement associated with RBBB. (C) A 70-year-old patient with COPD and severe arterial hypertension with a typical morphology of biventricular enlargement in the presence of advanced RBBB (see text).

tendency to develop complete atrioventricular (AV) block or elevated incidence of coronary heart disease. Some epidemiological studies (Schneider *et al.* 1980) indicate that the mortality in patients with advanced RBBB initiated in adulthood is greater than that of a control population group. However, when Kulbertus *et al.* (1980) studied a

series of patients with virtually no heart disease, the prognosis was not worse than that of a control group.

Patients with proximal RBBB secondary to surgery for Fallot's tetralogy are more likely to develop AV block (Horowitz *et al.* 1980). It has been demonstrated (Sung 1979) that the advanced RBBB that appears after corrective surgery for Fallot's Tetralogy is usually peripheral (normal V–RVA time) when it presents alone, and is generally proximal (lengthened V–RVA) when associated with superoanterior hemiblock. Most of the chronic advanced RBBBs unrelated to cardiac surgery have been considered proximal. However, other authors (Dancy *et al.* 1982) consider that peripheral advanced RBBB is also common.

Pre-existing RBBB was observed in 13% of patients that underwent TAVR increases risk for overall mortality after TAVR with a balloon-expandable valve (Watanabe *et al.* 2016).

Peripheral block appearing in adulthood has a poor prognosis that is related to a greater number of clinical complications/syncope and presyncope (Dancy *et al.* 1982). The appearance of wide final R in aVR in patients with LBBB and heart failure suggest associated delay of basal part of the right ventricle (Van Bommel *et al.* 2011).

Thirty percent of cases of advanced RBBB with normal PR have a lengthened HV interval (Narula 1979). If HV >100 ms, especially in the presence of symptoms (syncope), pacemaker implantation is indicated.

In the presence of advanced RBBB morphology, measurement of the HV interval and V–RV apex (distance from the onset of ventricular activation on the left side to the arrival of the impulse at the apex of the right ventricle) helps to locate the blockade site (see Figure 11.9). The block is truncal when HV is normal and the V–RVA is lengthened. It is peripheral when both HV and RVA are normal. However, in practice we usually do not perform

that, because as we have said the prognosis is related to associated disease.

An advanced RBBB pattern which appears during pulmonary embolism usually indicates that the pulmonary embolism is massive (see Figure 10.16).

In patients with acute infarction, RBBB usually occurs in cases of anterior infarction due to occlusion of proximal LAD because the right bundle is perfused by the first septal branch. Thus, it is accompanied by prolonged V–RVA (Mayorga-Costes *et al.* 1979).

First-degree (partial) right bundle branch block (Figures 11.14–11.17)
Activation
The location of the block can also be proximal or peripheral. **If proximal, the impulse is delayed in the right bundle branch trunk**, or, much less often, through the right side of the bundle of His. The delay is less than 0.06 sec. Two consequences ensue: (i) part of the right septum depolarizes transseptally, and (ii) the rest of the right septum and right ventricle depolarize normally, although late, and are the last parts of the heart to depolarize. The longer the delay, the more septum is depolarized transseptally and the larger the portion of right ventricle to depolarize last (Figure 11.14). In the last part of the QRS loop, the slurrings are directed right and forward. The shorter the delay, the less marked the slurrings. This is because the transseptal depolarization vector and the delayed final depolarization vector are directed forward, upward, and to the right. The duration of the QRS complex is always less than 0.12 sec.

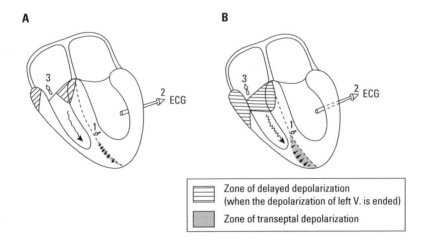

Figure 11.14 Diagram of ventricular depolarization in global but partial (first-degree) RBBB of proximal origin, less intense in (A) and more intense in (B). In this type of RBBB (see text), one part of the right septum (dotted area) depolarizes transseptally because when the impulse reaches the right septum from the left side, the impulse from the right bundle branch has still not arrived. The longer this impulse takes to reach the right septum, the larger the portion of it that depolarizes transseptally (B). This delay in the arrival of the impulse to the right ventricle means that a proportionate part of the right ventricle depolarizes later than the left ventricle (lined area), originating a final ventricular depolarization vector directed upward and to the front. It must be remembered that under normal circumstances a small portion of the right ventricle is the last to depolarize, and it produces a vector directed upward and backward. In partial RBBB, the vector is directed upward and a little forward, and it falls at the very least in the positive hemifield of V1 and aVR. It is also somewhat delayed. Therefore, an rSr′ or rsR′ morphology in V1 and a final r′ in aVR that is wider than normal but with QRS <0.12 sec is produced.

If the site of partial RBBB is peripheral, **right ventric- ular activation** is also slowed. A delayed right ventricular depolarization that is probably not transseptal presents with less delay than in the case of advanced peripheral block (see before). The morphology observed in atrial sep- tal defect (ASD) and in some cases of cor pulmonale (rsR' with QRS<0.12 sec) is mixed, partly due to RVE and partly due to the accompanying global non-advanced probably peripheral RBBB (De Micheli *et al.* 1983).

Ventricular repolarization is less opposed to QRS in proportion to the lesser degree of delayed right ventricu- lar depolarization seen.

ECG changes

The loop–hemifield correlation accounts for the morphol- ogies seen in either proximal or peripheral partial RBBB (Figures 11.15 and 11.16): I and V6 (narrow S), aVR (final R) and V1 (rsr') with greater r' height in proportion with

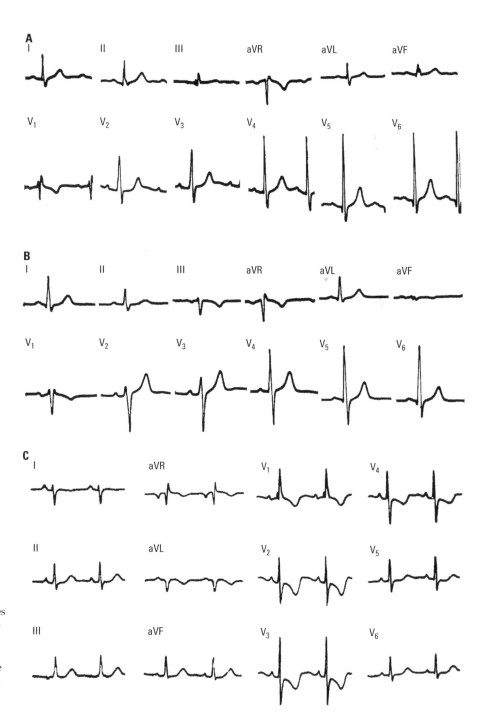

Figure 11.15 Three examples of first-degree RBBB morphology (QRS <0.12 sec) with different degrees of r'. (A and B) Two patients with no evident heart disease. (C) Postoperative ECG of a patient with Fallot's tetralogy. In the preoperative ECG, there was no rsR' in V1. In this case, the morphology is mixed (partial RBBB + RVE) (see text).

the degree of delay, resulting in more septum depolarizing abnormally and more free right ventricular wall depolarizing late, but always with a QRS narrower than 0.12 sec.

The induction of progressive RBBB morphologies (Figures 11.6 and 11.16) (Peñaloza *et al.* 1961; Piccolo 1981) demonstrates that before the r' morphology appears in V1, a globally more anterior QRS loop without final forces directed to the right and forward is usually seen in the horizontal plane (counterclockwise rotation). In this case, the QRS complex in V1 progresses from rS to Rs with slurring or RS, and finally to rsr'. As a result, partial RBBB can exist without r' in V1 (Figures 11.6 and 11.16). To avoid overdiagnosing partial RBBB, we continue to use r' morphology in V1 as a diagnostic criterion (see block of middle fibers).

Differential diagnosis and clinical implications

Generally speaking, the rsR' morphology with QRS <0.12 sec results more from RVE with some degree of RBBB than from isolated partial RBBB. It is often a more severe disorder due to associated RVE (chronic obstructive pulmonary disease (COPD) or other) with a worse prognosis than the pattern of isolated RBBB with QRS ≥ 0.12 sec morphology.

The rSr' morphology may also be due to a highly misplaced V1 electrode (Figure 11.17), thoracic malformation (*pectus excavatum*), or sport. In these cases, the rSr' pattern has no clinical significance. However, this ECG pattern has to be differentiated from the ECG pattern with r' in V1 corresponding to type II Brugada pattern. In Chapters 7 and 22, we describe the differential ECG patterns between *pectus excavatum*, athletes, and type II Brugada pattern (see Figure 7.16). Other explanations for prominent R or rSr' in V1 are shown in Table 10.3.

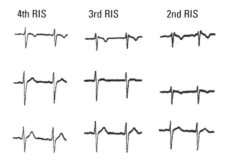

Figure 11.17 A very lean 15-year-old patient without heart disease. The rSr' morphology is due to a misplaced V1 electrode in the second right intercostal space (see negative P wave) and disappears when the electrode is properly positioned (fourth right intercostal space) (see text).

Table 11.3 Left bundle branch block (delayed left ventricular activation)

	The conduction delay zone can be situated at different levels of the His–Purkinje system (see text). The classical form is in the trunk of the left bundle
Global	• The ECG morphology depends especially on the grade of the block, not on its location (see VR1, V1, and V6). Some types of peripheral block present slightly different ECG characteristics (see text): Third-degree (advanced)—corresponds to type III of the Mexican School. First-degree (partial)—corresponds to types I and II of the Mexican School. Second-degree—corresponds to a special type of ventricular aberration
Zonal or divisional	• The block is located in the divisions of the left bundle branch. Superoanterior and inferoposterior hemiblocks (Rosenbaum *et al.* 1968) • Possible block of middle fibers (see text)

It is important to remember (see Chapter 9) that the P terminal in force V1 (PtfV1) may be considered abnormal a risk marker of AF, and even stroke. However, if the ±pattern presents as a consequence of bad placement of electrodes of V1 in a higher position, then the pattern ± is not considered abnormal.

Second-degree right bundle branch block (Figure 11.18)

This type of block usually located in the proximal right bundle branch trunk is responsible for the intermittent appearance of advanced or partial RBBB morphology (Figure 11.14). This relatively infrequent phenomenon can appear without changes in heart rate or without being conditioned by variations in heart rate (phase 3 achycardia-dependent block and phase 4 bradycardia-dependent block) (see Chapter 14). Its presentation can be either sudden (Mobitz type II block: abrupt appearance of advanced

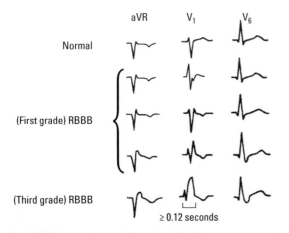

Figure 11.16 aVR, V1, and V6 morphologies in a normal case and in third- and first-degree RBBB. Note that in partial (first-grade) RBBB, three ECG patterns corresponding to three consecutives bigger grades of first-degree RBBB may be seen (see Figure 11.6).

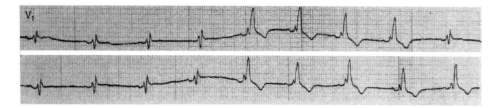

Figure 11.18 V1. Continuous recording. A 55-year-old patient with first-degree RBBB morphology (the first four complexes) who abruptly presented with advanced RBBB morphology (third-degree) for four complexes, with minimal changes in the RR interval. After four first-degree RBBB complexes, there were five advanced RBBB complexes. This is an example of second-degree RBBB (some impulses are completely blocked in the right bundle branch), although it stems from a first-degree RBBB morphology.

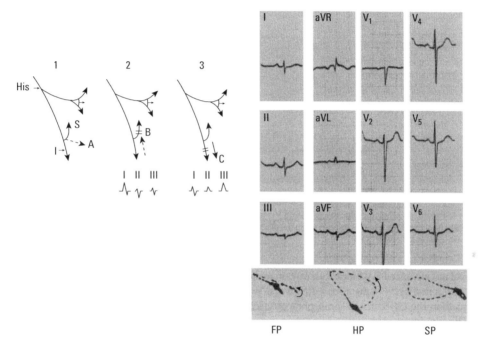

Figure 11.19 Left: Diagram of the morphologies that appear in anterosuperior (2) and inferoposterior (3) peripheral right ventricular zonal block. In the normally specialized conduction system (SCS) with right and left bundle branch divisions, the right bundle branch produces a resultant depolarization vector (A) oriented to the left and a little downward (1). If the right anterosuperior zone of right bundle is blocked (2), a final depolarization vector (B) directed toward the blocked zone is produced, which explains the SI, SII, SIII morphology. If the inferoposterior zone is blocked (3), a final depolarization vector (C) directed toward the blocked zone is produced, which accounts for the SI, RII, RIII morphology usually seen in this type of block. Right: An ECG–VCG example of right ventricle anterosuperior peripheral block. As indicated in the text, the same morphology can be seen in right ventricular enlargement and as a normal variant.

or partial RBBB morphology) or progressive (Mobitz type I block, a Wenckebach-type that is much more rare). In the latter, the RBBB pattern progressively appears in successive complexes of advanced degree. Second-degree block corresponds to a type of ventricular aberrancy (see Chapter 14).

Zonal or divisional right ventricular blocks

The number of peripheral divisions of the right bundle is not well-defined. From an anatomic point of view, it may be considered that there are three divisions (Uhley and Rivkin 1961). However, electrophysiologically only two divisions are usually considered (Marquez-Montes 1975;

Medrano and De Micheli 1975; Bayés de Luna *et al.* 1982). Experimentally, blocks of the anterosuperior subpulmonary and inferoposterior Purkinje network of the right ventricle (divisional or zonal blocks) produce, respectively, SI, SII, SIII, and SI, RII, RIII-type morphologies without conspicuous r' in V1 (Figure 11.19). The SI, SII, SIII morphology appears more frequently than the SI, RII, RIII.

With spatial velocity ECG techniques (Hellerstein and Hamlin 1960; Bayés de Luna *et al.* 1982, 1987), we have demonstrated in humans that SI, SII, SIII and also the SI, RII, RIII morphologies may reflect a right conduction delay, associated with RVE in patients with COPD, and also in healthy people. In the latter, the conduction delay probably expresses a decreased number or abnormal distribution of Purkinje fibers (Figures 11.19 and 11.20).

On rare occasions, these patterns, especially SI, SII, SIII, appear transiently in the case of pulmonary embolism or after the administration of some drugs.

ECG diagnostic criteria (Figures 11.19 and 11.20)

In view of these facts, we suggest the following diagnostic criteria for these two types of zonal block:
* **Superoanterior zonal block (SAZB)** (Bayés de Luna *et al.* 1982): (i) SI, SII, SIII morphology with SII ≥ SIII; (ii) if there is no SI, the RI is of low voltage; (iii) V1 = rS or rSr′; (iv) V6 = S wave.
* **Inferoposterior zonal block (IPZB):** The diagnostic criteria are: (i) S (I) R (II) R (III) morphology; (ii) rS, RS, or rSr′ morphology in V1; (iii) V6 with a very evident S wave.

We have already commented that in rare cases, these ECG patterns may occur transiently, which confirms that they correspond to a conduction delay (block) due to various causes (dilation of right ventricle, effect of drugs).

Differential diagnosis

Both blocks must be differentiated from other processes that can produce similar morphologies.

Superoanterior zonal block (SAZB)

The differential diagnosis should be made with the following:
* **Normal variant.** The SI, SII, SIII morphology is often seen in healthy subjects. We hypothesize (see above) that this pattern in healthy people is caused by an anomaly in the distribution of the Purkinje fibers (fewer and/or abnormal distribution of Purkinje fibers in the upper right ventricle, resulting in an activation delay but no pathological block). The classical explanation of this pattern in the normal population was a special rotation of the heart (Cabrera's back oriented apex) (Bayés de Luna *et al.* 1982) (see Chapter 7, Rotation on the transversal axis).
* **Left superoanterior hemiblock** (LSAH). Here, the SII, SIII morphology has SII < SIII, with SI usually absent (see Figure 11.21).
* **Right ventricular enlargement** (RVE). The morphology is the same as in normal variant and SAZB. In reality, many patients with right heart disease and SI, SII, SIII morphology also have RVE. We have demonstrated that in patients with SI, SII, SIII, and COPD, both processes (RVE and SAZB) are present (see Figure 11.19). The presence of a P wave of RAE favors the presence of RVE. Definitively, the clinical setting and echocardiography may assure the diagnosis.

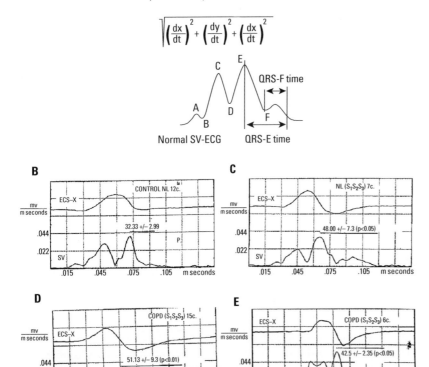

A

Spatial velocity ECG: Hellerstein Me

$$\sqrt{\left(\frac{dx}{dt}\right)^2 + \left(\frac{dy}{dt}\right)^2 + \left(\frac{dx}{dt}\right)^2}$$

Figure 11.20 (A) Diagram of the normal spatial velocity ECG. (B–E) Examples of spatial velocity ECGs in an individual with a normal ECG (B), in a normal SI, SII, SIII-type patient (C), in a patient with COPD (D), and SI, SII, SIII, and in another patient with COPD and SI, RII, RIII (E). In the three last cases, the increase in the duration of QRS-E and QRS-F time parameters in relation to the control group was statistically significant. This confirms that SI, SII, SIII pattern of any type and SI, RII, RIII pattern in patients with COPD present some zonal delay of conduction in the right ventricle (see text).

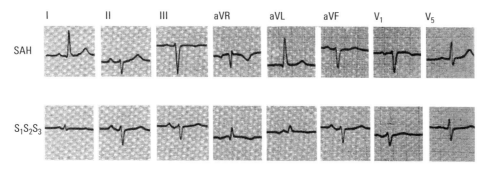

Figure 11.21 Comparison between a typical S$_1$ S$_2$ S$_3$ morphology (normal variant, right ventricular enlargement, right peripheral block) and superoanterior hemiblock (SAH) morphology. In the SI, SII, SIII morphology, S$_1$ is present and S$_2$>S$_3$, in contrast to SAH (see text).

• **Brugada syndrome** (BS). According to the neural crest theory (Elizari *et al.* 2007), in BS there is an activation delay of the right ventricle outflow tract (RVOT), and this explains the frequent SI, SII, SIII pattern that may be seen in this syndrome (≈40% cases) (see Chapter 21).

Inferoposterior zonal block (IPZB)
Differential diagnosis must be made with:
• **Normal variant**. The SI, RII, RIII morphology, with or without r′ in V1, is found in normal subjects with *pectus excavatus* or extremely vertical heart, and sometimes in normal individuals without these characteristics who probably present with some anomalies in the Purkinje network distribution (fewer Purkinje fibers than normal in the inferoposterior zone of the right ventricle).
• **Left inferoposterior hemiblock** (LIPH). This diagnosis requires the exclusion of very lean individuals, RVE, and any evidence that some pathology of left ventricle exists.
• **Right ventricular enlargement**. In most patients with right heart disease and SI, RII, RIII morphology, there is concomitant RVE (Bayés de Luna *et al.* 1982) (Figure 11.19). The electrocardiographic tracing alone does not show whether the morphology is caused by IPZB or RVE, or both. The clinical setting, the P wave morphology, and echocardiography may assure the diagnosis.

Clinical implications
It has to be considered that both patterns—SI, SII, SIII and SI, RII, RIII—may be seen both in normal people or as an expression of RVE or abnormal activation as in Brugada syndrome. This is a differential that we need to perform when we are faced with a patient with such ECG patterns. It is also important to perform the differential diagnosis with superoanterior and inferoposterior hemiblock (see Figure 11.21 and later).

Left bundle branch block (Tables 11.3 and 11.4)

This block produces a somewhat marked global delay in left ventricular activation. Like RBBB, the morphology depends more on the degree of block than on its location

(proximal or peripheral). Classically, it was considered that third-degree (or advanced) LBBB occurred when the QRS ≥0.12 sec with slurring in the plateau of the R wave; first-degree LBBB when the QRS <0.12 sec with solitary R in V6; and second-degree LBBB when the pattern is intermittent. However, these values may be currently a little different (Strauss *et al.* 2011) (see later) (see Table 11.4). Later, we will explain zonal or divisional left ventricular blocks, which include hemiblocks and the controversial block of the middle fibers.

Third-degree (advanced) LBBB
This can be produced by proximal block of the trunk or, rarely, the left hisian area, or peripheral block (Table 11.2). Peripheral block is caused by involvement of the entire left Purkinje network and produces ECG morphologies similar to those of proximal blocks, with some increase in the slurrings and usually a wider QRS (see later). Distal or proximal blocks of the two divisions of the left bundle can also produce a third-degree LBBB pattern, although they really are a type of bifascicular block (see Figure 11.3). However, the activation wave in this case could hypothetically reach the left ventricle via the middle fibers (Medrano *et al.* 1970).

Activation (Figures 11.22–11.24) (Wilson 1941; Grant and Dodge 1956; Sodi *et al.* 1964; Strauss *et al.* 2011)
Advanced LBBB of proximal origin
This is the most frequent LBBB. **The depolarization process** starts with the impulse descending through the right bundle branch normally, but not descending though the

Table 11.4 ECG features of advanced left branch bundle block.

• QRS ≥120 ms. Recent studies suggest ≥130 ms per women and 140 ms for men (Strauss et al. 2011)
• V1 QS or rS with tiny r. Positive asymmetric T wave
• V6 R exclusive with usually negative asymmetric T wave
• In all the leads, the ST is opposed to the polarity of QRS and is quickly followed by asymmetric T wave
• Presence of mid-QRS notching or slurring in ≥2 leads V1, V2, V5, V6, I, and aVL

left bundle branch, or descending with a delay of 0.06 sec or more. This delay lasts long enough for the whole septum to be depolarized transseptally from the right ventricle (Figures 11.22 and 11.23). This produces a prolongation of HV and QRS (Cannom *et al.* 1980).

The QRS loop undergoes alterations as a consequence of the change in cardiac depolarization from the onset of QRS occasioned by advanced LBBB. Activation commences at the base of the anterior papillary muscle of the right ventricle, then transseptally depolarizes the septum anteriorly to posteriorly before depolarizing the free left ventricular wall (Figure 11.22). This type of depolarization is completely abnormal, with a slow impulse conduction, and produces slurring of the QRS loop and QRS complex, especially in the middle part of QRS (median

slurrings). Projection of this loop on the frontal and horizontal planes accounts for the different lead morphologies according to the loop–hemifield correlation theory (Figure 11.22).

Projection of the loop in the horizontal plane shows the most important changes for the diagnosis of advanced LBBB. The loop is first directed to the left and forward, followed by a backward counterclockwise rotation and finally a forward clockwise rotation (Figure 11.22). **In the frontal plane, the loop** is directed mainly to the left from the beginning with middle slurrings, but its orientation in this plane presents little modification with respect to the previous orientation.

Like RBBB, advanced LBBB depolarization can be visualized as being represented by four vectors in order to

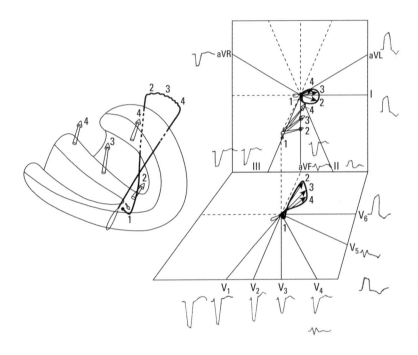

Figure 11.22 Left: QRS vectors and loops in advanced LBBB (third-degree). Right: projection of the four vectors on the two planes with formation of the respective loops and ECG morphologies most often seen in clinical practise (see text).

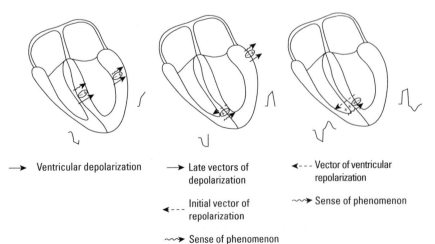

→ Ventricular depolarization

→ Late vectors of depolarization

⦗---⦘ Initial vector of repolarization

⤳ Sense of phenomenon

◄--- Vector of ventricular repolarization

⤳ Sense of phenomenon

Figure 11.23 Diagram of formation of dipole and the depolarization and repolarization vector in advanced LBBB.

understand these changes (Sodi *et al.* 1964) (Figure 11.22). Vector 1 is directed forward and to the left; Vectors 2 and 3 represent the transseptal depolarization forces and are oriented from right to left and forward to backward, with Vector 3 being less posterior; Vector 4 is oriented in a similar way to 2 and 3, but it is even less posterior and represents the depolarization of part of the upper septum and the free left ventricular wall.

The results of left ventricular activation with endocardial mapping in the case of LBBB (Vassallo *et al.* 1984; Auricchio *et al.* 2004) and with computer simulation of LBBB (Strauss and Selvester 2009; Strauss *et al.* 2011) show that the presence of mid-QRS notches with slurring in between is the result of abnormal activation of the left ventricle. The first notch occurs when the transseptal activation reaches the endocardium of the left ventricle (at 50 ms) and the second when the activation front reach the epicardium of the lateral wall (at 90 ms). All this process last ≥130 ms. Figure 11.24 shows how this process occurs.

The **repolarization process** is directed from left to right, as the result of a mechanism similar to that of advanced RBBB (see before) with the T loop and ST vector opposite in direction to QRS (Figure 11.23). This explains why the polarity of the T loop and T wave is opposite in direction to the slurrings. This also explains why the ST segment is slightly depressed in the leads with negative T, and somewhat elevated in leads with positive T.

These variations in the QRS and T loops account for the changes in ECG and VCG morphology observed in advanced LBBB discussed below (Figures 11.25–11.27).

Advanced LBBB of peripheral origin

The delay of conduction (depolarization) occurs in the distal part of the divisions or at the level of the Purkinje network. There are often greater or lesser degrees of block at proximal levels of the left ventricle. Therefore, the global left ventricular activation is delayed. The possibility that left ventricular activation may be done by the middle fibers, despite diffuse lesions distal to the two divisions of the left bundle branch, is very small (Medrano *et al.* 1970) (see before). In any case, the important delay of left ventricular activation explains how a great part of the left ventricle depolarizes from right to left through the Purkinje network of the right ventricle, and lower septum in a way similar to proximal LBBB, but at distal level.

ECG changes (Figures 11.22, 11.23, 11.25–11.28)
QRS duration

In proximal block, the duration of the QRS complex is longer than normal, because of the change in ventricular activation described above (transseptal depolarization of the left ventricle). It is probably longer (Strauss *et al.* 2011) than classically accepted (≥120 ms) (Table 11.4). **In peripheral block,** diffuse involvement of the Purkinje network

A Normal conduction

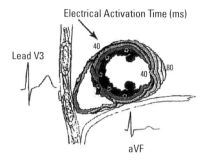

B Left bundle branch block

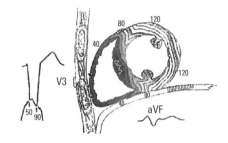

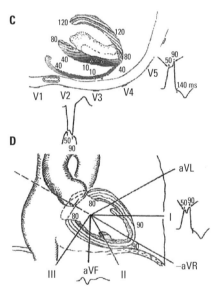

Figure 11.24 (A) Normal activation of left ventricle starts almost simultaneously at right and left side of the septum. (B) In the case of LBBB, the activation front spreads from right to left side through the septum. Each change of gray line represents successive 10 ms. (C and D) See the aspect of QRS pattern in horizontal plane and frontal plane (see text) (Reproduced with permission from Strauss *et al.* 2011).

occurs, and usually there is also a degree of proximal block. The QRS complex is generally 0.14 sec or more (Figure 11.28). If the QRS duration is longer than 0.14 sec, some degree of peripheral blocks or extreme left ventricular hypertrophy very probably exists.

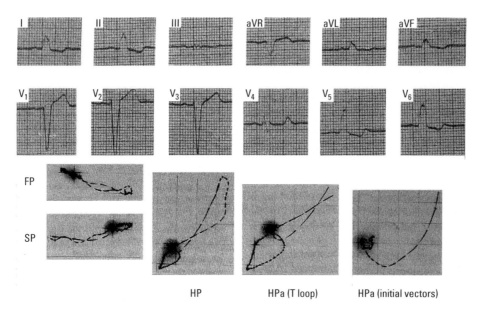

Figure 11.25 Advanced LBBB in a patient with no apparent heart disease. QRS>0.12 sec. Its morphology is consistent with those in Figure 11.22.

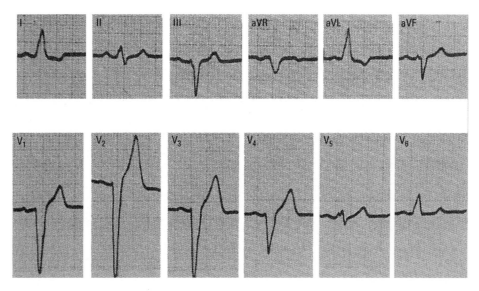

Figure 11.26 Advanced LBBB in a patient with no apparent heart disease. The T wave is positive in V6 but negative in I and aVL. This same morphology has persisted without change for 10 years. It corresponds to advanced LBBB without a wide QRS of 120 ms. In the case of QRS with this borderline width, the normal repolarization of the left ventricular wall may influence the T wave morphology. It must be remembered that the positive T wave in the left precordial leads in advanced LBBB with QRS>140 ms obliges us to exclude the possibility of coronary heart disease because in this case the abnormal repolarization of the septum dominates the repolarization of the left ventricular wall (see text).

ÂQRS in the frontal plane

Normally, the axis is not right-deviated or extremely left-deviated, but rather situated between −30° and +60°. Experimentally, Ribeiro (1968) demonstrated that in peripheral block, ÂQRS can be more deviated to the left or even upward.

- **Extreme left axis deviation** (morphology of third-degree LBBB, with rS or QS in II, III, and aVF) suggests the following possibilities:
  - Advanced LBBB with inferior infarction (QS pattern in II, III, and aVF).

- Associated SAH: the superoanterior zone depolarizes later than the inferoposterior zone (Figures 11.29B, 11.30, and 11.32) (Moreu 1985).
- Advanced peripheric LBBB with more delay activation in SA division (Figures 11.28 and 11.29A).
- Similar morphologies can also be seen in some types of classical and atypical pre-excitation (Bayés de Luna and Baranchuk 2017) and with pacemakers implanted in the right ventricle.

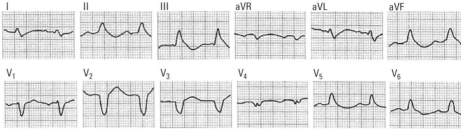

Figure 11.27 ECG of a patient with congestive heart failure and a morphology of advanced LBBB with right-deviated ÂQRS, low voltage in FP and QS pattern till V4.

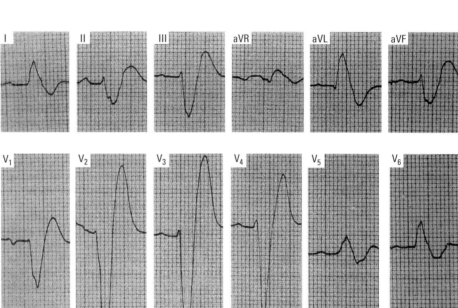

Figure 11.28 Patient with hyperkalemia (K = 7.5 mEq/l) and LBBB pattern with QRS of 0.16 sec, slurrings in all QRS and left-deviated axis. A diffuse and peripheric left intraventricular block exist more important in superoanterior division.

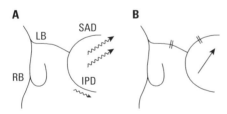

Figure 11.29 (A) Diagram of how the association of a delay activation more important in SA than in IP division can shift the ÂQRS up and leftward in presence of peripheral advanced LBBB. Note that the global LV depolarization is directed upward (see Figure 11.28). (B) The same upward direction is seen if a superoanterior hemiblock is associated to proximal LBBB. LB: left bundle; RB: right bundle; SAD: superoanterior division; IPD: inferoposterior division.

An ECG pattern of advanced LBBB with left axis deviation is often seen in patients with dilated cardiomyopathy. **Right axis deviation**, which usually does not exceed +90°, generates an atypical advanced LBBB morphology which can be attributed to:

• Extreme verticalization of the heart
• Acute right ventricular overload
• Right ventricular enlargement, generally associated with signs of congestive heart failure, in which case the change in precordial leads to an R pattern occurs very late (≈V5) (see Figures 11.27 and 11.31)
• Occasionally, left ventricular free wall infarction.

In all these cases, the inferoposterior zone depolarizes later than the superoanterior zone.

Sometimes, the ÂQRS has a SI, SII, SIII morphology. This occurs more often in peripheral blocks, usually in cases of heart failure and often with low voltage in frontal plane leads (Figure 11.31).

ECG diagnostic criteria

Proximal block

The most important ECG diagnostic criteria are listed in Table 11.4.

• **QRS complex (Table 11.4): Duration was classically considered to be ≥120 ms.** However, if we define LBBB duration in the era of resynchronization therapy, it is probably ≥130 ms for women and ≥140 ms for men (Strauss *et al.* 2011) (see Clinical implications).

With regard to morphology in the frontal plane:

• **Leads I and VL:** The onset of the loop to the left and the presence of mid QRS-notching or slurrings, in the middle part of the loop, due to slowing of the inscription of Vectors 2 and 3 justify the absence of "q" in the QRS complex in I and aVL. The morphology of QRS when the ÂQRS is not strongly deviated to the right is a solitary R with notching or slurring of the R plateau. If there are initial slurrings, the differential diagnosis with Wolff–Parkinson–White (WPW)-type pre-excitation may be difficult to achieve, especially if the PR interval is relatively short. Rarely in lead I, a complex in "M" or even qR with tiny "q" is sometimes observed in the absence of myocardial infarction.

• **Lead VR:** Here, the QRS complex is of the QS type. If a terminal R wave is found, a masked associated right ventricular delay exists due to partial truncal RBBB (Figure 11.32) or right ventricular dilation if heart failure is present (Figures 11.30A).

• **Lead III:** The QRS morphology is Rs, rS, or even QS.

• **Lead II and VF:** The morphology is conditioned by the position of the heart, but it is most often RS or Rs. An rS or QS-type morphology in these leads is the result of the causes already mentioned (left ÂQRS).

In patients with congestive heart failure, a QRS of low voltage (<20 mm, the sum of the voltage of six frontal plane leads) is frequently seen (Figures 11.27 and 11.31).

In the horizontal plane:

• **Lead V1: The QRS morphology** is often completely negative, with median slurrings (Vectors 2+3). Occasionally, a very small initial positivity is seen, a rS morphology with a very small "r" due to the influence of the depolarization of the free right ventricular wall. The presence of QR in aVR and evident r′ in V1 located in 2nd ICS suggest associated RV delay (in case of heart failure) (Figure 11.30A) or partial truncal RBBB (Figure 11.32).

• **Leads V2 and V3**: The morphology is usually rS. On occasions (right ventricular dilation, position change of electrodes, etc.), a QS or a very small r morphology is seen, most often in V2. We have reported (Bayés-Genís *et al.* 2003) that the morphology of S in V3 in patients with

LBBB due to cardiomyopathy and congestive heart failure has a much higher voltage and is without notches if the etiology is idiopathic cardiomyopathy compared with ischemic cardiomyopathy (Figures 11.31 and 22.6).

• **Lead V4:** The morphology is usually transitional, with more or less R (rS, rsr′, RS). In patients with congestive heart failure, the change to an R pattern may occur in V5–V6.

• **Leads V5 and V6:** There is commonly a solitary R morphology with notching/slurring in the plateau accompanied by a negative and asymmetric T. We have to remember that the ECG pattern of mid-left precordial leads may change from one day to another, from R/S to a solitary R wave with small changes in the location of the electrode. Sometimes, more frequently in presence of heart failure (dilated cardiomyopathy) but also occasionally in isolated LBBB, the RS pattern is seen until V6, even in the presence of a left-deviated ÂQRS (Figure 11.30A,B).

• **ST segment and T wave:** The T wave and ST segment (see above) in advanced LBBB are opposite in direction to the middle slurrings, and as such are positive in V1, V2, aVR and, generally, III, negative in I, V5, V6, and aVL, and variable in the other leads.

Nonetheless, in patients without left ventricular enlargement, ventricular repolarization may present with a flat or diphasic – +type T wave or even slightly positive T wave in V6 and/or I, aVL (Figure 11.26). This happens more often in women. Positive T in leads with solitary R wave (V5–V6, I) may be seen also in advanced LBBB in patients with right septal ischemia (ischemia vector moves from the ischemic area on the right and is recorded as positive T wave in the other side, V5–V6). In patients with important left ventricular enlargement and positive T in the ECG in the absence of LBBB, the repolarization of the left ventricular wall may predominate over that of the septum modified by LBBB and the pattern of LBBB may present with a positive T wave.

A

B

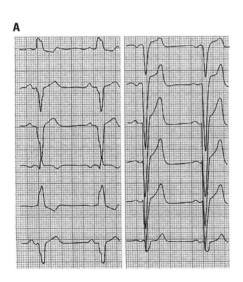 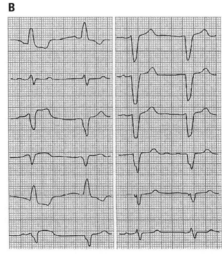

Figure 11.30 (A) ECG of a patient with idiopathic dilated cardiomyopathy with very low ejection fraction and LBBB. The ECG is similar to (B) that corresponds to an elderly patient with chronic obstructive pulmonary disease but without evident heart failure with LBBB at least in the last 20 years. The only difference is that in the first case, there is a QR pattern in aVR that is explained by late activation of right ventricle due to its dilation (see text and Figure 11.33).

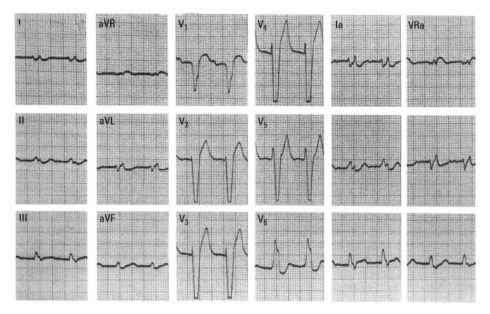

Figure 11.31 Patient with dilated cardiomyopathy and congestive heart failure. The QRS in the frontal plane is polymorphic (rsr′s′) in some leads and of low voltage. The P wave is of low amplitude in the majority of leads. a: amplified.

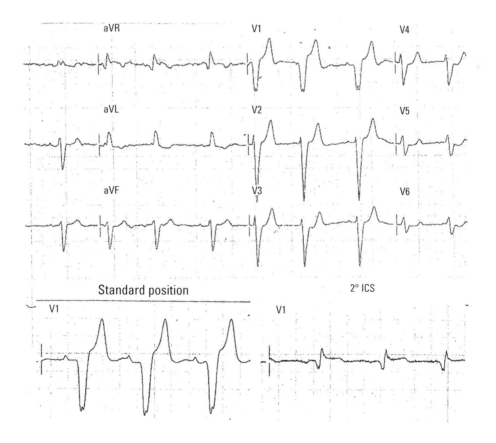

Figure 11.32 ECG of a patient without heart failure and very advanced left intraventricular block (QRS ≈160 ms) that in the standard ECG shows morphology of advanced LBBB with very left-deviated ÂQRS and QR in aVR suggestive of associated right ventricular delay (see Figure 11.30). Also in the second intercostal space lead V1 records a QR that has to be considered in a patient without heart failure probably due to partial truncal RBBB. There are also frequent premature atrial beats (see text: Masked block).

Peripheral block

The ECG morphology of advanced peripheral LBBB **is similar to that seen in proximal LBBB, but with some specific characteristics. The QRS is frequently wider,** especially in cardiomyopathy, electrolyte imbalances, such as hyperkalemia (Figure **11.28**), and as an effect of drugs. Occasionally, particularly in congestive heart failure, **the voltage in frontal plane leads is reduced** (Figure **11.27**). Moreover, in peripheral block, **slurrings are appreciated, not only in the middle part of QRS but also at the beginning and/or end,** which are the result of a diffuse conduction delay of all left ventricular conduction systems. The impulse, when transmitted from the right to the left side, encounters difficulties, not only in transseptal conduction, responsible for the presence of middle slurrings in advanced proximal LBBB, but also from the onset of depolarization (resulting in initial slurrings that can simulate a delta wave and create confusion with WPW syndrome) and at the end of depolarization, reflecting disturbances in the Purkinje network and left ventricular wall (parietal block) and producing final slurrings.

The presence of a small "q" wave in V6 in advanced LBBB in the absence of necrosis may be explained by conduction through the middle fibers, despite the fact that the superoanterior and inferoposterior fascicles are blocked (Medrano *et al.* 1970). However, the presence of evident "q" wave in I, V5, V6 that may be seen in advanced LBBB, is much probably due to the presence of associated myocardial infarction (see later).

The association of LVH plus superoanterior hemiblock may produce a similar pattern of complete LBBB with wide QRS, but without the typical mid QRS notching.

Association with other processes

Right ventricular enlargement (see Chapter 10)
This may be suggested when:
• **ÂQRS is right deviated**, although there are other explanations for this occurrence (see before: Right axis deviation);
• **the initial "r" in V1 is conspicuous** in the absence of necrosis;
• **the transition zone is displaced to the left** (V5–V6).

Left ventricular enlargement (see Chapter 10)
Anatomic correlation studies in autopsies show that patients with advanced LBBB have important LVE. According to Scott in 1973 (see Chapter 10), the sensitivity of the ECG criteria for LVE in the presence of global advanced LBBB is only slightly smaller than that in cases without conduction disturbances.

Other authors have reached similar conclusions from echocardiographic correlation. In fact, Kafka *et al.* (1985) found that using four LVE parameters produced a cumu-

lative sensitivity of 5% and a specificity of 90%. On the other hand, Lópes (1978) and Cokkinos *et al.* (1978) have shown that in intermittent left ventricular block, the Sokolow–Lyon index is hardly modified by the appearance of block because reduction of R in V5–V6 is compensated by the increase voltage of S in V1. In some cases of LVE associated with advanced LBBB, a higher than normal voltage is observed, and the vertex of the R wave may be more peaked because Vector 4 has greater magnitude (see Chapter 10).

Pre-excitation
This is discussed briefly in Chapter 12.

Ischemic heart disease
The associations between LBBB, acute ischemia, and chronic Q wave myocardial infarction are described in Chapters 13 and 20.

Differential diagnosis with LBBB-like morphology
When confronted with a possible morphology of partial or advanced LBBB, the following alternatives should be considered:
• **WPW type I or atypical-type pre-excitation** (Bayés de Luna and Baranchuk 2017) (see Figure 12.4);
• **left ventricular enlargement,** with no "q" in V5, V6, I, or aVL. In reality, there is probably always a certain degree of LBBB in these cases (Piccolo *et al.* 1979). We should remember that the same morphologies seen in partial LBBB (the absence of "q" in I, aVL, V5–V6 with no "S" in these leads) may appear in the presence of septal fibrosis (see Chapter 10; Bayés de Luna *et al.* 1983).

Clinical implications
Advanced LBBB is found in 0.1% of the normal population (Barret *et al.* 1981). Its **prognosis depends on whether there is any associated heart disease.** In the Framingham study (Schneider *et al.* 1985), it was shown that subjects with recently diagnosed advanced LBBB who were followed for 18 years had more heart diseases than normal controls. The ECG signs most often associated with poor prognosis and organic heart disease are: (i) interatrial conduction delay, (ii) ÂQRS leftward beyond 0°, (iii) negative T wave in V6, and (iv) abnormal ECG in the absence of LBBB. Advanced LBBB coexists more often with ischemic heart disease than advanced RBBB plus superoanterior hemiblock and therefore it should be considered to have a worse prognosis: 10 years after the appearance of LBBB, 50% of the subjects will have died of heart disease.

Between 60% and 90% of the individuals with advanced LBBB have a prolonged HV interval and often present with other abnormalities in the sinoatrial node or the His–Purkinje system (Narula 1979; Alboni 1981). The HV interval is lengthened because initiation of ventricular activation is slowed, the V–RVA distance is equal to zero because ventricular depolarization commences in the area of the right ventricular apex, and QRS ≥0.12 sec because of abnormal transseptal activation of the left ventricle (Figure 11.28).

During exercise testing, angina may appear coinciding with the appearance of LBBB. In few occasions (Candell-Riera *et al.* 2002), the presence of intermittent LBBB with or without exercise produces chest pain coinciding with the first LBBB complex. The pain ends suddenly when LBBB disappears. The coronarography is often normal and the cause of pain is unknown.

Advanced LBBB with an extremely left-deviated ÂQRS (Dihingra *et al.* 1978) is more common in the elderly, in patients with ischemia or cardiomyopathy, and in patients with congestive heart failure.

Patients with asymptomatic LBBB are at increased risk of developing CHF and of dying from cardiovascular diseases. Further study is warranted to determine if more diagnostic testing or earlier treatment in patients with asymptomatic LBBB can decrease cardiovascular morbidity or mortality (Azadani *et al.* 2012).

The incidence of mortality and evolution to AV block is in these cases higher. In two years of follow-up, 3 out of 50 cases (6%) with advanced LBBB plus extremely left-deviated ÂQRS presented with complete AV block, whereas this did not occur in any of the 50 cases with LBBB and normal ÂQRS.

Other authors (Moreu 1985) have found differences in the ejection fraction between cases with normal ÂQRS and cases with left axis deviation.

The results of Bogale *et al.* (2007) confirm previous observations showing substantially increased mortality in patients with bundle branch block pattern at baseline or occurring soon after acute myocardial infarction.

In cases of advanced heart failure, final R in aVR is frequently seen. In fact, it has been shown (Van Bommel *et al.* 2011) that combining two or three of the following ECG criteria (wide R in Avr, low voltage (<0.6 mV) in each of all frontal plane leads, and R/S<1 in V5) allows for accurate detection of right ventricular dilation in patients with heart failure and LBBB (Figure 11.30A). The QR in aVR is more due to delay of stimuli in the basal part of the right ventricle than to partial associated typical RBBB, as happens in the absence of heart failure (Figure 11.32).

After catheter aortic valve implantation (TAVI), LBBB pattern appears in 40% of cases and it is the strongest predictor of mortality in the follow-up (Van Gersse *et al.* 2011).

Patients with LBBB that present normal stress echocardiogram have a benign prognosis similar to those without LBBB and normal stress echocardiogram (Supariwala *et al.* 2015).

The patients with advanced LBBB had a higher mortality from heart disease (3.2% yearly) in comparison with the control group, although the difference was not statistically significant (Kulbertus *et al.* 1980). Also Rabkin (1980)

found that in the first 5 years after the onset of advanced LBBB, the incidence of sudden death is greater than in the control group without advanced LBBB.

We have already commented on other clinical implications that arise from the ECG pattern found, such as the **association between LBBB and right ÂQRS** as a possible sign of congestive heart failure and the possibility to diagnose the etiology of advanced LBBB by looking at the S wave in V3 (higher voltage favors idiopathic vs. ischemic cardiomyopathy) (Bayés-Genís *et al.* 2003).

Recently, it has been demonstrated (Baldesseroni *et al.* 2002; Vazquez *et al.* 2009) that the **association of LBBB + atrial fibrillation** in patients with congestive heart failure is a marker of bad prognosis.

Patients with **LBBB present with an abnormal depolarization of the left ventricle** that has hemodynamic consequences and may induce an **impairment of left ventricular function** and even heart failure. In recent years (Cazeau *et al.* 2001; Moss *et al.* 2009), it has been demonstrated that it is useful to correct this abnormality with resynchronization pacemakers (CRT), even in cases of mild heart failure, especially if the QRS measure ≥140 ms. Patients with heart failure and LBBB especially if LVEF is lower than 35% the association of resynchronization therapy (RT) to medical treatment is recommended, because the treatment with medicinals alone is often insufficient and the patients may be better served with earlier RT (Sze *et al.* 2018). Because of this, the diagnosis of advanced LBBB by the width of QRS from a clinical point of view should probably be considered that is 130 ms in women and 140 ms in men (Strauss *et al.* 2011) (see Table 11.4).

On the other hand, there are at least 10% of cases of isolated LBBB (primary disease of the LV conduction system) that has a good prognosis. Therefore, it is not well known if only permanent dyssynchronization of the LV may be sufficient in the absence of latent CM to induce LV failure in a long follow-up (Breithardt and Breithardt 2012).

First-degree (partial) left bundle branch block
Activation

The impulse slowly courses through the left bundle branch trunk, but the delay is less than 0.06 sec. In consequence, part of the left septum depolarizes abnormally from the right side by the transseptal route, while the rest of the left ventricle does so normally, although with a delay. The later the impulse from the left bundle branch arrives, the larger the part of septum depolarized anomalously from the right side (Figure 11.33). If slurrings appear, they are not in the middle or final parts of the QRS complex, which now depolarize normally, but in the R upstroke, where they occasionally simulate a delta wave. When the initial slurrings resembling a delta wave are prominent, a differential diagnosis with true pre-excitation can be difficult if the PR interval is relatively short (≈120 ms) or if the rhythm is not a sinus rhythm

A

B

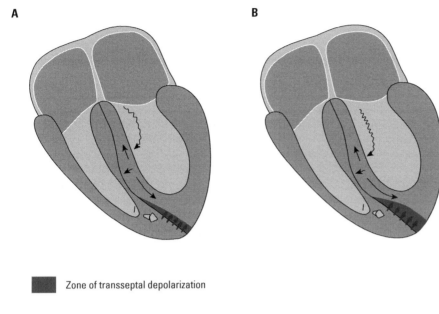

Zone of transseptal depolarization

Figure 11.33 Diagram of ventricular depolarization in first-degree LBBB. If the delay is short (A), there is small transseptal depolarization by the right bundle branch and the only ECG repercussion is the disappearance of the first vector due to the fact that the delay in its inscription causes it to cancel out the right forces. The T wave is positive except when there is associated disease. If the delay is greater (B), there is more anomalous septal depolarization, resembling more advanced LBBB, but the QRS does not reach 0.12 sec in duration and the T wave is positive or negative–positive in I, aVL, and/or V5 and V6.

A

B

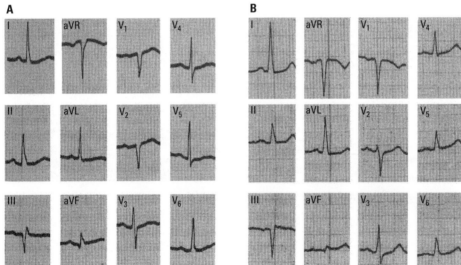

Figure 11.34 Two examples of partial LBBB. (A) A 55-year-old patient with mild hypertension. (B) A 75-year-old patient without clinical heart disease.

(the short PR cannot be evaluated in this case), as occurs in atrial fibrillation.

The QRS loop shows that the slurrings are not in the middle of QRS, and both the QRS loop and QRS complex, while of variable duration, are always less than accepted criteria for advanced LBBB (see Table 11.4). The initial abnormal depolarization explains the absence of "q" in the left precordial leads, I and aVL (Figure 11.34).

As repolarization becomes less opposed to QRS, less anomalous transseptal depolarization is found as well. As a result, the T wave, although it can be negative, is more often negative–positive or even completely positive in the leads facing the left ventricle (Figure 11.34).

ECG diagnostic criteria

The range of QRS widths is between 100 ms and <120 ms according to the classical criteria, but this may be modified after the last studies of Strauss *et al.* (2011).

In the lesser degree of partial LBBB, the ECG is almost normal because there is hardly any abnormal transseptal depolarization and the T wave is positive in I, aVL, V5, and V6. **It only becomes apparent though the disappearance of the first vector**, which is cancelled out by the right forces simultaneously inscribed. This is supported by **QS in V1 and a solitary R in V6 and I**. In V1, there may be a small "r" produced by the right septum or right ventricular wall activation.

Partial LBBB with more abnormal septal depolarization has a morphology more like that of advanced LBBB, but

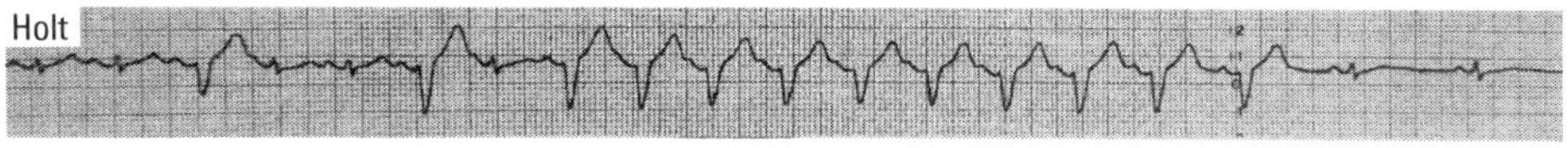

Figure 11.35 Intermittent LBBB. The third and sixth complexes manifest a LBBB morphology. The same occurs from the eighth complex to the seventeenth complex, after which rhythm becomes bradycardic and LBBB disappears.

the QRS complex width is less than 0.12 sec and the T wave is often less negative in the left precordial leads I and aVL, or is negative–positive or even completely positive when free left ventricular wall repolarization prevails over septal repolarization. We have already discussed how the negative–positive or completely positive T wave sometimes seen in advanced LBBB can be explained.

Differential diagnosis and clinical implications

The possibility of septal infarction (T wave usually negative in V1–V2), septal fibrosis, block of middle fibers (MacAlpin 2002), emphysema, and dextrorotation (in the last two instances, generally S in V6) must be considered, although often to assure the cause of ECG pattern is not easy.

Intracavitary ECG detects lengthened HV, V–ARV equal to zero, and widened QRS that is less marked than in advanced LBBB (Cannom *et al.* 1980).

Coronary patients with an ECG pattern of partial LBBB often present with involvement of the anterior descending coronary artery (Romanelli *et al.* 1980), although this same ECG pattern is seen in about 5% of adults without ischemic heart disease.

Second-degree left bundle branch block (Figure 11.33)

This corresponds to a type of ventricular aberrancy. In these cases, we can apply the same considerations used in second-degree RBBB (see above). This is usually a transitory form previous to a fixed block (Abben *et al.* 1979). Its presentation may be either abrupt (Mobitz II) or progressive (Mobitz I, Wenckebach type), which is very rare (Brenes *et al.* 2006) (see Figure 18.9).

The presence of a negative T wave when ventricular conduction is normal is relatively frequent, even with no evidence of heart disease (cardiac memory) (Denes *et al.* 1978) (see Figure 13.103).

Although second-degree LBBB is generally independent of myocardial ischemia, exercise-induced LBBB has been reported in relation to myocardial ischemia (Paleo 1984).

Left divisional blocks

Included in this section are the blocks of the superoanterior and inferoposterior divisions of the left bundle branch (**hemiblocks**), as well as the controversial block of middle fibers.

The electrocardiographic idea of hemiblocks was conceived by Rosenbaum *et al.* in 1968. Etymologically speaking, the term "hemiblock" is no longer the best one to use; it would be more exact to refer to it as the block of the superoanterior and inferoposterior fascicles of the left ventricle. We conserve the name in honor of Rosenbaum and Elizari, who first precisely defined this type of block and introduced this widely accepted terminology. According to these authors, the term hemiblocks refers to the expression of the delay in impulse conduction in the left bundle branch superoanterior fascicle or division (superoanterior hemiblock; SAH) or inferoposterior fascicle or division (inferoposterior hemiblock; IPH) (**trifascicular theory**) (see before and Chapter 4). If the delay is peripheral (i.e. located in the Purkinje area corresponding to one of the two divisions), the ECG morphology is similar, but it has more terminal slurrings. Rarely, lesions in the bundle of His or left bundle branch fibers destined for the respective fascicles have this ECG morphology, as demonstrated in SAH (Narula 1977; Sobrino *et al.* 1978; Castellanos *et al.* 1981). The superoanterior fascicle is longer and narrower than the inferoposterior fascicle (see Figures 4.11 and 11.1) and subject to more intense hemodynamic overload because it is located in the outflow tract of the left ventricle that bears the pressure of ejection, whereas the wider and shorter inferoposterior fascicle is situated in the left ventricular inflow tract. For these reasons, isolated superoanterior division block is frequent, while isolated inferoposterior division block is very rare. However, as with bundle branch block, the anatomic involvement is more extensive than the ECG expression.

The repercussions of hemiblocks are evidenced as QRS loop modifications mainly in the frontal plane, with the maximum loop vector directed upward (toward the blocked zone) in SAH and downward (also toward the blocked zone) in IPH (Figures 11.35 and 11.36). This delay alone can never produce a QRS complex of 0.12 sec or more.

As mentioned (see Chapter 4), there is anatomic evidence that in addition to the superoanterior and inferoposterior fascicles, groups of fibers between the two fascicles, fundamentally directed forward (midseptal fibers) and of heterogeneous anatomic distribution, exist (Kulbertus *et al.* 1976) (Figure 11.3). It seems evident that block of these fibers may produce electrocardiographic repercussions. Durrer's studies (1970), which demonstrate that ventricular depolarization starts simultaneously in three points (the high anterior point situated in the area of implantation of the superoanterior fascicle or division, the inferoposterior paraseptal point in the area of implantation of the inferoposterior division or fascicle, and the medial septal point in the area of the medial septal fibers) (Figure 4.12), also reinforce the theory of an intraventricular system formed by four input areas of ventricular activation (**the quadrifascicular theory**) (see Chapter 4).

We will principally deal with the superoanterior and inferoposterior division of fascicle blocks (SAH and IPH) and their associations (bifascicular and trifascicular block), which are concepts that are already very well established. We will also briefly comment on the concept of ECG patterns, which may be seen in the case of block of middle fibers, which is not a completely established concept (see later).

Superoanterior hemiblock (SAH)

With regard to this phenomenon, we refer now to advanced, **or third-degree, SAH**, assuming that the impulse is blocked in the fascicle itself. Some type of peripheral block may also be present (see before). Later, we briefly mention the concept of partial (first-degree) and intermittent (second-degree) hemiblocks.

Activation (Figure 11.36)

The blocked zone depolarizes later. As a result, the detention of the impulse in the superoanterior fascicle modifies the sequence of left ventricular depolarization and, consequently, the QRS loop.

The QRS loop begins with a vector directed forward, to the right and somewhat more downward than normal because when the superoanterior fascicle is blocked, the

vector resulting from the remaining inferoposterior and anteroseptal forces is directed downward (Figure 11.36 marked a+b). The forces of the right ventricle, depolarized at almost the same time, contribute to the somewhat more forward and right direction of the vector. Thus, the first vector represents the sum of depolarization of part of the right ventricle, the medial third of the septum, and the area of the left ventricular posterior papillary muscle (zone of implantation of the inferoposterior fascicle). Later, ventricular depolarization follows its route, the QRS loop rotating counterclockwise, depolarizing the lower left ventricular wall and apex, and finally, the lateral and anterior wall of the left ventricle. This produces a second, very powerful vector directed to the left, upward, and more or less backward (Figure 11.36). The final part of this loop is located in the apparent negative hemifield of lead I. However, there is no final S in this lead because the true lead I, according to Burger's triangle (see Figure 6.6), has to be located slightly upward and therefore the positive hemifield of lead I ends around −100° and not at −90° (see Figure 11.36 dotted line).

Projection of the resulting QRS loop on the frontal plane produces (Figure 11.36) a QRS loop directed sharply upward and rotated counterclockwise. On the horizontal plane, the QRS loop is oriented first forward and then backward, normally with more of the loop posterior than anterior. As such, SAH mainly affects the frontal QRS loop because the second vector in SAH is directed fundamentally upward and to the left, the blocked area being essentially superior.

The modifications in the ECG in advanced SAH, which are seen below, can be explained by the projection of a

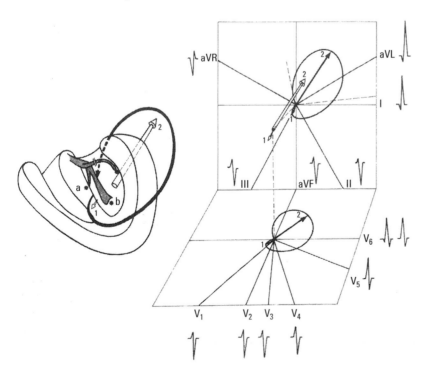

Figure 11.36 Diagram of the activation in superoanterior hemiblock. On the left are two vectors responsible for ventricular depolarization and the global QRS loop. The three stars represent the three entrances of the electric impulse in the left ventricle. On the right is the projection of the two vectors on the frontal and horizontal planes, with formation of the respective loops and the most common morphologies observed in clinical practice. The dotted line above lead I represents what is probably the most exact situation of the positive part of lead I. As such, the entire last part of the loop would be in the positive hemifield of I, justifying the absence of S in I, which normally occurs (a line perpendicular to the true I has been added to the sketch, delimiting the positive and negative hemifields of this lead and illustrating this point) (see Chapter 6).

QRS loop in the frontal and horizontal planes and the correlation with positive and negative hemifields of different leads (Figures 11.36 and 11.37).

The T loop shows no abnormal changes in isolated SAH.

ECG changes: diagnostic criteria (Figures 11.36–11.41) (Table 11.5)

QRS duration

Because activation delay is only intraventricular and not transseptal, it does not exceed 10 or 20 ms. Therefore, the duration of the QRS complex in isolated SAH is always less than 0.12 sec. Effectively, in intermittent SAH, it has been demonstrated that hemiblock prolongs QRS duration by a maximum of 10–20 ms.

ÂQRS in the frontal plane

Because of the special activation in SAH, ÂQRS in the frontal plane strongly deviates upward and to the left, and orientation is typically between −45° and −75°. However, between −30° and −45°, there is usually first-degree SAH, especially in very lean individuals. Nonetheless, when

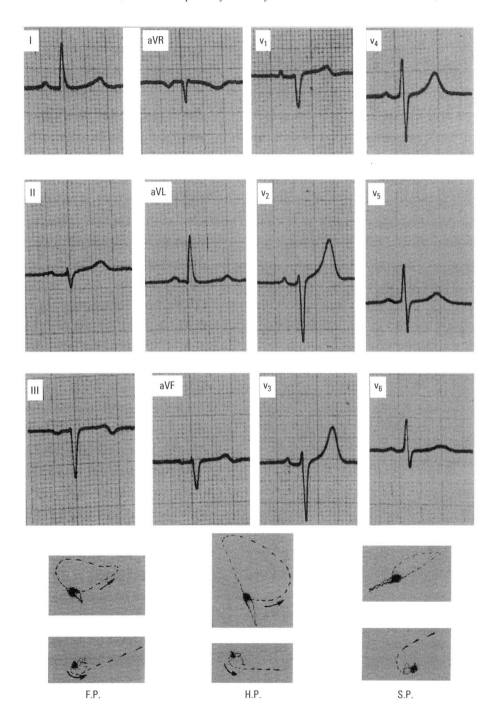

Figure 11.37 ECG–VCG of a patient with typical isolated superoanterior hemiblock. The morphology is that corresponding to Figure 11.36.

Table 11.5 ECG diagnostic criteria for advanced superoanterior hemiblock.

- ÂQRS sharply deviated to the left (especially between −45° and −75°). Other causes of extreme left deviation of ÂQRS must be excluded
- qR morphology in I and aVL, r or R terminal in aVR, rS in II, III, and aVF with SIII > SII and RII > RIII
- S wave until V6, with IDT V6 < IDT aVL, with IDT aVL ≥50 ms
- Occasionally, minimum "q" in V2–V3
- QRS complex <0.12 sec
- Slight midterminal slurrings in VL and sometimes in I (advanced cases)

ÂQRS is about −30°, it is difficult to distinguish between left deviation caused by the extreme horizontalization or left ventricular enlargement and that caused by first-degree SAH. Only the evolution of the morphology, and the transient nature of the changes, as shown in Figures 11.38, let us confirm that partial SAH exists.

QRS complex in the frontal plane

- **Leads I and aVL:** qR morphology (q = Vector 1, R = Vector 2) with fairly high R voltage. If R has a very low voltage, the addition of right ventricular enlargement, or superoanterior peripheral right ventricular block, which sometimes occurs in emphysematous patients, or even, lateral infarction, should be suspected. Due to the activation asynchrony between the lower (V6) and upper (aVL) left ventricle, intrinsicoid deflection time (IDT) in aVL is 15 ms longer than that of V6, and in advanced hemiblock is usually ≥0.05 sec.
- **Leads II, III, and VF:** rS morphology (r = Vector 1, S = Vector 2) with SII < SIII and RII > RIII, due to the fact that a larger portion of the loop remains in the negative hemifield of III when compared to lead II. The negativity of S in lead II should exceed the positivity of R as an expression of the ÂQRS deviation farther than −30°. The presence of SII > SIII, especially if SI is present, rules out SAH, suggesting instead right ventricular block in the peripheral zone, right ventricular enlargement, or a thoracic anomaly (SI, SII, SIII pattern) (Figure 11.21).
- **VR:** Usually, QR or Qr. The small final "r" is due to the fact that the final part of the loop remains in the positive hemifield of VR. The presence of evident final R waves suggests associated partial RBBB. In this case, a V1 lead located in the second intercostal space records a QR pattern (Rosenbaum *et al.* 1968) (see later).

QRS complex in the horizontal plane

- **Lead V6:** Rs or qRs morphology, with IDTV6 < IDTVL (asynchrony ≥15 ms), because the impulse now takes longer to reach the situation of aVL compared to V6, due to the fact that this lead records the lateroinferior aspect activated earlier by the inferoposterior fascicle.

- **The other precordial leads** show their normal morphologies, although sometimes a small "q" is seen in the right precordial leads, especially V1. This probably occurs because the electrode is situated higher than usual and faces the tail of the first vector, which in SAH is directed more downward than normal. When the electrode is moved down to the correct position, an initial "r" is recorded. This does not generally occur in septal necrosis, except in cases of very obese people (see Figure 13.93). As explained above, if there is associated partial RBBB, lead V1 located in a higher position will record an evident final "r" wave. In isolated SAH, V2 (left) more than V1 (right) located in a high position (2nd intercostal space) may record an evident final "r′" that disappears in the 4th left intercostal space.

ST segment and T wave

Because the T loop is normal in isolated SAH, the ST segment and T wave are also normal when associated heart disease is absent. However, the T wave is often a little different because the loop morphology and direction are slightly different from the T loop without SAH.

The ECG diagnostic criteria may be seen in Table 11.5.

Differential diagnosis

A differential diagnosis must be made with other causes of extreme left ÂQRS deviation, **such as the following:**

- Horizontal heart: ÂQRS does not reach −30°.
- Left ventricular enlargement: ÂQRS does not pass −30° in isolated LVE.
- Zonal anterosuperior RBBB: the morphology is SI, SII, SIII with SII > SIII (Figure 11.21).
- WPW syndrome: is accompanied by delta wave and short PR interval (see Chapter 12).
- Inferior infarction isolated or associated to SAH: signs of necrosis (QS, QR, qrS) (see Figure 13.97).
- Right ventricular pacemaker rhythm: a spike appears.
- In some congenital heart diseases (ostium primum-type ASD, tricuspid atresia, single ventricle, corrected transposition and double outlet of the right ventricle with infracristal ventricular septal defect), ÂQRS may be deviated farther than −30°, generally not because of true SAH, but because of congenital alterations in the SCS encompassing the superoanterior division.

Special characteristics

Special characteristics of SAH are as follows:

- **Partial SAH** presents with an ÂQRS between −30° and −45° or even less, deviated to the left. The evolution to advanced SAH (ÂQRS beyond −40°) assures the diagnosis (Figures 11.38 and 11.39) (see before).
- When there is **significant delay** situated less in the fascicle as **more in the corresponding parietal zone, evident slurrings (≥30 ms) appear in the descendent branch of R in aVL**, reflecting the final delay in inscription of the up

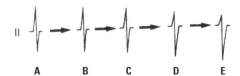

Figure 11.38 Evolution in time in a case of superoanterior hemiblock (SAH). Different drawings in QRS recording in lead II. In D and E, SAH is evident, but there must also be a certain degree of SAH in A and B, and especially in C.

and leftward directed loop. QRS may be ≥0.12 sec, especially if the block is mixed at both fascicular and parietal levels.

• Associated left ventricular enlargement is described before and in Chapter 10 (Figure 11.40).

• **Combined SAH and necrosis** is described in Chapter 13.

• **In SAH and partial LBBB**, the following may be seen:

i. global advanced LBBB morphology with ÂQRS at −60°;

ii. QRS ≥0.12 sec (because of the coexistence of both blocks);

iii. ÂQRS hyperdeviated to the left (because of SAH); there is absence of Q in I and aVL (because of first-degree LBBB). Similar morphologies can be explained by other circumstances (see LBBB: Differential diagnosis).

• Sometimes, **SAH is associated with delay in right ventricular activation caused by partial truncal RBBB, zonal RBBB, or RVE**. In this situation, as the last part of the loop is more to the right than normal, a small S wave is seen in I, with SIII > SII and usually without r′ in V1, but with evident final R in aVR (Figure 11.41). If heart failure exists, probably as happens in case of LBBB with left ÂQRS, the R wave in aVR may be explained by RV dilation. In V1 a terminal, "r" may be recorded if the electrode is placed at a high level in cases of partial RBBB (see before).

• **A prolonged HV interval** is observed in 30% of cases in series with predominantly elderly persons (Narula 1979).

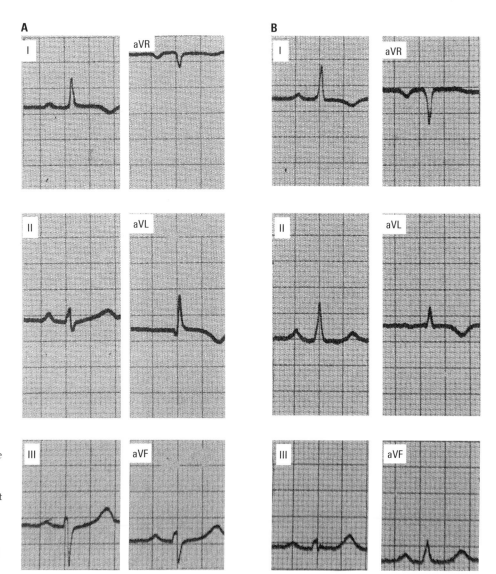

Figure 11.39 Patient in subacute phase of coronary syndrome. Left (A): The morphology of II is R = S, or even R > S, with ÂQRS at about −30°. The next day (right) (B), ÂQRS = +30°. Thus, we can suggest that a certain degree of superoanterior hemiblock existed in the first ECG.

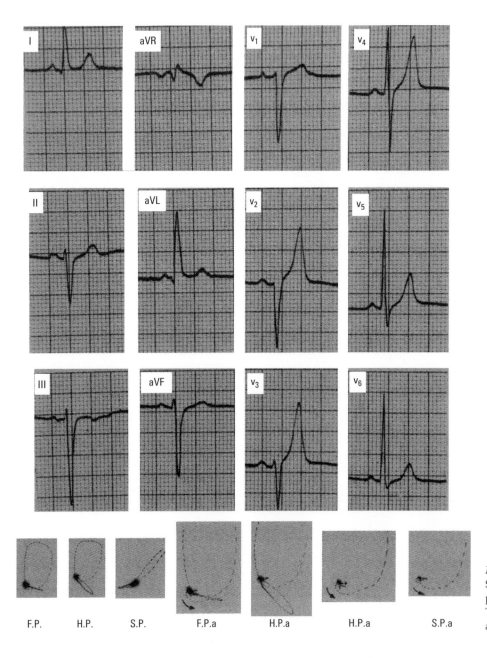

Figure 11.40 Typical example of SAH + LVH in a 55-year-old patient with severe hypertension. There is a high voltage in aVL, V5 and V6, II, III, and aVF.

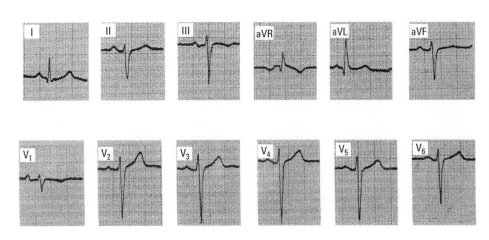

Figure 11.41 ECG of a 60-year-old patient with chronic obstructive pulmonary disease (COPD). The presence of SII < SIII indicates superoanterior hemiblock, and the S in I and terminal R in VR and rS in V6 suggest the association of partial RBBB and/or right ventricular enlargement.

Clinical implications

The prevalence in the normal population varies according to series and ranges from 0.9% to 1.4% (Barret *et al.* 1981). In the absence of associated heart disease, it should not be considered an important risk factor for cardiac morbidity or mortality. It does not worsen the prognosis of patients with heart disease. Although it should be considered an early sign of degenerative disease of the specialized conduction system, this process often evolves slowly. In some series, over 50% of patients with SAH do not present with associated heart disease.

The evolution of SAH to global advanced LBBB or complete AV block is very infrequent (Kulbertus *et al.* 1980) and the development of RBBB+SAH is infrequent but statistically significant when compared to a control group.

Inferoposterior hemiblock (IPH)

With regard to this phenomenon, we refer mainly to advanced or third-degree IPH, assuming that the impulse to be blocked is in the fascicle itself. Like SAH, the block is very rarely more proximal (in the corresponding part of the left bundle or bundle of His), but sometimes peripheral block may be present.

Activation (Figure 11.42)

The QRS loop begins with a first vector directed forward, upward, and to the left (in some cases to the right) because of the delay of the impulse in the inferoposterior fascicle,

representing the depolarization of the zone corresponding to the anterior papillary muscle of the left ventricle and of the middle third of the septum (a + b of Figure 11.42). From there, the impulse is propagated to the anterolateral wall of the left ventricle, the loop describing a clockwise rotation. Finally, the blocked zone that corresponds to the inferolateral wall of the left ventricle is depolarized. This produces a very powerful second vector directed to the right, backward, and downward.

The projection of the resulting QRS loop on the frontal plane (Figure 11.42) is oriented sharply downward and to the right, and rotated clockwise. On the horizontal plane, the QRS loop is directed first forward, then in a counterclockwise rotation backward and to the right. The IPH modifications appear mainly in the frontal QRS loop because the second vector in this case is directed mostly downward and somewhat to the right because of the predominantly inferior position of the inferoposterior fascicle.

Based on the projection of the loop in the frontal and horizontal planes (projection in the hemifields of different leads), these changes in the QRS loop explain **the ECG variations in advanced IPH** (Figures 11.42 and 11.43).

The T loop in isolated IPH falls within normal limits.

The diagnosis of IPH may only be made in the absence of RVE and very vertical heart. For some authors, it is necessary that the patient has left heart disease.

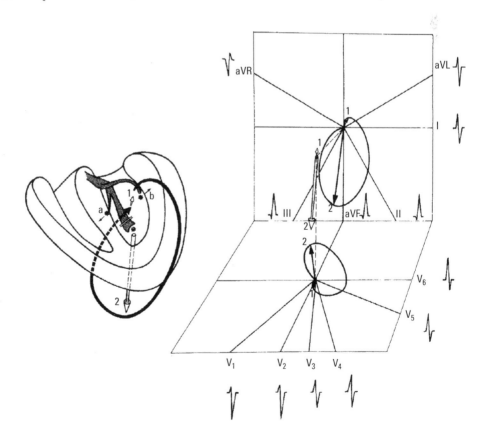

Figure 11.42 Diagram of activation in inferoposterior hemiblock. On the left are the two vectors that account for ventricular depolarization and the global QRS loop, and on the right, the projection of these vectors on the frontal and horizontal planes, with formation of the respective loops and the most common morphologies seen in practise.

A

B

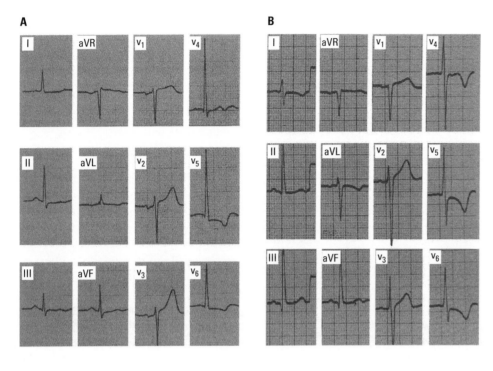

Figure 11.43 (A) ECG of a 55-year-old patient with arterial hypertension and coronary heart disease. (B) Unaccompanied by any clinical change, a month later the patient presented a striking ECG change (ÂQRS went from left to right, in aVF Rs passed to qR with IDT = 0.06 sec, and in V6 qR changed to Rs). All this may be explained by the appearance of inferoposterior hemiblock.

ECG changes: diagnostic criteria (Figures 11.42 and 11.43) (Table 11.6)

The above criteria alone may not be enough to perform the diagnosis.

QRS duration

The duration of the QRS complex is always less than 0.12 sec in isolated advanced IPH for the same reasons described earlier when dealing with SAH (see above).

ÂQRS in the frontal plane

Because of the special activation in IPH, ÂQRS in the frontal plane is deviated to the right and downward. It is usually situated between +90° and +140°, although there is evidence that in first-degree IPH, ÂQRS of <+90° can be seen (corresponding with the Rs or even low-voltage R morphology in I seen in these cases).

QRS complex in the frontal plane

• **Leads I and aVL:** rS, RS, or even Rs morphology (lesser degrees can probably be accompanied by solitary, but low-voltage, R in I).
• **Leads II, III, and aVF:** qR morphology (q = Vector 1, R = Vector 2) with prominent "q" wave, especially in III and aVF. IDT is generally ≥0.05 sec in VF in advanced IPH, and is delayed 15 ms or more with respect to IDT in aVL because aVF (and V6) records the inferior wall, with delayed activation in this case, and aVL explores the anterosuperior wall, which is depolarized earlier. As a consequence of the delayed activation of the inferior wall, midterminal slurrings are appreciated in these leads.
• aVR: QS or Qr morphology (see Figure 11.42).

Table 11.6 ECG diagnostic criteria for advanced inferoposterior hemiblock.

• ÂQRS extremely deviated to the right (between +90° and +140°, often >100°) in the absence of other factors that might explain this deviation
• RS or Rs in I and aVL and qR in II, III, and VF
• QRS complex <0.12 sec, IDT ≥ 50 ms in aVF and V6, and IDT >50 ms in aVL
• Slight midterminal slurrings in II, III, and aVF (advanced cases)

QRS complex in the horizontal plane
Precordial leads:
• **Lead V1:** rS or QS pattern.
• **Lead V6:** Rs, qRs, or solitary, low-voltage R. The IDT in V6 equals that of aVF, since both leads are low and record the same activation delay in the inferior wall of the left ventricle.

ST segment and T wave

Since the T loop falls within normal limits in isolated IPH, the ST segment and T wave are normal in the absence of associated heart disease. However, IPH is commonly accompanied by cardiac disease, which is the cause of the repolarization changes often encountered.

The ECG diagnostic criteria may be seen in Table 11.6.

The sudden appearance of compatible ECG pattern in decisive for assuring the diagnosis (Figure 11.43).

Differential diagnosis

Similar ECG morphology is observed in the following:
• **Right ventricular enlargement with posterior QRS loop.** In this case, the P wave may suggest right

heart disease. The onset of the loop is usually less superior and therefore the "q" wave in II, III, and aVF is generally smaller. Moreover, in IPH, there is usually less terminal "r" in aVR and less "S" in V6 (Figure 11.43).

• **Similar loops, although more closed,** appear in very lean individuals or persons with thoracic malformations, occasionally with increased IDT in aVF. The asynchrony between the IDT of aVF or V6 and that of aVL clearly reflects IPH.

It is thus necessary to exclude the possibility of right ventricular enlargement and asthenic constitution when diagnosing IPH (see before).

Special characteristics

• **Partial degrees of IPH** can be seen with ÂQRS somewhat inferior to +90° and probably without S in I or with Rs morphology.

• When there is an **important activation delay, situated more in the corresponding parietal zone than in the fascicle,** evident slurrings (≥30 ms) appears in the descendent branch of "R" in II, III, and especially aVF. They are the expression of the final delay in recording the down and rightward oriented vector. In this situation, the QRS can be ≥0.12 sec, especially if the block is mixed (both fascicular and parietal).

• **Combined IPH and necrosis** is described in Chapter 13.

• There is a **prolonged HV** interval in 40% of cases with isolated right axis deviation (Narula 1979).

Clinical implications

No large patient series has been studied to firmly establish the diagnosis of IPH and consequently the prognosis is not well known. Rajala *et al.* (1984) encountered a prevalence of IPH in very elderly subjects that was either isolated or associated with RBBB of less than 1%, while the prevalence of SAH, according to a different series, is from 8% to 20% in the elderly. In the normal population, the prevalence of IPH is less than 0.1% (Barret *et al.* 1981). IPH represents a more extensive ventricular conduction system disorder, considering that the inferoposterior division is much wider than the superoanterior division. Theoretically, the prognosis for IPH should be worse than that of SAH.

IPH is very rare if heart disease is absent, but it appears with relative frequency associated to myocardial infarction (see Figures 13.90, 13.92, 13.95, and 13.96) and occasionally in other situations like aortic regurgitation. In this latter instance, it is the result of an injury produced by the effect of the regurgitation jet on the inferoposterior fascicle. This explains some cases of severe aortic regurgitation in non-lean persons accompanied by right-deviated ÂQRS but no right heart involvement or failure due to valvular disease accounting for the right ÂQRS deviation.

Anteroseptal middle fiber block

It has been questioned whether a ECG diagnosis of anteroseptal middle fiber block exists. However, probably this may be done bearing in mind that the intraventricular conduction system may be considered quadrifascicular (see Chapter 4), it may be hypothesized that the block of middle fibers, which are located in an anteroseptal zone between superoanterior and inferoposterior fascicles (Figure 11.1), may produce an anterior displacement of the QRS loop in the horizontal plane, and this would account for a prominent R wave in V1–V2 (Hoffman *et al.* 1976; Nakaya *et al.* 1978; Moffa *et al.* 1997; De Padua *et al.* 2011). Other authors (MacAlpin 2002) postulate also other criteria (lack of septal "q" wave). The Brazilian School has outlined ECG criteria for this diagnosis emphasizing as a major criteria for the diagnosis of MFB the presence of prominent anterior force (RS in V1–V2 and Rs pattern in V6) (Pastore *et al.* 2009; Pérez Riera *et al.* 2011). This hypothesis is plausible especially if the pattern with prominent anterior forces is transient, as seen in cases of septal ischemia due to LAD occlusion (Figure 11.44) (Pérez Riera *et al.* 2008; Bayés de Luna and Baranchuk 2017).

However, before confirming that these transient ECG changes are caused by a block of left middle fibers, sometimes referred to with different names, **such as "left septal fascicle" (Pérez Riera *et al.* 2011) the following aspects should be borne in mind:**

a) the pathological studies of Demoulin and Kulbertus (1972) demonstrate that a true septal fascicle stemming from the left bundle branch is present in only 30% of cases] (see Figure 11.2) (Chapter 4).

b) The experimental data obtained after the section of these Middle Fibers (MF) show some discordant results (Dabrowska *et al.* 1978, Uhley and Rivkin 1964, Nakaya *et al.* 1981). The latter study demonstrates that after the section, the breakthrough of the apical area has disappeared and a small delay of activation is observed. Thus, the onset of LV activation is modified. Uhley presents relatively similar results (Figure 11.45). Dabrowska considers that the section of MF is either equivalent to partial truncal LBBB or does not present a big change in QRS morphology.

c) The diagnosis of MF block (MFB) may not be based on the loss of a septal "q" wave. In fact, this is a key criterion to diagnose truncal partial LBBB and therefore is no longer considered a major criterion for diagnosis of MFB.

d) It was demonstrated in humans by Peñaloza (1961) with catheter compression of RBB (Figure 11.6); by Piccolo *et al.* (1980) with programmed atrial stimulation (PAS) (Figure 11.46); and by Rosenbaum *et al.* (1968) with clinical tracings that an RS pattern appears transiently before the advanced RBBB pattern. Other authors (Cohen *et al.* 1967; Reiffel and Bigger Jr 1978) obtained with PAS

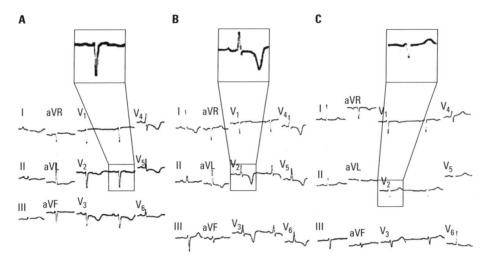

Figure 11.44 (A) ECG from an ischemic heart disease patient who, during an acute coronary syndrome (B), showed a significant morphology change in V2 (high transitory R), with very negative T wave in right precordial leads (left anterior descending coronary artery involvement), which disappeared after some hours (C). As there is no evidence of transient lateral ischemia, the transient pattern of V2 (tall R wave) (B) may be explained by either a block of the middle fibers of left bundle branch or partial right bundle branch block (see text).

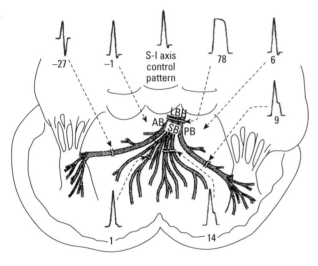

Figure 11.45 This drawing shows that the incision at the site of the middle fibers does not produce an evident change in the QRS morphology in the frontal plane axis leads but with a tendency to be oriented anteriorly and to the left (Modified from Uhley and Rivkin 1961).

the same results, but they consider, in our opinion wrongly, that the RS pattern in V1 did not correspond to a partial RBBB.

e) The RBB and MF are usually perfused by septal branches of the LAD coronary artery. Therefore, in cases of ischemia due to proximal occlusion of LAD, both RBB and MF will be under perfused. This may explain the transient presence of RS in V1–V2 due to block of one of both structures.

f) In patients with intraventricular conduction disturbances, the pathological involvement is much more extensive than what the ECG pattern indicates. Therefore, this may explain that the presence of RS pattern in V1–V2 in patients with heart disease coincides with important fibrosis of both RBB and MF in necropsy (Nakaya 1978).

g) The permanent RS or rs pattern in V1–V2 has been considered diagnostic evidence of block of both partial RBBB (Alboni 1981) or MFB (de Padua *et al.* 2011) (Figure 11.47). However, there are many other causes that may present similar patterns including many normal variants such as special rotation, chest anomalies, obesity, etc., and that does not evolve in a long follow-up to advanced right or left BBB (see Table 10.3).

Therefore, after all these arguments we may say that at present, the ECG pattern with RS in V1–V2 that is permanent cannot be considered a major criteria for the diagnosis of any type of intraventricular block. However, the presence of transient RS in V1–V2 although may be due to BMF may also often be explained by partial RBBB. Perhaps the most probable is that the injury of both RB and MF is present at the same time as was seen in the case studied at necropsy by Nakaya (1978). In fact, the Brazilian school emphasizes that BMF is frequently associated with RBBB (qR in V2).

To advance in the understanding whether RS patterns are due to BMF, or partial RBBB (or both), it would be advisable:

i) to perform more histologic studies (heart transplant, necropsy) of ventricular conduction system (CVS) in cases with RS pattern in V1–V2.

ii) to repeat with new methodology the experimental studies sectioning MF.

iii) to change the paradigma: do not try to demonstrate if the block of these fibers produces an ECG change, but to study with new imaging techniques (endocardial recording), if these ECG changes described by the Brazilian

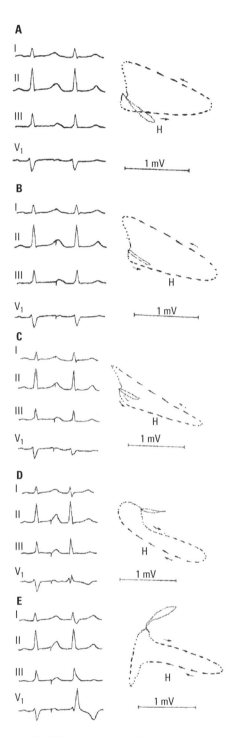

Figure 11.46 ECG from a 22-year-old man without structural heart disease. (A) Control tracing of I, II, III, and V1 and horizontal plane VCG loop (HP). (B–E) Programmed right atrial stimulation (PRAS) with progressive shortening of coupling interval (H1–H2 from 530 ms in B to 420 ms in E). See the progressive anterior displacement of HP–VCG loop conserving the CC rotation in B and C and small change of V1 (without r') (V2 is not recorded but in C, an RS pattern would be recorded) according to ECG–VCG correlation. When the VCG loop rotates clockwise, D and E, an rsR' pattern appears in E with important terminal slurrings and wide QRS (advanced RBBB) (see text) (Modified from Piccolo *et al.* 1980).

School (Moffa, Pastore, Perez Riera, Barbosa), correlates with a delay of activation in the zone of the LV that receive the activation through these fibers.

Combined blocks

We will now describe according the classification of Figure 11.3 the characteristic ECG features of bi- and trifascicular block, as well as the most important clinical implications of this phenomenon.

Bitruncal block: RBBB plus LBBB

If both blocks are truncal and advanced (third degree), this corresponds to an bilateral advanced AV block.

If one block is advanced and the other is first degree, a right or left BBB morphology is observed and the PR interval becomes somewhat prolonged, although it may still be within normal limits. Lengthening of the PR interval may also be due to a slowing of the conduction proximal to the bundle of His bifurcation. An ECG of the bundle of His can clarify. Figure 11.32 shows an example of LBBB with the QRS at −60° (or LAH + LV parietal block) showing a prominent terminal R in aVR and a QR pattern in high V1. This probably is explained in absence of important heart failure (see Figure 11.30) with associated partial RBBB.

If both blocks are not advanced, the QRS morphology is dominated by the more severe block and the PR interval becomes longer compared to the previous one.

If the extent of the block is the same on both sides—an event that is possible in theory but very rare in practise—the QRS morphology is normal and the PR interval is lengthened compared to the pre-block morphology.

The clearest example of bitruncal block is the presence of RBBB, with or without anterosuperior hemiblock, alternating with LBBB (Figure 11.48).

Bifascicular block

Figure 11.49 shows all possible combinations of bifascicular block whereby two of the four fascicles (see Figure 11.3) are involved and the block is either first or third degree. The electrocardiographic repercussions of the different bifascicular blocks are shown in this figure. We will discuss the most frequent and important bifascicular blocks, from clinical point of view that are advanced RBBB + SAH and advanced RBBB + IPH.

Right bundle branch block plus superoanterior hemiblock (Figures 11.50–11.53)

This association is frequent, among other reasons, because the two fascicles are close to each other and they are perfused by the same descending anterior coronary artery.

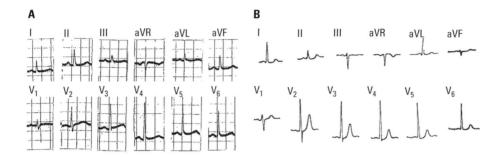

Figure 11.47 Two cases with very similar prominent R wave in V1–V2. (A) Case of prominent R in V1–V2 that in the absence of lateral myocardial infarction and right ventricular hypertrophy, the diagnosis of left septal fascicular block would be postulated (Adapted with permission from De Padua *et al.* 2011). (B) Case of prominent R in V2 that occurs before the appearance of advanced RBBB using premature atrial extra stimulus with shortening coupling intervals. It is considered that it corresponds to partial RBBB before the appearance of rSr′ in V1 (Based on Alboni 1981). These two examples show that the same morphology has been used to diagnose block of middle fibers (A) and partial RBBB (B) (see text).

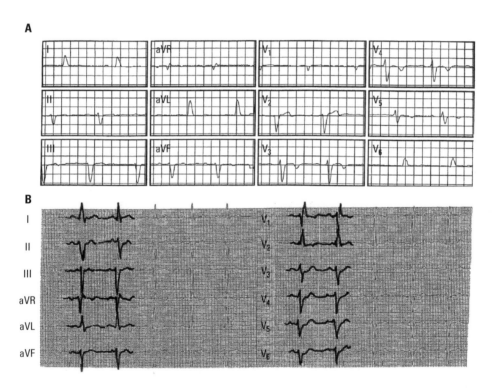

Figure 11.48 Typical bilateral block. (A) LBBB with left ÂQRS deviation pattern. (B) RBBB and superoanterior hemiblock (RBBB + SAH) pattern. The patient suffered from syncope and a pacemaker was immediately implanted.

Activation

The first part of ventricular depolarization is modified by SAH and the second part by RBBB. Consequently, the forces in the first half of the QRS are directed, as in SAH, first to the right, downward, and forward, and subsequently to the left, upward, and backward. In the second half, they are directed as in RBBB, to the right and forward. This represents an advanced degree of ventricular conduction disturbance, which in the majority of cases is accompanied by a prolonged HV interval.

ECG diagnosis criteria

- **QRS duration:** The QRS complex is ≥0.12 sec. The first part of ÂQRS is directed upward and to the left, as in SAH, and the second part upward and to the right, as in advanced RBBB.
- **ECG morphology: QRS complex in the frontal plane.** As a result of abnormal activation, typical cases present with the QRS morphologies shown in Figure 11.50.
- **QRS complex in the horizontal plane.** Since SAH has little effect on the horizontal plane, the morphologies are those of advanced RBBB (rSR′ in V1 and slurred qRs in V6).

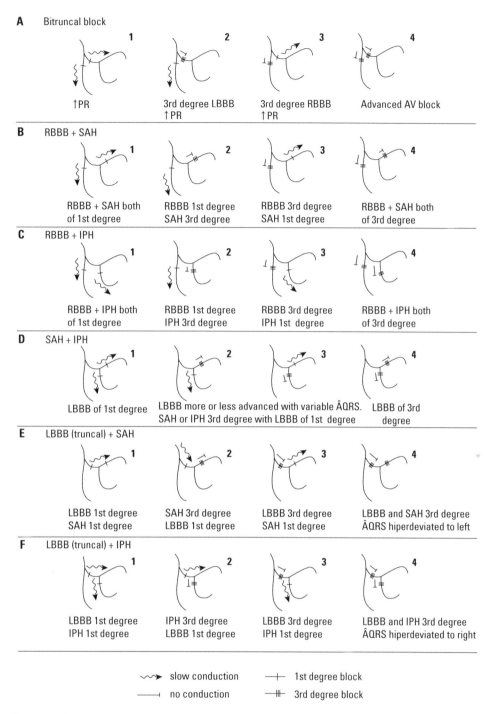

A Bitruncal block

1 ↑PR

2 3rd degree LBBB ↑PR

3 3rd degree RBBB ↑PR

4 Advanced AV block

B RBBB + SAH

1 RBBB + SAH both of 1st degree

2 RBBB 1st degree SAH 3rd degree

3 RBBB 3rd degree SAH 1st degree

4 RBBB + SAH both of 3rd degree

C RBBB + IPH

1 RBBB + IPH both of 1st degree

2 RBBB 1st degree IPH 3rd degree

3 RBBB 3rd degree IPH 1st degree

4 RBBB + IPH both of 3rd degree

D SAH + IPH

1 LBBB of 1st degree

2, 3 LBBB more or less advanced with variable ÂQRS. SAH or IPH 3rd degree with LBBB of 1st degree

4 LBBB of 3rd degree

E LBBB (truncal) + SAH

1 LBBB 1st degree SAH 1st degree

2 SAH 3rd degree LBBB 1st degree

3 LBBB 3rd degree SAH 1st degree

4 LBBB and SAH 3rd degree ÂQRS hiperdeviated to left

F LBBB (truncal) + IPH

1 LBBB 1st degree IPH 1st degree

2 IPH 3rd degree LBBB 1st degree

3 LBBB 3rd degree IPH 1st degree

4 LBBB and IPH 3rd degree ÂQRS hiperdeviated to right

∿➤ slow conduction   —┼— 1st degree block

—⊣ no conduction   —⊦⊦— 3rd degree block

Figure 11.49 Different possibilities of bifascicular block when assuming that four fascicles exist (right bundle branch trunk, left bundle branch trunk, and the superoanterior and inferoposterior divisions of the left bundle branch) and that the block is of first or third degree. The ECG repercussions in each situation have been shown (RBBB: right bundle branch block; LBBB: left bundle branch block; SAH: superoanterior hemiblock; IPH: inferoposterior hemiblock). (A) Bitruncal block. (B) RBBB + SAH. (C) RBBB + IPH. (D) SAH + IPH. (E) Truncal LBBB + SAH. (F) LBBB + IPH. In each case, 1, 2, 3, and 4 represent a combination of first- (I) and third- (III) degree block of two fascicles.

In V6, an S wave is more evident than in isolated advanced RBBB due to associated SAH. If there is emphysema, the q in V6 may disappear and the s in V1 may be minimal or non-existent.

• **Repolarization.** This morphology shows the modifications produced by advanced RBBB, although it is often accompanied by alterations produced by LVE or myocardial ischemia.

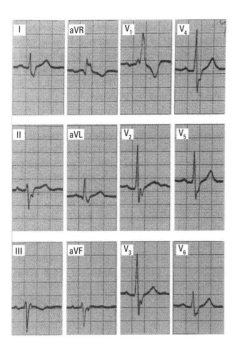

Figure 11.50 A 70-year-old patient with no apparent heart disease with a typical advanced RBBB + SAH morphology.

Masked block (Figure 11.51)

There are many different types of masked block. We will comment on just two types of masked blocks that are due to involvement of RB + SA division: RBBB + SAH mimicking RBBB pattern in horizontal plane (precordial leads) and LBBB pattern in frontal plane leads, and LBBB or SAH that masked RBBB.

RBBB + SAH with ECG pattern of RBBB in HP and LBBB in FP

When advanced RBBB is associated with advanced SAH and a certain degree of LBBB, and/or left ventricular

parietal block usually with important LVH, the right forces (RBBB) do not clearly prevail over the left forces (SAH + associations) and the resulting forces are therefore directed forward and upward, but to the left instead of the right (Figure 11.51). This is due to the balance between the final forces derived from the impulse delay in the free left ventricular wall, which would draw the loop backward and to the left, and the impulse delay on the right side occasioned by RBBB, which if alone would take the loop forward and to the right. For this reason, V1 continues to record dominant R morphology, because the final anterior part of the loop, although left, still falls within the positive hemifield of V1. In contrast, wide R or qR without S or with minimal "S" (Figure 11.51A,B) is observed in I and aVL, with rS or QS in II, III, and aVF, due to the fact that the final forces of the loop are directed to the left and upward. This type of block has been appropriately named "masked block," because it looks like right ventricular block in the horizontal plane and left ventricular block in the frontal plane.

This masked bifascicular block may be associated with left parietal block (if "q" is found in I and aVL) or first-degree left BBB (if R is solitary in I and aVL). The latter is in fact a trifascicular block, with a more frequently lengthened PR interval.

This masked block often terminates in advanced AV block (Bayés de Luna *et al.* 1988). We have described the appearance of this intermittent masked bifascicular block (Garcia Moll *et al.* 1994) (Figures 11.52 and 11.53).

Second type of masked RBBB

Sometimes, SAH may completely mask RBBB in conventional leads but not in high (2nd intercostal space) V1 where a final r′ of R′ is recorded (Rosenbaum

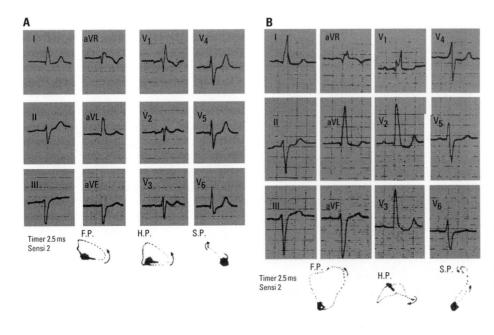

Figure 11.51 Two examples of classical bifascicular masked block, one (A) with a small S in I and counterclockwise rotation of the QRS loop in horizontal plane, and the other (B) with clockwise rotation and without S in I.

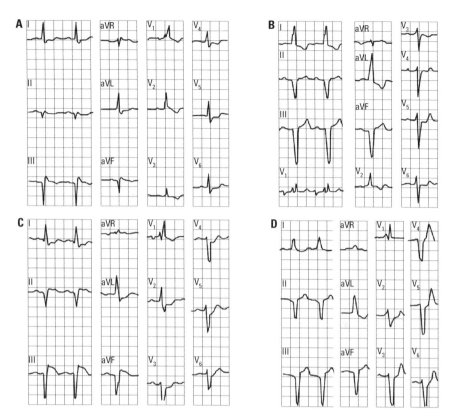

Figure 11.52 Different ECGs in the same patient presenting with intermittent masked bifascicular block (A to D). Note that the S wave disappears in I and aVL (B and D), coinciding with two crisis of pulmonary edema, and that the R wave in V1 is seen in all ECGs.

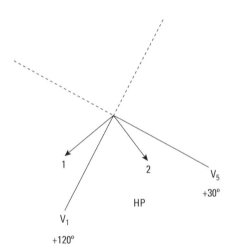

Figure 11.53 In the presence of masked block, the disappearance of the S wave in I, aVL, and sometimes V6 is due to the fact that the final activation vector (2) is directed forward, falling into the positive hemifield of V1 and thus originating an R in V1. As it is also directed leftward (due to the significant leftward final forces), it does not, however, produce an S wave in I and aVL. Vector 1 is the final vector seen in cases of normal bifascicular block and Vector 2 in cases of masked block.

et al. 1973). **This especially occurs when SAH is associated with LV parietal block and the QRS is ≥0.12 sec. In fact, the ECG pattern in conventional leads is similar (fewer middle slurrings) to advanced LBBB with left ÂQRS (Figure 11.32). The morphology with terminal R′**

(RBBB) is recorded in high position (2nd intercostal space) of V1. The RBBB usually is partial but may be also relatively advanced if the LV block is SAH+parietal block (not advanced LBBB) because in this case the left ventricular activation still may take place through the inferoposterior fascicle. In this block, a QR pattern is recorded in VR that may be due to truncal RBBB with delayed right ventricular wall or in case of heart failure the delay of right ventricular wall is due to right ventricular dilation (Van Bommel *et al.* 2011) (see before and Figure 11.30A).

Right bundle branch block plus inferoposterior hemiblock (Figure 11.54)

This association is less common. When it appears, it reflects a more important ventricular conduction disorder than in advanced RBBB with SAH because the inferoposterior division is relatively shorter and thicker than the superoanterior division, it has double perfusion (LAD + RCA or CX), and it is subject to less hemodynamic stress than the superoanterior division.

Activation

The first part of cardiac activation is modified by IPH, while the second part is modified by advanced RBBB. As a result, the first half of the QRS is upward and to the left, as in IPH, continuing downward and backward. The forces of the final part of QRS are directed as in advanced RBBB, to the right and forward.

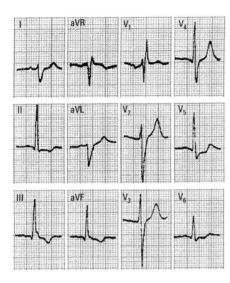

Figure 11.54 A 76-year-old patient with ischemic coronary heart disease and arterial hypertension, and with no right heart disease or asthenic constitution, who presented with a morphology typical of advanced RBBB + IPH (see text). The ST segment is depressed in the left precordial leads because of the underlying disease.

This represents an important ventricular conduction disturbance and is associated with 80–100% of cases with prolonged HV interval (Figure 11.54).

ECG diagnosis criteria

• **QRS duration:** The duration of the QRS complex exceeds 0.12 sec. The first part of the ÂQRS is directed downward, as in IPH, and the second part to the right and forward, as in advanced RBBB.

ECG morphology:

• **QRS complex in the frontal plane.** As a consequence of the activation just described, typical cases present with the morphologies depicted in Figure 11.54. The terminal "r" wave in VR is smaller than in isolated advanced RBBB or RBBB+SAH or may even be absent.

• **QRS complex in the horizontal plane.** Since IPH hardly changes the QRS morphology in this plane, it is the same as that of advanced RBBB (rsR' in V1 and slurred qRs in V6), with the S wave in this last lead usually less evident than in isolated advanced RBBB because of the accompanying IPH. Compared with isolated RBBB, the lower "r" voltage in aVR and of "S" in V6 are the most characteristic ECG signs of this bifascicular block (Masoni and Alboni 1982).

• **Repolarization.** This presents with the modifications occasioned by advanced RBBB. If ischemic heart disease also exists, as often is the case since this type of block frequently appears in the acute phase of myocardial infarction, the subsequent repolarization alterations are apparent.

Differential diagnosis

Right ventricular enlargement or very lean body habitus plus advanced RBBB can produce a similar morphology. For this reason, RBBB+IPH cannot be diagnosed in the presence of RVE or in very lean individuals.

Other types of bifascicular blocks

Superoanterior hemiblock plus inferoposterior hemiblock (Figure 11.49D)

If both blocks are advanced, the block is equivalent to that of an advanced LBBB pattern. Some authors (Medrano *et al*. 1970) believe that in these cases, the activation through the medial fibers may be responsible for the normal initiation of depolarization, although the rest of the left ventricular depolarization will occur transseptally much later. In this case, the ECG pattern will be of advanced LBBB, but often with "r" in V1 and "q" in V6.

If one block is advanced and the other is partial but relatively important, we find a somewhat advanced LBBB morphology with right ÂQRS deviation, if the most advanced block is in the inferoposterior fascicle, or left axis deviation, if it is in the superoanterior fascicle. If both hemiblocks are first degree, we will have different patterns of first-degree LBBB.

Left bundle branch block (trunk) with superoanterior or inferoposterior hemiblock (Figure 11.49E,F)

The transseptal depolarization of the left ventricle due to first-or third-degree LBBB is delayed in the Purkinje zone depending on the respective superoanterior or posteroinferior division. This results in a first- or third-degree LBBB morphology with ÂQRS hyperdeviated to the left or to the right. Due to the conjunction of both blocks, QRS usually is ≥0.12 sec.

Clinical implications of bifascicular block

Bifascicular block, the more frequent combined block, is present in about 0.1% of the general population.

Patients with advanced right BBB plus superoanterior hemiblock (RBBB + SAH) are not a homogeneous group. Although it is the most common manifestation of bifascicular block, the exact incidence of advanced AV block in these cases is not known because these data are conditioned greatly by clinical context. Advanced AV block and also trifascicular block (RBBB+alternating SAH and IPH) were frequently seen in the past in acute anterior infarction (5–10%). Now with current treatments, they occur much less frequently.

In approximately 80% of patients with RBBB + SAH or isolated RBBB or LBBB, an associated heart disease was found (Dihingra *et al*. 1978). In a three-year follow-up period of patients with bifascicular block, 5% of the cases with associated heart disease presented with second- or third-degree AV block, while only 1% of cases without heart disease presented with these types of block ($p < 0.05$). Another series (Chamberlain 1980) found that patients with advanced RBBB + SAH and heart disease presented with an annual rate of progression toward complete AV block of 4%. At the same time, Kulbertus' series (Kulbertus *et al.* 1980) demonstrated that like LBBB, cases with RBBB + SAH had a greater mortality (4.5% yearly) compared to a control group, although it was not statistically significant. In contrast, the HV interval is found to be shorter in patients without heart disease. What is not clear, however, is whether the prognosis is worse in cases with long HV, especially if no associated heart disease is found.

A recent study (Marti-Almor *et al.* 2009) demonstrated that the overall mortality rate in patients with chronic bifascicular block is lower than previously thought (a two-year mortality rate of 6%), and that the most important predictive factors for mortality are advanced heart disease and renal failure.

No consensus exists as to when a pacemaker should be placed in patients with RBBB + SAH or whether implantation of a pacemaker in symptomatic patients prolongs survival. In the end, the physician is required to take decisions considering the clinical setting. The following recommendations may be useful.

• In asymptomatic individuals with advanced RBBB + SAH with or without heart disease, we do not recommend electrophysiological study or pacemaker implantation, although periodic Holter controls may be indicated in some cases.

• We do not think it is necessary to implant a preventive pacemaker in patients with RBBB + SAH who are to undergo surgery, even if there is a slightly prolonged PR interval. Only the presence of clinical manifestations or the diagnosis of advanced AV block indicates this measure.

• There is probably no difference in prognosis between RBBB + SAH and RBBB + IPH, although the latter is infrequent and requires further study. In our experience regarding progression to advanced block, masked blocks (RBBB + SAH) have shown the poorest prognosis (Bayés de Luna *et al.* 1988).

• Patients with this type of masked blocks are usually of an advanced age and present conduction abnormalities at other points in the specialized conduction system, usually accompanied by severe heart disease. This is relatively frequent in Chagas cardiomyopathy, but rare in other heart diseases. In our experience, the prognosis is poor and the incidence of AV block is high (40% in the first year after diagnosis). The prognosis usually does not improve with pacemaker implantation due to the severe underlying heart disease (Bayés de Luna 1988).

• A Holter recording identifying major associated AV block or a very slow heart rate indicates urgent pacemaker implantation.

• In unclear cases where the cardiac origin of syncope or presyncope is not ascertained despite the use of a Holter recording, tilt test, and neurological study to rule out cerebral origin, performing an EPS may be useful. The existence of a long HV interval (>70 ms for some authors, >100 ms for others) (Figure 11.55) or the induction of infrahisian block by atrial pacing makes pacemaker implantation advisable (Narula 1979; Chamberlain 1980).

• We recommend consulting Bayés de Luna and Baranchuk (2017) and the ACC/AHA/ESC guidelines.

Trifascicular block

The variations of trifascicular block are numerous (Bayés de Luna 2012) (see Figure 11.2). The following are the most frequent trifascicular blocks:

• **All bifascicular blocks** mentioned in Figure 11.49 in which **alternance with blocks of other fascicles occur**. The most frequent case is the association of RBBB with SAH, alternating with RBBB and IPH. It merits the name **"Rosenbaum–Elizari's syndrome"** (Rosenbaum *et al.* 1968) because of the detailed description of the association made by these authors (Figure 11.56). This ECG pattern is equivalent to advanced AV block and indicates urgent pacemaker implantation.

• **Another possibility may be** bifascicular block with a long PR interval (e.g. RBBB + SAH and long PR, or RBBB + IPH and long PR) probably due to trifascicular block caused by a conduction delay in one of the two remaining fascicles.

• On occasion, advanced RBBB or LBBB with long PR or second-degree AV block may be a type of trifascicular block. An example of this is advanced global RBBB with

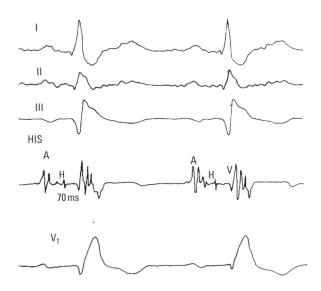

Figure 11.55 A patient with RBBB + IPH and inferior myocardial infarction. The bundle of His electrogram shows a prolonged HV interval (70 ms).

A   **B**

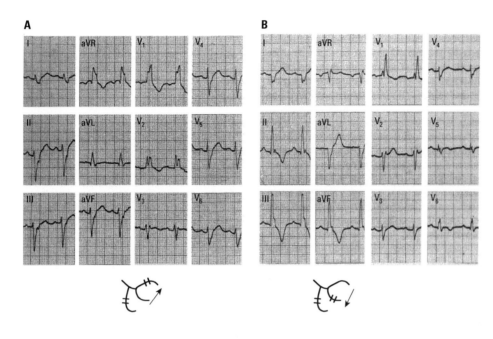

Figure 11.56 Typical example of trifascicular block. (A) RBBB+SAH. (B) The next day, the frontal ÂQRS passed from −60° to +130°, indicating the appearance of an inferoposterior hemiblock substituting the superoanterior hemiblock.

first-degree block of the superoanterior and inferoposterior fascicles that could account for a long PR.
• Some cases of masked block are in fact trifascicular blocks.
It must be remembered that the long PR interval may be due to a delay produced in the bundle of His. In this case, trifascicular block does not occur and consequently intracavitary recording must be made to determine exactly where the PR delay is being produced. However, in clinical practice this will not change the management of our patients.

Delayed diffuse intraventricular QRS activation

Some patients, especially those with IHD or cardiomyopathy but also has been found in studies performed with general population probably as a sign of subclinical disease, present with a QRS duration ≥110 ms, without any ECG pattern of bundle branch block. Recently, it has been demonstrated that these cases are associated with increased mortality even in the absence of overt heart disease (Aro *et al.* 2011).

References

Abben R, Rosen KM, Denes P. Intermittent left bundle branch block: anatomic substrate as reflected in the electrocardiogram during normal conduction. *Circulation* 1979;59:1040.

Aguilar LR, Cabades A, De la Hoz JC, *et al.* Bloqueo completo de rama derecha. Del haz de His durante la implantación de un catéter de Swan-Ganz. *Rev Esp Cardiol* 1977;30:309.

Alboni P. *Intraventricular Conduction Disturbances.* Martinus Nijhoff, 1981.

Aro A, Anttonen D, Tikkanen J, *et al.* Intraventricular conduction delay in 12 lead ECG as a predictor of mortality in general population. *Circ Arrhythm Electrophysiol* 2011;4(5):704–710.

Auricchio A, Fantoni C, Regoli F, *et al.* Characterization of left ventriuclar activation in patients with heart failure and left bundle-branch block. *Circulation* 2004;109:1133.

Azadani PN, Soleimanirahbar A, Marcus GM, *et al.* Asymptomatic left bundle branch block predicts new-onset congestive heart failure and death from cardiovascular diseases. *Cardiol Res* 2012;3:258.

Baldesseroni S, Operich C, Gorini M, *et al.* Left bundle branch block in associated with increased 1-year sudden and totally mortality death. *Am Heart J* 2002;143:398.

Barret PA, Peter CT, Swan HJ *et al.* The frequency and prognosis significance of ECG abnormalities in clinically normal individuals. *Prog Cardiovasc Dis* 1981;23:299.

Bayés-Genís A, Lopez L, Viñolas X, *et al.* Distinct left bundle branch block pattern in ischemic and non-ischemic dilated cardiomyopathy. *Eur J Heart Failure* 2003;5:165.

Bayés de Luna A. *Clinical Electrocardiography: A Textbook.* Willey-Blackwell, 2012.

Bayés de Luna A, Baranchuk A. *Clinical Arrhythmology,* 2nd edn. Wiley-Blackwell, 2017.

Bayés de Luna A, Cosín J, Carrió J, *et al.* Right ventricular peripheral blocks: diagnostic problems. In Masoni A, Alboni P (eds) *Cardiac Electrophysiology Today.* Academic Press, 1982, p. 401.

Bayés de Luna A, Serra Genís C, Guix M, *et al.* Septal fibrosis as determinant of Q waves in patients with aortic valve disease. *Eur Heart J* 1983;4(suppl E):86.

Bayés de Luna A, Carrió I, Subirana MT, *et al.* Electrophysiological mechanisms of the SI, SII, SIII electrocardiographic morphology. *J Electrocardiol* 1987;20:38.

Bayés de Luna A, Torner P, Oter R, *et al.* Study of the evolution of masked bifascicular block. *PACE* 1988;11:1517.

Bayés de Luna A, Platonov P, García-Cosio F, *et al.* Interatrial blocks. a separate entity from left atrial enlargement: a consensus report. *J Electrocardiol* 2012;45:445–451.

Bialostosky D, Medrano GA, Muñoz L, Contreras R. Vectorcardiographic study and anatomic observations in 21 cases of Ebstein's malformations. *Am J Cardiol* 1972;30:354.

Bogale N, Ørn S, James M, *et al*. Usefulnes of either or both left and right bundle branch block at baseline or during follow-up for predictiong death in patients following acute myocardial infarction. *Am J Cardiol* 2007;99:647.

Breithardt G, Breithardt OA. Left bundle branch block: Anold-new entity. *J Cardiovasc Transl Res* 2012;5(2):107–116. doi:https://doi.org/10.1007/s12265-011-9344-5.

Brenes JC, Brenes-Pereira C, Castellanos A. Wenckebach phenomenon at the left bundle branch. *Clin Cardiol* 2006;29:226.

Candell-Riera J, Gordillo E, Olla-Martinez S, *et al*. Long term outcome of painful left bundle branch block. *Am J Card* 2002;89:602.

Cannom DS, Wyman M, Goldreyer B. Initial ventricular activation in left-sided intraventricular conduction defects. *Circulation* 1980;62:621.

Castellanos A, Ramirez AV, Mayorga-Cortes A, *et al*. Left fascicular block during right heart catheterization using the Swan-Ganz catheter. *Circulation* 1981;64:1271.

Cazeau S, Leclercq C, Lavergne T, *et al*. Effects of multisite biventricular pacing in patients with heart failure and intraventricular conduction delay. *N Engl J Med* 2001;344:873.

Chamberlain DA. *Cardiac arrhythmias in the active population: prevalence, significance and management: proceedings of a conference held in Køge, Denmark, October 4–5, 1979, sponsored by the European, Danish, and Swedish Societies of Cardiology in collaboration with AB Hässle, Mölndal, subsidiary of AB Astra, Sweden Cardiac arrhythmias in the active population*. Mölndal, Hässle, 1980. ISBN:91-85520-18-7sidottu

Cohen SI, Lau SH, Haft JI, et al. Experimental production of aberrant ventricular conduction in man. *Circulation* 1967;36:673–685.

Cokkinos DV, Demopoulos JN, Heimonas T, *et al*. Electrocardiographic criteria of left ventricular hypertrophy in left bundle branch block. *Br Heart J* 1978;40:320.

Cooksey I, Dunn M, Massie E. *Clinical ECG and VCG*. YearBook Medical, 1977.

Dabrowska B, Ruka M, Walczak E. The ECG diagnosis of left septal fascicular block. *Eur J Card* 1978;6:347.

Dancy M, Leech G, Lentham A. Significance of complete right bundle branch block when an isolated finding. an echocardiographic study. *Br Heart J* 1982;48:217.

De Micheli A, Medrano GA, Martínez Ríos MA, *et al*. Despolarización y repolarización ventricular en las sobrecargas diastólica y mixta del ventrículo derecho. *Rev Esp Cardiol* 1983;38:113.

De Padua F, Pereirinha A, Marques N, Lopes MG, Macfarlane P. Conduction defects. In Macfarlane P, van Oosterom A, Pahlm O, Kligfield P, Janse M, Camm J (eds) *Comprehensive Electrocardiology*, Vol. 2. Springer-Verlag, 2011, p. 547.

Demoulin JC, Kulbertus HE. Histopathological examination of concept of left hemiblock. *Br Heart J* 1972;34:807.

Denes P, Pick A, Miller RH, *et al*. A characteristic precordial repolarization abnormality in patients with intermittent left bundle branch block. *Ann Intern Med* 1978;89:55.

Dihingra RC, Amat-Y-Leon F, Wyndham Ch, *et al*. Significance of left axis deviation in patients with chronic left bundle branch block. *Am J Cardiol* 1978;42:551.

Durrer D, Van Dam R, Freud G, *et al*. Total excitation of the isolated human heart. *Circulation* 1970;414:899.

Elizari MV, Levi R, Acunzo RS, *et al*. Abnormal expression of cardiac neural crest cells in heart development: a different hypothesis for the etiopathogenesis of Brugada syndrome. *Heart Rhythm* 2007;4:359.

Fontaine G, Frank R, Guiraudon G, *et al*. Significado del bloqueo ventricular en la displasia arritmogénica del ventrículo derecho. In: Piccolo E, Raviele D (eds) *Número monográfico sobre avances en Electrocardiología*. Revista Latina de Cardiología, 1987, Vol. 8, no. 2.

Frais M, Botvinick EH, Shosa DW, *et al*. Phase image characterization of ventricular contraction in left and right bundle branch block. *Am J Cardiol* 1982;50:95.

Garcia Moll X, Guindo J, Viñolas X, *et al*. Intermittent masked bifascicular block. *Am Heart J* 1994;127:214.

Grant RP, Dodge HT. Mechanisms of QRS complex prolongation in man: left ventricular conduction disturbances. *Am J Med* 1956;20:834.

Hellerstein HK, Hamlin R. QRS component of the spatial vectorcardiogram and of the spatial magnitude and velocity electrocardiograms of the normal dog. *Am J Cardiol* 1960;6:1049.

Hoffman I Mehta J, Hilsenrath J, *et al*. Anterior conduction delay: a possible cause for prominent anterior QRS forces. *J Electrocardiol* 1976;9:15.

Horowitz LW, Alexander JA, Edmunds LH. Postoperative right bundle branch block. Identification of three levels of block. *Circulation* 1980;62:319.

Kulbertus HE, de Leval-Rutten F, Casters P. Vectorcardiographic study of aberrant conduction. Anterior displacement of QRS: another form of intraventricular block. *Br Heart J* 1976;38:549.

Kulbertus HE, Leval-Rutten I, Dubois M, Petit JM. Sudden death in subjects with intraventricular conduction defects. In Kulbertus HE, Wellens HJJ (eds) *Sudden Death*. Martinus Nijhoff, 1980, p. 392.

Kafka E, Burggraf GV, Milliken JA. Electrocardiographic diagnosis of left ventricular hypertrophy in the presence of left bundle branch block: an echocardiographic study. *Am J Cardiol* 1985;55(1):103 doi:https://doi.org/10.1016/0002-9149(85)90308-x.

Laham J. *Les troubles de la conduction intraventriculaire*. Ed Les heures de France, 1980.

Lenegre J. Etiology and pathology of bilateral bundle branch block in relation to complete heart block. *Prog Cardiovasc Dis* 1964;6:409.

Lópes MG. The diagnosis ventricular hypertrophy in the presence of bundle branch block: an ECG/VCG and echocardiographic correlation. In Antaldezy Z (ed.) *Modern Electrocardiology*. Excerpta Medica, 1978, p. 423.

MacAlpin RN. In search of left septal fascicular block. *Am Heart J* 2002;144:948.

Macfarlane PW, Veitch Lawrie TD (eds). *Comprehensive Electrocardiography* (3 vols). Pergamon Press, 1989.

Marquez-Montes J. Bloqueo periférico de rama derecha del haz de His. *Rev Esp Cardiol* 1975;28:373.

Marti-Almor J, Cladellas M, Bazan V, *et al*. Long-term mortality predictors in patients with chronic bifascicular block. *Europace* 2009;11:1201.

Masoni A, Alboni P (eds) *Cardiac Electrophysiology Today*. Academic Press, 1982.

Mayorga-Costes A, Rozansky J, Sung R, *et al*. Right ventricular apical activation times in patients with conduction disturbances occurring during acute transmural myocardial infarction. *Am J Cardiol* 1979;43:913.

Medrano GA, De Micheli A. Contribución experimental al diagnóstico de los bloqueos periféricos fasciculares derechos. *Arch Inst Cardiol Mexico* 1975;45:704.

Medrano GA, Brenes C, De Micheli A, *et al*. El bloqueo simultáneo de las divisiones anterior y posterior de la rama izquierda del haz de His (bloqueo bifascicular) y su asociación con bloqueos de rama derecha (bloqueo trifascicular). *Arch Inst Cardiol Mexico* 1970;40:752.

Moffa PJ, Ferreira BM, Sanches PC, *et al*. Intermittent ântero-medial divisional block in patients with coronary disease. *Arq Bras Cardiol* 1997;68:293.

Moreu J. Left bundle branch block with left axis deviation. A not so different entity. *PACE* 1985;8:A-15.

Moss AJ, Jackson Hall W, Cannom DS, *et al*. Cardiac resynchronization therapy for the prevention of heart failure events. *N Eng J Med* 2009;361:1329.

Nakaya Y, Hiasa Y, Murayama Y, *et al*. Prominent anterior QRS force as a manifestation of left septal fascicular block. *J Electrocardiol* 1978;11:39–46.

Nakaya Y, Inoue H, Hiasa Y, *et al*. Functional importance of left septal Purkinje network in the LV conduction system. *Jap Heart J* 1981;22:364.

Narula OS. Longitudinal dissociation in the His bundle. Bundle branch block due to asynchronous conduction within the His bundle in man. *Circulation* 1977;56:996.

Narula OS. Intraventricular conduction defects: current concepts and clinical significance. In Narula OS (ed.) *Cardiac Arrhythmias. Electrophysiology, Diagnosis and Management*. Williams-Wilkins, 1979, p. 124.

Paleo P. Exercise induced left bundle branch block. *Am Heart J* 1984;108:1373.

Pastore CA, Pinho C, Germiniani H, *et al*. Directrices Soc. Brasileira Cardiologia sobre analisis ECG. *Arq Bras Card* 2009;93(3 Sup 2):1.

Peñaloza D, Gamboa R, Sime F. Experimental right bundle branch block in the normal human heart. *Am J Cardiol* 1961;8:767.

Pérez Riera A, Ferreira C, Ferreira Filho C, *et al*. Wellens-syndrome associated with prominent anterior QRS forces: an expression of left septal fascicular block? *J Electrocardiol* 2008;41:671.

Pérez Riera A, Ferreira C, Ferriera Filho C, *et al*. Electro-vectorcardiographic diagnosis of left septal fascicular block: anatomic and clinical considerations. *Ann Noninvasive Electrocardiol* 2011;16:196.

Piccolo E. *Elettrocardiografia e vectorcardiografia*. Piccin Edit, 1981.

Piccolo E, Raviele A, Delise P, *et al*. The role of left ventricular conduction in the electrogenesis of left ventricular hypertrophy. *Circulation* 1979;59:1944.

Piccolo E, Delise P, Raviele A, *et al*. The anterior displacement of the QRS loop as a right ventricular conduction disturbance. Electrophysiologic and vectorcardiographic study in man. *J Electrocardiol* 1980;13:267.

Rabkin SW. Natural history of left bundle branch block. *Br Heart J* 1980;43:164.

Rajala S, Kaltiala K, Haavisto M, *et al*. Prevalence of ECG findings in very old people. *Eur Heart J* 1984;5:168.

Reiffel JA, Bigger T, Jr. Pure anterior conduction delay: a variant "fascicular" defect. *J Electrocardiol* 1978;11:315–319.

Ribeiro C. Les blocs intraventriculaires gauches: Le role de la paroi libre dans la genese de leurs morphologie électro-vectorcardiographique. *Arch Mal Cœur* 1968;59:1665.

Romanelli R, Willils WH, Mitchell WA, *et al*. Coronary arteriograms and myocardial scintigrams in the ECG syndrome of septal fibrosis. *Am Heart J* 1980;100:617.

Rosenbaum M, Elizari M, Lazzari E. *Los hemibloqueos*. Edit Paidos, 1968.

Rosenbaum M, Yesuron J, Lazzari J, *et al*. Left anterior hemiblock obscuring the diagnosis of right bundle branch block. *Circulation* 1973;48:298.

Rotman N, Frietwaser J. A clinical and follow-up study of right and left bundle branch block. *Circulation* 1975;51:477.

Schneider JF, Emerson Thomas H, Kreber BE, *et al*. Newly acquired right bundle branch block. *Ann Intern Med* 1980;92:37.

Schneider JF, Thomas HE Jr, McNamara PM *et al*. Clinical electrocardiographic correlates of newly acquired left bundle branch block: the Framingham study. *Am J Cardiol* 1985;55:1332.

Sobrino JA, Sotillo JF, Del Río A, *et al*. Fascicular blocks within the His bundle. *Chest* 1978;74:215.

Sodi D, Bisteni A, Medrano G. *Electrocardiografía y vectorcardiografía deductivas*, Vol. I. La Prensa Médica Mexicana, 1964.

Strasberg B. M-mode echocardiography in left bundle branch block: significance of frontal QRS-axis. *Am Heart J* 1982;104:775.

Strauss DG, Selvester RH. The QRS complex—a biomarker that "images" the heart: QRS scores to quantify myocardial scar in the presence of normal and abnormal ventricular conduction. *J Electrocardiol* 2009;42:85.

Strauss DG, Selvester RH, Wagner GS. Defining left bundle branch block in the era of cardiac resynchronization therapy. *Am J Cardiol* 2011;107:927.

Sung RJ, Tamer DM, García DL, *et al*. Analysis of surgically-induced right bundle branch block pattern using intracardiac recording techniques. *Circulation* 1976;54:442.

Supariwala AA, Ricardo J, Mohareb S, *et al*. Prevalence and long-term prognosis of patients with complete bundle branch block (right or left bundle branch) with normal left ventricular ejection fraction referred for stress echocardiography. *Echocardiography* 2015;32:483.

Sze E, Samad Z, Dunning A, *et al*. Impaired recovery of left ventricular function in patients with cardiomyopathy and left bundle branch block. *JACC* 2018;71:306.

Uhley HN, Rivkin L. ECG patterns following interruption of main and peripheral branches of the canine right bundle. *Am J Cardiol* 1961;7:810.

Uhley H, Rivkin L. Electrocardiographic patterns following interruption of the main and peripheral branches of the canine left bundle of His. *Am J Cardiol* 1964;13:41.

Van Bommel R, Marsan N, Delgado V, *et al*. Value of the surface ECG in detecting right ventricular dilatation in the presence of left bundle branch block. *Am J Cardiol* 2011;107:736.

Van Dam R, Janse M. Ventricular activation in canine and human bundle branch block. *Circulation* 1974;50:III:82.

Van Gersse L, Houthuizen P, Poels T, *et al*. Left bundle branch block induced by transcatheter aortic valve implantation increases risk of 1-year all cause mortality. *Circulation* 2011;124:A11770.

Vanderburg B, Sagar K, Romhilt D. ECG criteria for the diagnosis of left ventricular hypertrophy in the presence of complete right bundle branch block. *J Am Coll Cardiol* 1985;5:511.

Vassallo JA, Cassidy DM, Marchlinski FE, *et al*. Endocardial activation of left bundle branch block. *Circulation* 1984;69:914.

Vazquez R, Bayes-Genis A, Cygankiewicz I, *et al*. The MUSIC Risk score: a simple method for predicting mortalityin ambulatory patients with chronic heart failure. *Eur Heart Failure* 2009;30:1088.

Watanabe Y, Kozuma K, Hioki H, *et al*. Pre-existing right bundle branch block increases risk for death after transcatheter aortic valve replacement with a balloon-expandable valve. *J Am Coll Cardiol* 2016;9:2210.

Wilson FN. Concerning the form of the QRS deflections of the electrocardiogram in bundle branch block. *J Mount Sinai Hosp NY* 1941;9:1110.

Windham C, Smith T, Hersh S, *et al*. Epicardial activation in patients with left bundle branch block. *Circulation* 1978;58:II:156.

Chapter 12
Ventricular Pre-excitation

Concept and types of pre-excitation

The term "ventricular pre-excitation" implies that the myocardium depolarizes earlier than expected if the stimulus follows the normal pathway through the specific conduction system (Wolff *et al.* 1930). In fact, this is not really what happens before excitation (pre-excitation). Instead, it refers to ventricular excitation occurring earlier than expected.

Three types of pre-excitation have been defined:
- **Wolff–Parkinson–White pre-excitation (WPW)** (Table 12.1 and Figures 12.1 and 12.2), in which the early excitation is caused by muscular connections composed of working myocardial fibers that connect the atrium and ventricle, bypassing the atrioventricular (AV) nodal conduction delay. These comprise the accessory AV pathways that are known as Kent bundles.
- **Atypical pre-excitations**, encompassing different long anomalous pathways or tracts showing decremental conduction, localized on the right side of the heart. This type of pre-excitation includes the classical Mahaim fibers (Sternick and Wellens 2006) (see Atypical pre-excitation, below).
- **Short PR pre-excitation** (Lown *et al.* 1957), where the early excitation is due to an accelerated conduction through the AV node and, in some cases, is due to the presence of an atriohisian tract (Figure 12.2) (see Short PR interval pre-excitation). Currently, it is widely accepted that there are no "specific" tracts but rather an accelerated conduction over the AV node and "proper" terminology should be "enhanced AV node conduction."

WPW-type pre-excitation (type 1)

Concept and mechanism
WPW-type pre-excitation occurs by means of the presence of accessory AV pathways (Kent bundle) (Figure 12.3).

In general, only one accessory pathway (AP) exists (>90% of cases) and conduction is usually fast and in both directions (anterogradely and retrogradely) (≈2/3 of cases). On certain occasions (20%), the conduction of the AP occurs only retrogradely (concealed WPW). Other WPW-type pre-excitations are less frequent (Table 12.1).

These APs can integrate a circuit (specific conduction system (SCS)–ventricle–AP–atrium–SCS) with anterograde or retrograde conduction, which constitutes the anatomic substrate of reentrant arrhythmias that are frequently observed in the presence of WPW-type pre-excitation (WPW syndrome). Table 12.1 shows the most characteristic ECG morphologies in sinus rhythm and during a tachycardia episode, according to the anatomic and functional properties of the different types of pre-excitation (anterograde and/or retrograde conduction, and fast or slow conduction).

ECG characteristics
The ECG changes in sinus rhythm are only observed when anterograde conduction exists. They consist mainly of a short PR interval and an abnormal QRS complex with initial slurring (delta wave) which is a manifestation of ventricular fusion, due to simultaneous activation through the accessory pathway and the AV node–His system.

The short PR interval occurs because the sinus stimulus reaches the ventricles through the AP sooner than through the SCS. The presence of an abnormal QRS complex is the result of the ventricular activation taking place through two pathways: the normal AV conduction and the AP (a Kent bundle). These result in slightly early activation of the ventricles in subepicardial zones where there are very few Purkinje fibers. This explains not only the early QRS complex (short PR interval), but also the delta wave as the result of the slow activation of the myocardial tissue. The rest of the myocardial mass is activated through the normal pathway (SCS). The QRS complex is thus a genuine fusion complex.

Clinical Electrocardiography: A Textbook, Fifth Edition. Antoni Bayés de Luna, Miquel Fiol-Sala, Antoni Bayés-Genís, and Adrián Baranchuk.
© 2022 John Wiley & Sons Ltd. Published 2022 by John Wiley & Sons Ltd.

Table 12.1 Pre-excitation types: (1) WPW-type pre-excitation; (2) atypical pre-excitation; (3) short PR-type pre-excitation. Surface ECG rate and characteristics in sinus rhythm and during paroxysmal tachycardia episodes, according to the functional characteristics of the different types of pre-excitation

	Accessory pathway	Frequency	ECG in sinus rhythm	ECG during tachycardia
Type 1	(a) Fast conduction in both ways: AV accessory pathway (classical Kent bundle) (see Figures 9.1–9.7)	60–65%	Short PR δ wave	No δ wave RP′ < P′R
	(b) Fast conduction in the AV accessory pathway (only in retrograde direction) (concealed pre-excitation)	20–30%	Normal PR No δ wave	No δ wave RP′ < P′R
	(c) Fast conduction in the AV accessory pathway (only in anterograde direction) (frequently two or more bundles involved)	5–10%	Short PR δ wave	Wide QRS due to an anterograde conduction of the stimuli through the accessory pathway (antidromic tachycardia)
	(d) Only retrograde and slow conduction through AV accessory pathway	≈5%	Normal PR No δ wave	Frequently incessant tachycardia with RP′ > P′R
	(e) Presence of >1 accessory pathway	5–10%	May switch from one to another QRS morphology qrs or qRs in V1 This diagnosis is generally difficult based only on a surface ECG	Antidromic tachycardia or alternating antidromic/orthodromic tachycardia Alternation of short and long PR Morphology changes in ectopic P wave Electrophysiological studies confirm this diagnosis
Type 2	Slow anterograde conduction, generally through a long atriofascicular tract (distal right branch), without retrograde conduction (including classical Mahaim[a] fibers–node ventricular or fascicle ventricular-)	Rare	Non-existent or slight pre-excitation (i.e. no Q in V5–V6, with borderline PR and uncertain δ wave, and rS in III) This is due to the slow conduction through the abnormal tract. Globally the ECG is normal or presents different grades of LBB pattern	Antidromic tachycardia with anterograde conduction through the right atriofascicular tract and retrograde conduction through the RBB. Therefore, it features a LBBB morphology. Compared with the antidromic tachycardias (generated due to anterograde conduction through a right AV accessory pathway—Type C in this table), features a narrower QRS complex and a delayed transition to RS in precordial leads (compare Figures 15.16 and 16.18)
Type 3	AV node accelerated conduction, sometimes due to an atriohisian tract (short PR pre-excitation)	Rare	Short PR interval No δ wave	Normal QRS complex No δ wave

[a] Today, it is believed that the classical Mahaim fibers (nodoventricular and fasciculoventricular fibers) initiate paroxysmal tachycardias less frequently than the right atriofascicular tracts. Currently, it is considered that they are not involved in the circuit which triggers the tachycardia, which is usually due to a right atriofascicular tract, as previously mentioned.

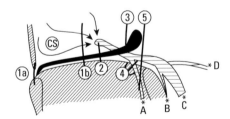

*A, B, C, D. Points of onset of ventricular activation
▨▨▨ Cardiac muscle
■ Central fibrous body
1. Bundle of Kent (A) ventricular wall (b)
2. AV node
3. Atriohisian
4. His/fascicle
5. Atrium fascicle
Coronary sinus (CS)

Figure 12.1 Right lateral view of the accessory pathways.

Depending on what myocardial areas are activated through one pathway or the other, the QRS complex will show a greater or lesser degree of pre-excitation.

In the rare cases of type 2 pre-excitation (Table 12.1), the baseline ECG may have morphologies varying from normal to subtle evidence of minimal pre-excitation that looks like cases with left bundle branch block (LBBB) pattern (see Atypical pre-excitation, below). In type 3 pre-excitation, the only anomaly of the ECG is the short PR interval (see Short PR interval pre-excitation, below).

PR interval

This generally ranges from 0.08–0.11 sec. Cases with normal PR interval are rare. They may occur due to the presence of a long left AV AP Kent bundle type with delayed atrial conduction. In this scenario, even though the ventricular activation is performed through a classical Kent

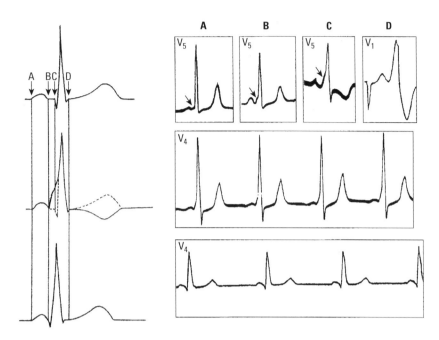

Figure 12.2 Left top panel: Diagram of the P–QRS relationship in normal cases. AB: P wave; BC: PR segment; CD: QRS. Middle panel: WPW-type pre-excitation (the broken line represents the QRS complex if no pre-excitation occurred). AD distance is the same as under normal conditions, with a wide QRS complex in detriment to the PR segment (BC distance), which partially or totally coincides with the delta wave. Lower panel: in cases of short PR segment, the QRS complex is shifted forward because the PR segment is shortened or may even disappear. Top right: four examples of delta wave (arrow) by increasing order of relevance. (D) Atrial fibrillation patient in whom the first QRS is conducted over the normal pathway, while the second QRS is conducted over the accessory pathway with maximum pre-excitation. Middle panel: example of four complexes with pre-excitation, with an average-sized delta wave. Lower panel: four complexes in a case of short PR pre-excitation.

bundle, the PR interval is usually at the lower limit of normality (0.12–0.13 sec), and therefore is not considered short. It is, however, shorter than when no pre-excitation occurs, as conduction through the normal pathway would have a longer PR interval.

A normal PR interval may also exist in the following cases: atypical long atriofascicular/atrioventricular anomalous tracts (currently termed "enhanced AV node conduction," see above) with slow conduction or other atypical tracts, including the classical Mahaim fibers (very rare). These tracts may partially or completely prevent the slow intranodal conduction (Sternick and Wellens 2006) (see Atypical pre-excitation, below).

Ventriculogram alterations (Figures 12.4 and 12.5)

The QRS complexes show an abnormal morphology wider than the baseline QRS complex (frequently ≥ 0.11 sec) with characteristic initial slurring (delta wave) due to the activation being initiated at the working contractile myocardium in an area with few Purkinje fibers. The degree of abnormality of the QRS complex depends on the amount of ventricular myocardium that has been depolarized through the AP (Figure 12.1, arrow from A–D).

The QRS complex morphology in the different surface ECG leads depends on which epicardial area is excited earliest. Studies correlating surface ECGs, vectorcardiography (VCG), and epicardial mapping performed during surgical ablation of APs by the Gallagher group (Tonkin *et al.* 1975) have shown the value of studying delta wave polarity to identify the site of earliest ventricular epicardial excitation. The first 20 ms vector in the ECG (first delta wave vector that can be measured on the ECG) is situated in different places on the frontal plane (in the horizontal plane it is always directed forward), depending on the site of earliest ventricular epicardial excitation. These studies precisely locate the AP according to the surface ECG findings, at 10 sites around the AV ring (Gallagher *et al.* 1978). There is an electrophysiological statement (Cosio *et al.* 1999) to standardize the terminology of APs around the AV junction.

Milstein *et al.* (1987) (see Figure 12.6) described an algorithm that allows the correlation of the alterations found in the surface ECG with four ablation zones. From a practical point of view, the WPW-type pre-excitation may be classified into four types based on these findings: anteroseptal, right ventricular (RV) free wall, inferoseptal, and left ventricular (LV) free wall (Bayés de Luna and

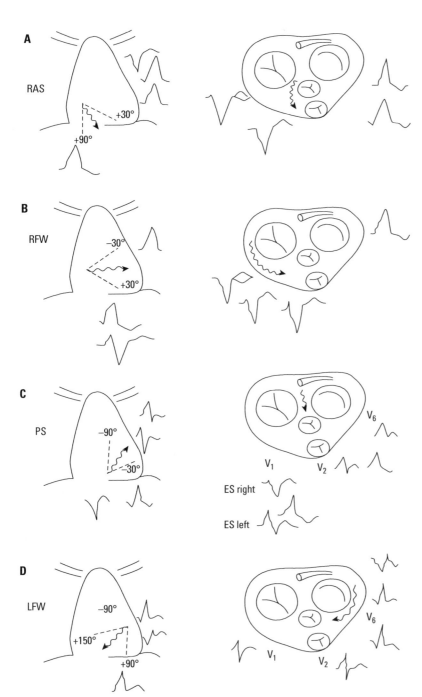

Figure 12.3 WPW-type pre-excitation morphologies according to the different localization of the AV accessory pathway: (A) Right anteroseptal area (RAS); (B) right ventricular free wall (RFW); (C) inferoseptal area (IS); and (D) left ventricular free wall (LFW).

Baranchuk, 2017) (Figure 12.3). A complete electrophysiologic study (EPS) should be carried out to precisely identify the exact location of the AP before performing an ablation.

In Figures 12.7–12.8, we can see examples of QRS morphologies in these four electrocardiographic modalities of WPW-type pre-excitation. **Types I and II mimic a LBBB**, with a more deviated left axis (ÂQRS beyond +30°) in type II, whereas in type I the ÂQRS is usually between +30° and +90°. **In type III,** the QRS is predominantly negative in inferior leads, especially in III and aVF, with R or RS morphology in V1 or V2, and the ÂQRS is between −30°

and −90°. **Type IV** has a predominantly negative morphology in lateral leads (I, aVL) and a generally high R wave in leads V1 or V2, with a right axis deviation (ÂQRS beyond +90° up to +150°).

Type IV is the most frequent (≈50% of cases) followed by inferoseptal (25%). The APs in close proximity to the bundle of His are located in the anteroseptal zone, close to the anteroseptal and midseptal tricuspid annulus (Arruda *et al.* 1998). The prevalence is low (1–2%), but it is important to localize them precisely by electrophysiologic studies (WPS) because they may present with AV block during the ablation procedure.

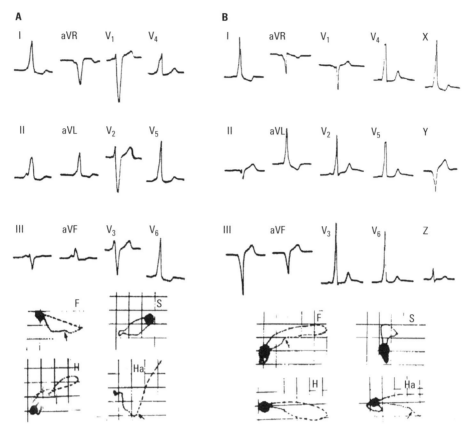

Figure 12.4 (A) ECG–VCG of a patient with WPW type II (Ha: amplified horizontal plane). The arrows indicate the end of the delta wave. (B) Another ECG–VCG of a patient with WPW type II.

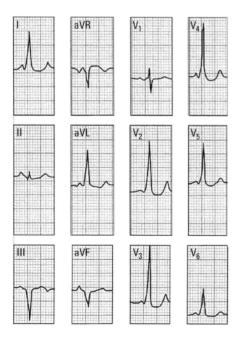

Figure 12.5 A WPW patient with the accessory pathway located in the inferoseptal heart wall (type III WPW). This case may be mistaken for an inferior infarction, right ventricular hypertrophy, or right bundle branch block (RBBB).

Other algorithms have been published (Lindsay *et al.* 1987; Chiang *et al.* 1995; Iturralde *et al.* 2006). Yuan *et al.* (1992) carried out a comparative study of eight algorithms, some of which allow for a better identification of the different types of septal pathways. They are difficult to memorize, and they are neither sensitive nor specific for all the cases. Later, Basiouny *et al.* (1999) reviewed 10 algorithms and found that the PPV was lower in those algorithms aimed at reaching a more precise localization (>6 sites), whereas PPV was found to be higher (>80%) when the AP was located on the left side. Because their reproducibility is not very high, it is advisable that each center become more familiar with the algorithm they consider best suited to their needs. A complete EPS should, therefore, be carried out to precisely identify the exact location of the AP before performing an ablation.

Repolarization alterations

Repolarization is altered except in those cases with minor pre-excitation. These changes are secondary to depolarization alterations, and become more pathologic (more significant opposing polarity when compared with that of the R wave) as the degree of pre-excitation increases (Figure 12.2).

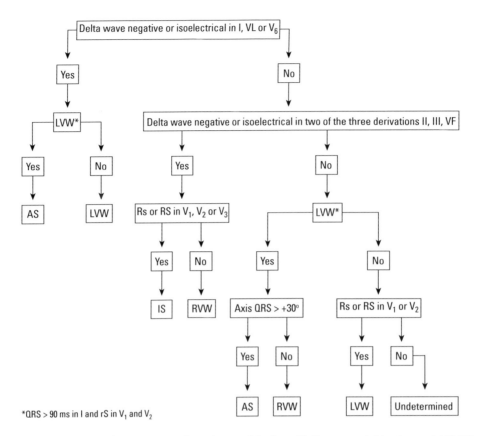

Figure 12.6 Algorithm used to localize the accessory pathway in one of the four ablation areas: right anteroseptal (RAS); right ventricular free wall (RFW); inferoseptal area (IS); and left ventricular free wall (LFW) (see text).

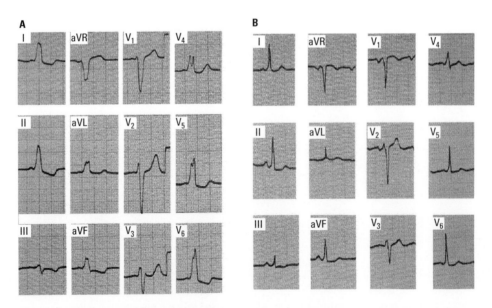

Figure 12.7 Two examples of WPW type I pre-excitation. (A) Important pre-excitation in a 65-year-old patient with intermittent WPW. (B) Slight pre-excitation in a 25-year-old patient with mitral stenosis. Observe in both cases the short PR and the positive delta wave in every lead except VR, where it is negative, and V1 where it is positive. The case on the left (A) can be confused with advanced LBBB and the case on the right (B) with not advanced LBBB.

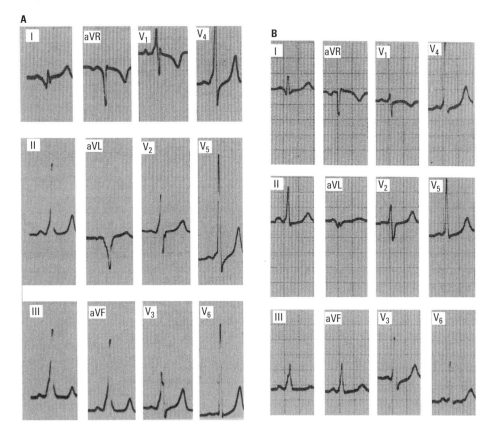

Figure 12.8 Two cases of WPW patient with the accessory pathway located in the left ventricular free wall (type IV WPW). These cases may be mistaken for a lateral infarction, right ventricular hypertrophy, or right bundle branch block.

When pre-excitation is intermittent, the complexes conducted without pre-excitation may show repolarization alterations (negative T wave), which are explained by an electrical "electrical memory phenomenon" (Chatterjee *et al.* 1969; Nicolai *et al.* 1981; Rosenbaum *et al.* 1982).

ECG diagnosis of more than one accessory pathway (Wellens *et al.* 1990)

Approximately 5–10% of cases involve more than one AP. This may be clinically suspected when the patient suffers from syncope or malignant ventricular arrhythmia, or wide QRS complex paroxysmal tachycardia (antidromic tachycardia).

Some ECG data are indicative of this association, both in sinus rhythm and during tachycardia. These are as follows:

• **I sinus rhythm**: (i) QrS or qRs morphology in lead V1; and (ii) morphology changes from one to the other type of pre-excitation (Figure 12.10).

• **During tachycardia:** (i) wide QRS complex or alternating wide and narrow QRS complexes; (ii) alternating long and short RR; and (iii) changes in the P' wave morphology.

In general, this diagnosis suspicion should be confirmed with intracavitary electrophysiologic study (EPS).

How to confirm or exclude the presence of pre-excitation

Some patients are referred with suspected WPW pre-excitation when none exists and others have a genuine pre-excitation and are considered normal. Using a selective AV node blocking agent, such as adenosine, may confirm or exclude the presence of pre-excitation (Belhassen *et al.* 2000). Its rapid action, and fast degradation, makes Adenosine the best choice to confirm the presence of "hidden" accessory pathways in the EP lab.

On the other hand, the presence of the septal Q wave in V6 is considered to be evidence that excludes minimal pre-excitaton in doubtful cases (Bogun *et al.* 1999).

Finally, Eisenberger *et al.* (2010) has shown a stepwise approach that is very sensitive and specific for excluding or confirming WPW pre-excitation.

Differential diagnosis of WPW-type pre-excitation

• **WPW type I and II** pre-excitation may be mistaken for **LBBB** (Figures 12.4 and 12.5A). We have already seen that in type II pre-excitation, a left axis deviation of ÂQRS beyond +30° is observed.

• **Type III** pre-excitation requires differential diagnosis with **inferior myocardial infarction, a right bundle**

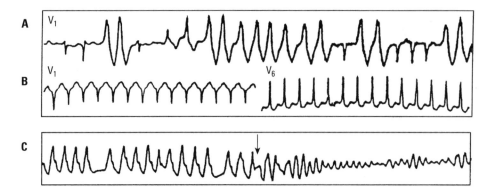

Figure 12.9 Atrial fibrillation episode (A) and supraventricular paroxysmal tachycardia (B) in the same patient with WPW syndrome. See the typical ECG patterns in both cases. (C) Patient with WPW syndrome presenting with a very fast atrial fibrillation triggering a ventricular fibrillation (arrow). This was treated with electrical cardioversion.

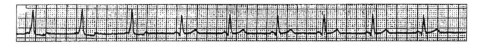

Figure 12.10 Intermittent pre-excitation. In the first three complexes, the PR interval is short (80 ms) and the delta wave is observed. In the rest of the tracing, the delta wave disappears, but a short PR interval is still observed (100 ms). Thus, this surface ECG suggests the presence of two types of pre-excitation, one of which short circuits the AV node (short PR, QRS with no delta wave), while the other is a pathway located in the ventricular myocardium (Kent bundle), since the PR interval is very short and a clear delta wave is seen.

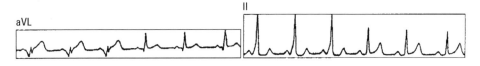

Figure 12.11 Intermittent type IV pre-excitation: the pattern is similar to that observed in a lateral infarction (see aVL).

branch block (RBBB), or a **right ventricular hypertrophy** (Figure 12.6).

• **Type IV** pre-excitation should be distinguished from a **lateral myocardial infarction, RBBB, or right ventricular hypertrophy** (Figures 12.8 and 12.11).

Associated ischemic heart disease

It is important to recognize the different signs that allow us to suspect the presence of acute or chronic ischemia when pre-excitation is present. However, this occurs very rarely because the presence of WPW pre-excitation is less prevalent, especially in adults.

In the acute phase, the repolarization changes, especially the ST segment elevation, may lead us to suspect acute coronary syndrome (ACS) with ST elevation. It is more difficult to make the correct diagnosis in ACS without ST elevation. In the chronic phase of Q wave myocardial infarction, the association may sometimes be suspected when repolarization shows more symmetrical T waves (Fiol-Sala *et al.* 2020). Sometimes, echocardiography imaging is required to establish the presence of localized wall motion abnormalities.

In any case, the presence of a short PR interval and/or a delta wave, always keeping in mind the possibility of

WPW-type pre-excitation, are key ECG data for the correct diagnosis of this condition.

Associated with bundle branch block

The presence of short PR and delta wave indicates pre-excitation. Therefore, in practice the association is usually only diagnosed when pre-excitation is transient. However, there are cases with borderline PR interval or pseudo-delta wave such as in cardiomyopathy or distal bundle branch block in which the association may be suspected if the bundle branch block is contralateral to the pre-excited ventricle (Pick and Fisch 1958, Denes *et al.* 1975). This results in QRS complexes that may show an early pre-excitation delta wave and also a terminal slurring due to BBB (i.e. left anomalous pathway + RBBB). On the contrary, the presence of BBB with ipsilateral pre-excitation results in masking the BBB due to premature depolarization of the blocked ventricle by the anomalous pathway. Patients with Ebstein disease present frequently right anomalous bundle and RBBB. Iturralde *et al.* (1996) demonstrated that RBBB pattern is usually masked by pre-excitation. After ablation and pathway removal, a clear pattern of RBBB may be seen.

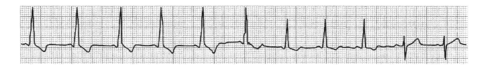

Figure 12.12 "Concertina" effect. The five first complexes are identical and show short PR and pre-excitation. In the next four complexes, pre-excitation decreases with a shorter PR = 0.12 sec. The three last complexes do not show any pre-excitation and the PR = 0.16 sec.

Holt.

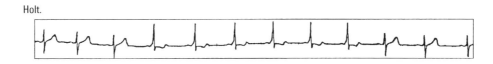

Figure 12.13 Conduction occurs via both the normal and the accessory pathway. When the stimulus is conducted over the accessory pathway, the PR interval is shorter than when the stimulus is conducted over the normal pathway (0.15 sec).

Spontaneous or induced changes of the abnormal morphology

Pre-excitation may be intermittent (Figures 12.10, 12.11, and 12.13). Sometimes the degree of pre-excitation changes progressively ("concertina" effect) (Figure 12.12).

Pre-excitation may increase if stimulus conduction through the AV node is depressed (vagal maneuvers, some drugs such as digitalis, beta blockers, calcium antagonists, adenosine, etc.) and vice versa (full "pre-excitation is obtained when the stimulus travels predominantly through the accessory pathway"). It may decrease when the AV node conduction is facilitated (i.e. through exercise etc.) (Figure 12.13). Historically, intermittent pre-excitation was associated with "benign" pathways, but this concept is currently under revision (Jastrzębski *et al.* 2017).

We have already commented on how the presence of sudden changes in the QRS complex morphology with the delta wave remaining present, or changes from the typical WPW pattern to short PR interval alone, suggests that two pathways of pre-excitation could coexist (Figure 12.10).

Arrhythmias and WPW–type pre-excitation: Wolff–Parkinson–White syndrome (Figure 12.9)

Patients with WPW pre-excitation can present paroxysmal reentrant tachycardia using an AP (AVRT) (slow–fast type), accounting for 50% of all supraventricular paroxysmal tachycardias (see Figures 15.11–15.13). In this case, during tachycardia, ventricular depolarization usually occurs through the normal pathway (AV node–His), and the AP serves as the retrograde limb of the macro-reentrant circuit. For this reason, the QRS complex does not show pre-excitation at this time (orthodromic tachycardia).

In fewer than 10% of cases of paroxysmal tachycardia, antegrade ventricular depolarization takes place over the

AP, depicting a very wide QRS complex (antidromic tachycardia) (see Figure 15.16). Antidromic tachycardia can also occur through two accessory WPW-type pathways, one with anterograde conduction and the other with retrograde conduction. When antidromic tachycardia is the result of an atypical pre-excitation (long atriofascicular pathway with decremental conduction) (type 2 pre-excitation in Table 12.1), the QRS complex morphology of the tachycardia presents some differences with respect to the QRS morphology in cases of typical AV (Kent bundle) antidromic tachycardia. The differences particularly concern the R/S transition in precordial leads, which is delayed beyond V3 in atypical pre-excitation (compare Figures 15.16 and 16.18).

The rare cases of incessant reentrant AV junctional tachycardias are explained by a circuit involving an accessory pathway with slow retrograde conduction (fast-slow type) (Farré *et al.* 1979; Critelli *et al.* 1984) (see Figure 15.15).

Patients with WPW-type pre-excitation can present with atrial fibrillation and flutter episodes more frequently than the general population (Figures 15.31 and 15.41). This happens because patients with WPW often present with a shorter atrial refractory period and higher atrial vulnerability (Hamada *et al.* 2002). All these properties favor the triggering of atrial fibrillation (AF). Occasionally, a fast retrograde conduction of a premature ventricular complex over the AP falls in the atrial vulnerable period (AVP), or a paroxysmal reentrant tachycardia triggers atrial fibrillation (Peinado *et al.* 2005).

In the presence of rapid atrial fibrillation, more stimuli are conducted to the ventricles through the AP than through the normal pathway. If one of them falls in the vulnerable ventricular period, it may trigger ventricular fibrillation (VF) and sudden death (Figure 12.9C) (Castellanos *et al.* 1983). This phenomenon accounts for some cases of sudden death, especially in young people, although this is fortunately rare. Figure 15.41 shows a patient with WPW syndrome and an atrial fibrillation (top) and atrial flutter (bottom) episodes. In both cases, the differential diagnosis with ventricular tachycardia (VT) is difficult, even more in cases of atrial flutter because the heart rate is regular (see Chapter 15, Atrial fibrillation: ECG findings). In cases of atrial fibrillation, the diagnosis is based on the irregularity of the rhythm and the presence of narrow QRS complexes, sometimes premature and sometimes late, whereas in VT the rhythm is regular and, if narrow QRS complexes are present, they are always premature (captures) (see Figure 16.15). However, in a 2:1 atrial flutter with pre-excitation, these key points for differential diagnosis do not exist. We have to take into consideration other clinical and ECG data (history taking, AV dissociation, etc.). Figure 12.9A,B shows a patient with both a paroxysmal tachycardia and an atrial fibrillation episode.

> - The WPW-type pre-excitation is characterized by specific ECG changes.
> - The WPW syndrome is a combination of the WPW ECG pattern (the result of the WPW-type pre-excitation) and different arrhythmias.

Clinical implications

The significance of WPW-type pre-excitation may be seen in two ways:
- If it is not correctly diagnosed, it may be mistaken for different and serious problems (myocardial infarction, bundle branch block and/or ventricular hypertrophy) (see before).
- Its relationship with supraventricular arrhythmias and SD. Approximately 10–20% of paroxysmal AV node reentrant tachycardias are caused by a circuit including an AP (AVRT) (see Chapter 15, Junctional reentrant (reciprocating) tachycardia; Figures 15.11–15.13). Paroxysmal tachycardia episodes in patients with WPW syndrome may lead to important hemodynamic alterations, although generally they have a good prognosis. They are, however, potentially dangerous because they may trigger fast atrial fibrillation which may lead exceptionally to SD (Figure 12.9C).

It should be remembered that antidromic tachycardia could involve the presence of two WPW-type APs, one with anterograde conduction and the other with retrograde conduction; however, more frequently the AV node serves as the retrograde limb of the reentrant macro-circuit.

Electrocardiographic criteria have been described to allow for the identification of patients at higher risk for SD during an atrial fibrillation episode or other supraventricular tachyarrhythmia episodes. They include the following (Klein *et al.* 1979; Torner-Montoya *et al.* 1991):
- a very short RR interval (≤220 ms) during spontaneous or induced atrial fibrillation;
- the presence of two or more types of supraventricular tachyarrhythmia;
- the presence of underlying heart disease;

- the presence of permanent pre-excitation during a Holter recording, exercise test, and after the administration of certain drugs;
- the presence of more than one AP. This could be seen in the presence of antidromic AVRT.

Nowadays, performing ablation of the AP with radiofrequency techniques is very successful (≈90%) and recommended, not only in cases of patients meeting high-risk criteria for developing malignant arrhythmias (see before), but also in any patient who experiences paroxysmal arrhythmias and in some cases of asymptomatic WPW (Santinelli *et al.* 2009) (Pappone *et al.* 2012).

Atypical pre-excitation

Concept and mechanism

This group includes those cases of pre-excitation not included in the classical Kent bundle group (AV APs), or the short type PR pre-excitation group.

It has been observed that long anomalous tracts, with slow anterograde decremental conduction only, exist from the right atrium to the right ventricle, known as atriofascicular and atrioventricular tracts, which constitute 80% of atypical tracts. Short bundles with slow decremental conduction (nodoventricular or fasciculoventricular Mahaim-type) formed by Mahaim fibers have also been described (Table 12.1) (Sternick and Wellens 2006).

ECG characteristics

In sinus rhythm, most atypical pre-excitation cases present with a normal ECG or an ECG with subtle evidence of minimal pre-excitation (absence of "q" wave in V6 and I and presence of rS morphology in III lead) that looks like LBBB.

During tachycardia, in general slow decremental right atriofascicular or rarely atrioventricular tracts participate in reentrant antidromic tachycardias. Anterograde conduction is usually over the abnormal tract, whereas retrograde conduction is through the right bundle, depolarizing the whole left ventricle through the septum. This accounts for the morphology of wide QRS complexes with LBBB and left axis deviation of ÂQRS. Characteristically, a late R/S precordial transition is observed (V5–V6) (see Figure 15.16). Meanwhile, in cases of antidromic WPW-type tachycardia (AV AP) (Kent bundle), the precordial R/S transition occurs earlier (V3) (see Figure 16.18).

If the long tract is atriofascicular, the QRS of the tachycardia is relatively narrow (<140 ms). In the rare cases when the long tract is atrioventricular, the QRS is wider because the tract inserts directly into the ventricular muscle and the LBBB pattern is less characteristic.

Clinical implications

Today, it is thought that even in the absence of definite anatomic correlations, the long right atriofascicular tracts with only anterograde conduction probably account for most antidromic tachycardias with LBBB morphology, which until recently were considered to be related to classical Mahaim fibers (Table 12.1, type 2).

It is currently believed that classical nodoventricular or fasciculoventricular fibers described by Mahaim, although they exist, are not involved in the tachycardia circuit, which, in most cases, comprises a long right AV pathway (Table 12.1, type 2).

The best treatment in these patients with paroxysmal tachycardia is ablation of the anomalous tract (Cappato *et al.* 1994).

Short PR interval pre-excitation (Lown *et al.* 1957) (Figures 12.14–12.16)

Concept and mechanism

The short PR interval is generally caused by the presence of a hyperconductive AV node, usually related to an anomaly in the AV node that allows rapid conduction to occur.

Occasionally, it may be caused by the presence of an anomalous atriohisian bundle that short circuits the slow conduction zone of the AV node. Unlike the WPW syndrome, characterized by an AP (Kent bundle) that is implanted in the ventricular working myocardium, in this case the anomalous bundle is implanted in the bundle of His (Figure 12.1). Lack of anatomical isolation of such tracts has led terminology to evolve into "enhanced AV node conduction."

The likelihood that reentrant paroxysmal arrhythmias are generated is lower than in WPW-type pre-excitation.

ECG characteristics

The only ECG manifestation is a short PR interval (Figure 12.15 and Table 12.1). Based on the surface ECG, it is impossible to confirm that the short PR is caused by a genuine pre-excitation from an atriohisian tract or an

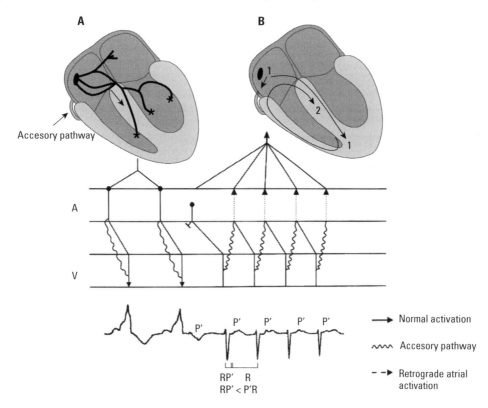

Figure 12.14 Scheme of a heart with a right accessory AV pathway, which leads to faster than normal AV conduction (short PR) and early activation of part of the ventricles and appearance of abnormal QRS morphology (delta wave) (A). All this may be observed in the first two PQRS complexes of the scheme. The QRS is a summation complex due to initial depolarization through the accessory AV pathway (curved tracing) and the rest of depolarization through the normal AV pathway (rectilinear tracing). The third P wave is premature (atrial ectopic P′) that finds the accessory AV pathway in the refractory period. Due to this, the impulse is only conducted by normal AV conduction (rectilinear tracing in AV node) usually with a longer than normal P′R interval, because the AV node is in a relative refractory period. This stimulus produces a normal QRS complex (1) and, due to the fact that the accessory AV pathway is already out of the refractory period, it enters from behind and is conducted retrogradely to the atria, generating an evident P′ after the QRS complex. In case of reciprocal intranodal tachycardia AVNRT, the P′ is within the QRS complex or can be seen in its final part, modifying the QRS morphology. At the same time, the impulse reenters and is conducted down to the ventricles via normal AV conduction (B-2). Due to this macro-reentry circuit, the reciprocating tachycardia is maintained. The conduction in this circuit is retrograde via accessory AV pathway (curved tracing) and anterograde via the normal AV conduction (rectilinear tracing). The RP′ interval is smaller than the P′R interval, which is typical of the reciprocating tachycardia that involves an accessory AV pathway (WPW).

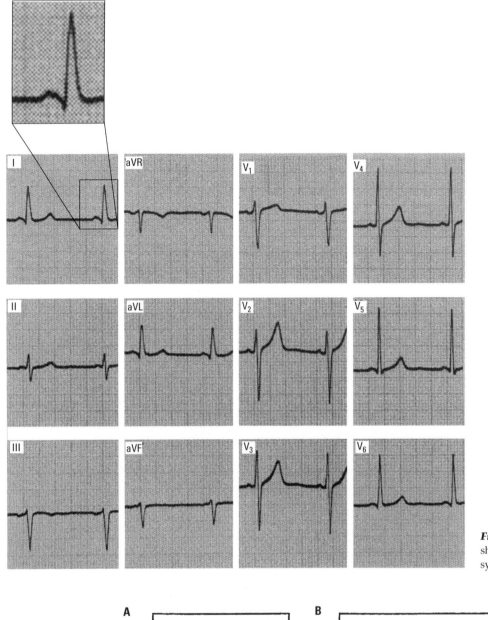

Figure 12.15 Example of typical short PR interval pre-excitation syndrome (0.10 sec).

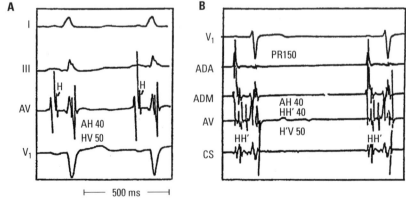

Figure 12.16 (A) A hisiogram showing a typical case of short PR syndrome. The PR shortening is caused by the AH interval shortening (40 ms). (B) In this case, the AH is also short but due to the presence of long HV (HH' + H'V = 90 ms) the PR interval is normal (150 ms) (concealed short PR syndrome).

accelerated conduction through the AV node, as is the case with some subjects (with or without heart disease) (sympathetic overdrive).

Intracavitary ECG shows a short atrio-His (AH) interval (see Figure 15.16) in the presence of accelerated AV conduction, whereas in the case of an atriohisian tract, it shows a short hisian–ventricular (HV) deflection, or no inscription of the H deflection.

If AH interval is short but the HV interval is long, the PR interval will be normal in the surface ECG (concealed short PR) (Figure 12.16B) (Ruiz-Granell *et al.* 2000).

When confronted with a short PR interval, we should rule out other causes that may initiate such a pattern. In exceptional cases, generally with important electrolytic disorders, it may be caused by a disturbance in the atrial muscle activation (sinoatrial block) in the presence of a normal sinus–AV node conduction through the atrial bundles. This is known as **sinoventricular conduction**, in which the QRS complex is recorded at time, although the P wave onset is delayed, resulting in a shorter PR interval that is not caused by an accelerated AV conduction but rather by the late inscription of the P wave (see Figure 7.2).

Clinical implications

Short PR-type pre-excitation is also associated with arrhythmias, mainly reentrant supraventricular arrhythmias, and occasionally with atrial fibrillation that, given AV conduction characteristics, may be very rapid.

In comparison with WPW-type pre-excitation, fewer cases of reentrant paroxysmal tachyarrhythmias are observed and the risk of sudden death is probably lower, although the occurrence of atrial fibrillation with rapid ventricular response is a potential risk.

The hyperconductive AV node may sometimes be controlled with beta blockers. Patients with an anomalous atriohisian bundle and atrial flutter or fibrillation with rapid ventricular response require urgent treatment with drugs or catheter ablation.

References

Arruda M, McCleland J, Wang, *et al.* Development and validation of an algorithm identifying accessory pathway ablation site in WPW syndrome. J Cardiovasc Electrophysiol 1998;9:2.

Basiouny T, De Chillou C, Fareh S, *et al.* Accuracy and limitations of published algorithms using the twelve-lead electrocardiogram to localize overt atrioventricular accessory pathways. J Cardiovasc Electrophys 1999;10:1340.

Bayés de Luna A, Baranchuk A. *Clinical Arrhythmology.* 2nd edn. Wiley-Blackwell, 2017.

Belhassen B, Fish R, Viskin S, *et al.* Adenosine-5′-triphosphate test for the noninvasive diagnosis of concealed accessory pathway. J Am Coll Cardiol 2000;36:803.

Bogun F, Kalusche D, Li YG, *et al.* Septal Q waves in surface electrocardiographic lead V6 exclude minimal ventricular preexcitation. Am J Cardiol 1999;84:101.

Cappato R, Schlüter M, Weiss C, *et al.* Catheter-induced mechanical conduction block of right-sided accessory fibers with Mahaim-type preexcitation to guide radiofrequency ablation. Circulation 1994;90:282.

Castellanos A, Bayés de Luna A, *et al.* Risk factors for ventricular fibrillation in preexcitation syndromes. Pract Cardiol 1983;9:167.

Chatterjee K, Harris AM, Davies JG, *et al.* T-wave changes after artificial pacing. Lancet 1969;1:759.

Chiang C, Chen S, Teo W, *et al.* An accurate stepwise ECG algorithm for localization of accessory pathway during sinus rhythm. Am J Cardiol 1995;76:40.

Cosio FG, Anderson RH, Kuck KH, *et al.* Living anatomy of the atrioventricular junctions. a guide to electrophysiologic mapping. Circulation 1999;100:31.

Critelli G, Gallagher JJ, Monda V, *et al.* Anatomic and electrophysiologic substrate of the permanent form of junctional reciprocating tachycardia. J Am Coll Cardiol 1984;4:601.

Denes P., Goldfinger P, Rosen K. Left bundle branch block and intermittent type a preexcitation. Chest 1975;68:356.

Eisenberger M, Davidson NC, Todd DM, *et al.* A new approach to confirming or excluding ventricular pre-excitation on a 12-lead ECG. Europace 2010;12:119.

Farré J, Ross D, Wiener I, *et al.* Reciprocal tachycardias using accessory pathways with long conduction times. Am J Cardiol 1979;44:1099.

Fiol-Sala M, Birnbaum Y, Nikus K, Bayés de Luna A. *Electrocardiography in Ischemic Heart Disease. Clinical and Imaging Correlations and Prognostic Implications.* 2nd edn. Willey-Blackwell, 2020.

Fisch Ch. Ventricular preexcitation in the presence of bundle branch block. Am Heart J 1958;55:504.

Gallagher J., Pricchett Sealy W, *et al.* The preexcitation syndrome. Prog Cardiovasc Dis 1978;20:285.

Hamada T, Hiraki T, Ikeda H, *et al.* Mechanisms for atrial fibrillation in patients with Wolff-Parkinson-White syndrome. J Cardiovasc Electrophysiol 2002;13:223.

Iturralde P, Araya-Gómez V, Colin L, *et al.* A new ECG algorithm for the localization of accessory pathways using only the polarity of the QRS complex. J Electrocardiol 1996;29:289.

Iturralde P, Nova S, Sálica G, *et al.* Clinical electrocardiographic characteristics of patients with Ebstein's anomaly before and after ablation of an accessory atrioventricular pathway. J Cardiovasc Electrophysiol 2006;17:1332.

Jastrzębski M, Kukla P, Pitak M, Rudziński A, Baranchuk A, Czarnecka D. Intermittent preexcitation indicates "a low-risk" accessory pathway: time for a paradigm shift? Ann Noninvasive Electrocardiol. 2017;22:12464

Klein GJ, Bashore T, Sellers T, *et al.* Ventricular fibrillation in the WPW syndrome. N Engl J Med 1979;301:1080.

Lindsay BD, Crossen KJ, Cain ME. Concordance of distinguishing electrocardiographic features during sinus rhythm with the location of accessory pathways in the Wolff-Parkinson-White syndrome. Am J Cardiol 1987;59:1093.

Lown B, Ganong W, Levine S. The syndrome of short PR interval, normal QRS and paroxysmal rapid heart rate. Circulation 1957;5:693.

Milstein S, Sharma AD, Guiraudon GM, Klein GJ. An algorithm for the ECG localization of accessory pathway in the WPW syndrome. Pacing Clin Electrophysiol 1987;10:555.

Nicolai P, Medvedowsky JL, Delaage M, *et al.* Wolff-Parkinson-White syndrome: T wave abnormalities during normal pathway conduction. J Electrocardiol 1981;14:295.

Pappone C, Santinelli V, Rosanio S, *et al.* Usefulness of invasive electrophysiologic testing to stratify the risk of arrhythmic events in asymptomatic patients with Wolff-Parkinson-White pattern: results from a large prospective long-term follow-up study. J Am Coll Cardiol 2003;41(2):239–244.

Peinado R, Merino JL, Gnoatto M, *et al.* Atrial fibrillation triggered by postinfarction ventricular premature beats in a patient with Wolff-Parkinson-White syndrome. Europace 2005;7:221.

Pick A, Fisch Ch. Ventricular preexcitation in the presence of bundle branch block. Am Heart J 1958;55:504.

Rosenbaum MB, Blanco HH, Elizari MV, *et al.* Electrotonic modulation of the T wave and cardiac memory. Am J Cardiol 1982;50:213.

Ruiz-Granell R, Garcia Civera R, Morel S, *et al. Electrofisiologia cardíaca clínica.* McGraw-Hill, 2000.

Santinelli V, Radinovic A, Manguso F, *et al.* The natural history of asymptomatic ventricular pre-excitation a long-term prospective follow-up study of 184 asymptomatic children. J Am Coll Cardiol 2009;53:275.

Sternick E, Wellens H. *Variants of Ventricular Preexcitation.* Blackwell-Futura, 2006.

Tonkin A, Wagner G, Gallagher J, *et al.* Initial forces of ventricular preexcitation in WPW syndrome. Circulation 1975;52:1030.

Torner-Montoya P, Brugada P, Bayés de Luna A, *et al.* Ventricular fibrillation in the WPW syndrome. Eur Heart J 1991;12:144.

Wellens H, Attie F, *et al.* The ECG in patients with multiple accessory pathways. J Am Coll Cardiol 1990;16:745.

Wolff L, Parkinson J, White PD. Bundle branch block with short PR interval in healthy young people prone to paroxysmal tachycardia. Am Heart J 1930;5:685.

Yuan S, *et al.* Comparative study of 8 sets of ECG criteria for localization of the accessory pathway in the WPW syndrome. J Electrocardiol 1992;25:203.

Chapter 13
Ischemia and Necrosis

Concept

Myocardial ischemia is defined as the sudden decrease or even stop of the flow of oxygenated blood that in normal conditions perfuse the myocardial tissue. The presence of myocardial ischemia initiates a cascade of events (Nesto and Kowaldruk 1987), as summarized in Figure 13.1, that ends with the appearance of symptoms—angina or the equivalent—and often evolves into myocardial infarction (MI). Recently, however, Kenigsberg *et al.* (2007) have demonstrated that delay of repolarization (QT lengthening and peaked and symmetric T wave) appears after a few seconds of coronary occlusion. This probably means that the electrical disturbances may be present at the same time or even before mechanical alterations. Frequently, arrhythmias appear and these may even lead to sudden death.

The ECG alterations appear as a consequence of the electrophysiological and pathological changes that transient or long-lasting ischemia induces in the myocardial cells.

Experimental mechanisms of ischemia

Here, we comment on the results obtained using different methodologies to occlude coronary arteries, and experiments induced by cooling (equivalent to ischemia) and warming different zones of the left ventricle wall. We consider that these experiments are very helpful in clarifying and understanding the mechanisms that explain ECG changes in human beings.

ECG changes after experimental occlusion of a coronary artery

In the 1940s, Bailey *et al.* (1944) conducted open chest experiments in dogs in which the left anterior descending (LAD) coronary artery was occluded, with the electrodes located in the pericardial sac. It was found (Figure 13.2A)

that the first ECG change recorded in the area with induced ischemia was a negativity of the T wave. This was called **an ECG pattern of ischemia.** If the ischemia persisted, it was followed by an ST elevation that was called **an ECG pattern of injury.** Finally, a Q wave of necrosis appeared, which Bayley called an **ECG pattern of necrosis** (see Figure 13.2A). This terminology was accepted by several groups (Sodi and Calder 1956; Chou *et al.* 1974) and used in clinical practice. Therefore, it was considered that in patients with ischemic heart disease (IHD), the presence of a negative T wave represented a grade of acute ischemia that was less severe and/or persistent than an ST segment elevation.

Later on, Lengyel *et al.* (1957) found that **when the experiment to occlude the artery was performed in awake dogs with a closed chest**, and the ECG was recorded with a 12-lead surface ECG, the changes in the ECG (Figure 13.2B) were similar to those that occurred in coronary spasm or transmural MI in humans. This means that the negative T wave only appeared as a late manifestation, when the acute ischemia was already vanishing or had already disappeared. In Chapter 20, we will comment that clinically negative T wave never appears during the acute phase of ischemia (pain). It may be seen during the evolving phase of STEMI if the artery opens, and in the evolution of Q-wave MI, as a deep negative T wave, or in some phases of NSTEMI as a mild negative T wave (less than 2 mm).

Various studies (Khuri *et al.* 1975; Franz 1983) have recorded unipolar ECG and transmembrane action potentials (APs) during regional ischemia produced by temporary coronary occlusion in open chest dogs, both in subepicardial and in subendocardial zone (with the deepest intramyocardial electrode), and also in the vicinity of the ischemic area. In all ischemic areas, the AP shows a progressive decrease of its rate of rise and its amplitude (low-quality AP). However, the TAP remains normal outside the cyanotic border (the ischemic area). The unipolar ECG taken in various ischemic areas records successively

Clinical Electrocardiography: A Textbook, Fifth Edition. Antoni Bayés de Luna, Miquel Fiol-Sala, Antoni Bayés-Genís, and Adrián Baranchuk.
© 2022 John Wiley & Sons Ltd. Published 2022 by John Wiley & Sons Ltd.

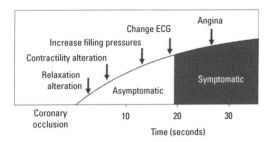

Figure 13.1 Ischemic cascade. The figure shows the sequence of events in asymptomatic period before angina starts (Modified from Nesto and Kowaldruk 1987) (see text).

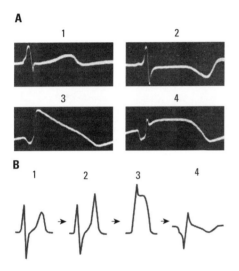

Figure 13.2 (A) Recordings in the case of experimental occlusion of left anterior descending (LAD) coronary artery in a dog with open heart. (1) Control. (2) ECG pattern of ischemia (negative T wave). (3) ECG pattern of injury (ST segment elevation). (4) Appearance of ECG pattern of necrosis (Q wave) (Based on Bailey *et al.* 1944). (B) Electrocardiographic–pathological correlations after the occlusion of a coronary artery in an experimental animal with its thorax closed. (1) Control. (2) It changes from a subendocardial ischemia pattern (tall and peaked T wave) to a pattern of an ST segment elevation when the acute clinical ischemia is more severe and transmural (3). Finally (4), the "q" wave of necrosis develops, accompanied as time passes by an increasingly evident pattern of negative T wave (see text) (Based on Lengyel *et al.* 1957).

the positivity of the T wave followed by ST elevation and the appearance of Q with a negative T wave, but the AP changes record the local electrophysiological changes more precisely, which demonstrates that they express the changes induced by ischemia better than unipolar ECG recordings (Franz 1983).

Experimental cooling and warming the epicardial zone

On the other hand, in experimental models or anesthetized dogs with the heart exposed through a sternetomy and with electrodes pulled over its surface, Burnes *et al.* (2001) induced a delay of repolarization of the AP of the epicardial zone submitted to cooling that overcame the duration of the AP of mid-endocardium. This explains that the T wave becomes negative (see Figure 13.3A-3). In this model, warming the same subepicardial zone produces a shortening of AP of this zone and a more positive and peaked T wave arises (Figure 13.3A-2). The same difference in the duration of AP of the subepicardium (shorter), and mid-subendocardium (longer), could theoretically also be obtained by cooling the subendocardial area. Thus, the longer AP of mid-subendocardium may explain the wider and peaked T wave observed at the onset of subendocardial ischemia. In the experiment, the evaluation of 12-lead ECGs during cooling and warming shows changes similar to those seen in epicardial electrograms (see Figure 13.3B and C).

Correlation with electrophysiological and ECG changes

We will now summarize the correlation of these different types of ischemia or similar damage with electrophysiological and surface ECG changes.

Changes in transmembrane action potential

According to the importance and duration of ischemia or similar damage (cooling the area or the effect of some toxins), experimental studies (Coksey *et al.* 1960; Horan *et al.* 1971; Burnes *et al.* 2001) have demonstrated that the APs of myocardial cells present changes in both repolarization and depolarization:
- **Changes of repolarization**: (Lengthening of AP that corresponds to lengthening of QT and primary T wave changes). The changes of shape of AP caused diastolic depolarization of the ischemic tissue that explains the changes of ST.
- **Changes of depolarization:** Lack of formation of AP that explains the presence of the Q wave in the surface ECG.

Changes in the surface ECG (Fiol-Sala *et al.* 2020; Nikus *et al.* 2010) (see later)

The classical ECG changes due to ischemia are the following:

Changes of repolarization
- **Primary T wave changes** include T wave wider, peaked, and/or taller in the first stage of acute ischemia. The appearance of T wave flat or negative is a consequence of ischemia (post-ischemic reperfusion changes) (see later).
- **Primary ST deviations** include ST segment deviations (up and down shifts) from baseline that represents acute ischemia with ST elevation (transmural involvement) or with ST depression (non-transmural involvement).

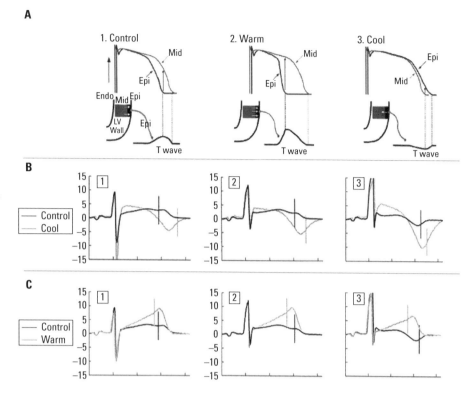

Figure 13.3 (A) Transmembrane action potential (AP): control (1) and after warming (2) and cooling (3) the epicardium. It is seen that after cooling (3), equivalent to ischemia, there is a delay of AP of subepicardium that explains the negativity of the T wave. After cooling the mid-endocardium area, there is probably a delay of AP of this area that explains the existence of a voltage gradient similar to what would exist in the presence of warming the epicardium (2), which explains the appearance of a taller and wider T wave with longer QT interval. B and C show the ECG changes in surface ECG after cooling (B) (negative T wave) and warming (C) (positive T wave) the epicardium (1, 2, and 3 surface ECG leads) (Reproduced with permission from Burnes *et al.* 2001.)

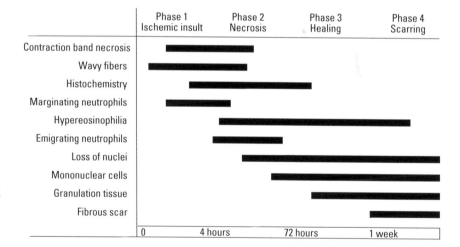

Figure 13.4 The different morphological features that appear after coronary occlusion (Reproduced with permission from Fallon 1996).

Changes of depolarization

These include the **Q wave of necrosis** and reciprocal patterns, and changes in the mid-late part of QRS (**fractionated QRS**).

Other changes

Other changes include lengthening of QT interval (this is, in fact, the first change according to Kenigsberg *et al.* (2007)), QT dispersion, changes of P wave, increase in duration and distortion of QRS, active and passive arrhythmias, and sudden death (see Chapter 20 and Fiol-Sala *et al.* 2020).

Correlation with pathologic changes

The occlusion of a coronary artery leading to MI represents a pathological process that **may be divided into four phases** (Fallon 1996): (i) ischemic insult, (ii) coagulation necrosis, (iii) healing, and (iv) scarring. Figure 13.4 shows the most important morphological features of each phase. **ECG changes appear very early and last throughout this process.** This includes ST/T changes and the appearance of Q of necrosis. Figure 13.5 shows the sequence of appearance of these ECG patterns. First the peaked, symmetric, and usually taller T wave and after the shifts of ST (ST/T changes) corresponds to

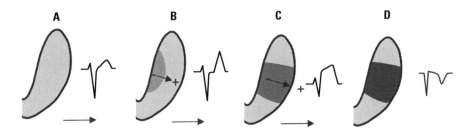

Figure 13.5 Observe how different degrees of ischemia that appear sequentially after total coronary occlusion in a heart without previous ischemia (A) explain the ECG morphologies. (B) Ischemia predominant in the subendocardial area (T wave symmetric and usually taller than normal with longer QT interval). (C) In the presence of more severe ischemia evolving to transmural injury, ST segment elevation is present. (D) If the ischemia persists, transmural necrosis expressed as Q wave of necrosis and a negative T wave appears.

the phase of ischemic insult, and the appearance of pathologic Q waves with negative T waves indicates the phase of necrosis. The evolution of Q wave–MI corresponds to phases 3 and 4 of Fallon's classification.

Correlation between ECG changes, the coronary artery involved, and the affected left ventricular walls

We will comment throughout this chapter and in Chapter 20 on the correlations between the ECG changes, the site of the occluded artery, the area at risk (ST/T changes), and the final necrotic area (Q wave or equivalent). We will always have in mind the importance of the direct and mirror patterns (see Figures 13.13 and 13.35–13.39).

All ECG changes induced by ischemia (T wave, ST segment, and Q wave) in the left ventricle are located **in the four walls of the left ventricle** that are in agreement with the statement of the Imaging Societies of the US (Cerqueira *et al.* 2002), and the statement of the International Society for Holter and Noninvasive Electrocardiology (ISHNE) (Bayés de Luna *et al.* 2006a; Fiol-Sala *et al.* 2020), are named: **anterior, septal, inferior, and lateral** (see Chapter 3). The old posterior wall coincides with the inferobasal segment of the inferior wall (Thygesen *et al.* 2019). Furthermore, this segment rarely bends upward to become a true posterior position. Usually it remains flat and is the posterior part of the inferior wall but not a true posterior wall (see Figures 4.1–4.6).

In this chapter, we will focus on the changes in T wave, ST segment, and QRS complex that are induced by experimental and clinical ischemia and their electrophysiologic mechanism in the presence of narrow and wide QRS complexes. Later, in Chapter 20, the ECG changes that appear during the evolution of different clinical settings of IHD, their diagnostic criteria, and the most important clinical and prognostic implications of QRS–ST–T ECG changes and other changes already mentioned will be discussed.

Changes of repolarization: T wave

Experimental electrophysiological mechanisms

The electrophysiologic explanation of the changes in the T wave caused by experimental ischemia or similar damage (cooling the area) that produces delay of repolarization in the affected zone (prolonged action potential -AP-), without change in the shape of it may be explained by two theories (Sodi and Calder 1956; Cabrera 1958; Coksey *et al.* 1960; Franz 1983; Burnes *et al.* 2001; Fiol-Sala *et al.* 2020).

The first theory is based on AP summation. The same reasoning has also been used to explain the appearance of a normal ECG (see Chapter 5). Figure 13.6 shows how the sum of the APs of the subendocardium and subepicardium, when the delay of repolarization due to ischemia is in the subendocardium or in the subepicardium, respectively, may explain the appearance of a taller or wider T wave (**ECG pattern named subendocardial ischemia**) (Figure 13.6B) or a flat or negative T wave (**ECG pattern named subepicardial ischemia**) (Figure 13.6C,D). Both cases are caused by delay of repolarization in the affected area and present with a lengthening of the QT interval.

The second theory is the theory of the ischemic vector. According to this theory, the area with delayed TAP (named the ischemic area), either in the subendocardium (Figure 13.7B) or in the subepicardium (Figure 13.7A), was not fully repolarized at the time when the other area was already repolarized. Therefore, it still presents with negative changes. As repolarization starts in the zone that is less ischemic, the sense of repolarization (〜〜►) will face the more ischemic zone. However, as this zone still has negative changes, **a flow of current having a vectorial expression is generated going from more ischemic to less ischemic area**. Therefore, the ischemic vector directed away from the ischemic area **produces a more positive T wave in experimental subendocardial ischemia and a flat or negative T wave in experimental subepicardial ischemia**. Note that the vector of necrosis is also directed

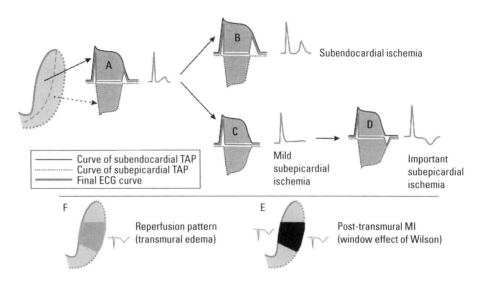

Figure 13.6 Explanation of how the sum of the transmembrane action potentials (APs) from the subepicardium and the subendocardium explain the ECG, both in the normal situation (A), in the case of experimental subendocardial ischemia (B) (tall and peaked T wave), and in mild (C) and severe (D) experimental subepicardial ischemia (flattened or negative T waves). This is the consequence of the repolarization delay in ischemic areas and the more prolonged AP. Clinically, ischemia is never exclusively subepicardial. Negative T wave related to ischemia may be seen in post Q-wave MI (E), and also when the surface ECG records the gradient of voltage between the transmural involved area probably due to edema (Based on Migliore *et al.* 2011) (longer AP) and the rest of the left ventricular wall (F) (see text, Figure 13.7, and Chapter 20).

away from the necrosis area (see Figure 13.62), but in contrast, the vector of ischemia is directed toward the injured area (Figure 13.24).

Changes of T wave in patients with ischemic heart disease (see Table 13.1 and Chapter 20)

The normal T wave (see Chapter 7) is asymmetric and is positive in all leads apart from aVR and often V1, and on occasion in III, aVF, and rarely II and even aVL in the case of vertical heart with rS or QS, and usually negative P wave. The normal negative T wave is of low voltage (except aVR) and asymmetric. Therefore, the appearance of a flattened or negative and symmetric T wave in other leads (V2–V6, I, II, and in general V2 and aVL) is **abnormal**, and also is a suspicious, positive, tall, and symmetric T wave, and its presence in V1 is also abnormal.

Table 13.1 shows the current ECG criteria for T changes due to ischemia. However, in our opinion, T inversion usually is a sign of reperfusion and therefore is not due to acute ischemia (post-ischemic change) (Birnbaum *et al.* 2020a, 2020b) (see later) and Chapter 20—ECG in NSTEMI).

Peaked, symmetrical, wider, and/or taller T wave (Figure 13.10)

Mechanism

As a consequence of occlusion, the first effect is subendocardial involvement in the left ventricle (Figure 13.5B). As a result of the delay of repolarization in this area

(prolonged AP without change of its shape) (Figure 13.6B and 13.7B), a peaked, wide, and usually tall T wave appears, accompanied by QT lengthening (**T wave of subendocardial ischemia**). It has been suggested that this tall T wave also reflects a release of K (Katz 2001). In fact, the subendocardium is more vulnerable to ischemic damage than the subepicardium. Different factors explain the susceptibility of the subendocardium to the development of ischemia. These include the characteristics of subendocardial coronary flow, the greater dependence of this region on diastolic perfusion, and the greater degree of shortening and therefore of energy expenditure of this area during systole (Bell and Fox 1974). Epicardial stenosis is associated with reduction in the subendocardial to subepicardial flow ratio. This first prolongs the AP of the zone (positive T wave) and if the reduction is greater, the AP changes its shape (ST depression) (Dunker *et al.* 1998; Figure 13.8).

Thus, in the subendocardium after epicardial coronary occlusion, the wave front of ischemia starts (Reimer *et al.* 1981). If more important subendocardial ischemia exists, the AP of the area will present not only longer duration but also smaller area. The sum of two AP of the subendocardium and the subepicardium (Figure 13.5C) explains the ECG pattern with mild/moderate ST depression and tall T wave that is seen sometimes in the acute phase of STEMI due to LAD subocclusion (De Winter *et al.* 2008) (Figure 20.7). Also, it has been demonstrated with CV magnetic resonance (CE-CMR) (Marholdt

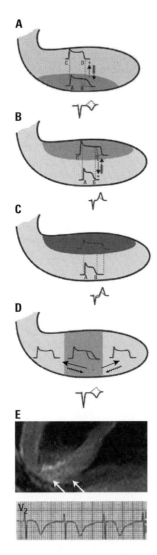

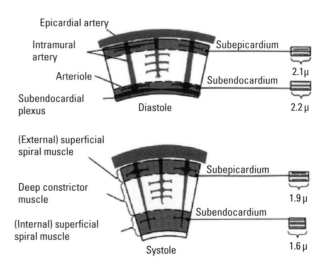

Table 13.1 ECG manifestations of acute myocardial ischaemia (in the absence of left ventricular hypertrophy and left bundle branch block).

ST elevation	New ST elevation at the J-point in two contiguous leads with the cut-point: ≥1 mm in all leads other than leads V2–V3 where the following cut-points apply: ≥2 mm in men ≥40 years; ≥2.5 mm in men <40 years, or ≥1.5 mm in women regardless of age[a]
ST depression and T-wave changes	New horizontal or downsloping ST depression ≥0.05 mV in two contiguous leads; and/or T inversion ≥0.1 mV in two contiguous leads with prominent R wave or R/S ratio >1

[a] When the magnitudes of J-point elevation in leads V2 and V3 are registered from a prior electrocardiogram, new J-point elevation ≥1 mm (as compared with the earlier electrocardiogram) should be considered an ischemic response.
From Thygesen *et al.* (2019).

Figure 13.8 Cross-section of the left ventricular wall in diastole and systole. Factors involved in the susceptibility of the subendocardium to the development of ischemia include the greater dependence of this region on diastolic perfusion and the greater degree of shortening—and therefore of energy expenditure—of this region during diastole (Reproduced with permission from Bell and Fox 1974).

Figure 13.7 (A) Subepicardial experimental ischemia. Subendocardial repolarization is complete, but the transmembrane action potential (AP) in the subepicardium still shows negative charges and is longer than normal (AP prolongation further beyond the dotted line) because the subepicardium is not completely repolarized yet. Thus, the vector of ischemia that is generated between the already polarized area in the subendocardium with positive charges and the subepicardial area still with an incomplete repolarization (with negative charges) due to the ischemia in that area, is directed from the subepicardium to the subendocardium, with the head of the vector coinciding with the positive charge of the dipole of repolarization. Therefore, the subendocardium is faced with the vector head (positive charge of the dipole), which explains why the T wave is negative in the subepicardium. (B) In subendocardial ischemia (experimental and clinical), a similar but inverse phenomenon occurs, which explains the development of peaked, longer, and positive T waves (see also Figure 13.6). If more important subendocardial ischemia exists, the AP of the area will present not only longer duration but also smaller area. The sum of two AP explains the ECG pattern with some ST depression and tall T wave (C) (see text). In D, the AP of involved transmural area due, at least sometimes, to edema (E transmural edema seen in CV magnetic resonance) is longer but with similar shape of the rest of LV. The recording electrode faces the tail of ischemic vector and records negativity (deep negative T wave sometimes seen in the evolving phase of STEMI) (D and E) (Migliore *et al.* 2011).

et al. 2005) that the first area where appears a wave front of necrosis starts in the subendocardium (Figure 13.9).

Morphology and duration

The positive T wave seen in the hyperacute phase of ischemia is symmetrical and peaked, and often presents with high voltage and is usually preceded by a clear ST segment, because the T wave arises in the second phase of repolarization (Figures 13.6 and 13.7). This is especially seen in case of LAD involvement (Figure 13.10C). The ST segment in V1–V2 to V4–V5 may be depressed (Figure 13.10E). However, often there is no ST depression, probably because it is already in the first stage of ongoing ST elevation (Figure 13.10B,D). It is not always easy to detect these changes of T wave (peaked T wave) because

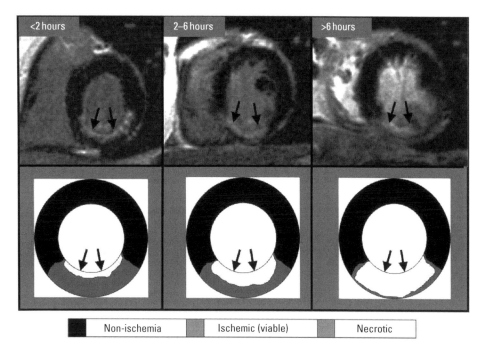

Figure 13.9 The typical pattern of ischemic heart disease can be explained by the pathophysiology of ischemia studied with contrast-enhanced cardiovascular magnetic resonance (CE-CMR). Little or no cellular necrosis is found until about 15 minutes after occlusion. After 15 minutes, a "wavefront" of necrosis begins subendocardially and grows toward the epicardium over the next few hours. During this period, the infarcted region within the ischemic zone increases continuously toward a transmural infarction (Reproduced with permission from Marholdt *et al.* 2005).

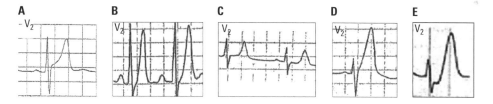

Figure 13.10 A normal variant tall T wave. B to E morphologies of taller than normal T wave in patients with ischemic heart disease. (A) Normal variant. (B) T wave very tall not preceded by rectified ST segment: this morphology is frequently observed as a transitory form to ST elevation. (C) A tall T wave, very symmetric and with rectified ST segment completely abnormal in V2 lead, which may be frequently observed in a hyperacute phase of STEMI before ST segment elevation (see Figure 20.4). (D) V2 lead: T wave with very wide base and straight ascendant slope of T wave that can be seen in a patient with an acute myocardial infarction. This pattern is transitional between the typical pattern of tall T wave of subendocardial ischemia to ST elevation. (E) Very tall and peaked T wave preceded by mild but evident ST depression. In spite of the presence of mild ST depression, this is a pattern of evolutive ST segment elevation acute coronary syndrome (STEMI) (see Figure 20.7) (Based on Wackers *et al.* 1978).

they are sometimes minor. The earliest change is that the T wave becomes symmetric.

Usually this tall and peaked T wave pattern is very transient (see Figure 20.4B-1). **However, sometimes** the peaked and symmetric T wave, with or without mild ST depression, **persists** for hours and remains unchanged until it evolves into Q-wave MI, often with clear ST elevation (Sagie *et al.* 1989, De Winter *et al.* 2008) (Figures 20.4B-2 and B-3). This was clearly seen in the cases described by Dressler and Roesler (1947) (see Figure 20.7). According to Birnbaum *et al.* (1993b), the cases of persistent tall T wave correspond to grade I of ischemia, although in the series reported by De Winter *et al.* (2008), there is at least a moderate increase of biomarkers. These cases have tight or

even total LAD occlusion, but without transmural involvement due to collaterals/preconditioning. The amount of necrosis at this time is probably at least moderate but we can presume that this pattern does not represent at this moment complete transmural involvement. However, if not treated, it will usually develop into transmural homogeneous involvement with ST elevation Q-wave MI (Dressler and Roesler 1947; Sagie *et al.* 1989) (Figures 20.6 and 20.7) (see Chapter 20).

As mentioned earlier, the results of studies on the experimental occlusion of coronary arteries in animals with closed chest (Lengyel *et al.* 1957) agree with the ECG changes that often appear in various clinical settings of transmural ischemia and that are a consequence of coronary occlusion, such as coronary spasm (see Figure 20.46), hyperacute phase of STE-ACS (Figure 20.4B) and PCI (see Figures 20.13 and 20.14), and also occasionally during exercise test (Table 25.6). In many cases, after a short period of peaked T wave with QT prolongation, if ischemia persists, an evident ST segment elevation appears and, later on, the ECG pattern evolves to Q-wave MI (Figure 13.32 and 20.4B1).

In addition, a tall, positive, and symmetrical T wave is frequently seen in V1–V3 in the chronic phase of lateral or inferolateral Q-wave MI. This is not an expression of the subendocardial ischemia, it is a mirror pattern of a negative T wave seen in opposed leads as a window effect of Wilson (Figures 3.6E and 13.13).

Flat or negative T wave
Mechanism
In clinical setting, the presence of flat/negative T wave is never present; except in myopericarditis, only a subepicardial involvement. Therefore, the theories that explain the presence of flat/negative T waves in experimental ischemia (see Figures 13.3–13.7) as a result of anoxia or similar damage in subepicardial area have a limited value in the clinical setting. The mechanism that explains the presence of T wave may be different according to the clinical situation: in post-Q-wave MI (see Figure 13.6E) or in the evolving course of an STEMI without Q-wave MI (Figure 13.6F and 13.7D,E), or in NSTEMI (see later).

According to the new universal definition of MI (Thygesen *et al.* 2019) (see Table 13.1 and later), the presence of T inversion ≥0.1 mV in two contiguous leads with prominent R or R/S ratio >1 is considered to be an ECG manifestation of clinical acute myocardial ischemia. It is true that during acute episode of chest discomfort, the pseudonormalization of previous inverted T wave may indicate acute ischemia (Figure 13.11), but the presence of a persistent negative T wave **is an expression of a post-ischemic change more than of acute ischemia**.

The following observations are in favor of the suggestion that a negative T wave does not appear during acute ischemia and that it corresponds to a post-ischemic change (Nikus *et al.* 2010; Fiol-Sala *et al.* 2020).

• The morphology of **deep negative T wave** appears in the **resolution process of Q-wave MI** (Figure 20.1). Sometimes the negative T wave is very deep but decreases or even may disappear with time (Figures 13.32 and 20.36). The appearance of a negative T wave in Q-wave MI is explained by the recording of intra LV ECG ("window effect") of Wilson (see Figure 13.6E and Q-wave of necrosis).

• **A negative T wave, which is also usually deep, appears** after fibrinolytic treatment or PCI **when the acute pain vanishes and is the manifestation of an open artery** (see Figure 20.11).

• **A negative T wave**, frequently very deep, **may appear in V1–V4** when the pain has already disappeared **in the evolution phase of STE-ACS due to LAD tight subocclusion** but without evolving to Q-wave MI (Figure 13.11). This situation in patients with ACS was considered a marker of impending MI (De Zwan *et al.* 1982). In fact, if

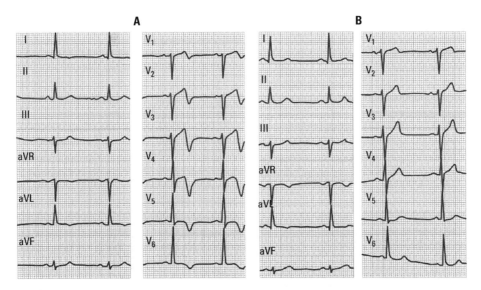

Figure 13.11 (A) ECG with a quite negative T wave in V1–V2 to V5, with extension to I and aVL in a patient with ACS, without chest pain, corresponding to a critical lesion in the proximal part of the left anterior descending (LAD) coronary artery that practically normalizes during a chest pain crisis (B). This corresponds to an atypical pattern of ST segment elevation acute coronary syndrome (STE-ACS) (see Figure 20.4C). The normalization of this pattern is an intermediate situation between the negative T wave and the ST segment elevation that would appear if the chest pain were more intense and prolonged. It is quite important to bear this in mind and to perform sequential ECGs, as the normal ECG during the angina crisis can provide quite confusing and dangerous information.

the patient is in the acute phase of an ACS, the artery may still reocclude and evolve to complete transmural involvement and Q-wave MI (see Figure 20.4C). Currently, with the new treatment of acute phase, this usually does not occur. **The presence of this negative T wave is the expression of an at least partially open artery**, or even if it is totally closed, there is no total transmural involvement because of the presence of very good collateral circulation and/or preconditioning. Therefore, it is necessary to perform PCI but not as an emergency. In these cases, the affected LV area is transmurally involved and its AP is longer than the rest of LV. Therefore, this transmural zone not yet polarized presents more negative changes and the ischemic vector leaves this zone and faces the rest of LV and the electrode located in the epicardial surface records negativity (Figure 13.7D). Recently, it has been shown by CMR (Migliore *et al.* 2011) that in some cases, transmural involvement is due to edema that disappears when the negative T wave normalizes (Figure 13.7E).

• **A negative/flat T wave may also be seen in the evolution phase of non-ST segment elevation ACS (NSTE-ACS)** (Figures 13.12 and 20.25) (see Chapter 20) (Cannon 2003). The morphology of the T wave is usually symmetric and not deep (<2 mm) and is usually seen in leads with R/S>1 but also in some cases with rS morphology (Figure 13.12). In fact, patients with NSTE-ACS and negative T waves have better prognosis, probably because this indicates that the clinical acute phase of ischemia is over. However, coronary subocclusion, even tight, may still exist (see Figure 13.12). Therefore, it is necessary to check the clinical data carefully and in the course of NSTE-ACS, non-emergency PCI is often also recommended in these cases. It is not well known the electrophysiological explanation of this type of negative/flat T wave. Probably, there is a difference in the length between the AP of the area with negative/flat T wave with transmural involvement (longer) and the AP of the rest of LV (shorter), and this may explain the ECG pattern.

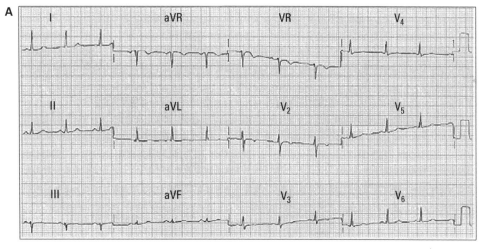

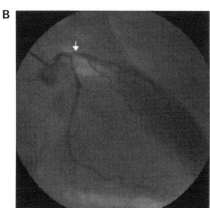

Figure 13.12 ECG of a 55-year-old man without chest pain and with non-ST segment elevation acute coronary syndrome (NSTE-ACS) (unstable angina) and ECG with symmetric and mild negative T wave from V1 to V3. The coronarography shows important left anterior descending (LAD) proximal subocclusion.

• **A flat/negative T wave may be seen for years as a residual pattern in chronic IHD** with or without Q-wave MI (Figure 13.13). Characteristically, this presents as a **mirror pattern in the frontal plane** (i.e. if negative in II, III, and aVF, is positive in I and aVL). It is important to perform differential diagnosis with the negative T wave of pericarditis, which usually does not present with a mirror pattern (see Figure 13.17).

• A positive T wave never becomes negative during angina crisis or positive exercise testing. The change is always ST depression, which, if it is very prominent, includes a T wave that is seen as negative or just with minor final positivity (see Figures 13.26, 20.16, and 20.17).

Morphology and duration

Negative T waves are abnormal if present in at least **two contiguous leads** (Thygesen *et al.* 2019) and may be located in different areas of the left ventricle according to the previously mentioned established correlations with different leads. In V1–V2, a peaked T wave may be seen as an expression of a mirror pattern of the lateral wall (see above).

The morphology of negative T wave is **symmetric** and shows a **mirror pattern** in the frontal plane leads (Figure 13.13). Usually a well-defined isoelectric ST segment is observed and sometimes only the second part of the T wave is negative (±) (Figure 13.11) because the T wave originates in the second phase of the repolarization. In general, the **depth of a negative T wave depends on the intensity of the previous ischemia** and on the extension of transmural homogeneous involvement. Therefore, it is much deeper (>4–5 mm in some leads) in the resolution of STE-ACS without Q-wave MI (Figure 13.11) or after evolved Q-wave MI, or even after fibrinolysis than in cases of NSTE-ACS (<1–2 mm or even flat T wave) (Figure 13.12).

However, **its duration is in relation to the reversibility of the left ventricular damage**. In the case of coronary spasm, the depth of the negative T wave that appears after the crisis is an expression of the severity of the ischemia (grade III ischemia), but it is very transient (non-irreversible damage) and disappears very soon (ischemia-reperfusion pattern) (Figure 20.45). In contrast, after Q-wave MI, the T wave may be more or less deep in different leads according to the intensity of the damage, but the duration may last forever (Figure 13.13). The disappearance of a negative T wave in these cases is a sign of good prognosis (Figure 13.32).

Nevertheless, do not forget that the sudden pseudonormalization of a negative T wave in the evolution of ACS is always abnormal and represents an intermediate transient situation to an evolving ST elevation (see Figures 13.11 and 20.4C).

Diagnosis of negative primary T wave due to ischemia or other causes in patients with left ventricular hypertrophy and/or wide QRS

The association of negative T wave due to **primary alteration** of repolarization (ischemia, drugs, electrolyte disturbances, etc.) **with secondary alterations** due to left ventricular enlargement (LVE) with strain, and/or left bundle branch block (LBBB), produces a **mixed pattern**. In these cases, the resultant negative T wave frequently appears more symmetric (Figure 13.14) (see Chapter 7, abnormalities of repolarization, and Chapter 10, LVH strain).

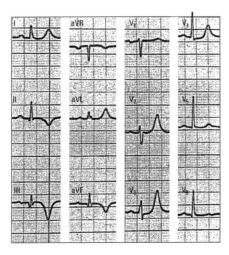

Figure 13.13 ECG with a typical pattern of chronic negative T wave in the leads facing the inferior wall (negative T wave in II, III, and aVF) and the lateral wall (positive peaked T wave in V1–V2). There is a necrosis in inferior wall with QR complex in II, III, and aVF. CE-CMR shows that the affected area of lateral wall was the basal zone. Due to that, there is no RS pattern in V1.

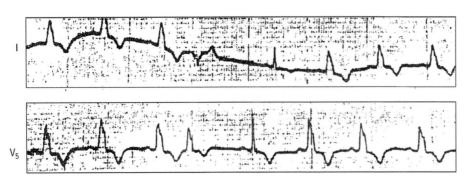

Figure 13.14 Symmetric negative T wave (see leads I and V5) in a patient with hypertension and intermittent complete left bundle branch block, who presents with symmetric T wave when the LBBB disappears after a ventricular extrasystole. This is a mixed pattern (ischemia + LVH). Also the T wave of complexes with LBBB shows more symmetric morphology than in cases of isolated LBBB.

Changes in T wave in clinical practice in patients with ischemic heart disease

Peaked, wider, and/or taller T waves
• These are usually the **initial changes** in the case of occlusion of a coronary artery and sometimes are accompanied by ST depression usually mild.

• In general, the ECG pattern is very **transient** and is explained because the ischemia first has an effect in the subendocardium, which produces a delay of repolarization (AP) in this area (long QT interval). The pattern is more persistent, meanwhile there is no total transmural involvement (collateral circulation or preconditioning).

• The appearance in the course of ACS of sudden pseudonormalization of a previously inverted T wave is clearly suggestive of acute ischemia (Figures 13.11 and 20.4C).

• These may also be seen in the chronic phase of IHD as a mirror pattern of negative T wave.

Flat or negative T waves
• **The depth of the negative** T wave is variable (less deep in NSTE-ACS), and the morphology is symmetric and with mirror pattern in the frontal plane.

• **Negative T waves do not represent acute active ischemia**, but rather are the expression of **post-ischemic changes.** In the presence of an isolated negative T wave without ST depression when it is present in patients with ACS, the pain has already vanished.

• Acute ischemia (ACS or exercise testing) never induces the appearance of negative T wave without ST depression.

• The deep negative T wave that appears in the chronic phase of Q-wave MI is an intraventricular LV pattern (Figure 13.6E).

• The ECG changes in STE-ACS are always from normal ECG to more positive T wave and ST elevation, and in NSTE-ACS, directly from normal T wave to ST depression, which sometimes includes the negativity of a previously positive T wave.

• Figures 13.6 and 13.7 explain the mechanism of changes T wave when a localized ischemia (or similar damage) is experimentally produced in the subepicardium or subendocardium. These figures also explain the ECG pattern of negative T wave when it is seen in a clinical setting when the ischemia has produced transmural irreversible (MI) or not (edema) damage (see text).

T wave changes in other heart diseases and situations
Differential diagnosis
Taller T wave
A long list of conditions, other than IHD, may present with changes in the T wave (symmetric, wide, and/or taller than normal) (Fiol-Sala *et al.* 2020). Table 13.2 summarizes the most important conditions, and Figure 13.15 illustrates some striking examples.

Flat or negative T wave
Table 13.3 lists the more frequent causes of flattened or negative T wave aside from IHD. Figure 13.16 shows some striking examples.

The most negative T waves usually appear in some cases of hypertrophic cardiomyopathy (HCM) (see Figure 21.2) and in some strokes or metabolic shock with long QT.

Chronic pericarditis is the most important condition for a clinical differential diagnosis because this disease also presents with pain in the acute phase and even may present mild increase of biomarkers. The negative T wave of chronic pericarditis (see Figure 13.17) is usually more extensive, does not present mirror pattern in the frontal plane, and is less intense (negative) than in cases of IHD, especially in post-Q-wave MI. However, especially when **associated myocarditis** exists, the pattern may be more striking than a case of IHD (Figure 13.18). In fact, some type of epicardial involvement often exists in pericarditis. In this case, the pattern of flat/negative T wave is a result of clear subepicardial involvement (Figures 13.6 and 13.7).

Table 13.2 Causes of taller-than-normal T wave (aside from ischemic heart disease; Figure 13.15).

1. **Normal variants**: Children, black ethnicity and hyperventilation, women (right precordial leads), etc. May sometimes be diffuse (global T-wave inversion of unknown origin). More frequently observed in women.
2. **Pericarditis**: In the convalescent phase of pericarditis, diffuse T-wave inversion can be seen, but T-wave negativity is generally mild.
3. *Cor pulmonale* **and pulmonary embolism**.
4. **Myocarditis (perimyocarditis)** (Figure 13.24) and **cardiomyopathies**
5. **Alcoholism**
6. **Stroke**: Not frequent.
7. **Myxoedema**
8. **Athletes**: With or without ST segment elevation. Hypertrophic cardiomyopathy, especially the apical type, must be ruled out.
9. **Drugs** (prenylamine and amiodarone) (flattened T wave).
10. **Hypokalemia**: The T wave can be flattened.
11. **Post-tachycardia**
12. **Abnormalities secondary** to left ventricular hypertrophy or to left bundle branch block.
13. **Intermittent left bundle branch block** and other situations of intermittent abnormal activation [pacemakers, Wolff–Parkinson–White syndrome].

It is also important to know that flat or mildly negative T waves may appear transiently after alcohol ingestion (see Figure 23.18) or even after the administration of some drugs (see Figure 23.13).

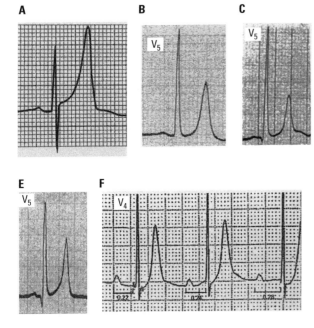

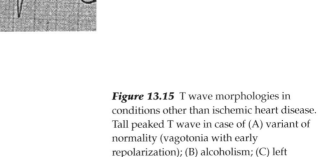

Figure 13.15 T wave morphologies in conditions other than ischemic heart disease. Tall peaked T wave in case of (A) variant of normality (vagotonia with early repolarization); (B) alcoholism; (C) left ventricular enlargement; (D) stroke; (E) hyperkalemia; (F) congenital atrioventricular block.

Table 13.3 Causes of negative or flattened T waves (aside from ischemic heart disease) (Figure 13.16).

1. Normal variants: Children, pertaining to Black race, hyperventilation, women (right precordial leads), etc. May sometimes be diffuse (global T wave inversion of unknown origin). More frequently observed in women
2. Pericarditis: in this condition, the pattern is usually extensive, but generally the negativity of T wave is not very important
3. Cor pulmonale and pulmonary embolism
4. Myocarditis (perimyocarditis) and cardiomyopathies: sometimes deep (Figure 13.18)
5. Alcoholism
6. Stroke: not frequent
7. Myxedema
8. Sportsmen: with or without ST segment elevation. Hypertrophic cardiomyopathy, especially apical type, must be ruled out
9. After the administration of certain drugs: prenylamine and amiodarone (flattened T wave)
10. Hypokalemia: the T wave can be flattened but usually the ST segment depression is more evident
11. Post-tachycardia
12. Abnormalities secondary to left ventricular hypertrophy or to left bundle branch block (asymmetric)
13. Intermittent left bundle branch block and other situations of intermittent abnormal activation (pacemakers, Wolff–Parkinson–White syndrome) (asymmetric)

Changes of repolarization: ST segment

Experimental electrophysiologic mechanisms

The area of the left ventricular myocardium subepicardium or subendocardium or the zone of tissue (wedge preparation of left ventricular muscle) or a single heart muscle cell close to or far from the recording electrodes **with significant and persistent ischemia (called the area of injury,** term that we believe not very lucky because it means transmural ischemia) present due to different grades of depolarization during systole and diastole, **two currents generated as a consequence of this important ischemia—one occurring during systole and the other during diastole** (Hellerstein and Katz 1948; Cabrera 1958; Janse 1982; Franz 1983; Coksey *et al.* 1960) (Figures 13.19 and 13.20) (for more information, consult Fiol-Sala *et al.* 2020). However, **the ischemic current generated during systole is the only one considered here** because ECG equipment is adjusted by alternating current (AC) amplifiers to maintain a stable isoelectric baseline during diastole, despite the existence of diastolic depolarization. Without this adjusted mechanism, the changes in the ECG generated by the transmural ischemia would be the sum of TQ plus ST deviations (depression or elevation) depending on whether the ECG faces the ischemic area or is in the opposite wall (Figure 13.20).

Currently, in the surface ECG, we only recognize the consequences of this systolic depolarization by the modification that, according to the membrane response curve (Singer and Ten Eick 1971) (Figure 13.21), is induced in the AP of the affected area, which is converted to a **"low-quality" AP (slower upstroke, lower voltage, smaller area, etc.) (systolic ischemic current).** This change in AP expression of the systolic ischemic current is responsible for the ST changes found in the surface ECG.

The ST segment changes (ST deviations) caused by this important and persistent experimentally induced ischemia that produces a "low-quality" TAP in the involved area varies depending on the location of the ischemia. **An ST segment depression is observed if the ischemia affects the subendocardium** or area far from the recording electrode, **whereas an ST segment**

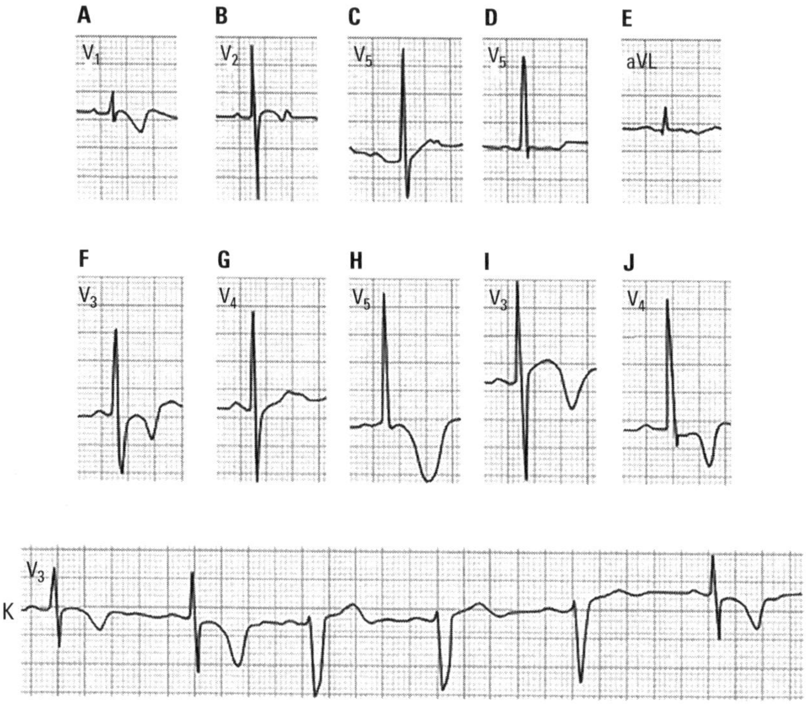

A　B　C　D　E

F　G　H　I　J

K

Figure 13.16 T wave morphologies in conditions other than ischemic heart disease. Some morphologies of flattened or negative T wave: (A,B) V1 and V2 of a healthy 1-year-old girl; (C,D) alcoholic cardiomyopathy; (E) myxedema; (F) negative T wave after paroxysmal tachycardia in a patient with initial phase of cardiomyopathy; (G) bimodal T with long QT frequently seen after long-term amiodarone administration; (H) negative T wave with very wide base, sometimes observed in stroke; (I) negative T wave preceded by ST elevation in an apparently healthy tennis player rules out HCM; (J) very negative T wave in a case of apical cardiomyopathy; and (K) negative T wave in a case of intermittent left bundle branch block in a patient with no apparent heart disease.

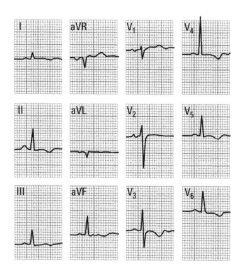

Figure 13.17 A patient with chronic constrictive pericarditis. The T wave is negative in many leads, but not quite deep, without the "mirror pattern" in the frontal plane. The T wave is only positive in aVR and V1 because, as this is a diffuse subepicardial ischemia, they are the only two leads in which the ischemic vector that is directed away from the ischemic area is approaching the exploring electrode.

elevation is recorded if the experimental transmural ischemia affects the subepicardium or area close to the exploring electrode.

Two theories have been suggested to provide an electrophysiologic explanation of these injury patterns found in areas with low-quality TAP due to experimental

subepicardial or subendocardial injury (Coksey *et al.* 1960; Samson and Scher 1960; Fiol-Sala *et al.* 2020):

- **The first theory is based on summation of the APs.** According to this theory (Figure 13.22), the sum of the APs of the subendocardium and the subepicardium with a AP with slower upstroke and smaller area in the ischemic zone may explain the presence of ST segment depression following subendocardial ischemia (zone with low-quality AP) (**ECG pattern named subendocardial injury or transmural subendocardial predominance ischemia**), or of ST segment elevation after transmural ischemia (zone with low-quality AP in the subepicardium) (**ECG pattern of subepicardial injury or transmural ischemia**). Figure 13.22D shows how this theory may explain the ST elevation in a clinical setting when transmural involvement, not only subepicardial involvement, exists.

- **The second theory is the theory of the ischemic vector** (Figure 13.23). According to this theory, when the zone with low-quality AP (ischemic zone) is on the subendocardium, at the end of depolarization (end of systole), this zone has fewer negative charges because the ischemic area undergoes earlier repolarization. Consequently, **a flow of current exists from the zone with more negative charges (subepicardium) to the low-quality AP zone with fewer negative charges (subendocardium). This produces an ischemic vector with lower negative charge (relatively positive) in the head, which points to the zone with low-quality AP, or the ischemic zone.** Therefore, the ischemic vector points toward the

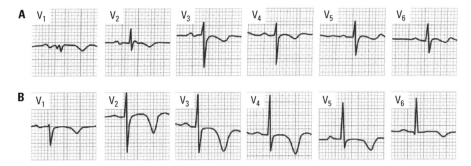

Figure 13.18 (A) ECG of a patient with chronic ischemic heart disease. (B) ECG of a patient with myopericarditis. The ECG does not aid in this case in establishing the differential diagnosis. Even, the patient with myopericarditis shows more negative and deeper T waves.

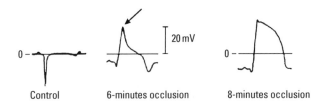

Figure 13.19 Local DC extracellular ECGs from the left ventricular subepicardium of an isolated pig heart before (control) and 6 and 8, minutes after coronary artery occlusion. Horizontal lines indicate zero potential. Note decrease in resting potential (TQ segment depression in extracellular complex) and reduction in action potential upstroke velocity with the appearance of ST segment elevation. After 8 minutes of occlusion, the ECG shows monophasic morphology. (There is a TQ depression and huge ST segment elevation.) After an hour, the ischemic zone becomes permanently unexcitable. Characteristically, some time before the ischemic cells become unresponsive, they showed electrical alternance of amplitude and duration of action potential (Adapted from Janse 1982).

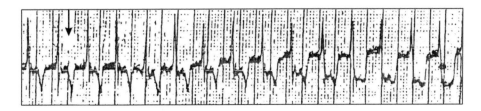

Figure 13.20 The electrode located in the epicardium of anterior cardiac wall records a simultaneous ST segment depression and T–QRS elevation after subepicardial ischemia of the lateral wall (arrow) is produced (Source: Adapted with permission from Hellerstein and Katz 1948).

subendocardium (ischemic zone) and is expressed as an ST segment depression in the surface leads (Figure 13.23A-1). Likewise, when the ischemic zone is on the subepicardium, this zone is also relatively less negative (relatively positive) than the normal zone, and the ischemic vector points toward this zone and is recorded as an ST segment elevation (Figure 13.23B-1). Figure 13.23B-2 shows the explanation of ST elevation in the clinical setting when transmural involvement and not just subepicardial involvement exists. The transmural LV ischemic wall is relatively less negative than the rest of nonischemic LV wall, and the ischemic vector faces the surface electrode and records an ST elevation (see later).

ST segment deviations in patients with ischemic heart disease (see Tables 13.1 and 20.2)

In Chapter 7, we commented on the limits of ST segment elevation and depression found in a normal population (see Figures 7.12–7.17). **In the clinical setting, the ECG manifestation of acute ischemia in the absence of left ventricle hypertrophy or left bundle branch block, in respect to ST segment (elevation or depression), according to the new universal definition of MI (Thygesen *et al.* 2019), is described in Table 13.1.** We will refer to this throughout this chapter and also in Chapter 20.

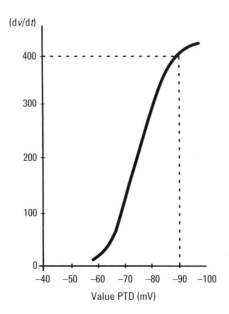

Figure 13.21 Note the relationship between the value of the transmembrane diastolic potential (TDP) in millivolts and the velocity of response (response dV/dt).

Table 20.2 summarizes the clinical, electrophysiological, coronarographic, and pathological findings that usually differentiate STE-ACS from NSTE-ACS (Sclarovsky 1999; Wellens *et al.* 2003; Fiol-Sala *et al.* 2020).

ST segment depression (Figures 13.22–13.30)
Mechanism

ST segment depression in clinical practice usually appears because the subendocardium is more vulnerable to ischemic damage than the rest of the ventricular wall, and thus, it may be affected without transmural involvement if the occlusion is subtotal although the ischemia usually extends beyond the limits of anatomic subendocardium (Figure 13.23A-2). When the subendocardial/subepicardial ratio is reduced to approximately 40%, the flow ratio decreases dramatically. This occurs during exercise and mental stress and also in other situations with increased left ventricular end-diastolic pressure (Nikus *et al.* 2010). In these cases, the AP of the subendocardium due to extensive and already usually existent ischemia shows a fundamental change in its shape (see above T wave: experimental electrophysiologic

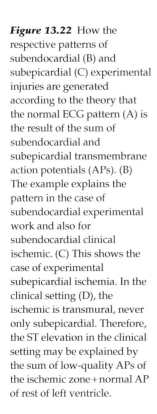

Figure 13.22 How the respective patterns of subendocardial (B) and subepicardial (C) experimental injuries are generated according to the theory that the normal ECG pattern (A) is the result of the sum of subendocardial and subepicardial transmembrane action potentials (APs). (B) The example explains the pattern in the case of subendocardial experimental work and also for subendocardial clinical ischemic. (C) This shows the case of experimental subepicardial ischemia. In the clinical setting (D), the ischemic is transmural, never only subepicardial. Therefore, the ST elevation in the clinical setting may be explained by the sum of low-quality APs of the ischemic zone + normal AP of rest of left ventricle.

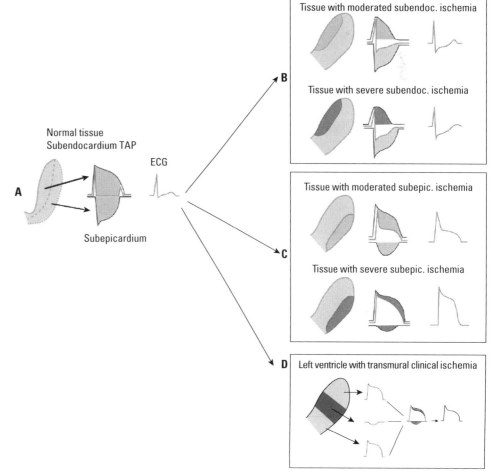

Experimental   Clinical

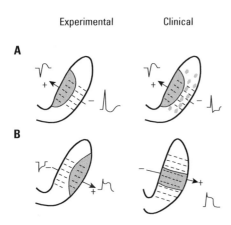

Figure 13.23 (A) In significant experimental subendocardial ischemia (1) (ischemic zone), the ischemic vector is directed from the non-injured zone (with more negative electric charges) toward the ischemic zone (with fewer electric negative charges, being relatively positive in comparison with the non-injured area). The ischemic vector faces the ischemic zone, while the ischemia and necrosis vectors are directed away from the involved area. Therefore, when significant experimental ischemia (injury) is located in the subendocardium (A-1), the vector is directed from the subepicardium to the subendocardium and generates ST segment depression in the ECG leads facing the subepicardium. **In clinical subendocardial ischemia,** this is predominantly but not exclusively subendocardial (A-2) and the ST depression may be explained by the same mechanism. (B) In the case of significant experimental subepicardial ischemia (ischemic zone (B-1), the ischemic vector is directed toward the subepicardium because, in this case, the current flow runs from the subendocardium to subepicardium because the subepicardium shows less negative changes, and is relatively positive. This generates ST segment elevation in the ECG leads facing the subepicardium. In clinical practice, exclusive subepicardial ischemia does not exist.

mechanism) and because of that an ST depression appears as a consequence of the summation of the AP of subepicardium and subendocardium (Figure 13.22B) and in the leads facing the tail of the ischemic vector (Figure 13.23A-2). When the number of involved leads is important, there are some leads with a mirror pattern (see Figures 13.28 and 13.29) (see Chapter 20).

The ST depression appears in relation to the following mechanisms:

• **ST depression in V1 to V3–V4 as a mirror pattern of transmural ischemia in lateral wall** due to total occlusion of the left circumflex artery (LCX) with transmural homogeneous involvement. **This is true STE-ACS (STE-ACS equivalent).** This pattern is the most striking ECG finding in some of these cases of total occlusion of LCX, with sometimes ≥3–4 mm of ST depression, and in the acute phase without or with only mild positive final T wave and often only mild or even non-existent ST elevation in inferior or lateral leads (Figure 20.5). After some time, final positive T wave appears as the expression of evolving STE-ACS (mirror pattern of negative T wave in back

leads). This is important because in cases of ST depression due to LAD subocclusion (NSTE-ACS) in the acute phase (when it is necessary to take the decision to activate the cath-lab), there is usually already a final tall T wave (see Chapter 20).

The ischemia that first is subendocardial, soon becomes transmural. In this case, the surface ECG records the pattern as ST elevation (B-2) because all the left ventricular transmurally ischemic walls are relatively less negative than the other zones of LV farthest from the electrode (see text).

• **Pattern of NSTE-ACS. In general, the ST depression corresponds to a pattern of NSTE-ACS. This occurs in** patients usually with pre-existent IHD who present with **non-total occlusion of the artery**. Often an ulcerated and a ruptured plaque is present, often with angiographic evidence of thrombus that increases the occlusion but without total occlusion of the artery, and with no transmural involvement. In these cases, there is important impairment of subendocardial flow as a consequence of sudden but not total decrease of flow. Some cases with NSTE-ACS and ST depression in V1–V4 **may present with total occlusion of LAD** (around 1% of all patients with ACS enrolled in the Triton 38 TIMI trial) (Pride *et al.* 2010) (Figure 20.22 group A) but due to collaterals/preconditioning probably **do not have homogeneous transmural involvement** and therefore do not present with ST elevation. Thus, in spite of a totally occluded artery, ECG signs of NSTE-ACS are seen. In these cases of tight proximal LAD occlusion with ST depression usually presents final positive T wave (De Winter *et al.* 2008) and in spite that are cases of NSTEMI as usually evolves quickly to ST elevation and Q-wave MI it is probably necessary to activate the catheterization laboratory (see Chapter 20). An even smaller number of cases in the same trial present with ST depression in inferior leads with an occluded artery (see Figure 20.1).

• **Patients with IHD during exercise or stress (Figures 13.26 and 13.27) present with an increased demand of flow** that cannot be supplied because they already have a fixed stenosis with decreased subendocardial flow. In these cases, different types of ST segment depression may appear (Figure 13.26). As the stenosis is fixed, there is no total occlusion and no transmural ischemia, and therefore there is no ST elevation unless a coronary spasm exists (very rarely) (see Figure 20.50).

• The STE in ACS appears when complete transmural involvement exists with total/near-total coronary occlusion.

• However, in the presence of total coronary occlusion, if there is collateral circulation/preconditioning, there is no complete transmural involvement, and the ECG pattern is of NSTEMI (see Table 2, Chapter 20).

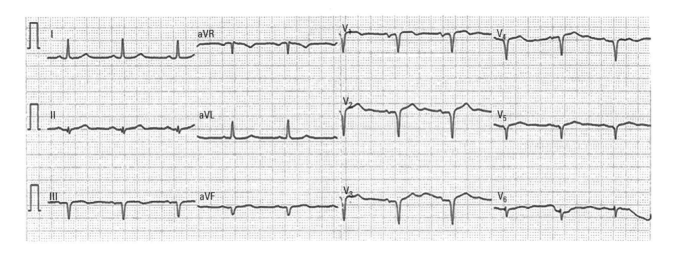

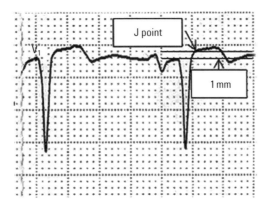

Figure 13.24 Observe how an amplified ECG (4×) of lead V1 allows the proper assessment of ST segment deviation. The patient had a previous anterior myocardial infarction, and there is mild ST segment elevation in the right precordial leads.

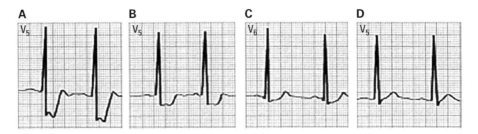

Figure 13.25 Evolution of non-Q-wave myocardial infarction with important ST segment depression at the beginning which normalizes in few weeks (A–D).

Morphology and duration

In the surface ECG, new ≥0.5 mm of ST depression horizontal or downsloping found in two consecutive leads measured at J point are sufficient to be considered pathological in patients with possible NSTE-ACS (chest pain) (Table 13.1). It is important to record an amplified (×4) ECG to better assess these small ST changes (Figure 13.24). The morphology is usually flat or downsloping, and not quickly upsloping (Figures 13.25–13.30).

The ST segment depression tends to normalize from the acute to subacute phase (Figure 13.25). If the ST depression is small, it is most probably a case of unstable angina. However, the distinction between unstable angina and non-Q-wave MI is shown by the biomarkers.

The number of leads with ST depression and the coronary artery involved in patients with NSTE-ACS

We comment these aspects more extensively in Chapter 20 (see Table 20.4). Patients with NSTE-ACS can be divided in two groups according to the number of leads with ST segment depression:

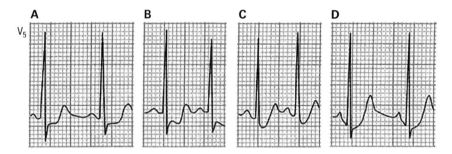

Figure 13.26 Various types of subendocardial ischemia patterns may appear in the course of an exercise test: (A) horizontal displacement of the ST segment, (B) descendant displacement of the ST segment, (C) concave displacement, and (D) ST segment depression from J point with ascendant morphology and rapid upslope. This usually is seen in normal cases. The coronary angiography was abnormal in A, B, and C, and normal in D. These changes are especially visible in leads with dominant R wave, especially V3–V4 to V5–V6, I, and aVL, and/or inferior leads present with dominant R wave.

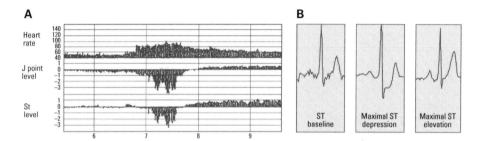

Figure 13.27 Changes of the ST segment in a patient with exercise angina. (A) The trend of ST segment changes and heart rate; (B) the different morphologies of ST.

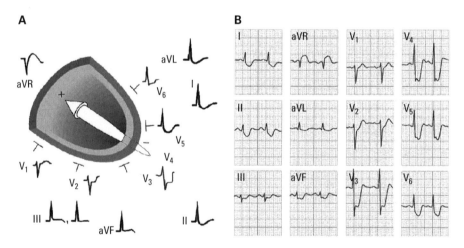

Figure 13.28 (A) In the case of diffuse subendocardial circumferential injury due to tight subocclusion of the left main trunk (LMT) in a heart with previous important subendocardial ischemia, the ischemic vector that points to the circumferential subendocardial area is directed from the apex toward the base, from forward to backward and from left to right. This explains the typical morphology of ST segment depression in all the leads except aVR and V1, with maximal ST segment depression in V3–V5. As the ischemic vector faces more aVR than V1, the ST segment elevation is aVR>V1. (B) Typical ECG of LMT critical subocclusion. The ST segment depression is higher than 6 mm in V3–V5 and there is no final positive T wave in V4–V5.

• ST depression in seven or more leads (extensive involvement) and

• ST depression in fewer than seven leads (regional involvement).

We comment on the ECG usually recorded during anginal pain. In around 50%, in the absence of pain, the ECG is normal/near normal.

ST depression in seven or more leads (extensive involvement)

The more striking ST depression is found in V3–V5, V6 with or without final positive T wave and usually with evident positive ST elevation in aVR as a mirror pattern (Figures 13.28 and 13.29, 20.17, 20.19, and 20.20) (see legends, and Chapter 20).

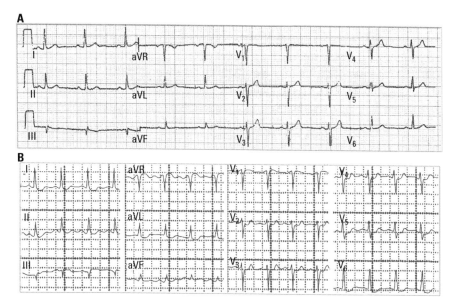

Figure 13.29 (A) Normal control ECG of a patient with chronic ischemic heart disease. (B) During non-ST segment elevation ACS (NSTE-ACS), diffuse and mild ST segment depression is seen in many leads, especially in I, V5, and V6 with small ST segment elevation seen in III, VR, and V1. The coronary angiography shows three-vessel disease with important proximal obstruction in the left anterior descending (LAD) and left circumflex artery (LCX).

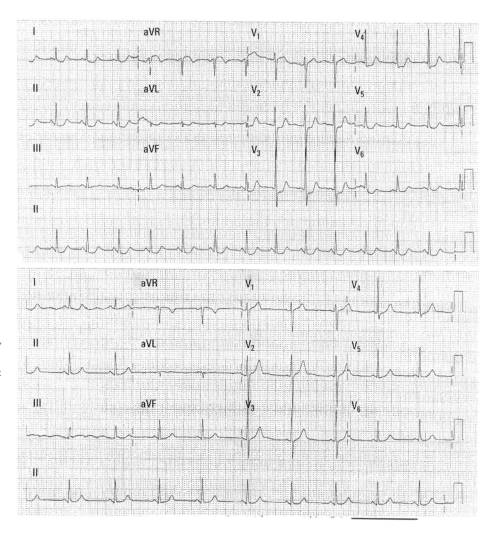

Figure 13.30 Top panel. This ECG was recorded during an episode of chest pain in a patient with single-vessel coronary artery disease. On angiography, there was a 95% stenosis of the midpart of the left circumflex artery (LCX). The ST segment is depressed in leads I, II, aVF, aVL, and V2–V6. These leads with ST depression show positive T waves. The ST segment is elevated in leads aVR and V1. Bottom panel. A second ECG recorded when the patient was pain free showed no significant ST changes.

This abnormal ECG pattern is recorded in patients with **left main coronary artery subocclusion or equivalent (2–3 proximal vessels disease)**, and also in cases of very **proximal subocclusion of long LAD**, even without important compromise of other arteries, or rarely in proximal subocclusion of dominant LCX.

To identify, with some limitation, the involved (culprit) artery, we have to look especially to aVR (check ST elevation) (remember that aVR = I + II/2) (Chapter 7), and **mid precordials leads** (Table 20.4 and Chapter 20).

• **aVR:** In severe LM/3VD, the ST elevation in aVR is usually >1 mm (ST elevation aVR > ST elevation V1) (Kosuge *et al.* 2011). In tight isolated proximal LAD subocclusion, the ST elevation is usually <1 mm.

• **In mid precordial leads,** the ST depression in cases of severe LM disease is usually important (>2–3 mm) without final positive T wave or only small final T wave (Figure 20.17). The ST segment depression in V2–V3 is not accompanied by ST elevation in inferior leads (except sometimes III), and should not be confounded with inferoplateral "mirror image" transmural ischemia due to LCX occlusion (usually maximal ST depression in V1–V4) (Figure 13.31)

In cases of severe 2/3 vessel disease, the ECG pattern may be similar but frequently either the ST depression is less deep or the final T wave is more positive (Figure 20.19).

In tight LAD subocclusion, the ECG pattern presents less ST depression and taller T wave. Furthermore, in aVR, the ST elevation is usually <1 mm (Figure 20.21).

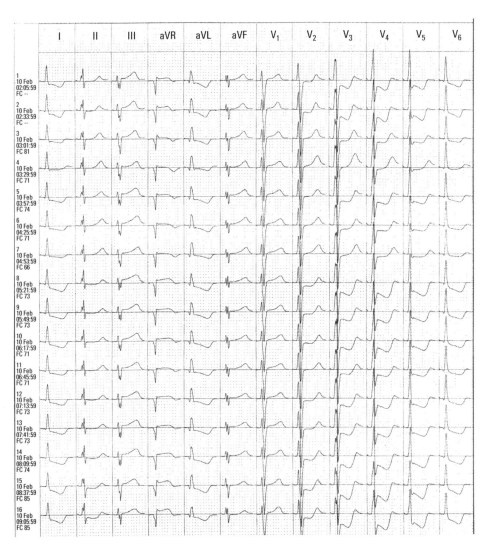

Figure 13.31 Patient with subocclusion of the LMT. The figure shows the sequence of progressive changes of the ST segment and the T wave obtained through monitoring with the MIDA system (Ortivus Medical AB, Sweden), pending coronary angiography. When the patient experienced anginal pain, an increase of the ST segment depressions was seen in I, aVL, and from V2 to V6 with a final negative T wave in V5–V6. There is also mild ST segment elevation in III during almost the entire sequence (somewhat less when the patient was pain free, row 4). At the time of maximal pain, the ST of aVR was higher than in V1. The first and second rows show a pattern of circumferential subendocardial ischemia. Rows 3–7 show some resolution with less ST segment depression and positivization of the terminal part of the T waves, but after that the situation worsened.

Finally, in rare cases, a tight proximal subocclusion of long LCX shows an ECG pattern usually with prominent R wave and ST depression is usually not very deep (Figure 20.21).

ST depression in fewer than seven leads (regional involvement) (Figure 13.30)

In Chapter 20, Table 20.4 lists the different groups of ECG pattern that may be found. Although it is, in general, difficult to identify which is the culprit artery, may be useful to remember the following:

• In the case of RCA or LCX, usually the number of leads involved is limited to some precordials, in general mid-left precordial leads, with a final positive T wave, and sometimes some leads of frontal plane (Figure 13.30).

• LAD subocclusion is not severe or the occlusion is distal and often affects V1–V4 if is proximal and V4–V6 if is distal.

• Two/three-vessel disease usually presents with ST depression in some frontal and horizontal plane leads, and often the basal ECG is normal with only small changes appearing during exercise testing.

• In general, cases with the worst prognosis present with ST depression in the left lateral leads without final T wave (Birnbaum and Atar 2006) (see Chapter 20).

It should be remembered that **ST depression in V1, V3–V4 may be an expression of true ST elevation myocardial infarction (STEMI equivalent) (mirror pattern) in the case of LCX total occlusion with transmural involvement** (see above) (see Figure 20.5).

ST segment elevation: evolving STEMI (Figures 13.32–13.52) (see Chapter 20)

Mechanism (Figures 13.22, 13.23, 13.32, and 13.33)

These patients present with transmural involvement but usually do not have a previous important ischemia. The surface electrodes record an ECG pattern of ST elevation (Figures 13.22D and 13.23B-2).

The mechanisms that explain the ECG pattern of subepicardial injury in clinical setting are based on the theory of summation of AP of transmural affected zone and the rest of the LV and, in theory, of injury vector which have been explained before (see Figures 13.22D and 13.23B-2).

To explain the presence of a tall T wave in the early phase (see above) (Figures 13.3, 13.6, 13.7, 13.10, and 20.4B), we have to consider that before the injured zone is transmural, the effect of ischemia is exclusively or predominantly subendocardial. This explains the presence of a tall, usually transient, T wave, which in a few number of cases (1–2% of ACS) is more or less persistent (Figures 20.7 and 20.9).

Because **the ischemic patterns develop at the end of the depolarization**, which corresponds to the end of QRS at the beginning of repolarization, the ECG expression of

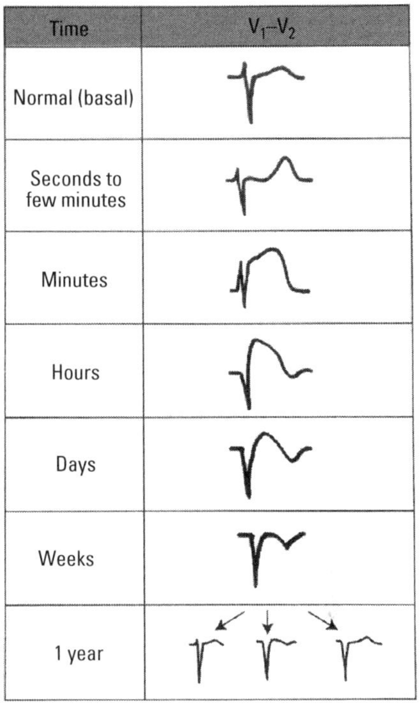

Time	V$_1$–V$_2$
Normal (basal)	
Seconds to few minutes	
Minutes	
Hours	
Days	
Weeks	
1 year	

Figure 13.32 A flow chart drawing of the ECG changes in case of Q-wave anterior myocardial infarction: records in V1–V2 from the very onset (rectified ST and positive T wave) until the different evolution patterns that may be present throughout a year in the case where no treatment has been administered.

injury starts during the first part of the ST segment. In contrast, the ischemia pattern appears in the second part of repolarization, after a clear ST segment. Therefore, in cases of relevant ischemia, the final part of QRS (S wave) is pulled up, which is followed by striking ST segment elevation (Figures 13.34 and 20.3C) (see later "Distortion of Q wave" and Chapter 20).

An ST segment elevation may also be recorded in other clinical settings of ischemia that are not related to atherothrombosis, such as isolated coronary spasm (see Figure 20.47) and Tako–Tsubo syndrome (Figure 20.44) (see Chapter 20).

Morphology and duration

The ST segment elevation that appears in the course of ACS with ST elevation will evolve to Q-wave MI if it is not aborted (see Chapter 20). Before the ST elevation, a tall and wide T wave usually exists for a short period. The ST segment elevation tends to normalize from the acute to the chronic phase (Q-wave MI) if the MI is not aborted with treatment (Figures 13.32–13.34 and 20.36) (see Chapter 20, Acute coronary syndrome with narrow QRS).

In these cases, it is very important to note the presence of mirror patterns (Figures 13.35–13.37). The leads that face the head of the vector of ischemia in transmural acute ischemia record an ST segment elevation, whereas the

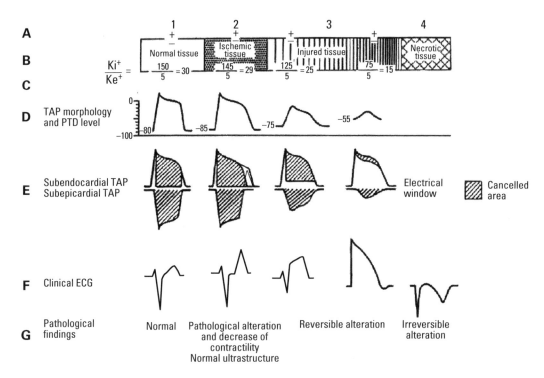

Figure 13.33 Different types of tissues (normal, ischemic, injured, and necrotic—from 1 to 4) (A) and (B). In each of them the corresponding electrical charges are shown—decreasing in steady fashion. Levels of Ki$^+$/Ke$^+$ (C), transmembrane action potential (AP) morphologies and the level of the transmembrane diastolic potential (DP) (D), the subendocardial and subepicardial AP (E), the corresponding patterns that are recorded in the ECG (F), considering that it is a transmural involvement and the pathological findings that are found (G). Note that necrotic tissue is non-excitable (does not generate an AP) due to the marked diastolic depolarization that it shows.

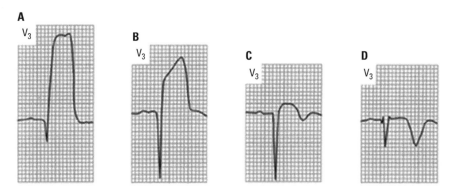

Figure 13.34 Acute infarction of anteroseptal zone with ST segment elevation in the pre-fibrinolytic era. Evolutionary phases: (A) at 30 minutes, (B) 1 day later, (C) 1 week later, and (D) 2 weeks later.

leads facing the tail of the ischemic vector record an ST segment depression. The global study of direct and mirror images of the ST deviations in different leads is crucial to correctly diagnose the location of the ischemia in the different walls of the heart (see later) and to understand the corresponding prognostic implications (Chapter 20).

Location of occlusion in STE-ACS

Different authors (Birnbaum *et al.* 1993a; Engelen *et al.* 1999; Chia *et al.* 2000) have described the value of ECG in localizing the occlusion site in STE-ACS. Figure 13.38 shows an algorithm that allows us to predict

the site of the LAD occlusion in the case of ACS with ST elevation in the precordial leads (Fiol *et al.* 2009) and Figure 13.39 shows an algorithm that we follow in the case of ACS with ST elevation in the inferior leads to distinguish between RCA or RCX occlusion (Fiol *et al.* 2004a, 2004b). Other algorithms, including one with "allcorners" with STEMI have also been published with good results (Tierala *et al.* 2009). The statistical power of these criteria in our experience (Fiol-Sala *et al.* 2020) and other studies (Birnbaum *et al.* 1993a; Engelen *et al.* 1999; Tierala *et al.* 2009) is very high (see Figures 13.38 and 13.39).

Figure 13.35 In an acute coronary syndrome with ST segment elevation in V1–V2 to V4–V6 as the most striking pattern, the occluded artery is the left anterior descending coronary artery (LAD). The correlation of the ST segment elevation in V1–V2 to V4–V5 with the ST morphology in II, III, and aVF allows us to know whether it is an occlusion proximal or distal to 1st diagonal. If it is proximal, the involved muscular mass in the anterior wall is large and the ischemic vector is directed not only forward but also upward, even though there can be a certain inferior wall compromise because of long left anterior descending (LAD). This explains the negativity recorded in II, III, and aVF. In contrast, when the involved myocardial mass in the anterior wall is smaller, because the occlusion is distal to 1st diagonal, if the LAD is long, as usually occurs, the ischemic vector in this U-shaped infarction (inferoanterior) is of course directed forward, but often somewhat downward instead of upward, and so it generally produces a slight ST segment elevation in II, III, and aVF (see Figure 13.38).

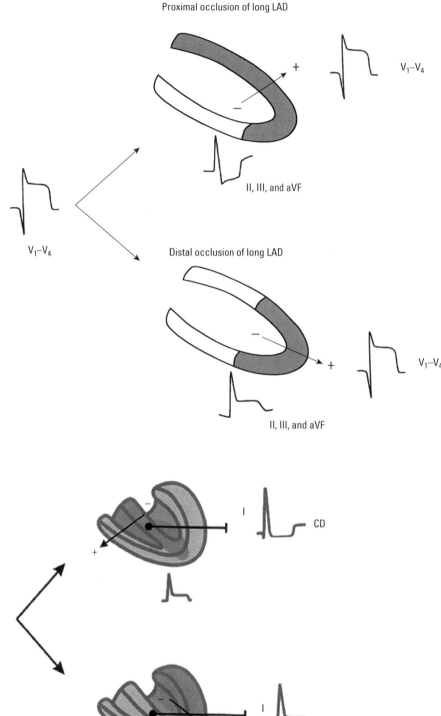

Figure 13.36 In an acute coronary syndrome with ST segment elevation in II, III, and aVF as the most striking abnormality, the study of the ST segment elevation and depression in different leads will allow us to determine whether the occluded artery is the right coronary artery (RCA) or the left circumflex artery (LCX) and even the site of the occlusion and its anatomical characteristics (dominance, etc.). This figure shows that the presence of ST segment depression in lead I means that this lead is facing the ischemic vector tail that is directed to the right and, therefore, the occlusion is located in the RCA. In contrast, when the occlusion is located in the LCX, lead I faces the ischemic vector head and, in this case, it is directed somewhat to the left and will be recorded as an ST segment elevation in lead I. To check the type of ST segment deviation in lead I is the first step of the algorithm for identification of the occluded artery (RCA or LCX) in the case of acute coronary syndrome with ST segment elevation predominantly in inferior leads (see Figure 13.39).

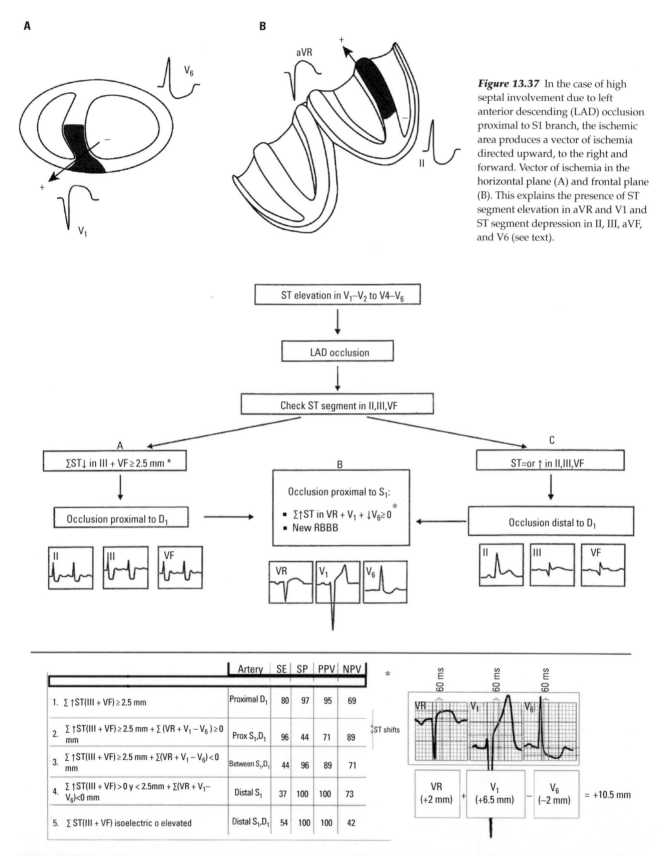

A

B

Figure 13.37 In the case of high septal involvement due to left anterior descending (LAD) occlusion proximal to S1 branch, the ischemic area produces a vector of ischemia directed upward, to the right and forward. Vector of ischemia in the horizontal plane (A) and frontal plane (B). This explains the presence of ST segment elevation in aVR and V1 and ST segment depression in II, III, aVF, and V6 (see text).

ST elevation in V_1–V_2 to $V4$–V_6

LAD occlusion

Check ST segment in II,III,VF

A

$\Sigma ST\downarrow$ in III + VF ≥ 2.5 mm *

Occlusion proximal to D_1

B

Occlusion proximal to S_1:
- $\Sigma\uparrow ST$ in VR + V_1 + $\downarrow V_6 \geq 0$ *
- New RBBB

C

ST= or ↑ in II,III,VF

Occlusion distal to D_1

	Artery	SE	SP	PPV	NPV
1. $\Sigma\uparrow ST(III + VF) \geq 2.5$ mm	Proximal D_1	80	97	95	69
2. $\Sigma\uparrow ST(III + VF) \geq 2.5$ mm + $\Sigma (VR + V_1 - V_6) \geq 0$ mm	Prox S_1,D_1	96	44	71	89
3. $\Sigma\uparrow ST(III + VF) \geq 2.5$ mm + $\Sigma(VR + V_1 - V_6) < 0$ mm	Between S_1,D_1	44	96	89	71
4. $\Sigma\uparrow ST(III + VF) > 0$ y < 2.5mm + $\Sigma(VR + V_1 - V_6) < 0$ mm	Distal S_1	37	100	100	73
5. $\Sigma ST(III + VF)$ isoelectric o elevated	Distal S_1,D_1	54	100	100	42

*

60 ms   60 ms   60 ms

VR V_1 V_6

$\frac{\text{VR}}{(+2 \text{ mm})}$ + $\frac{V_1}{(+6.5 \text{ mm})}$ − $\frac{V_6}{(-2 \text{ mm})}$ = +10.5 mm

Figure 13.38 Algorithm to precisely locate the left anterior descending (LAD) occlusion in the case of an evolving myocardial infarction with ST elevation in precordial leads. See inside the figure the sensitivity, specificity, and positive predictive value (PPV) of all these criteria (Based on Fiol *et al.* 2004b).

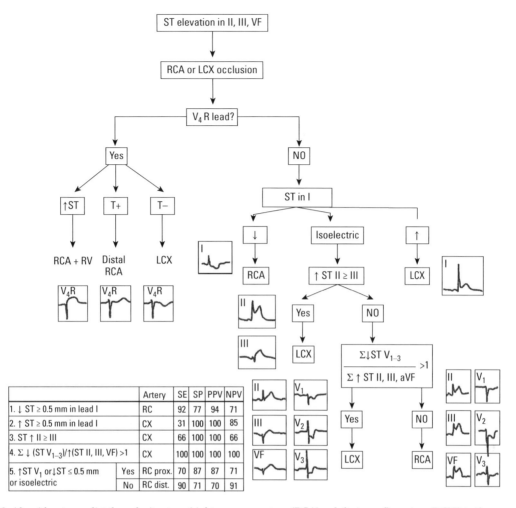

Figure 13.39 Algorithm to predict the culprit artery (right coronary artery (RCA) or left circumflex artery (LCX)) in the case of evolving myocardial infarction with ST elevation in inferior leads (see the text for details). See inside the figure the sensitivity, specificity, and positive predictive value (PPV) of all these criteria (Based on Fiol *et al.* 2004b).

In the case of **RCA occlusion,** there are increased chances of a **proximal occlusion and right ventricle involvement** if an ST elevation in the right precordial leads V3R–V4R is present (Wellens 1999). In our experience, we found that the presence of isoelectric or elevated ST in V1 is also useful (Fiol *et al.* 2004a, 2004b). Furthermore, in the case of occlusion of very long RCA occlusion (extra-large RCA), an ST elevation in V5–V6 is usually seen. ST elevation may even be seen in proximal occlusion of the RCA (ST elevation in V1–V3) due to proximal occlusion and in V4–V6 due to very long RCA (Eskola *et al.* 2004). In small number of these cases, the ST elevation may be seen in all the precordial leads (Garcia Niebla *et al.* 2009) (Figure 13.40).

Cases of complete occlusion of the left main trunk are very infrequent, and usually present as cardiogenic shock or cardiac arrest due to ventricular fibrillation. However, the survivors present an ECG with ST elevation similar to cases of proximal LAD occlusion but without ST elevation in V1 because this is balanced by the ST depression due to LCX involvement. The ECG often presents also RBBB and/or SA hemiblock (occlusion before first septal branch) (see Figure 20.3).

The correlation between the precordial leads with ST elevation and site of occlusion has some limitations (Huang *et al.* 2011, 2016). This may be for several reasons, such as differences in the location of the precordial leads, different terminologies used, cancellation of vectors, presence or not of small or large conal branch of the RCA, which, if large, may supply alternative blood to the high septum during occlusion of LAD (Ben-Gal *et al.* 1998), different lengths of coronary artery (Zhong-Qu *et al.* 2009), rapid changes from one to another ECG pattern in relation to the sudden change of the location and intensity of

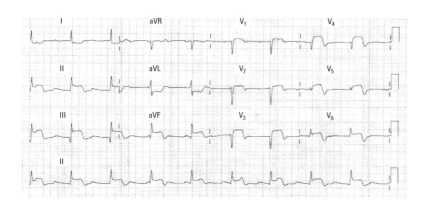

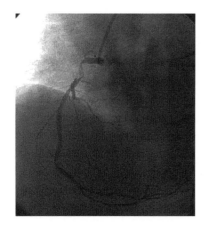
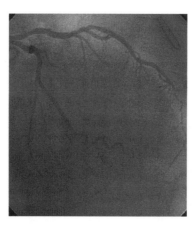

Figure 13.40 ECG and coronarography of a patient with ST elevation myocardial infarction (STEMI) due to proximal occlusion of dominant the right coronary artery (RCA). See ST depression in I and aVL (aVL > 1) and ST elevation in II, III, aVF (III > II), and all precordials (V1–V3–V4 for right ventricular infarction and V5–V6 for dominant RCA).

the occlusion (see Figure 20.9), that we comment with some extension in Chapter 20 (see ECG patterns in STEMI. Location of occlusion).

Nevertheless, taking all these factors into consideration, we believe that the correlation we have shown by just taking a glance the surface ECG has an extraordinary value to stratify risk and take the best decision in many cases of STE-ACS (see Chapter 20).

Figures 13.41–13.52 illustrate some examples of how the **changes of ST segment correlate with the area at risk, the coronary artery involved, and the site of occlusion in the presence of STE-ACS**, with the limitations just explained (see legends for explanation) and Figures 13.38 and 13.39. We do not show coronariography for limitation of space (for more details including coronariography of all these cases, consult Fiol-Sala *et al.* 2020).

Diagnosis of ST segment changes as a result of ischemia in patients with left ventricular enlargement and/or wide QRS

In cases of left ventricular hypertrophy (LVH) with strain pattern and/or wide QRS complex, **the ECG** diagnosis of transmural ischemia pattern is frequently more difficult, especially in the presence of an LBBB or pacemaker.

However, in the course of ACS, especially those secondary to the total proximal occlusion of an epicardial coronary artery, ST segment elevation are clearly seen **in**

ST changes (see Table 13.1)

• **ST depression is recorded in patients presenting with an abrupt decrease of blood flow without total occlusion and no transmural involvement, such as in NSTE-ACS, and in patients who present with ischemia due to increased demand, such as an exercise angina.** The ECG pattern is explained by important and predominant ischemia in the mid-subendocardium that induces an important change of the shape of the TAP in this area (ST depression).

• **ST elevation** is mainly recorded in patients with abrupt decreased blood flow that usually presents as total coronary occlusion, but especially with **global transmural involvement such as in STE-ACS**. The ECG pattern is explained in the presence of transmural clinical ischemia, because the transmurally affected zone presents less negative changes when is compared with the rest of LV and the surface electrode located at this zone, is less negative (relatively positive), faces the head of ischemic vector (+), and records ST elevation (Figure 13.23B-2).

• The same pattern may also be recorded in cases of **transient acute global transmural ischemia** with or without atherothrombosis (e.g. coronary spasm).

---

the presence of complete RBBB (Figure 13.53). Also, the presence of complete **LBBB or pacemaker** in the case of STE-ACS often allows us to visualize the ST segment

A

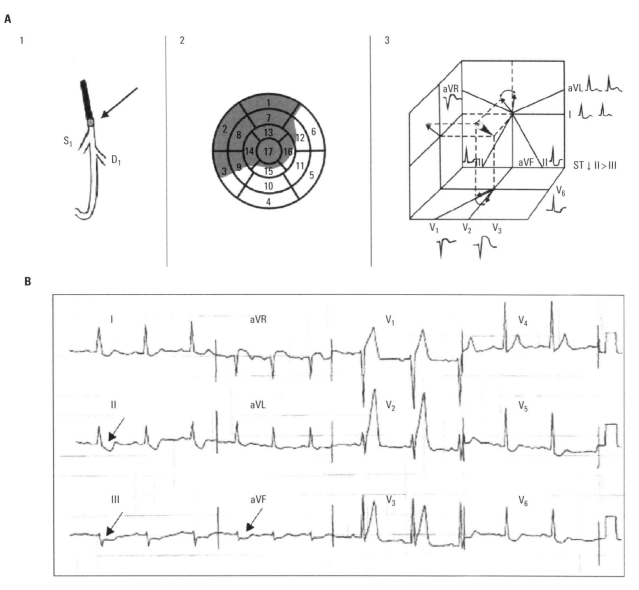

Figure 13.41 ST segment elevation acute coronary syndrome (STE-ACS) due to left anterior descending (LAD) occlusion proximal to D1 and S1. (A-1) Site of occlusion. (A-2) Myocardial area at risk with the involved segments marked in gray in "bull's-eye" projection. (A-3) Vector of injury and its projection in three planes: frontal, horizontal, and sagittal. The injury vector is directed somewhat to the right because the occlusion is proximal not only to D1 but also to S1. (B) The ECG in STE-ACS due to LAD occlusion proximal to D1 and S1 in a hyperacute phase. An evident ST segment elevation from V1 to V3 and aVR is recorded. Also ST segment depression in II, III, aVF (more evident in II) and in V5–V6 is present. This may be explained by LAD occlusion proximal to D1 but also to S1 that generates an injury vector directed upward to the right and forward.

elevation clearly (Figures 13.54–13.56). Sgarbossa *et al.* (1996a) have reported that in cases compatible with acute MI, a diagnosis of evolving infarction associated with a complete LBBB is supported by the following criteria (Figures 13.54 and 13.55): (i) ST elevation >1 mm concordant with the QRS complex; (ii) ST depression >1 mm concordant with the QRS complex; (iii) ST elevation >5 mm non-concordant with the QRS complex (e.g. in V1–V2). This last criterion is of less value when the QRS complex has an increased voltage (Madias *et al.* 2001). Concordant ST elevation has proved to be the single-most specific

criterion for the diagnosis of acute MI in the presence of LBBB, and improves the detection of this "STEMI equivalent" (Lopes *et al.* 2011).

These criteria have been studied by other authors, who have confirmed that they are highly specific (100%), especially in the presence of concordant ST segment elevation or depression, though they are not very sensitive (10–20%).

Recently, it has been reported (Wong *et al.* 2005, 2006a, 2006b) that patients with RBBB or LBBB and STEMI have different prognoses, depending on the ST segment morphology and QRS duration.

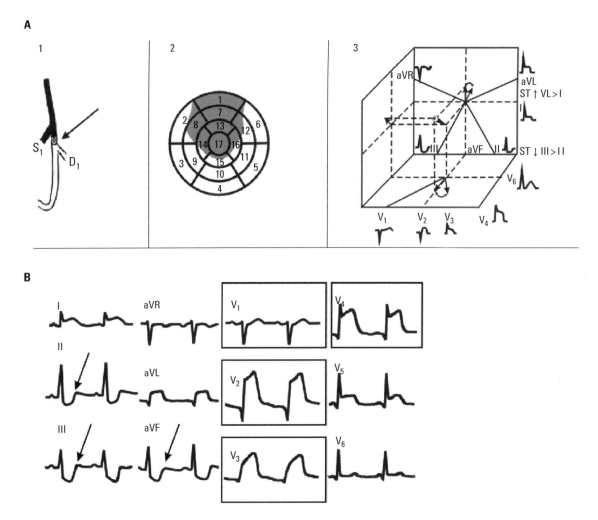

Figure 13.42 ST segment elevation acute coronary syndrome (STE-ACS) due to left anterior descending (LAD) occlusion proximal to D1 but distal to S1. (A-1) Site of occlusion. (A-2) Myocardial area at risk and "bull's-eye" polar map with involved segments. Very often, the apex is involved because the LAD is frequently long. (A-3) Ischemic vector in the acute phase is directed somewhat to the left, as the high part of septum is not involved. (B) The ECG showing ST elevation in V2 to V5, I, and aVL (not in V1 and aVR) with clear ST depression in inferior leads.

Similar criteria are also useful for the diagnosis of infarction in the presence of a pacemaker (Sgarbossa *et al.* 1996b) (Figure 13.56).

Occasionally, the presence of an intermittent RBBB (Figure 13.57) or LBBB allows the visualization of the underlying repolarization abnormality, such as ST segment deviation, or a negative T wave. Therefore, the evidence that there is a somewhat different repolarization pattern, with a generally more symmetric and deeper T wave, in the presence of a bundle branch block, is very much in favor of mixed origin of the ECG pattern.

In cases of LVH with strain pattern, often also some type of mixed patterns may be seen. The diagnosis, however, may usually be performed if sequential changes appear (increase in ST segment depression already present during pain) (Figure 13.58).

ST changes in other heart diseases and situations
Differential diagnosis

The list of conditions that, apart from IHD, may present with an ST segment elevation or depression is large. Table 13.4 summarizes the most frequent conditions that may present with ST elevation mimicking an STE-ACS, and Figure 13.59 shows some of the most characteristic examples. Note that there are some normal variants that present with ST segment elevation. In the first phase of pericarditis, a disease that also presents with chest pain, the most striking change is sometimes an elevation of the ST segment (see Figure 22.9).

Table 13.5 and Figure 13.60 show the same in the case of ST depression. Many conditions present with an ST segment depression, although it is usually small. Occasionally, a very evident ST depression is seen in cases with normal coronary circulation (Color Plate 3).

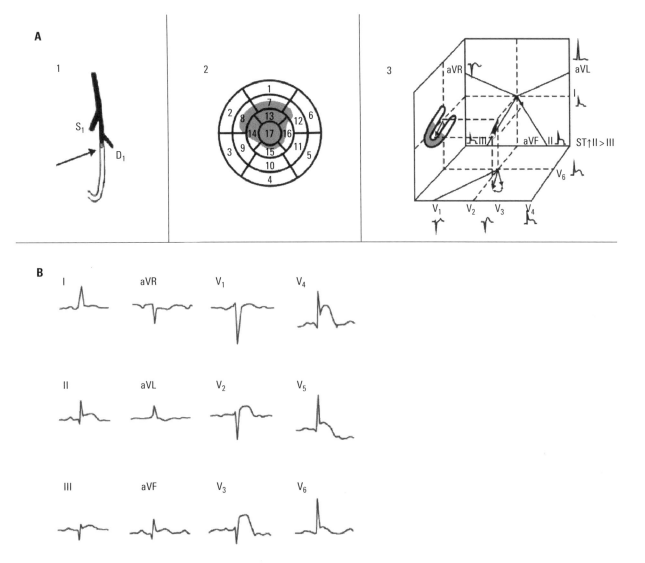

Figure 13.43 ST segment elevation acute coronary syndrome (STE-ACS) due to occlusion of long left anterior descending (LAD), distal to D1 and S1. (A-1) Site of occlusion. (A-2) Myocardial area at risk, and involved segments in "bull's-eye" projection. (A-3) Ischemic vector directed forward but somewhat downward and to the left, resulting in ST segment elevations in frontal and horizontal plane leads (V2–V6) and with ST segment elevation in II > III. (B) The ECG non-ST segment elevation ACS (NSTEMI) due to LAD occlusion distal to D1 and S1. Observe the ST segment elevation from V2 to V5–V6 with somewhat ST segment elevation in II, III, aVF (II > III) and ST depression in aVR.

The most important factor to take into account is the correlation of the clinical symptoms with the deviations of the ST segment (see Chapter 20).

Other changes of repolarization

Prolongation of QT interval

This may be considered a part of the changes of the repolarization. In fact, it is present in the first moments of acute transmural ischemia as in PCI (Kenigsberg *et al.* 2007), when due to an increase in the duration of AP

of the endocardium, the T wave is wider and taller and the QT interval is lengthened (see Figure 20.13).

Changes of U wave

Occasionally, ischemia may induce changes of U wave. The most frequent is the presence of negative T wave in precordials that are found in NSTEMI in some cases of LAD occlusion. These changes are usually found in the absence of pain (see Figure 20.15) but may also be an expression of active ischemia and may be seen in the evolving course of atypical patterns of STEMI or coronary spasm when the ECG evolves from deep negative T wave

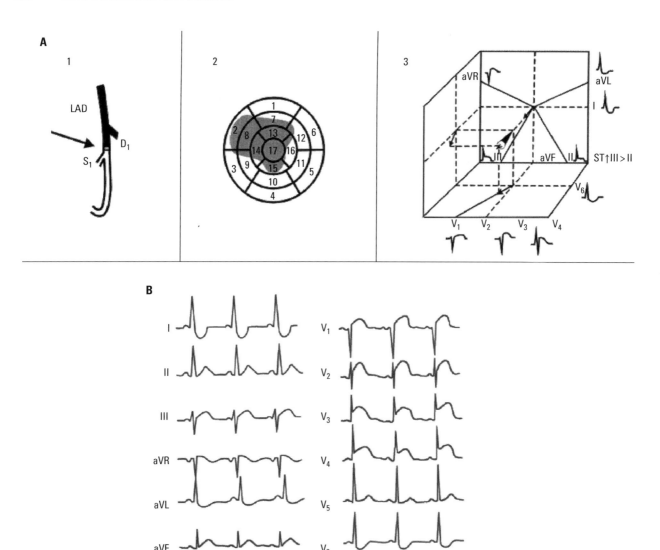

Figure 13.44 ST segment elevation acute coronary syndrome (STE-ACS) due to left anterior descending (LAD) occlusion proximal to S1 but distal to D1. (A-1) The site of occlusion. (A-2) Myocardial area at risk and "bull's-eye" polar map with involved segments. (A-3) Ischemic vector directed to the right and forward due to occlusion proximal to S1. In case of a long LAD involving also inferior wall, the vector can be directed somewhat downward due to relatively small myocardial area of anterior wall involved in case of occlusion distal to D1. The occlusion distal to D1 explains the ST segment elevation from V1 to V3–V4 and ST segment elevation in II, III, and aVF (III > II) and the occlusion proximal to S1—the ST segment elevation in aVR and ST segment depression in V6, I, and aVL due to ischemic vector directed somewhat to the right. (B) Typical example of ECG in ACS with LAD occlusion proximal to S1 and distal to D1. Observe ST segment elevation in II, III, and aVF (III > II) due to occlusion distal to D1 and ST segment elevation in aVR and V1 with ST segment depression in V6 due to occlusion proximal to S1.

to pseudonormalization of T wave and often to ST elevation (see Figure 20.26) (see Chapter 20).

Changes in QRS

We will comment first on the changes that ischemia produce in QRS in the chronic phase of Q-wave MI, in the case of a basal narrow QRS complex (**Q wave of necrosis and fractioned QRS**). Later, we will discuss how Q-wave MI may be diagnosed in the presence of intraventricular block, pacemaker, or pre-excitation.

Diagnosis of Q-wave MI in the presence of narrow QRS

Q wave of necrosis

Electrophysiologic mechanisms

The activation of the subendocardial area is very fast because the density of Purkinje fibers is so great that the electrodes located in this area do not record any positive deflection (1 and 2 in Figure 13.61A). Later on, the subsequent activation of the other part of the left ventricle wall records progressively greater R waves until a unique R wave is recorded from the epicardium (6 in Figure 13.61A).

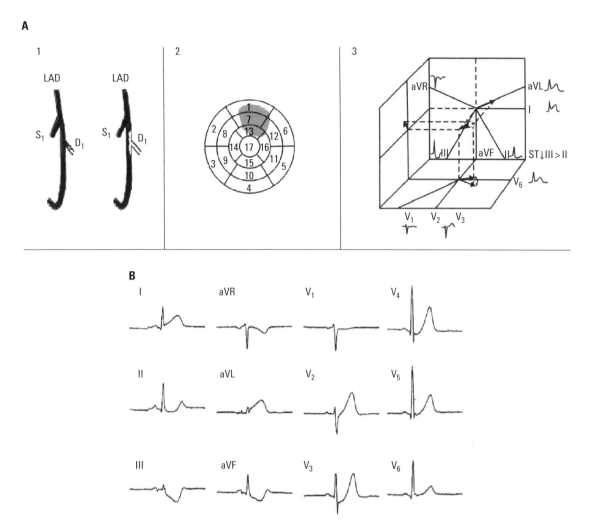

Figure 13.45 ST segment elevation acute coronary syndrome (STE-ACS) due to occlusion of D1 or incomplete occlusion of the left anterior descending (LAD) artery involving D1. (A-1) Site of occlusion. (A-2) Myocardial area at risk and "bull's-eye" polar map with involved segments. (A-3) Ischemic vector with its projection in frontal and horizontal planes and the corresponding ECG patterns. (B) ECG with clear ST segment elevation in I and aVL, and ST segment depression in II, III, and aVF. This strongly supports D1 occlusion. The presence of mild ST segment depression in V2–V3 (in contrast to what usually happens in D1 occlusion) may be due to an association of RCA or LCX occlusion, as in this case (70% distal RCA occlusion) (see text).

In the presence of MI, the diastolic depolarization in the infarcted area is so important that it cannot be excited and does not produce an AP. Therefore, a Q wave is generated opposite the R wave when the infarcted area surpasses the subendocardium and affects part of the myocardium that is responsible for generating the beginning of the QRS complex (R wave). This happens within the first 40–50 ms of QRS.

The generation of a Q wave of necrosis may be explained by two theories:

• **According to the theory of electrical window of Wilson,** the transmural infarcted area acts as an electrical window and, consequently, the electrode that faces the area records the negativity of the intracavitary QRS (Q wave of necrosis) (see Figure 13.61A).

• **According to the theory of the infarction vector (Figure 13.62B,C)** the infarcted area generates a vector (infarction vector) that has the same magnitude but opposite direction to the one that would have been generated in the same zone in the absence of infarction. Therefore, the infarction vector moves away from the infarcted area (see Figures 13.63 and 13.64). As we have stated, the ventricular depolarization changes that produce the Q wave occur when the infarction area is depolarized within the first 40 ms of ventricular activation.

Q versus non-Q wave myocardial infarction
It used to be considered that MIs located in subendocardial areas did not produce Q waves, as discussed in Figure 13.61, and that Q-wave MI occurs when some part of subepicardial area is affected. Today, thanks to

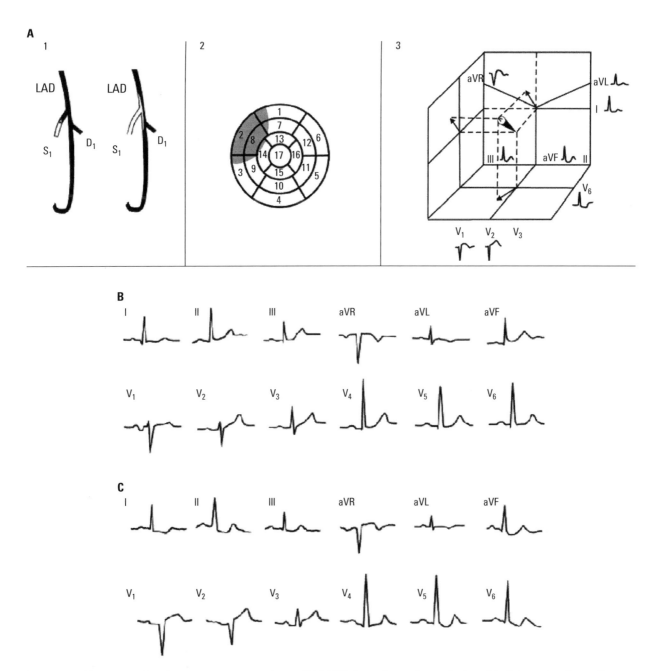

Figure 13.46 ST segment elevation acute coronary syndrome (STE-ACS) due to incomplete occlusion of the left anterior descending (LAD) artery involving the septal branches but not the diagonal branches. In exceptional cases, only S1 or S2 occlusion may be found. (A-1) Site of the occlusion. (A-2) Myocardial area at risk and involved segments in a "bull's-eye" projection. (A-3) Ischemic vector projected on frontal, horizontal, and sagittal planes and the corresponding ECG patterns. (B) Control ECG. (C) Typical ECG pattern in the case of occlusion of a large S1 artery during a percutaneous coronary intervention (PCI) procedure with involvement of the basal and probably also mid-septal part. Observe the ST segment depression in the inferior leads (II > III) and V6, and ST segment elevation in aVR and V1.

CE-CMR correlations it is known (Marholdt *et al.* 2005) that after epicardial coronary artery occlusion, the ischemic area begins in the subendocardium and grows toward the epicardium (Figure 13.9). Therefore, infarctions are never exclusively present in the mid/epicardial layer of the left ventricle. In a correlation study with CE-CMR, Moon *et al.* (2004) showed that infarctions with predominant subendocardium involvement exhibit a Q wave

of necrosis in approximately 30% of cases. Furthermore, they demonstrated that a similar number of transmural infarctions were found in non-Q wave infarctions. From the CE-CMR standpoint, 50% of the infarctions had been at some point transmural, but almost all of them had predominantly subendocardium extension in some zones. Therefore, Q waves are present in cases of only subendocardial necrosis, and are absent in some cases of

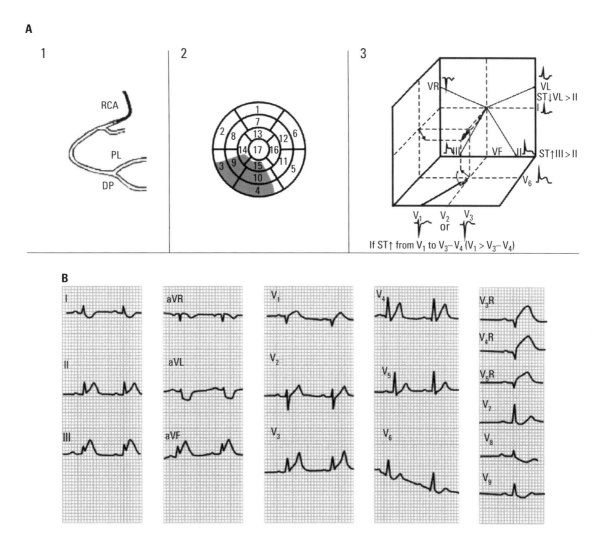

Figure 13.47 ST segment elevation acute coronary syndrome (STE-ACS) due to right coronary artery (RCA) occlusion proximal to right ventricle branches (arrow). (A-1) Site of occlusion and myocardial area at risk. (A-2) Polar map in "bull's-eye" projection with the most involved segments marked in gray. (A-3) Ischemic vector projected on frontal, horizontal, and sagittal planes with corresponding ECG patterns. Observe that the injury vector due to right ventricular involvement is directed more forward usually in the positive hemifield of V1 than in case of RCA occlusion distal to right ventricular branches. (B) Typical ECG in case of STE-ACS due to proximal RCA occlusion with right ventricular involvement. Observe ST segment elevation in II, III, and aVF with III > II, ST segment depression in I, and isoelectric or elevated in V1–V3 as well as in V3R–V4R leads with positive T wave.

transmural necrosis. However, although **Q waves of necrosis are not always present in transmural MI, they are expressions of larger MI. Therefore, differentiating between an MI with and without Q wave is important because the former involves a larger area, irrespective of whether it is or is not transmural.**

Though **the terms Q-wave MI and non-Q-wave MI are no longer accepted in the acute phase**, it is true that in the subacute and especially in the chronic phases of MI, there are infarctions with and without Q waves. **The higher the number of Q waves or their equivalent, the worse the prognosis.**

Characteristics of "necrosis Q wave" or equivalent

Table 13.6 shows the characteristics that are considered expressions of chronic MI in the presence of an adequate clinical setting. The evolution from ST elevation to Q-wave MI has been discussed before (see ST segment elevation: evolving STEMI). Figures 13.34 and 13.65, and more extensively in Chapter 20 (ACS with narrow QRS and ST elevation).

The appearance of the Q wave of necrosis in the evolutionary changes of STE-ACS shows that the patient has evolved to MI, involving an area that was thought surpasses the subendocardium (Figure 13.61). However, CE-CMR has demonstrated that this is not true (see above). Furthermore, a Q wave is not always an

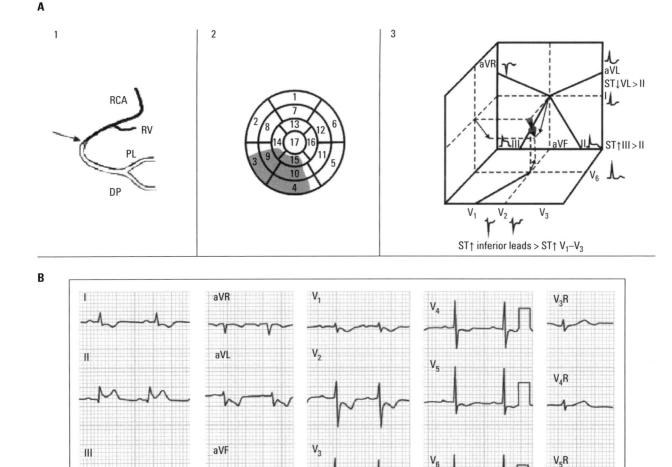

Figure 13.48 Typical case of ST segment elevation acute coronary syndrome (STE-ACS) due to right coronary artery (RCA) occlusion after right ventricular branches (arrow). (A-1) Site of occlusion. (A-2) Myocardial area at risk with the polar map in "bull's eye" projection with the most affected segments marked in gray. (A-3). (B) Typical ECG in the case of STE-ACS due to RCA occlusion distal to right ventricular branches. Observe the ST segment elevation in II, III, and aVF (III > II) with ST segment depression in I. ST segment depression exists in the right precordial leads (V1–V2). The right precordial leads also favor RCA occlusion after right ventricular branches (Figure 13.39).

irreversible pattern. In fact, in a few cases, such as in aborted MI and in Prinzmetal angina (coronary spasm), the presence of Q waves may be transient.

Diagnostic criteria

Table 13.7 shows the ECG changes associated with prior MI according to the new universal definition of MI (Thygesen *et al.* 2019). We will discuss some of the new criteria that have been defined after this classification in recent years, such as the new criteria of lateral MI (Bayés de Luna *et al.* 2008) and the concept of fractioned QRS (Das *et al.* 2006) (see throughout the chapter and in Chapter 20).

As with changes in the T wave and ST segment deviations, the presence of a **mirror image of the Q wave** of necrosis is also very important for diagnostic purposes. It is especially evident that, in patients with IHD, the presence of a prominent R wave in V1 may be the only manifestation of abnormality as a mirror pattern of Q waves in opposed leads. It is currently known that this R wave is a result of a lateral, not posterior MI (Bayés de Luna *et al.* 2006a, 2006b, 2008) (see below) (Figure 13.76).

Furthermore, **occasionally a cancellation of two necrosis vectors may not reflect the two** necrosis areas because the two Q waves are opposed and are cancelled (Color Plate 4).

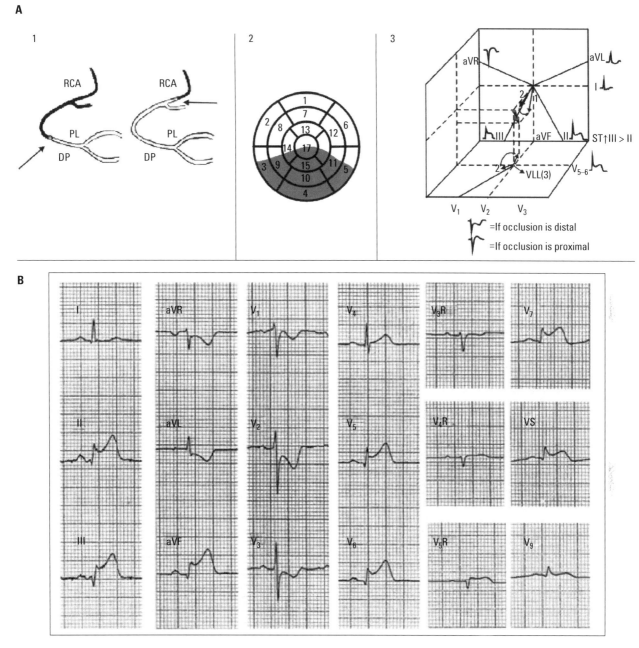

Figure 13.49 ST segment elevation acute coronary syndrome (STE-ACS) due to occlusion of very dominant right coronary artery (RCA). (A-1) Site of occlusion that may be before or after the right ventricular branches. (A-2) Myocardial area at risk and polar map in "bull's-eye" projection with the most involved segments. (A-3) Ischemic vector projected in frontal and horizontal planes. (B) Typical ECG in the case of STE-ACS due to occlusion of very dominant RCA distal to right ventricular branches. Observe the ST segment elevation in the inferior leads (III>II) and ST segment depression in V1–V3 (occlusion distal to the take-off of right ventricular branches). Furthermore, the ST segment elevation in V6–V8. The arrow shows the place of distal occlusion.

Location of Q wave myocardial infarction

Until recently, the accepted correlations of Q waves in different leads with the location of MI in ventricular walls were as follows (Surawicz *et al.* 1978): (i) Q waves in V1–V2 correspond to a septal wall; (ii) those in V3–V4 correspond to an anterior wall; (iii) those in I–aVL and/or V5–V6 correspond to the lateral wall (upper and/or lower, respectively); (iv) those in the II, III, aVF correspond

to the inferior wall; (v) the reciprocal pattern of R in V1–V2 corresponds to a posterior wall (after Perloff 1964).

However, a statement from the International Society for Holter and Noninvasive Electrocardiology (Bayés de Luna *et al.* 2006a) presented a new classification of Q-wave MI based on the correlation between the Q wave and the infarcted area as assessed by CE-CMR published by our group (Bayés de Luna *et al.* 2006a, 2008) and others (Rovai

A

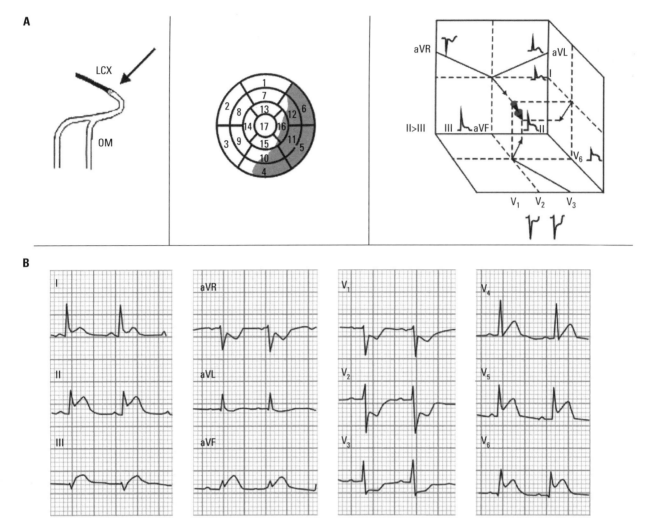

B

Figure 13.50 ST segment elevation acute coronary syndrome (STE-ACS) due to occlusion of the left circumflex artery (LCX) artery proximal to the obtuse marginal branch. (A-1) Site of occlusion. (A-2) Myocardial area at risk and polar map in "bull's-eye" projection with the most involved segments marked in gray. (A-3) Ischemic vector directed backward and somewhat to the left as projected in frontal, horizontal, and sagittal planes and the corresponding ECG patterns. (B) Typical example of ECG in a case of STEMI due to complete occlusion of proximal LCX. Observe the ST elevation in II, III, aVF (II > III), and V5–V6, and ST depression in V1–V3 more evident the ST elevation in inferior leads.

et al. 2007; Van der Weg *et al.* 2009; Allencherril *et al.* 2018). We would like to remind readers that this was already suggested by pathologic (Dunn *et al.* 1956) and isotopic correlations (Bough *et al.* 1984). We based this new classification (Figure 13.66 and Table 13.8) on the following.

The heart is divided into four walls (septal, anterior, inferior, and lateral). The correlation between ECG leads and these walls has been explained above (see Anatomic and pathological point of view). These four walls encompass two regions (see Figure 4.7): the anteroapical, perfused by the LAD, and the inferolateral, perfused by the RCA or the LCX. Evidently, these two regions are not equal, according to the anatomic variations of the arteries perfusing them (e.g. length, dominance).

The inferobasal segment of the left ventricle (former posterior wall), which corresponds to segment 4 of the statement of the AHA imaging societies (Cerqueira *et al.* 2002) (see Figures 4.4, 4.5, and 5.18), depolarizes after 40–50 ms. Therefore, this cannot produce an R wave in V1 that would be equivalent to the Q wave in the back of the heart because the beginning of QRS has already started.

We have demonstrated that **the inferobasal segment rarely bends upward**, and therefore, a true posterior wall hardly ever exists (see Figure 4.2). Furthermore, even in the case that this vector exists, which may happen in very lean individuals, the vector of necrosis of this area faces V3–V4 and not V1.

A

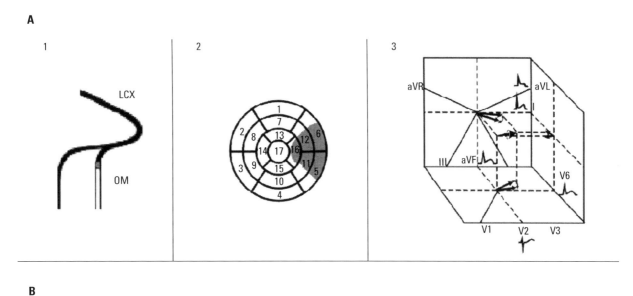

B

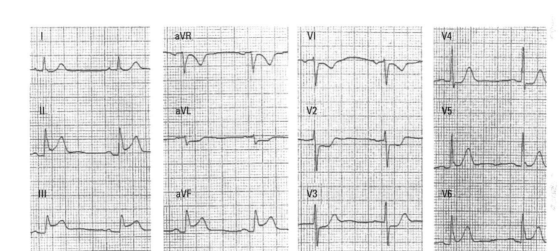

Figure 13.51 ST segment elevation acute coronary syndrome (STE-ACS) due to occlusion of the obtuse marginal branch (OM). (A-1) Site of the occlusion. (A-2) Myocardial area at risk and polar map of the involved area. (A-3) Ischemic vector that is directed to the left (approximately 0° to +20° in the frontal plane) and somewhat backward. Occasionally, if small, it hardly produces any ST segment deviations. If they occur, the ST segment elevation is observed in some lateral and inferior leads especially in I, II, aVF, and V6, with a usually slight ST segment depression in V2–V3. (B) ECG that shows slight elevation in II, III, and aVF, and ST segment depression in V1–V3 with isodiphasic ST in lead I. It is not easy in this case to decide from the ECG if the occlusion is in the RCA or LCX (OM). This case demonstrates that occasionally, especially when the changes of ST are not striking, it may be difficult to identify the culprit artery through ST segment changes. However, the ACS with small changes usually corresponds to a LCX occlusion.

Therefore, the oblique position of the heart in the thorax explains why the infarction vector of the lateral wall faces V1 (see Figures 4.3, 13.75, and 13.76).

It is clear that the posterior wall usually does not exist and, even when it does exist, it cannot produce a prominent R wave in V1 when necrosed.

The ECG can clearly distinguish between MIs of the anteroapical and inferolateral zones (see Figure 13.66). The specificity of these criteria is very high, especially in MIs of the inferolateral zone, although the sensitivity is lower, especially for MIs of the lateral wall. One factor that makes it difficult to distinguish MI of the anterolateral zone, especially type A1 and A2 of Figure 13.66 (septal and anteroapical), is that the precordial leads are not always located in the correct place (Fiol-Sala *et al.* 2020; Garcia Niebla *et al.* 2009) (Figure 13.76).

Figures 13.67–13.73 show examples of the new ECG classification of Q-wave MI with CE-CMR, the probable location of occlusion, the infarction area, and the VCG loops and ECG criteria.

Figure 13.74 shows that in the case of apical–anterior MI, the presence of a Q wave in the inferior leads depends on the importance of inferior wall involvement.

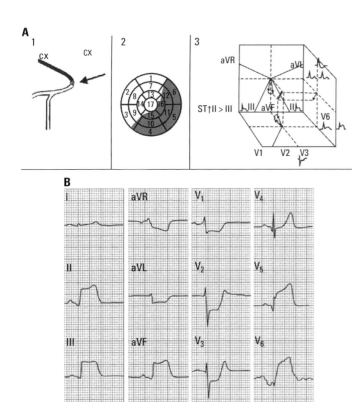

Figure 13.52 ST segment elevation acute coronary syndrome (STE-ACS) due to proximal occlusion of a very dominant left circumflex artery (LCX). (A-1) Site of occlusion. (A-2) Myocardial area at risk and polar map in "bull's-eye" projection with the most involved segments marked in gray. (A3) Important ischemic vector that is directed more backward than downward and less to the left or even a little to the right as projected in frontal, horizontal, and sagittal planes, and the corresponding ECG patterns of ST segment depression and elevation. (B) The ECG in the case of STE-ACS due to complete proximal occlusion of a very dominant LCX artery. Observe the criteria of LCX occlusion. ST segment elevation in II > III in the presence of isoelectric ST in I (second step of Figure 13.49). In aVL, there is ST segment depression due to LCX dominance. In the normal cases of LCX occlusion, there is no ST segment depression in aVL (isoelectric or elevated) (Figure 13.49). There is also a huge ST segment elevation in V5–V6 more evident than in the case of very dominant RCA (Figure 13.49). On the other hand, the sum of ST segment deviations is much higher than in the case of proximal occlusion of a non-dominant LCX (Figure 13.50).

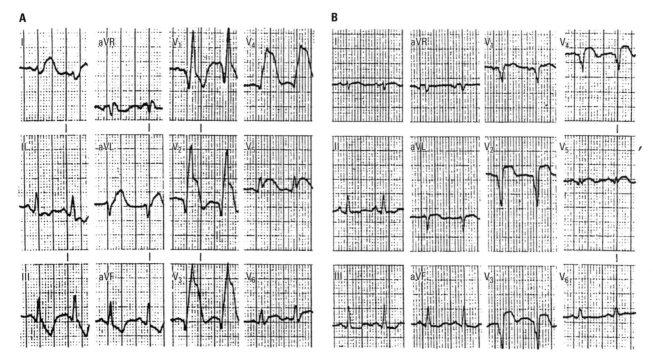

Figure 13.53 (A) Acute phase of evolving Q wave myocardial infarction of the anteroapical zone. There is a huge ST segment elevation, especially in I, aVL, and from V2 to V5, QRS >0.12 sec and morphology of complete right bundle branch block (RBBB) that was not present in the previous ECG. (B) Twenty-four hours later, the RBBB has disappeared and subacute anterior extensive infarction becomes evident. There is ST segment elevation from V1 to V4. The transient presence of new complete RBBB (RBB is perfused by S1) suggests that the occlusion of the left anterior descending artery (LAD) is proximal to S1 and D1.

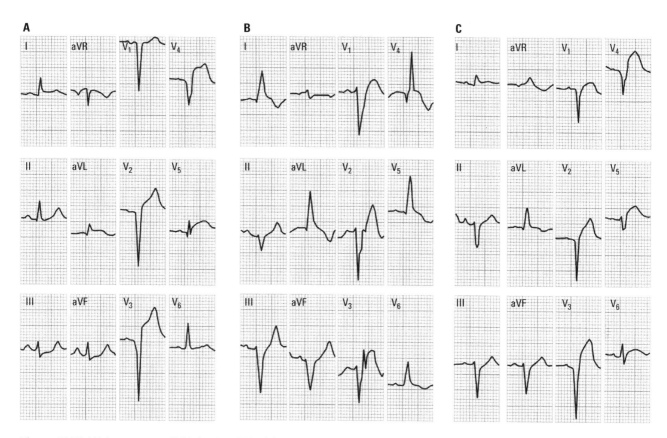

Figure 13.54 (A) Acute myocardial infarction (MI) of the anteroapical zone due to occlusion of the left anterior descending (LAD) artery proximal to D1 (ST segment depression in III and aVF) but distal to S1 (non-ST segment elevation in aVR and V1 and non-ST segment depression in V6). (B) After some hours, complete left bundle branch block (LBBB) appears (See q in I, aVL, and V4 and polyphasic morphology in V3) (see the Sgarbossa criteria, concordant ST segment elevation, in I, aVL, V4–V6). (C) The complete LBBB disappears but superoanterior hemiblock remains with the clear evidence of apical anterior MI (QS from V1 to V4 without "q" in aVL and I) (see Figure 13.68).

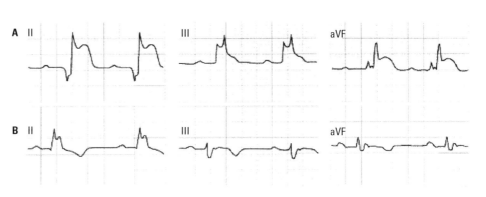

Figure 13.55 (A) Acute phase of an infarction in a patient with complete left bundle branch block. Note the clear ST segment elevation. In the chronic phase (B), the symmetrical T wave in III (mixed pattern of repolarization abnormality) leads to the suspicion of associated ischemia.

Lastly, in Figures 13.75 and 13.76, we show the new criteria and the three types of RS morphology seen in the case of lateral MI (Bayés de Luna *et al.* 2008; Fiol-Sala *et al.*, 2020).

The most important conclusions of these correlations are as follows:

- **R/S ≥ 1 in V1 is never a result of MI of the inferobasal segment (old posterior wall) but instead, it is always a**

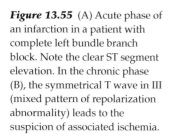

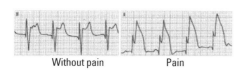

Figure 13.56 Patient with pacemaker and acute ST segment elevation acute coronary syndrome (STE-ACS). During an angina pain crisis of Prinzmetal type, a marked transient ST segment elevation is seen.

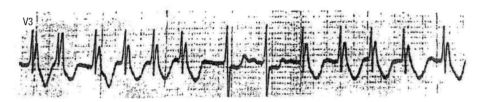

Figure 13.57 The ECG of a patient with rapid atrial fibrillation and right bundle branch block (RBBB). In the seventh and eighth complexes can be seen the disappearance of tachycardia-dependent RBBB, and then the morphology of subendocardial injury pattern appears. The complexes with RBBB also show a typical mixed pattern.

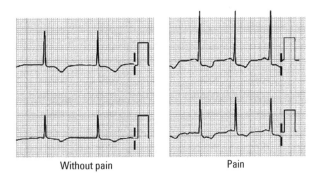

Without pain   Pain

Figure 13.58 A 62-year-old patient with hypertension presenting with a non-ST segment elevation acute coronary syndrome (NSTE-ACS). Left: without pain, there is a mixed pattern of left ventricular hypertrophy with strain + negative T wave. Right: during pain, a clear ST segment depression appears.

Table 13.4 Most frequent causes of ST segment elevation (apart from ischemic heart disease) (Figure 13.59).

1. Normal variants. Chest abnormalities, early repolarization, vagal overdrive. In vagal overdrive, ST segment elevation is mild, and generally accompanies the early repolarization image. T wave is tall and asymmetric
2. Sportsmen. Sometimes an ST segment elevation exists that even mimics an ACS with negative T wave, at times more prominent than ST elevation (Figure 23.8). No coronary involvement has been found, but this image has been observed in sportsmen who die suddenly; thus its presence implies the need to rule out hypertrophic cardiomyopathy
3. Acute pericarditis in its early stage and myopericarditis
4. Pulmonary embolism
5. Hyperkalemia. The presence of a tall, peaked T wave is more evident than the accompanying ST segment elevation, but sometimes it may be evident
6. Hypothermia
7. Brugada syndrome
8. Arrhythmogenic right ventricular dysplasia
9. Dissecting aortic aneurysm
10. Left pneumothorax
11. Toxicity secondary to cocaine abuse, drug abuse, etc.

result of MI of the lateral wall (100% specificity) (Figure 13.75). Other new criteria for lateral MI (R/S > 0.5 in V1 and an S wave < 3 mm in V1) maintain

Table 13.5 Most frequent causes of ST segment depression (apart from ischemic heart disease) (Figure 13.60).

1. Normal variants (generally slight ST depression). Sympathetic overdrive. Neurocirculatory asthenia, hyperventilation, etc.
2. Drugs (diuretics, digitalis, etc.)
3. Hypokalemia
4. Mitral valve prolapsed
5. Post-tachycardia
6. Secondary to bundle branch block or ventricular hypertrophy. Mixed images are frequently generated.

good specificity with an increase of sensitivity (Bayes de Luna *et al.* 2008) (Figure 13.76).

• **Exclusive MI of the inferior wall, including the inferobasal segment (old posterior wall), never present with prominent R waves in V1** (Figure 13.72). Therefore, **a new concept of inferior, lateral, and inferolateral infarction arises, which supercedes the diagnosis of posterior MI** (Figure 13.77).

• **Q wave in VL (and sometimes in I and small q in V2–V3) is not caused by high lateral MI perfused by LCX but by mid-anterior MI due to occlusion of the first diagonal** (Figure 13.70).

• In the presence of MI of the anteroseptal zone with Q wave beyond V2, **the presence of Q in I and/or aVL suggests that the infarction is more extensive** than the apical zone (Figure 13.69). What is more difficult is to differentiate the MI of the anteroseptal zone, especially when the location depends on the presence or not of Q wave in V3–V5. This is because the location of electrodes in the appropriate place in these leads may change if the person that performs the ECG does not follow the same methodology for the location of electrodes. Because of this, the sensitivity and specificity of Q wave to differentiate distinct MIs of the anteroseptal area may change unless a strict methodology of location of electrodes is used (Garcia Niebla *et al.* 2009; Fiol-Sala *et al.* 2020) (Figure 13.78).

Fractioned QRS

From an electrocardiographic point of view, the **Q wave has been considered to be the only specific finding in chronic MI**. MI without Q wave in the chronic phase does not show any specific ECG signs that allow its identification. However, in coronary patients, it is already known

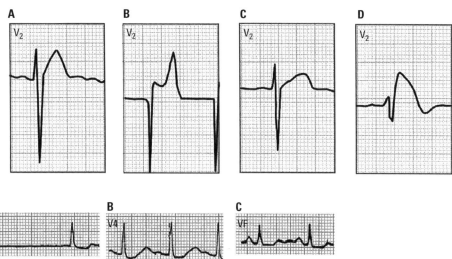

Figure 13.59 (A) The most frequent cases of ST segment elevation apart from ischemic heart disease. (A) Pericarditis; (B) hyperkalemia; (C) athletes; (D) typical Brugada pattern with coved ST segment elevation. The saddle-type variant of Brugada syndrome has to be differentiated from normal variant.

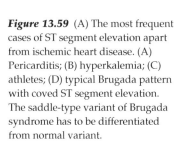

Figure 13.60 Non-ischemic ST segment depression. (A) ST segment depression secondary to digitalis effect: note the typical digitalis "scooped" pattern with a short QT interval in a patient with slow atrial fibrillation. (B) Example of hypokalemia in a patient with congestive heart failure who was receiving high doses of furosemide. What seems to be a long QT interval is probably a QU interval (T + positive U waves). (C) Case of mitral valve prolapse with ST segment depression in inferior leads.

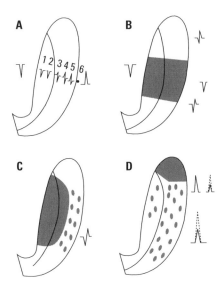

Figure 13.61 (A) Normal ventricular depolarization, being very rapid in the subendocardium, does not generate detectable potentials as this zone is full of Purkinje fibers (QS in 1 and 2). Starting from the border zone with subepicardium (3), morphologies with an increasing R wave (rS, RS, Rs) are registered (3–5) up to exclusive R wave in epicardium (6). As a consequence, in case of an experimental necrosis, the Q wave will be recorded only when it reaches the subepicardium and then will produce Q waves of higher or lower voltage according to the extension of necrosis. A morphology qR will be recorded in 3, QR in 4 and 5, up to QS if the necrosis is transmural. (B) This explains, according the theory of the electrical window of Wilson, how clinical transmural infarction produces QS morphology while (C) an infarction affecting the subendocardium and a part of the subepicardium may give rise to QR morphology without being necessarily transmural. Finally, (D) an infarction affecting basal areas or a part of myocardial wall, but in the form of patches, with necrosis-free zones, allows early formation of depolarization vectors that will be recorded as R waves but with slurrings, or small voltage (fractioned QRS).

from many years (Horan *et al.* 1971) that some changes in the mid-late part of QRS are also specific signs of chronic MI. These changes have now been reviewed (Das *et al.* 2006) and named **fractioned QRS**, to include **morphologies** such as low R in V6, rsr in some leads (I, II, precordial leads), notches and slurrings in the QRS, in at least two contiguous leads (Figures 13.79, 13.80, and 20.34). However, polyphasic QRS (rsr') in one inferior lead as an isolated finding may often be seen in normal individuals (see Figure 7.11).

These anomalies in the mid to late part of QRS correspond to a necrotic area that does not involve the whole wall or affect basal areas of the left ventricle transmurally, which, because they have recently been depolarized cannot produce pathological Q waves. These correspond to basal segments according to standardized myocardial segmentation nomenclature (Cerqueira *et al.* 2002). The fractioned QRS may appear either isolated or in the presence of a pathological Q wave.

MI with a fractioned QRS forms part of the MI without Q wave which will be discussed in Table 20.5. As we have said, it has been reported (Das *et al.* 2006) that the presence of **fractioned QRS** provides a more accurate criterion for the diagnosis of necrosis than the existence of a Q wave. However, it is necessary to match these morphologies with the clinical setting because they may also be seen in normal subjects.

Pathologic Q waves or fractioned QRS in patients without ischemic heart disease

The specificity of the pathologic Q wave for diagnosing myocardial necrosis is relatively high; however, it must be noted that similar "Q" waves are seen in other processes (Table 13.9). Figures 10.24 and 13.81 show two examples

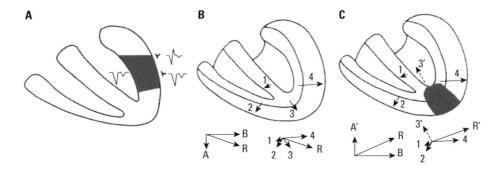

Figure 13.62 (A) Under normal conditions, the overall QRS vector (R) is made up of the sum of the different ventricular vectors (1 + 2 + 3 + 4). (B) When a necrotic (infarcted) area exists, the vector of infarction has the same magnitude as the previous vector, but has an opposite direction (3′). This change of direction of the initial depolarization electrical forces of a portion of the heart, the necrotic (infarcted) area, also implies the change of the overall vector direction (R′). (C) The development of a necrosis Q wave when a transmural infarction with homogeneous involvement of the left ventricle exists may be explained because the necrotic tissue, which is non-activable, acts as an electrical window, and allows for the recording of the left ventricular intracavitary QRS (which is a QS complex) from outside. The QS complex in the left ventricle is explained because the normal activation vectors—1, 2, and 3—are moving away from the infarcted zone.

Table 13.6 Characteristics of the "necrosis Q wave" or its equivalent[a].

---

1. Duration: ≥30 ms in I, II, III[c], aVL[b], and aVF, and in V3–V6. Frequently presents with slurrings. The presence of a Q wave is normal in aVR. In V1[b] and V2, all Q waves are pathologic, usually also in V3, except in case of extreme levorotation (qRs in V3). However, the presence in two consecutive leads is necessary

2. Q/R ratio: lead I and II > 25%, aVL > 50%, and V6 > 25% even in the presence of low R wave[c]

3. Depth: above the limit considered normal for each lead (i.e. generally 25% of the R wave) (frequent exceptions, especially in aVL, III, and aVF)

4. Presents even a small Q wave in leads where it does not normally occur (for example, qrS in V1–V3)

5. Q wave with decreasing voltage from V3–V4 to V5–V6

6. Equivalents of a Q wave: V1: R wave duration ≥40 ms, and/or R wave amplitude >3 mm and/or R/S ratio > 0.5

---

[a] The changes of mid to late part of QRS (low R wave in lateral leads and fractioned QRS) are not included in this list, which mentions only the changes of the first part of QRS (Q wave or equivalent).
[b] The presence of isolated Q in lead III usually is non-pathologic. Check changes with inspiration. Usually in III and aVF, Q/R ratios are not valuable when the voltage of R wave is low (<5 mm).
[c] QS morphology may be seen in VL in a normal heart in special circumstances (e.g. very lean individuals with vertical heart), and in V1, sometimes an absent of embryonic r wave may be seen in case of septal fibrosis (no q in V6).

of Q wave not due to IHD. The first case is an HCM and the second one a myocarditis. In the presence of pathologic Q waves, the diagnosis of acute MI is based not only on ECG findings, but also on the clinical setting, as well as on enzymatic changes. The presence of ST/T alterations accompanying a pathologic Q wave gives support to an IHD as the cause for this ECG pattern. However, in 5–25%

of infarctions (higher incidence in inferior infarction), the Q wave may disappear with time (Figure 13.32).

Thus, the sensitivity of the ECG for detecting old infarctions is not very high due to:
• the large number of MIs without Q wave (MI of the basal parts of the heart, etc.) (see Chapter 20);
• the presence of confounding factors—ventricular blocks, pacemakers, WPW;
• cases where the Q waves disappear due to improvement (collaterals) (Figure 13.32 and 20.35);
• the presence of new infarction (lateral plus septal) (Color Plate 4) (see Chapter 20).

Furthermore, fractioned QRS also arises in other diseases or circumstances, such as ventricular aneurysm (Das *et al.* 2006) and the Brugada syndrome (Morita *et al.* 2008).

Diagnosis of Q-wave MI in patients with intraventricular blocks pacemaker of WPW

Complete right bundle branch block (Figures 13.82–13.84)

The start of the cardiac activation is normal in the presence of a complete RBBB and, consequently, in the course of an infarction. ECG changes occur in the first part of the QRS complex, as in normal conditions. This causes an infarction Q wave that usually makes a distortion in the general morphology of the bundle branch block. For example, in the course of an **extensive infarction of the anteroseptal zone,** not only a Q wave appears in precordial leads but also a QS pattern because of the large infarcted area (Figure 13.82). In this figure, good correlation of Q waves with the infarcted area detected by CE-CMR may be seen. The basal segments, especially of the

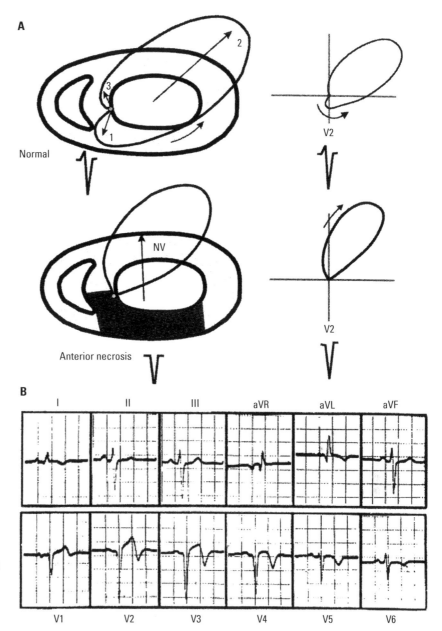

Figure 13.63 (A) Comparison between normal activation and the activation in the case of an extensive anterior infarction. The vector of infarction is directed backward and a loop–hemifield correlation explains the appearance of the Q wave in the anterior leads. (B) Example of myocardial infarction of the anteroapical zone.

Table 13.7 QRS ECG changes associated with prior myocardial infarction.

- Any Q-wave in leads V2–V3 ≥ 0.02 sec or QS complex in leads V2 and V3
- Q-wave ≥ 0.03 sec and ≥ 0.1 mV deep or QS complex in leads I, II, aVL, aVF, or V4–V6 in any two leads of a contiguous lead grouping (I, aVL, V6; V4–V6; II, III, and aVF)
- R-wave ≥ 0.04 sec in V1–V2 and R/S ≥ 1 with a concordant positive T wave in the absence of a conduction defect

---

From Thygesen *et al.* (2019).

lateral area, are spared. However, despite the lack of high lateral infarction, a QS morphology is seen in VL (and almost in lead I), due to the large mid-low anterior infarction with mid-low lateral extension. It has already been discussed (see above) that the QS morphology in VL is not caused by high lateral infarction (OM occlusion) but by mid-anterior infarction (diagonal occlusion). As the LAD is not very long, the infarcted inferior area is small (see A and D) and therefore, the Q wave of inferior infarction is not recorded.

When the MI involves the inferolateral wall, Q in inferior leads and/or an isolated R wave in V1–V2 with the notches in mid-late with depressed ST of concave morphology and often positive T wave, all expressions of lateral ischemia/infarction may be present (Figures 13.83 and 13.84).

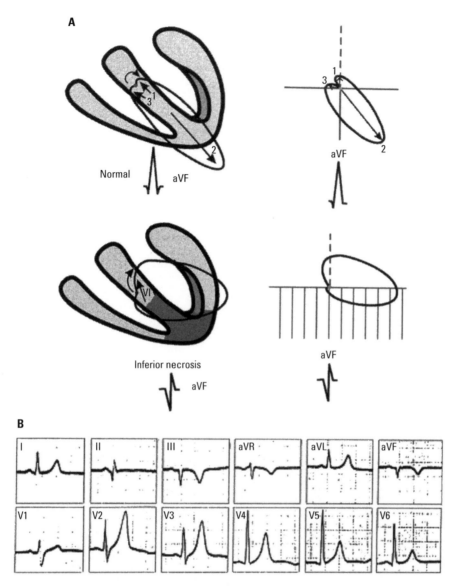

Figure 13.64 (A) Comparison between normal activation and activation in the case of inferolateral infarction. The vector of infarction is directed upward and a loop–hemifield correlation explains the appearance of a Q wave in the inferior leads. (B) Example of myocardial infarction of the inferolateral zone.

Also in the acute phase, the ST segment may be more or less elevated in V1–V2 (Figure 13.53) instead of isodiphasic or mildly depressed in V1 as it is in isolated RBBB (Figure 11.8).

Complete left bundle branch block (Figures 13.85–13.88)

In the presence of complete LBBB, even when large ventricular areas are infarcted, the general direction of the depolarization often does not change too much. This occurs because the vectors are still directed from right to left, and Q waves are often not recorded (Figure 13.85).

The QRS loop that is normally directed initially somewhat anteriorly and leftward, and then posteriorly, may be directed exclusively posteriorly and/or with an anomalous rotation (Figures 13.85–13.87). However, if we look with great detail at the ECG, we may find small changes that may suggest an associated infarction. For example, there may be a "q" wave in I and aVL (Figure 13.88) that is not recorded in the isolated LBBB. In other cases, Figure 13.81 (A) Patient with acute myocarditis and ECG with signs of RBBB plus superoanterior hemiblock (SAH) and Q wave of necrosis in many leads. After the acute phase (B), the Q waves practically disappear and also the SAH. In many leads a mild and diffuse pattern of subepicardial ischemia is still present. Note the low voltage in both ECGs.

In the 1950s, the Mexican School (Sodi Pallares and Rodríguez 1952) described ECG signs based on the changes of the QRS morphology with or without the

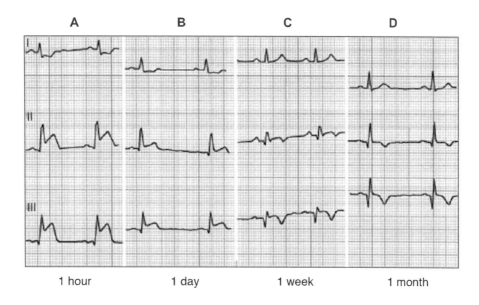

Figure 13.65 Evolution of a patient with acute myocardial infarction (MI) of the inferior wall due to occlusion of the right coronary artery. From A to D note the evolution of ST elevation and the appearance of Q wave and negative T wave.

development of Q waves (Sodi and Calder 1956; Cabrera 1958). Studies assessing the correlation between ECG and scintigraphy have proven that most of these signs were not very sensitive, even though they were specific (Wackers *et al.* 1978) (Table 13.10). The most specific QRS criteria (≈90%), even though they show a low sensitivity (30%), are the following (Figures 13.86–13.88 and Table 13.10):

• An abnormal Q wave (QS or QR morphology) in leads I, aVL, V4–V6, III, and aVF (Figure 13.87).

• Notches in the ascendant limb of R wave or qrS in I, aVL, V5, and V6 (Chapman's criterion) (Figure 13.87).

• Notches in the ascending limb of the S wave in the intermediate precordial leads V2–V4 (Cabrera's criterion) (Figure 13.87).

• The presence of an R wave (rS and RS) in V1 and RS in V6.

CE-CMR confirms often the location of necrosis in case of Q-wave MI (Figure 13.88) shows that in the presence of LBBB, the presence of a Q wave in lead I and aVL with notches in the ascending limb of S in the precordial leads, is due to infarction caused by a proximal occlusion of LAD above the diagonal branches involving all the anterior and septal walls, with also mid-lateral wall involvement.

With respect to **chronic repolarization abnormalities**, the negative T wave is more symmetric than that in the isolated complete LBBB (Figures 3.16 and 13.54B). In clinical practice, a positive T wave in V5 and V6 is usually seen when the LBBB is not too advanced (QRS < 130 ms), and septal repolarization does not predominate completely over left ventricular repolarization. In some cases of very advanced LBBB, this may be the expression of changes of repolarization polarity induced by right septal ischemia (Sodi and Calder 1956).

Hemiblocks

The location of two classical divisions of the left bundle— superoanterior and inferoposterior—with the middle fibers are also usually present in the sagittal view and in the left ventricular cone. We will now examine the following aspects of the associations between MI and block of the two classical divisions of the left bundle (hemiblocks) (Rosenbaum *et al.* 1968). We will refer to the diagnosis in the chronic phase. The hemiblocks do not alter the repolarization changes that can be observed in the acute phase of MI.

The late activation of some areas of the left ventricle due to the presence of hemiblocks explains the finding that sometimes the late QRS complex forces are opposed to the infarction Q wave. This association was recognized for many years before the concept of hemiblocks was coined, and was seen as part of the concept of "per infarction block." Because hemiblocks are diagnosed mainly by changes in the vector's direction in the frontal plane, the ECG changes secondary to the association with MI will be particularly noted in the frontal plane leads. However, the hemiblocks do not modify the diagnosis of MI of the anteroseptal zone in the precordial leads (horizontal plane), but may modify the presence or appearance of Q waves in the inferior leads (inferior MI) and in VL (midanterior MI or extensive MI involving mid-anterior area).

	Name	Type	ECG pattern	Infarction area (CE-CMR)	Most probable place of occlusion
A n t e r o s e p t a l z o n e	Septal	A1	Q in V1–V2 SE: 100% SP: 97%	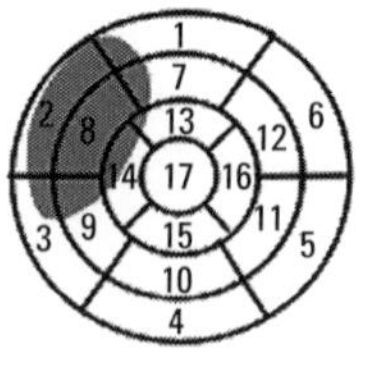	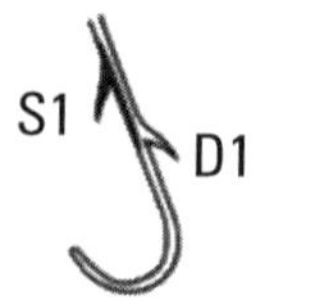 LAD S1 D1
	Apical–anterior	A2	Q in V1–V2 to V3–V6 SE: 85% SP: 98%	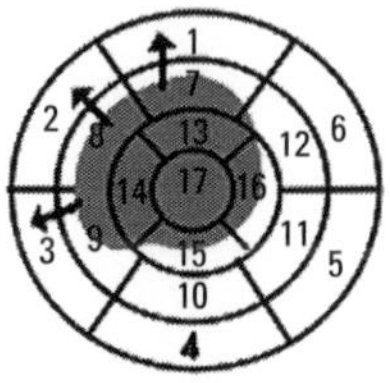	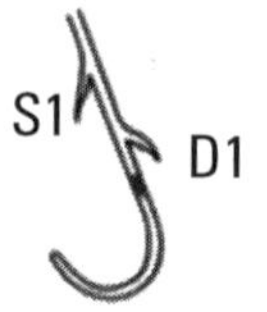 LAD S1 D1
	Extensive anterior	A3	Q in V1-V2 to V4-V6, I and aVL SE: 83% SP: 100%	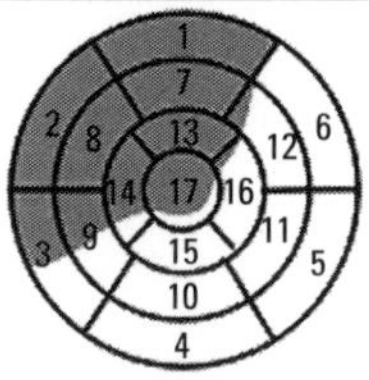	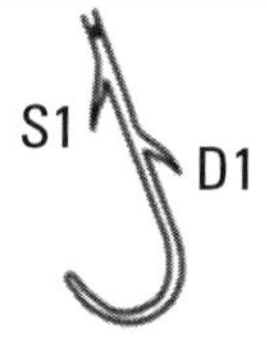 LAD S1 D1
	Mid–anterior	A4	Q (qs or qr) in aVL (I) and sometimes in V2–V3 SE: 67% SP: 100%	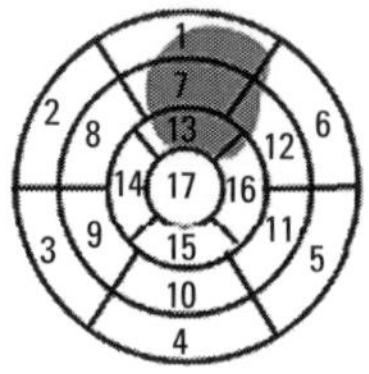	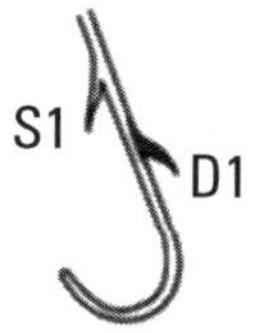 LAD S1 D1
I n f e r o l a t e r a l z o n e	Lateral	B1	RS in V1–V2 and/or Q wave in leads I, aVL, V6 and/or diminished R wave in V6 SE: 67% Sp: 99%	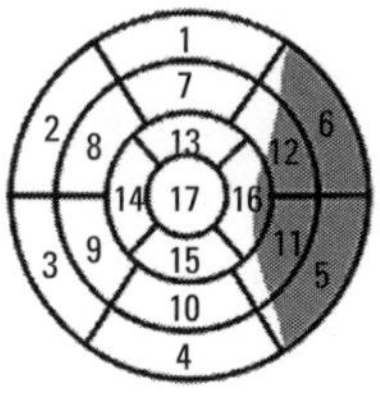	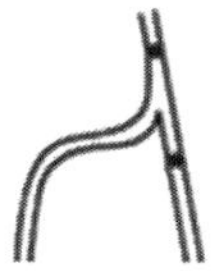 LCX
	Inferior	B2	Q in II, III, aVF SE: 88% SP: 97%	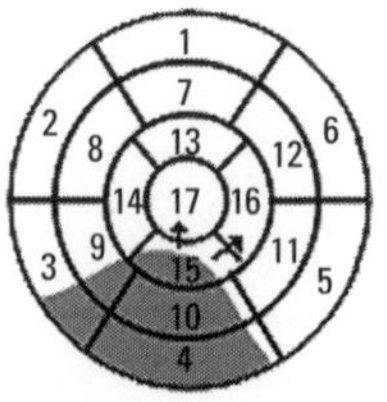	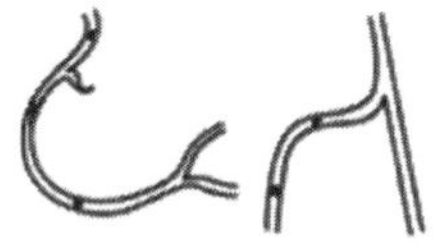 RCA LCX
	Infero-lateral	B3	Q in II, III, Vf (B2) and Q in I, VL, V5–V6 and/or RS in V1 (B1) SE: 73% SP: 98%	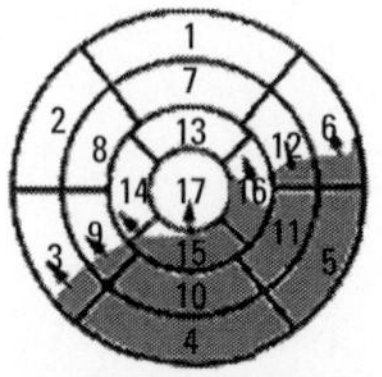	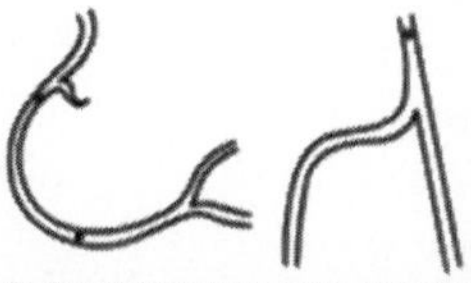 RCA LCX

Figure 13.66 Correlations between the different types of MI with their infarction area assessed by CMR, ECG pattern, name given to the infarction, and the most probable location of coronary artery occlusion. If coronary angiography is performed in the subacute phase, the angiogram does not necessarily show the actual location of the occlusion caused by the MI. The gray zones seen in bull's-eye view correspond to infarction areas and the arrows to its possible extension. As pointed out previously, recent findings by Allencherril *et al.* (2018) do not support existence of isolated basal anteroseptal or septal infarction. "Anteroapical infarction" is a more appropriate term than "anteroseptal infarction" (see text) (Modified from Bayés de Luna *et al.* 2006a).

Table 13.8 Proportions of agreement between patterns and contrast-enhanced cardiovascular magnetic resonance for the different myocardial infarction locations and their 95% confidence interval.

Myocardial infarction location		Proportions of agreement		95% Confidence interval	
CE-CMR location	ECG pattern[a]	Expected by chance	Observed	Lower limit	Upper limit
Septal	A-1	0.07	0.75	0.35	0.95
Apical-anterior	A-2	0.09	0.7	0.35	0.92
Extensive anterior	A-3	0.04	0.8	0.30	0.99
Mid-anterior	A-4	0.030	1	0.31	1.0
Lateral	B-1	0.045	0.8	0.30	0.99
Inferior	B-2	0.11	0.81	0.48	0.97
Infero-lateral	B-3	0.15	0.8	0.51	0.95
	Composite	0.17	0.88	0.75	0.95

CE-CMR, contrast-enhanced cardiovascular magnetic resonance.

[a] ECG pattern: A-1: Q in V1–V2; A-2: Q in V1–V2 to V3–V6; A-3: Q in V1–V2 to V4–V6, I and aVL; A-4: Q (qs or qr) in aVL (I) and sometimes in V2–V3; B-1: RS in V1–V2 and/or Q wave in leads I, aVL, V6 and/or diminished R wave in V6; B-2: Q in II, III, aVF; B-3: Q in II, III, Vf (B2) and Q in I, aVL, V5–V6 and/or RS in V1 (B1). Reproduced with permission from Bayes de Luna *et al.* (2006a).

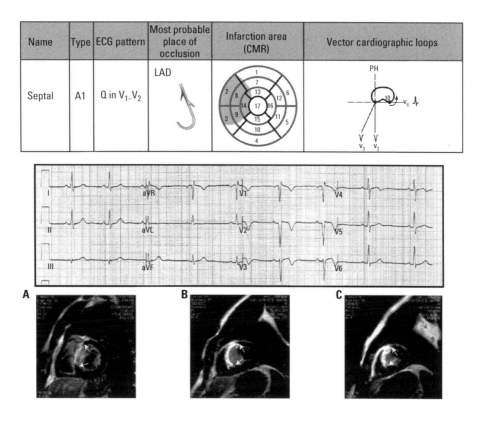

Figure 13.67 Example of large septal myocardial infarction (type A-1): ECG criteria (Q in V1–V2 with rS in V3), most probable site of occlusion, contrast-enhanced cardiovascular magnetic resonance (CE-CMR) images and vectorcardiographic (VCG) loops. The septal infraction is very extensive, encompassing the most of the septal wall at all levels—basal (A), mid (B), and apical (C) on the transverse plane. There is small extension toward the anterior wall at mid and apical levels (arrows).

In the following sections, we discuss: (i) diagnosis of the association; (ii) hemiblocks masking Q wave; (iii) hemiblocks concealed by Q wave; and (iv) pseudonecrosis pattern induced by hemiblocks.

Diagnosis of the association

• **Infarction of the inferior wall associated with a superanterior hemiblock (SAH) or an inferoposterior hemiblock (IPH):** Figures 13.89 and 13.90 show two

Name	Type	ECG pattern	Most probable place of occlusion	Infarction area (CMR)	Vector cardiographic loops	
Apical-anterior	A2	Q in V$_1$_V$_2$ to V$_3$_V$_6$	LAD		FP	PH

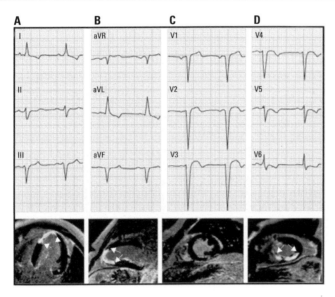

Figure 13.68 Example of apical-anterior myocardial infarction (Q wave beyond V2). In the horizontal plane (A), the septal and apical involvement is seen. The sagittal plane (B) shows that the inferior involvement is even larger than the anterior involvement, and in the mid and low transverse transections, especially in D, septal and inferior involvement is seen.

Name	Type	ECG pattern	Most probable place of occlusion	Infarction area (CMR)	Vector cardiographic loops	
Extensive anterior	A3	Q in V$_1$_V$_{2'}$ to V$_4$_V$_6$ I and VL	LAD		FP	HP

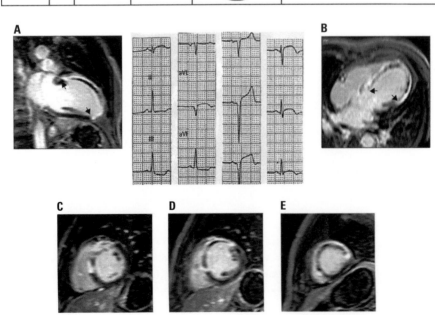

Figure 13.69 Example of extensive anterior myocardial infarction (type A-3) (Q in precordial leads and aVL, with qrs in L), most probable site of occlusion, contrast-enhanced cardiovascular magnetic resonance (CE-CMR) images and vectorcardiographic (VCG) loops. CE-CMR images show the extensive involvement of the septal, anterior, and lateral walls, less the highest part of the lateral wall (see B and C). The involvement of segments 7 and 12 explain that in this MI there is a Q in VL that is not present in MI of apical-anterior type. (A) Oblique sagittal view. (B) Longitudinal horizontal plane view. (C–E) Transverse views. The inferior wall is the only spared. The LAD is not very large and therefore the inferior involvement is not extensive (see A). Due to that there is QS in aVL and R in II, III, and aVF together with Q in V1–V5.

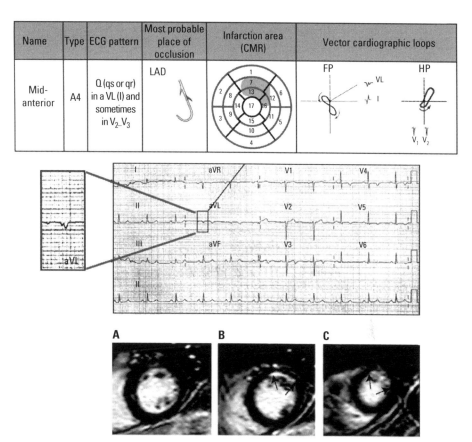

Figure 13.70 Example of mid-anterior myocardial infarction (type A-4) (QS in aVL without Q in V5–V6), most probable place of occlusion, contrast-enhanced cardiovascular magnetic resonance (CE-CMR) images and vectorcardiographic (VCG) loops. CE-CMR images show in transverse plane mid-low-anterior and lateral wall involvement (B,C).

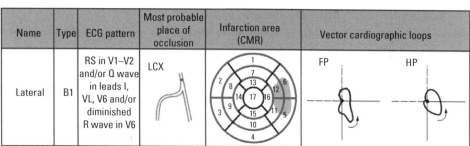

Figure 13.71 Example of lateral myocardial infarction (MI) with RS in V1 (type B-1). See the most probable place of occlusion, the contrast-enhanced cardiovascular magnetic resonance (CE-CMR) image, and the VCG loops. The CE-CMR images show that in this case the MI involves especially the basal and mid part of the lateral wall (A–C) (longitudinal horizontal and transverse planes) but not the apical part (D).

Name	Type	ECG pattern	Most probable place of occlusion	Infarction area (CMR)	Vector cardiographic loops
Inferior	B2	Q in II, III, VF	RCA		

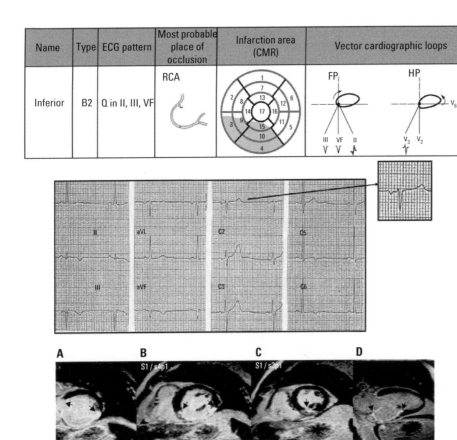

Figure 13.72 Example of inferior myocardial infarction (MI) with Q in II, III, and aVF and rS in V1. See the most probable place of occlusion, the contrast-enhanced cardiovascular magnetic resonance (CE-CMR) images, and the VCG loop. CE-CMR shows involvement of segments 4 and 10 and part of 15 and 3 and 9 (septal-inferior involvement) (A–C). The lateral wall is practically sparse. The most apical part of the inferior wall is not involved (D). In spite of the clear involvement of segment 4 (see A and D), the morphology of V1 is rS. Therefore, in the presence of MI of segment 4 (old posterior wall) without involvement of the lateral wall, there is no RS in V1.

Name	Type	ECG pattern	Most probable place of occlusion	Infarction area (CMR)	Vector cardiographic loops
Infero lateral	B3	Q in II,III,VF (B2)+Q in I, VL$_1$,V$_5$–VL$_6$ and/or RS in V$_1$(B1)			

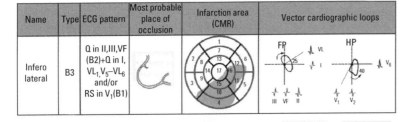

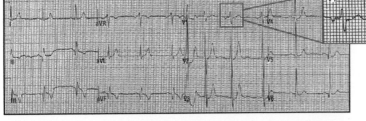

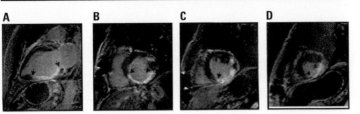

Figure 13.73 Example of inferolateral myocardial infarction (MI) (Q in II, III, and aVF, and RS in V1), most probable place of occlusion (RCA), the contrast-enhanced cardiovascular magnetic resonance (CE-CMR) images, and the corresponding VCG loops. The CMR shows involvement of the inferior wall and also part of the lateral wall. (A) Sagittal-like transection showing the involvement of the inferior wall. (B–D) Transverse transections at basal, mid, and apical level showing the lateral involvement, especially at mid and apical levels.

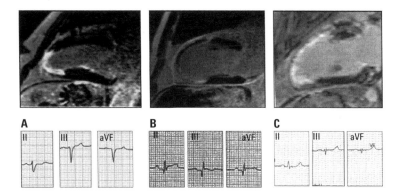

Figure 13.74 (A, B) Example of apical-anterior infarction with inferior involvement equal to or greater than the anterior. There is Q wave in the inferior leads that is not usually seen in cases of apical-anterior MI with anteroseptal involvement greater than the inferior involvement (C).

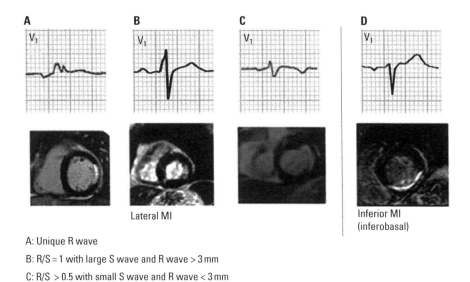

A: Unique R wave

B: R/S = 1 with large S wave and R wave > 3 mm

C: R/S > 0.5 with small S wave and R wave < 3 mm

Figure 13.75 The three typical patterns of R in V1 in lateral myocardial infarction (MI) (A–C) compared with inferior MI (D).

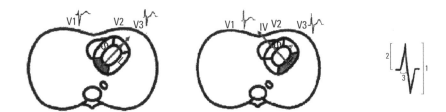

Figure 13.76 (A,B) Direction of necrosis vector in the case of myocardial infarction (MI) of inferobasal segment (old posterior wall) that does not produce RS in V1 and necrosis vector of lateral myocardial infarction (MI) that produces this pattern. (C) The new ECG criteria of lateral MI in V1 (R/S > 0.5, R amplitude > 3 mm, and duration > 40 ms, and S ≤ 3 mm).

typical examples of these associations with the scheme of the infarcted area, the QRS loop that shows the change in direction of depolarization, and the ECG–VCG correlation (see legends).

- **Anterior infarction associated with an SAH** (Figure 13.91) or **IPH** (Figure 13.92). Again, the legends are self-explanatory.

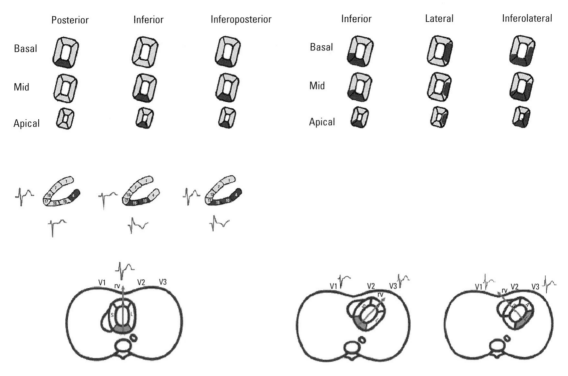

Figure 13.77 Left: The involved area in the case of inferior, posterior, and inferoposterior myocardial infarction (MI) with the classical ECG patterns in the chronic phase according to the old concept; right side shows that with the new concept exposed in this book, the name posterior disappears. The RS pattern in V1 is explained by lateral MI and the MI of the inferobasal segment of inferior wall (classically posterior wall) does not generate Q wave because it is a zone of late depolarization. Therefore, the MIs of the inferolateral zone are clustered in three groups: inferior (Q in II, III, and aVF), lateral (RS in V1 and/or abnormal Q in lateral leads), and inferolateral (both patterns).

Hemiblocks masking Q waves

The presence of a hemiblock can also mask the presence of a coexistent infarction. We will briefly discuss some examples.

• **An SAH may mask the Q wave of infarction.** For example, **in the case of a small inferior infarction** (Figure 13.93), if no SAH existed, the entire loop would rotate clockwise, first above and generally below, the axis of lead X, and would be recorded as a Qr complex in some inferior leads (Figure 13.97A–C). In the presence of a small inferior MI, the area that starts the left ventricular activation in the case of SAH is spared and may produce a small initial "r" even in the presence of inferior MI. The "r" wave in III being higher than the "r" wave in II supports the diagnosis of added inferior infarction (see legend).

• **In the case of a small septal infarction**, the SAH may mask the infarction in horizontalized hearts (Figure 13.94). In that figure, it is seen that a high positioning of the V1–V2 leads in the third intercostal space may be necessary in obese patients to check for a QS morphology, which would suggest the presence of an associated septal infarction (see legend of the Figure 13.94).

• **An IPH may mask a Q wave of infarction. In the case of a small mid-anterior infarction** (Figure 13.95), the area where the depolarization begins in the IPH (B in Figure 13.95) is spared. This initial depolarization vector (1) partially counteracts the vector of infarction (in vector) and gives rise to an initial, sometimes slurred, "r" wave in III and aVL that masks the mid-anterior infarction (see legend).

• **In the case of a small infarction of the septal area**, the IPH may mask the infarction in vertical hearts (Figure 13.96). In this figure, it is seen that in the case of IPH, the first vector in vertical heart, the beginning of QRS, is recorded as positive (rS pattern) in the fourth intercostal space (Figure 13.96B), because these leads are higher than those in the normal heart (Figure 13.96A). They should be positioned in the fifth intercostal space to record a QS morphology in V1–V2 so that the diagnosis may be confirmed.

• **In the case of a large inferior infarction**, the association of an IPH may convert the morphology QS or Qr in inferior leads in QR or even qR and therefore the IPH may partially mask the inferior MI (Figure 13.90).

Q waves of infarction masking hemiblocks

The following cases may occur:

• **Q wave of infarction masking an SAH**: On certain occasions, large inferior infarctions may make the diagnosis of hemiblock difficult. This occurs because the rS

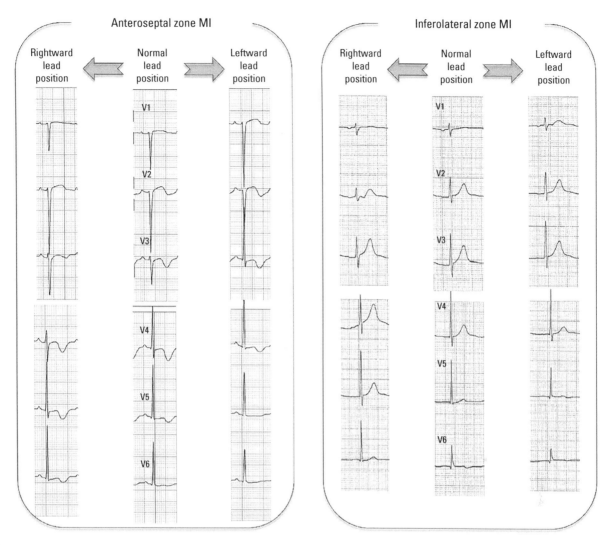

Figure 13.78 On the left a patient with myocardial infarction of the anteroapical zone (previously named anteroseptal) in the subacute phase: normal lead position displays negative T-waves up to V5. Small changes in the placement of precordial leads have significantly modified the morphology of QRS and T wave. On the right, a patient with an infarction of the inferolateral zone: moving the precordial leads a little to the right or left makes the negative T-wave inV6 to disappear.

morphology disappears and a QS morphology is seen in all the inferior wall leads (Figure 13.89). In a mid-anterior infarction, the RS morphology in the inferior wall may make the diagnosis of SAH more difficult (Figure 13.91).

• **Q wave of infarction masking an IPH**: In large anterior infarctions associated with an IPH, a QS morphology is seen in VL (instead of an rs morphology in the isolated IPH) (Figure 13.92) and in inferior infarctions, a QR morphology (instead of qR morphology) (Figure 13.90). In these cases, the hemiblocks may be masked to some degree because the typical IPH morphology has changed due to the infarction.

False Q wave patterns due to hemiblocks

When the V1–V2 electrodes are positioned very high, an initial "Q" wave may be recorded in SAH, due to the first activation vector, which is directed downward. This

suggests the false pattern of septal infarction that disappears when the electrodes are located more inferiorly. It has already been stated that in obese or very lean individuals, the higher or lower positioning of electrodes V1–V2 may be required to find patterns of added true septal infarction (Figures 13.94 and 13.96) (see Hemiblocks masking Q waves).

Q wave in the case of left-deviated ÂQRS with and without SAH (Figures 13.89, 13.93, and 13.97–13.99)

In spite of the left-deviated ÂQRS, Figures 13.96A–C and 13.99 show that there is no SAH associated with the inferior infarction, since the RS loop is always rotating in a clockwise direction. With the surface ECG we can suspect that there is no coexisting SAH because a Qr morphology is seen at least in some inferior leads (see Figure 13.97A–C). The final "r" wave is explained by the

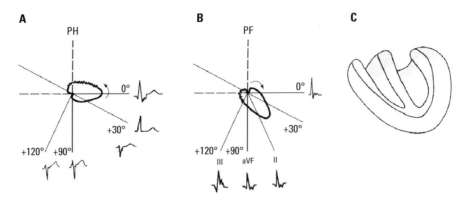

Figure 13.79 If the necrosis affects the areas of late ventricular depolarization (gray in C), instead of pathologic Q wave, it will result in a change of the direction of the vectors of the second part of QRS, which is presented as "slurrings" in the terminal part of QRS in II, III, aVF, and V5–V6 or as rr′ or r′ of a very low voltage in precordial leads and/or I or II, or even slurrings in the beginning of ST segment (A,B). These morphologies are considered as QRS (Based on Das *et al.* 2006).

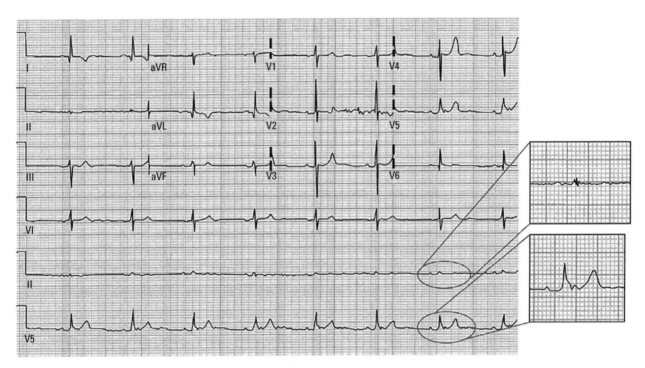

Figure 13.80 The ECG of a patient that has suffered two myocardial infarctions (MIs) of the inferolateral zone and a two-bypass grafting surgery. The patient presents with important left ventricular aneurysm. Observe the presence of RS in V1, q in lateral leads, and abnormal morphology of QRS (fractioned QRS) in several leads (see amplified leads II and V5).

fact that as the loop rotates only in the clockwise direction, the final portion is at least in the positive side of lead II (Figure 13.97C). Occasionally, in the case of an **inferior infarction without the coexistence of SAH**, the loop that makes an entire clockwise rotation is completely above the axis of lead X (Figure 13.98). In this situation, a QS morphology can be recorded in III and aVF, and even rS in III, but at least a **terminal small "r" wave exists in II**.

In the case of associated SAH, the final part of the loop rotates counterclockwise and this explains why in lead II a QS or qrs morphology may be seen without final "r"

(Figures 13.97D–E and 13.98). In isolated inferior MI, the loop is only clockwise and the morphology in II is qR but not qrS (Figure 13.99). Thus, although the VCG was thought to be the only technique that could assure the presence or not of an associated SAH (Benchimol *et al.* 1972), the correct incorporation of the information taken from VCG–ECG curves virtually allows us to rule out this association due to the presence of a final "r" wave (Qr) in the inferior leads, at least in II, and the absence of a final r in aVR (see Figure 13.97D–E compared with A–C and Figures 13.98 and 13.99). In turn, the absence of a

Table 13.9 Pathologic Q wave not secondary to myocardial infarction.

1. During the evolution of an acute (ischemic or not) disease involving the heart
1.1. Acute coronary syndrome with an aborted infarction
1.2. Coronary spasm (Prinzmetal angina type)
1.3. Presence of transient apical dyskinesia that also shows ST segment elevation and a transient pathologic "q" wave. Probably, corresponds to an aborted infarction
1.4. Acute myocarditis
1.5. Pulmonary embolism
1.6. Miscellaneous: toxic agents, etc.
2. Chronic pattern
2.1. Recording artifacts
2.2. Normal variants: aVL in the vertical heart and III in the dextrorotated and horizontalized heart
2.3. QS in V1 (hardly even in V2) in septal fibrosis, emphysema, the elderly, chest abnormalities, etc.
2.4. Some types of right ventricular hypertrophy (chronic cor pulmonale) or left ventricular hypertrophy (QS in V1–V2, or slow increase in R wave in precordial leads, or abnormal "q" wave in hypertrophic cardiomyopathy) (septal hypertrophy) sometimes deep but narrow and usually with normal repolarization
2.5. Left bundle branch conduction abnormalities
2.6. Infiltrative processes (amyloidosis, sarcoidosis, tumors, chronic myocarditis, dilated cardiomyopathy, etc.)
2.7. Wolff–Parkinson–White syndrome
2.8. Congenital heart diseases (coronary artery abnormalities, dextrocardia)
2.9. Pheochromocytoma
3. Presence of prominent R in V1 not due to a mirror pattern Q equivalent of lateral MI (see Table 10.3)

terminal "r" wave (slurred QS or sometimes qrs morphology) in II, III, and aVF with a final "r" in aVR virtually confirms the presence of an SAH associated with the inferior infarction (compare Figures 13.97A–E, 13.98, and 13.99).

Wolff–Parkinson–White-type pre-excitation (Figure 13.100)

It is difficult, and sometimes impossible, to confirm the association of a Q wave infarction in the presence of a Wolff–Parkinson–White-type (WPW-type) pre-excitation. In Figure 13.100, we observe that no Q wave is seen in the complexes with pre-excitation, despite the existence of an apical infarction (second QRS in each lead). When the pre-excitation disappears (first complex in each lead), the presence of Q wave from V1 to V4 is clear. However, during the pre-excitation, the presence of evident repolarization abnormalities may suggest the coexistence of IHD (symmetric and negative T wave from V2 to V6). We need to remember as well that intermittent conduction by the right anomalous bypass tract, intermittent complete LBBB, and intermittent right ventricular stimulation may be accompanied by a negative T wave when the conduction is made via the normal pathway, which can be explained by a "cardiac memory" phenomenon (Rosenbaum *et al.* 1982).

The possibility that a WPW-type pre-excitation may mask the infarction depends on the type of WPW. When the infarct is located contralaterally to the anomalous pathway, it is most probable that the infarction is masked. However, when the infarction is located ipsilaterally, it is most probably detected (Wellens 2006).

Pacemakers (Figures 13.101–13.103)

As discussed previously (Chapter 11), patients with intermittent right ventricular stimulation, when the stimulus is conducted via the normal path (Figure 13.101), may show a "cardiac memory" phenomenon (lack of adequacy of the repolarization to the depolarization changes), which explains the anomalous repolarization (negative T wave) that is sometimes observed in sinus rhythm in the absence of IHD. It has been demonstrated that in this situation the T wave is negative in the precordial leads but is positive in I and aVL.

In the chronic phase, the presence of a qR morphology after the pacemaker spike (St–qR) from V4 to V6, I, and aVL (Figure 13.102) is quite useful, being highly specific, but less sensitive for the diagnosis of associated MI (Barold *et al.* 1987). Besides, the presence of St–rS morphology in aVR has been described as quite a sensitive sign, but with a low specificity, for the diagnosis of an inferior infarction. Finally, an interval between the pacemaker stimulus and the beginning of the QRS complex has also been described in patients with associated MI (Figure 13.103). This occurs when the pacemaker stimulates the fibrotic infarcted area (latency) (Wellens *et al.* 2003).

Other changes

Ischemia may induce many other changes, including prolongation of QT interval, changes of U wave or P wave, distortion of QRS complex, and arrhythmias.

Changes in P wave

These may be seen in atrial infarction (see Chapters 9 and 20; Figure 9.33).

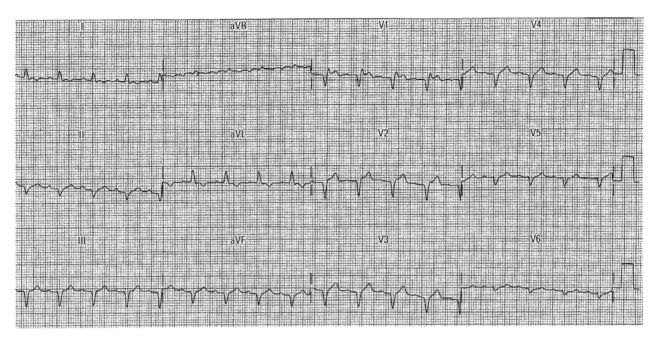

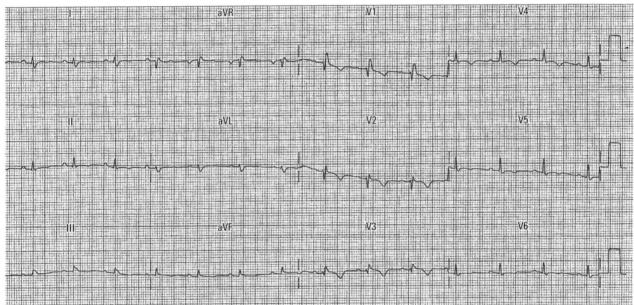

Figure 13.81 (Above) Patient with acute myocarditis and ECG with signs of RBBB plus superoanterior hemiblock (SAH) and Q wave of necrosis in many leads. After the acute phase (below), the Q waves practically disappear and also the SAH. In many leads a mild and diffuse pattern of subepicardial ischemia is still present. Note the low voltage in both ECGs.

Distortion of QRS complex

This may occur especially in very acute severe transmural ischemia, such as grade III ischemia, in which case the ST elevation brings the S wave upward (see Figure 20.3).

Arrhythmias

The appearance of different types of bradyarrhythmias (sinus bradycardia and AV block) and **tachyarrhythmias** (especially atrial fibrillation and ventricular arrhythmias)

is frequent in acute ischemia. Ventricular fibrillation usually appears without previous ventricular tachycardia and, **unfortunately, if it occurs outside the cardiac care unit, it leads to sudden death** (see Ischemia and sudden death, and Arrhythmias in Chapter 20).

Intraventricular block also occurs, especially in RBBB when the LAD occlusion is proximal to the first septal branch that perfuses the right bundle. Less frequently, LBBB appears because of double perfusion (LAD and LCX).

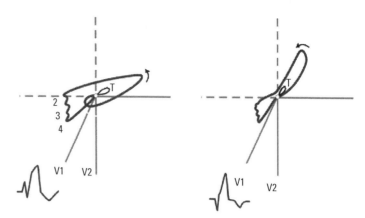

Figure 13.82 ECG–VCG correlation in the case of isolated right bundle branch block (RBBB) (left) and RBBB plus anteroseptal myocardial infarction (MI) (right).

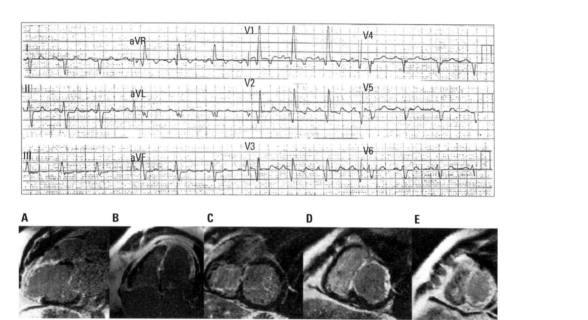

Figure 13.83 Patient with complete right bundle branch block (RBBB) and myocardial infarction type A-3 (extensive anterior myocardial infarction (MI) due to proximal LAD occlusion). Observe the Q wave in precordial leads and the QS morphology in aVL. Contrast-enhanced cardiovascular magnetic resonance (CE-CMR) images (A–E) show important involvement of lateral, anterior, and septal walls, and even the lower part of inferior wall (E). The lateral involvement (B, D, and E in white) is more important than in the apical-anterior MI even when there is an anteroseptal extension, but the basal lateral segments are spared because they are perfused by the circumflex artery. The QS in aVL is due to left anterior descending (LAD) artery occlusion before the first diagonal.

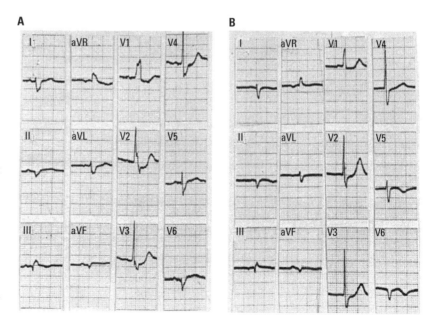

Figure 13.84 (A) Patient with complete right bundle branch block (RBBB) in acute phase of inferolateral infarction. ST segment depression is seen in V1, V2, and V3 with final positive T wave and Q wave in inferior leads. The high localization of the "notch" on the upward slope of the R wave supports the involvement of lateral wall. (B) The diagnosis of inferolateral infarction is confirmed when the RBBB resolves after a few days (Q in II, III, aVF and R in V1, and QS in V6).

A

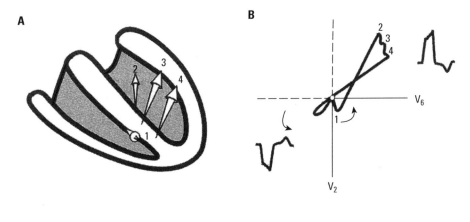

B

C

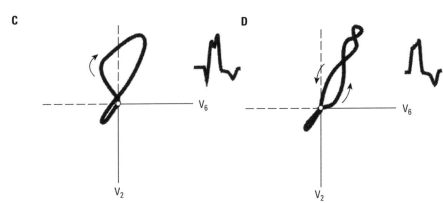

D

Figure 13.85 (A, B) Ventricular activation in the case of left bundle branch block (LBBB) and how this activation explains the LBBB morphology according to the ECG–VCG correlation. (C) However, when the infarcted area is extensive, it may produce changes in the direction of the vectors and in the morphology of the loop that explains the appearance of Q waves in the ECG. (D) The association of infarction frequently produces changes in the QRS loop that usually do not modify the ECG pattern of chronic infarction.

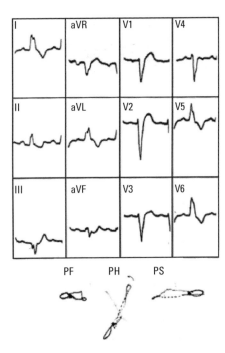

Figure 13.86 Example of the usefulness of vectorcardiography (VCG) to diagnose associated necrosis. In the case of left bundle branch block (LBBB), the loop shows a figure-of-eight morphology. In the horizontal plane that is abnormal and suggests the presence of associated necrosis in a patient with ischemic heart disease. The ECG does not suggest evident signs of necrosis, as the QRS is practically normal, although the presence of r ≥ 1 mm in V1 and symmetric T wave in I, aVL, and V5 is not usually seen in isolated LBBB.

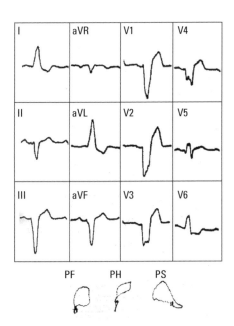

Figure 13.87 ECG–VCG of complete left bundle branch block (LBBB) with signs suggesting associated infarction. This might be suspected from the morphology in V5 (qrs) and evident slurrings in V2–V4 (Cabrera's sign). Also, the initial forces are posterior in the VCG, which is abnormal and clearly suggests associated myocardial infarction.

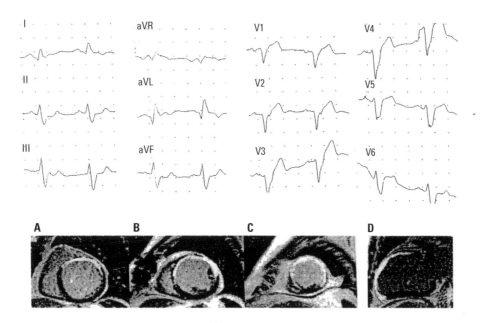

Figure 13.88 The ECG of a patient with complete left bundle branch block (LBBB) and associated infarction. There are ECG features suggestive of extensive anterior myocardial infarction (qR in I, QR in VL, and low voltage of S in V3–V6 with notches suggestive of myocardial infarction (MI) of the anteroseptal zone). The cardiovascular magnetic resonance (CMR) images (A–D) demonstrate the presence of an extensive infarction of anteroapical zone (type A-3) (proximal LAD occlusion). The inferior wall is free of necrosis (see D), because the LAD does not wrap around the apex. In the transverse transection in CMR (A–C), it can be seen that the MI involves most of the anterior and septal walls with also lateral extension, but the high lateral wall is spared (A), because it is perfused by LCX, and the inferior wall because the LAD is not long.

Table 13.10 Sensitivity, specificity, and predictive values of various ECG criteria[a] for patients with acute myocardial infarction, in relation to the specific infarction localization detected by 201 thallium scintigraphy.

ECG Criteria AMI	Sensitivity %				Specificity %	Predictive value %			
	All	AS		I	All	All	AS	A	I
	Controls	A	AMI						
Cabrera's sign[b]	27	47	—	20	87	76	47	12	18
Chapman's sign[c]	21	23	34	—	91	75	33	41	—
Initial (0.04 sec) notching of QRS in II, III, and precordial leads	19	22	13	27	88	67	17	17	34
RS in V$_6$	8	18	—	—	91	50	50	—	—
Abnormal Q in I, aVL, III, aVF, and V$_6$	31	53	27	13	91	83	50	22	11
QV$_6$, RV$_1$	—	20	—	—	100	—	100	—	—
ST elevation[d]	54	76	40	47	97	96	48	22	46
Positive T in leads with positive QRS	8	—	7	20	76	33	—	8	25

[a] Positive response for at least two observers. A: anterior (lateral) infarction; AMI: acute myocardial infarction; AS: anteroseptal infarction; I: interior (posterior) infarction.

[b] Notching of 0.05 sec in duration in the ascendant limb of the S wave in V$_3$–V$_4$.

[c] Notching of ascendant limb of R wave in I, aVL, V$_5$, or V$_6$.

[d] More than 2 mm concordant with main QRS deflection or >7 mm discordant with main deflection.

Adapted with permission from Wackers *et al.* (1978).

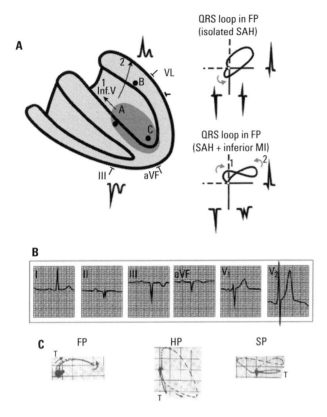

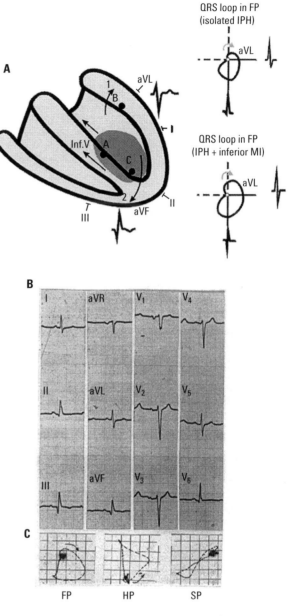

Figure 13.89 Inferior infarction associated with superoanterior hemiblock (SAH). (A) When the necrosis is rather large and comprises the area where ventricular depolarization is initiated in the case of SAH (point A+C), the first vector of ventricular depolarization (1) is neutralized by the infarction vector and the loop first goes directly upward and then, due to the SAH (see lower frontal plane image) instead of rotating in the clockwise direction downward, it rotates in the counterclockwise direction upward (2). Consequently, a QS morphology often develops with slurrings and generally with a negative T wave in III, aVF, and even lead II, but without a terminal "r" wave because the final portion of the loop falls in the negative hemifield of these leads. In the isolated inferior infarction, there is a terminal "r" wave (at least in II), because the final part of the loop that rotates in the clockwise direction is usually in the positive hemifield of inferior leads (at least of lead II). (B,C) ECG–VCG example of the inferior infarction in the presence of SAH.

For further information, see Chapters 14–16 and 20 (also consult Bayés de Luna and Baranchuk 2017; Fiol-Sala *et al.* 2020).

Figure 13.90 Inferior infarction associated with an inferoposterior hemiblock (IPH). (A) The vector of the first part of the activation (the sum of the normal activation initiating vector in the case of an IPH (see B-I) plus the infarction vector moves away from the inferior wall more than would be seen in an isolated IPH and is opposite to the final vector of ventricular depolarization that is directed downward because of the IPH (vector 2). This explains why the QRS loop is moving further upward and opens more than normal, generating the qR (QR) morphology in III and aVF and RS in I and Rs in aVL.

A

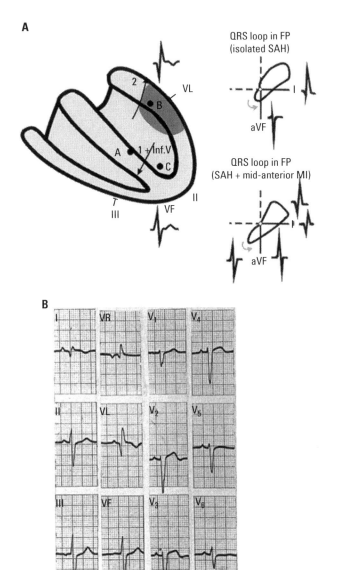

B

Figure 13.91 Mid-anterior infarction associated with superoanterior hemiblock (SAH). (A) The vector of the first part of the activation (that is the sum of vector 1, which is generated in A+C, plus the infarction vector (which moves away from VL) is opposite to the final vector of the ventricular depolarization due to the SAH (vector 2). This explains why the initial part of the QRS loop moves more rightward and downward and generates an RS morphology in II, III, and aVF with RIII > RII and QR in aVL and I. (B) ECG example of mid-anterior infarction (type A-4) plus an SAH.

A

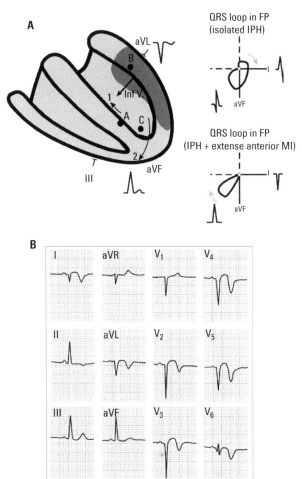

B

Figure 13.92 Extensive anterior infarction including mid-anterior wall associated with inferoposterior hemiblock (IPH). (A) The first ventricular depolarization vector (1) generated in A+B areas in case of isolated IPH is directed upward. However, in the case of extensive anterior infarction plus IPH, the infarction vector (Inf.V) is more important than the first depolarization vector and all the loops move away from the infarcted area in the same direction of the second vector of depolarization (2). Consequently, all the activation (loop) is moving away from aVL and I, which explains the QS morphologies in aVL and sometimes I, with a dominant R wave, generally pure R wave in II, III, and aVF (see the drawings of isolated IPH and IPH + associated anterior myocardial infarction (MI)). (B) ECG of extensive anterior infarction associated with an IPH.

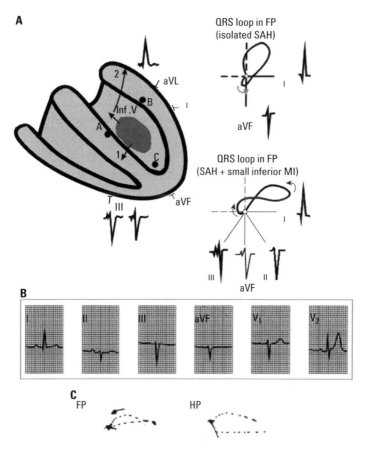

Figure 13.93 Superoanterior hemiblock (SAH) may mask a small inferior infarction. (A) In this situation, when in the presence of an SAH, the area initiating the ventricular depolarization (A–C) is spared by the necrosis, vector 1 that is directed downward and rightward can be only partially counterbalanced by the relatively small infarction vector. This allows the loop to initiate its movement downward and rightward, and then rotates immediately upward. The loop (see the low right side of A) can mask the inferior infarction pattern (QS in III and aVF) and may show as slurred rS morphology and often rIII > rII. (B) ECG–VCG of small inferior infarction plus SAH (see the rotation of QRS loop in the frontal plane that explains the rIII > rII).

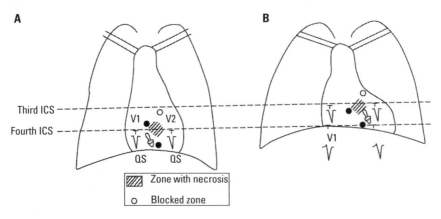

Figure 13.94 (A) Normal habitus. In the presence of small septal infarction with superoanterior hemiblock (SAH), the infarction vector is directed newly backward for the necrosis and downward for the SAH, and in V1 and V2, as in patients without SAH, a QS pattern is recorded. (B) In an obese patient, the same area of necrosis with SAH can produce an rS morphology in V1 and V2, because although the vector is oriented backward and downward, since it is above the normal V1 and V2 due to obesity, the leads at this place record the head of the first vector as positive. In this case, a higher V1–V2 lead (third intercostal space) records the tail of the first vector as QS and confirms the diagnosis of small septal infarction associated with SAH. The two black points represent the onset of depolarization.

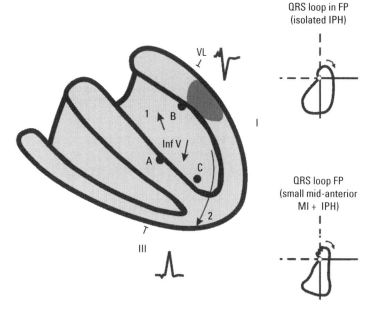

Figure 13.95 Inferoposterior hemiblock (IPH) may mask small mid-anterior infarction. In this situation, when in the presence of an IPH, the ventricular depolarization initiating area (A+B) is spared by the small necrosis, the first vector of depolarization vector 1, which is directed upward, can counteract the relatively small infarction vector (Inf.V). This allows the initial part of the loop to show slurred conduction but directed as in the isolated IPH. This loop (see the right side of the figure) can mask the mid-anterior infarction pattern (QS in aVL and sometimes in lead I) and explains a slurred "r" S morphology in aVL with slurred qR pattern in the inferior leads.

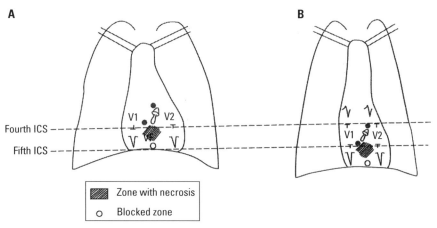

Figure 13.96 (A) Normal habitus. In the presence of small septal infarction with inferoposterior hemiblock (IPH), the infarction vector is directed backward for the necrosis and upward for IPH, and in V1 and V2, as in patients without IPH, a QS pattern is recorded. (B) In a very lean patient, the same area of necrosis in the presence of IPH can generate an rS morphology in V1 and V2, in spite of the backward and upward direction of the vector. These leads record the head of the first vector as positive because they are in a higher position than the normal V1 and V2 due to lean body habitus. In this case, a lower V1–V2 (fifth interspace) records the tail of the first vector as QS and confirms the diagnosis of a small septal infarction associated with IPH. The two black points represent the onset of depolarization.

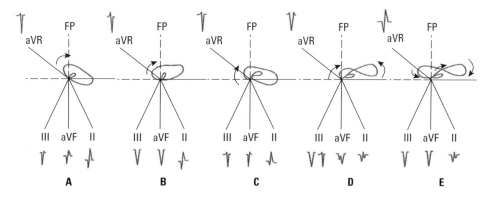

Figure 13.97 Vectorcardiography (VCG) loops in the case of inferior myocardial infarction (MI), in D and E associated with superoanterior hemiblock (SAH). In these latter cases due to a special rotation of the QRS loop, the final part of the loop always falls in the negative hemifield of II. Therefore, the morphology QS (qrs) without terminal r in II, III, and aVF (although a qrs morphology may be seen) and with the presence of terminal r in aVR, favors the presence of associated SAH. In the absence of SAH, even if the entire VCG loop falls above the "x" axis (lead I) (B), there would be always terminal r at least in II, but never terminal r in aVR (A–C).

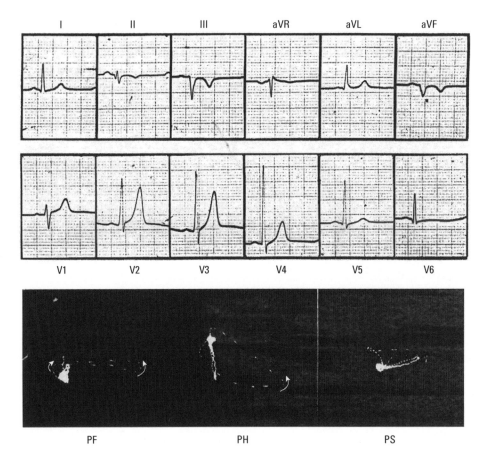

Figure 13.98 ECG–VCG example of inferior myocardial infarction (MI) + superoanterior hemiblock (SAH). There is q wave in II, III, and aVF without terminal r wave (qrs in II and QS in III and aVF). VCG loop in frontal plane rotates first clockwise and then counterclockwise. This explains the final small "r" in aVR (see Figure 13.97). The R in V1 > 3 mm suggests associated lateral MI.

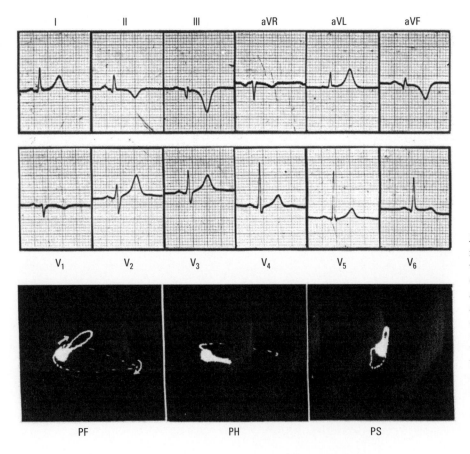

Figure 13.99 ECG–VCG example of inferior myocardial infarction (MI) without superoanterior hemiblock (SAH). There is qR in II, and qr in III and aVF. VCG loop in the frontal plane always rotates clockwise but is directed a little bit more downward than usual in the case of inferior MI. The last part of the QRS loop fails below the "X" axis; lead X is an orthogonal lead, equivalent to lead I. If all the loops rotating clockwise are above the X-axis, the ECG pattern in lead II is qr and not qR, as happens in this figure.

Figure 13.100 Above: ECG of a patient with an intermittent Wolff–Parkinson–White syndrome. In all the leads, the first complex shows no pre-excitation, while the second complex does. In the ECG without pre-excitation, the existence of an apical myocardial infarction can be observed, while in the ECG with pre-excitation, the primary characteristics of repolarization can be seen (symmetric T wave from V2 to V4). Note how the ischemic T wave in the absence of pre-excitation is flat or negative in I and aVL, in contrast to what happens in the absence of ischemic heart disease (Chapter 12). Below: Lead I with progressively pre-excitation activation (concertina effect).

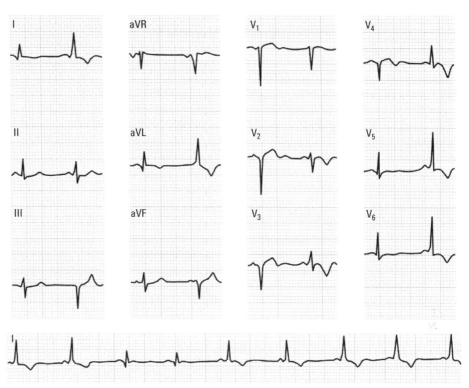

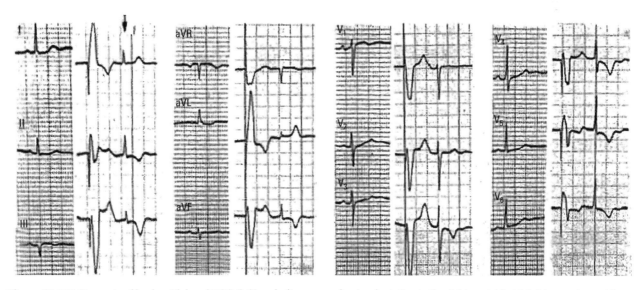

Figure 13.101 Four sets of leads with basal ECG (left) and after pacemaker implantation in the right ventricle (right) in a patient without ischemic heart disease. Note the negative T wave in sinus rhythm complexes after implantation due to "cardiac memory" phenomenon. Characteristically, in the case of "cardiac memory" repolarization, abnormalities in patients without ischemic heart disease, as happens in this case, the T wave is positive in I and aVL in the presence of inverted T waves in the precordial leads.

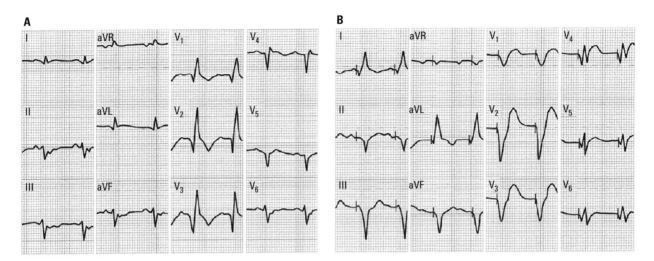

Figure 13.102 (A) Acute anterior myocardial infarction plus complete right bundle branch block (RBBB). (B) The implanted pacemaker still allows for the visualization of the necrosis (spike-qR in I, aVL, and V4–V6).

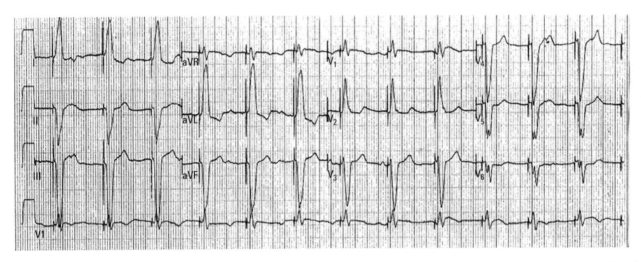

Figure 13.103 A 72-year-old man with previous apical-anterior myocardial infarction (MI) with anteroseptal extension with an implanted pacemaker due to paroxysmal atrioventricular block. There is a clear latency between the stimulus of pacemaker and the QRS complex.

References

Allencherril J, Fakhri Y, Enblom H, *et al.* Appropriateness of anteroseptal myocardial infarction nomenclature evaluated by late gadolinium enhancement cardiovascular magnetic resonance imaging. J Electrocardiol 2018;51:2018.

Bailey RH, LaDue JS, York DJ. Electrocardiographic changes (local ventricular ischemia and injury) produced in the dog by temporary occlusion of a coronary artery, showing a new stage in the evolution of myocardial infarction. Am Heart J 1944;25:164–169.

Barold SS, Falkoff MO, Ong LS, *et al.* Electrocardiographic diagnosis of myocardial infarction during ventricular pacing. Cardiol Clin 1987;5:403.

Bayés de Luna A, Wagner G, Birnbaum Y, *et al.* A new terminology for left ventricular walls and location of myocardial infarcts that present Q wave based on the standard of cardiac magnetic resonance imaging: a statement for healthcare professionals from a committee appointed by the International Society for Holter and Noninvasive Electrocardiography. Circulation 2006a;114:1755.

Bayés de Luna A, Baranchuk A. *Clinical Arrhythmology*, 2nd edn. Wiley-Blackwell, 2017.

Bayés de Luna A, Cino JM, Pujadas S, *et al.* Concordance of electrocardiographic patterns and healed myocardial infarction location detected by cardiovascular magnetic resonance. Am J Cardiol 2006b;97:443.

Bayés de Luna A, Cino J, Goldwasser D, *et al.* New electrocardiographic diagnostic criteria for the pathologic R waves in leads V1 and V2 of anatomically lateral myocardial infarction. J Electrocardiol 2008;41:413.

Bell J, Fox A. Pathogenesis of subendocardial ischemia. Am J Med Sci 1974;268:2.

Ben-Gal AT, Herz I, Solodky A, *et al.* Acute anterior myocardial infarction entailing ST elevation in V1: ECG and angiographic correlations. Clin Cardiol 1998;21:395.

Benchimol A, Desser KB, Shumacher J. Value of the vectorcardiogram for distinguishing left anterior hemiblock from inferior infarction with left axis deviation. Chest 1972;61:74–76.

Birnbaum Y, Atar S. Electrocardiogram risk stratification of non ST elevation acute coronary syndrome. J Electrocardiol 2006;39:558.

Birnbaum Y, Sclarovsky S, Solodky A, *et al.* Predicition of the level of left anterior descending coronary artery obstruction during anterior wall acute myocardial infarction by the admission electrocardiogram. Am J Cardiol 1993a;72:823.

Birnbaum Y, Sclarovsky S, Blum A, *et al.* Prognostic significance of the initial electrocardiographic pattern in a first acute anterior wall myocardial infarction. Chest 1993b;103:1681.

Birnbaum Y, Fiol M, Nikus K, *et al.* A counterpoint paper: comments on the electrocardiographic part of the 2018 Fourth Universal Definition of Myocardial Infarction. J Electrocardiol 2020a; 60: 142.

Birnbaum Y, Fiol M, Nikus K, *et al.* A counterpoint paper: comments on the electrocardiographic part of the 2018 Fourth Universal Definition of Myocardial Infarction endorsed by the International Society of Electrocardiology and the International Society for Holter and Noninvasive Electrocardiology. Ann Noninvasive Electrocardiol 2020b; 00:e12786.

Bough E, Boden W, Kenneth K, Grandsman E. Left ventricular asynergy in electrocardiograhic "posterior" myocardial infarctoin. J Am Coll Cardiol 1984;4:209.

Burnes JE, Ghanem RN, Waldo AL, *et al.* Imaging dispersion of myocardial repolarization, I. Comparison of body-surface and epicardial measures. Circulation 2001;104:1299–1305.

Cabrera E. *Teorí ay práctica de la electrocardiografía.* L La Prensa Médica Mexicana, 1958.

Cannon CP (ed). *Management of Acute Coronary Syndromes,* 2nd edn. Humana, 2003.

Cerqueira MD, Weissman NJ, Disizian V. Standardized myocardial segmentation and nomenclature for tomographic imaging of the heart: a statement for healthcare professionals from the Cardiac Imaging Committee of the Council onClinical Cardiology of the American Heart Association. Circulation 2002;105:539.

Chia B, Yip J, Tan HC, *et al.* Usefulness of ST elevation II/III ratio and ST deviation in lead I for identifying the culprit artery in inferior wall acute myocardial infarction. Am J Cardiol 2000;86:341.

Chou TCH, Surawicz B, Knilans TK. *Electrocardiography in Clinical Practice.* Grune & Stratton, 1974.

Coksey J, Massie E, Walsh T. *Clinical ECG and Vectocardiography.* Year Book Medical, 1960.

Das MK, Khan B, Jacob S, *et al.* Significance of a fragmented QRS complex versus a Q wave in patients with coronary artery disease. Circulation 2006;113:2495.

De Winter R, Wellens H, Wilde A. A new ECG sign of proximal LAD occlusion. N Engl J Med 2008;359:2071.

De Zwan C, Bär H, Wellens HJ. Characteristic ECG pattern indicating a critical stenosis high in left anterior descending coronary artery in patients admitted because of an impending infarction. Am Heart J 1982;103:730.

Dressler W, Roesler H. High T waves in the earliest stage of myocardial infarction. Am Heart J 1947;34:627.

Dunker D, Traverse J, Ishihashi Y. Effect of NO on transmural distribution of blood flow in hyptrophed LV during exercise. Am J Phys 1998;27:H1305.

Dunn W, Edward J, Puitt R. The electrocardiogram in infarction of the lateral wall of the left ventricle: a clinicopathological study. Circulation 1956;14:540.

Engelen DJ, Gorgels AP, Cheriex EC, *et al.* Value of the electrocardiogram in localizing the occlusion site in the left anterior descending coronary artery in acute anterior myocardial infarction. J Am Coll Cardiol 1999;34:389.

Eskola MJ, Nikus KC, Niemela KC, Sclarovsky S. How to use ECG for decision support in the catheterization laboratory. Cases with inferior ST elevation myocardial infarction. J Electrocardiol 2004;37:257.

Fallon J. Pathology of myocardial infarction in atherosclerosis and coronary heart disease. In Fuster V, Ross R, Topol E (eds). *Atherosclerosis and Coronary Artery Disease.* Lippincott–Raven Press, 1996. Vol. I, p. 791

Fiol M, Carrillo A, Cygankiewicz I, *et al.* New criteria based on ST changes in 12 leads surface ECG to detect proximal vs distal right coronary artery occlusion in case of an acute inferoposterior myocardial infarction. Ann Noninvasive Electrocardiol 2004a;9:383.

Fiol M, Cygankiewicz I, Bayés Genis A, *et al.* The value of ECG algorithm based on "ups and downs" of ST in assessment of a culprit artery in evolving inferior myocardial infarction. Am J Cardiol 2004b;94:709.

Fiol M, Carrillo A, Cygankiewicz I, *et al.* A new electrocardiographic algorithm to locate the occlusion in left anterior descending coronary artery. Clin Cardiol 2009;32:E1.

Fiol-Sala M, Birnbaum Y, Nikus K, Bayés de Luna A. *Electrocardiography in Ischemic Heart Disease. Clinical and Imaging Correlations and Prognostic Implications,* 2nd edn. Willey-Blackwell, 2020.

Franz MR. Long-term recording of monophasic action potentials from human endocardium. Am J Cardiol 1983;51:1629.

Garcia Niebla J. Llontop-García P, Valle-Racero JI, *et al.* Technical mistakes during the acquisition of the electrocardiogram. Ann Noninvasive Electrocardiol 2009;14:389.

Hellerstein A, Katz C. The electrical effects of injury at various myocardial locations. Am Heart J 1948;36:184.

Horan LG, Flowers NC, Johnson JC. Significance of the diagnostic Q wave of myocardial infarction. Circulation 1971;43:428.

Huang H, Tran V, Jneid H, *et al.* Comparison of angiographic findings in patients with acute anteroseptal versus anterior wall ST-elevation myocardial infarction. Am J Cardiol 2011;107:827.

Huang X, Ramdhany SK, Zhang Y, Yuan Z, Mintz GS, Guo N. New ST-segment algorithms to determine culprit artery location in acute inferior myocardial infarction. Heart 2016;102:1396

Janse MJ. Electrophysiological changes in acute myocardial ischemia. In Julian DG, Lie KI, Wihelmsen L (eds). *What Is Angina? Astra,* 1982, p. 160.

Katz R. *Electrophysiology of the Heart.* Mosby Co., 2001.

Kenigsberg D, Kanal S, Kowalski M. Prolongation of the QTc interval is seen uniformly during early transmural ischemia. J Am Coll Cardiol 2007;49:1299.

Khuri SF, Flaherty JT, O'Riordan JB, *et al.* Changes in intramyocardial ST segment voltage and gas tensions with regional myocardial ischemia in the dog. Circ Res 1975;37:455.

Kosuge M, Ebene T, Hubi K, *et al.* An early and simple predictor of severe left main and/or three-vessel diseases in patients with non-ST segment elevation acute coronary syndrome. Am J Cardiol 2011;107:495.

Lengyel L, Caramelli Z, Monfort J, et al. Initial ECG changes in experimental occlusion of the coronary arteries in non-anesthetized dogs with closed thorax. Am Heart J 1957;53:334.

Lopes RD, Siha H, Fu Y, et al. Diagnosing acute myocardial infarction in patients with left bundle branch block. Am J Cardiol 2011;108:782

Madias J, Sinha A, Ashtiani R. A critique of the new ST-segment criteria for the diagnosis of acute myocardial infarction in patients with left bundle-branch block. Clin Cardiol 2001;24:652.

Marholdt H, Wagner A, Judd RM, et al. Delayed enhancement cardiovascular magnetic resonance assessment of non-ischaemic cardiomyopathies. Eur Heart J 2005;26:1461.

Migliore F, Zorzi A, Perazzolo Marra M, et al. Myocardial edema underlies dynamic T-wave inversion (Wellens' ECG pattern) in patients with reversible left ventricular dysfunction. Heart Rhythm 2011;8:1629.

Moon JC, De Arenaza DP, Elkington AG, et al. The pathologic basis of Q-wave and non-Q-wave myocardial infarction: a cardiovascular magnetic resonance study. J Am Coll Cardiol 2004;44:554.

Morita H, Kusano KF, Miura D et al. Fragmented QRS as a marker of conduction abnormality and a predictor of prognosis of Brugada syndrome. Circulation 2008;118:1697.

Nesto R, Kowaldruk G. The ischemic cascade: temporal sequence of hemodynamic, electrocardiographic, and symptomatic expressions of ischemia. Am J Cardiol 1987;57:23C.

Nikus K, Pahlm O, Wagner G, et al. Electrocardiographic classification of acute coronary syndromes: a review by a committee of the International Society for Holter and Non-Invasive Electrocardiology. J Electrocardiol 2010;43:91.

Perloff J. The recognition of strictly posterior myocardial infarction by conventional scalar elelctrocardiography. Circulation 1964;30:706.

Pride Y, Tung P, Mohanavelu S, et al. Angiographic and clinical outcomes among patients with acute coronary syndrome with isolated anterior ST depression: A TRITON TIMI 38 Substudy. J Am Coll Cardiol 2010;3:806.

Reimer KA, Hill ML, Jennings RB. Prolonged depletion of ATP and the ademine nucleotide pool due to delayed resynthesis of adenine nucleotides following reversible myocardial ischemic injury in dogs. J Mol Cell Cardiol 1981;13:229.

Rosenbaum MB, Elizari MV, Lazzari JO. *Los Hemibloqueos*. Editorial Paidos, 1968.

Rosenbaum MB, Blanco H, Elizari MV, et al. Electrotonic modulation of the T wave and cardiac memory. Am J Cardiol 1982;50:213.

Rovai D, Di Bella G, Rossi G, et al. Q-wave prediction of myocardila infarct location, size and transmural extent at magnetic resonance imaging. Coron Artery Dis 2007;18:381.

Sagie A, Sclarovsky S, Strasberg B et al. Acute anterior wall myocardial infarction presenting with positive T waves and without ST segment shift. Electrocardiographic features and angiographic correlation. Chest 1989;95:1211.

Samson W, Scher A. Mechanisms of ST segment alterations during myocardial injury. Circulation 1960;8:780.

Sclarovsky S. *Electrocardiography of Acute Coronary Syndrome*. Martin Dunitz Ltd., London, 1999.

Sgarbossa EB, Pinski SL, Barbagelata A et al. Electrocardiographic diagnosis of evolving acute myocardial infarction in the presence of left bundle branch block. GUSTO-1 (Global Utilization of Streptokinase and tissue Plasminogen Activator for Occludded Coronary Arteries) Investigators. N Engl J Med 1996a;334:481.

Sgarbossa E, Pinski S, Gates KB, Wagner GS. Early ECG diagnosis of acute MI in the presence of ventricular paced rhythm. Am J Card 1996b;77:42.

Singer DH, Ten Eick RE. Aberrancy: elecrophysiologic aspects. Am J Cardiol 1971;28:381.

Sodi Pallares D, Rodríguez H. Morphology of the unipolar leads recorded at the septal surface: its application to diagnosis of left bundle branch block complicated by myocardial infarction. Am Heart J 1952;43:27.

Sodi D, Calder N. *New Basis of Electrocardiography*. Mosby, 1956.

Surawicz B, Uhley H, Brown R, et al. Task force I: standarization of terminology and interpretation. Am J Cardiol 1978;41:130.

Thygesen K, Alpert JS, Jaffe LS, et al. Fourth universal definition ofmyocardial infarction (2018). Eur Heart J 2019;40:237–269.

Tierala I, Nikus K, Sclarovsky S, et al. (HAAMU Study Group). Predicting the culprit artery in acute ST-elevation myocardial infarction and introducing a new algorithm to predict infarct-related artery in inferior ST-elevation myocardial infarction: correlation with coronary anatomy in the HAAMU Trial. J Electrocardiology 2009;42:120.

Van der Weg K, Bekkers SCAM, Winkens B, et al. on behalf of MAST. The R in V1 in non-anterior wall infarction indicates lateral rather than posterior involvement. Results from ECG/MRI correlations. Eur Heart J 2009;30(suppl):P2981K.

Wackers F, Lie KL, David G, et al. Assessment of the value of the ECG signs for myocardial infarction in left bundle branch block by thallium. Am J Cardiol 1978;41:428.

Wellens HJ. The value of the right precordial leads of the electrocardiogram. N Engl J Med 1999;340:381.

Wellens HJ. Recognizing those ECG that distinguish you as a smart clinician. Cardiosource Rev J 2006;15:71.

Wellens HJ, Gorgels A, Doevendans PA. *The ECG in Acute Myocardial Infarction and Unstable Angina*. Kluwer Academic, 2003.

Wong CK, French JK, Aylward PE, et al. HERO-2 Trial Investigators. Patients with prolonged ischemic chest pain and presumed-new left bundle branch block have heterogeneous outcomes depending on the presence of ST-segment changes. J Am Coll Cardiol 2005;46:29.

Wong CK, Gao W, Raffel OC, et al. HEERO-2 Investigators. Initial Q waves accompanying ST-segment elevation at presentation of acute myocardial infarction and 30-day mortality in patients given streptokinase therapy. An analysis from HERO-2. Lancet 2006a;367:2061.

Wong CK, Gao W, Stewart RA, et al. Hirulog Early Reperfusion Occluson (HERO-2) Investigators. Risk stratification of patients with acute anterior myocardial infarction and right bundle-branch block: importance of QRS duration and early ST-segment resolution after fibrinolytic therapy. Circulation 2006b;114:783.

Zhong-Qu Z, Wer W, Jun-Feng W. Does the LAD acute occlusion proximal to the first septal perforator counteract ST elevation in leads V5-V6?. J Electrocardiol 2009;42:52.

Part 4
Arrhythmias

Chapter 14
Mechanisms, Classification, and Clinical Aspects of Arrhythmias

Concept

Arrhythmias are defined as **any cardiac rhythms other than the normal sinus rhythm.** Sinus rhythm originates in the sinus node. **The ECG** characteristics of normal **sinus rhythm are as follows:**
• A sinus stimulus generated in a sinus node and subsequently is transmitted at appropriate rates of conduction transmitted through atria (P wave), the atrioventricular (AV) junction, and the intraventricular specific conduction system (ISCS). It initiates a positive P wave in I, II, aVF, V2–V6, and positive or +– in leads III and V1.
• In adults, in the absence of pre-excitation, the PR interval ranges from 0.12 to 0.20 sec.
• At rest, the sinus node discharge cadence ranges from 60 to 80 beats per minute (bpm) and tends to be regular, although it shows generally slight variations, which are not evident by palpation or auscultation. Under normal conditions, however, and particularly in children, it may show slight to moderate changes depending on the phases of respiration, with the heart rate increasing with inspiration. Thus, the evidence of a completely fixed heart rate both during the day and at night is suggestive of alterations of the heart rhythm, usually associated to certain degree of autonomic nervous system (ANS) dysfunction.

It is important to remember that:
• **The term arrhythmia does not mean rhythm irregularity**, as regular arrhythmias can occur, often with absolute stability (i.e. atrial flutter, paroxysmal atrial tachycardia, etc.), sometimes presenting with heart rates in the normal range, as is the case of atrial flutter with 4:1 AV conduction. On the other hand, some irregular rhythms should not be considered arrhythmias (mild to moderate irregularity in the sinus discharge, particularly when linked to respiration, as already stated, also known as sinus respiratory arrhythmia).
• **A diagnosis of arrhythmia in itself does not mean pathology**. In fact, in healthy subjects, the sporadic presence of certain arrhythmias, both active (premature complexes) and passive (escape complexes, certain degree of AV block, sinus respiratory arrhythmia, etc.), is frequently observed.

Classification

There are various ways to classify cardiac arrhythmias.
• **According to the site of origin:** Arrhythmias are divided into supraventricular (including those having their origin in the sinus node, the atria, and the AV junction), and ventricular arrhythmias.
• **According to the underlying mechanism:** Arrhythmias may be explained by: (i) abnormal formation of impulses (increased automaticity and triggered activity); (ii) reentry of different types; (iii) decreased automaticity; and (iv) disturbances of conduction (see later).
• **From the clinical point of view**: Arrhythmias may be **paroxysmal, incessant, or permanent.** The first occurs suddenly and usually disappears spontaneously (i.e. AV junctional reentrant paroxysmal tachycardia or paroxysmal AV block), **permanent** are always present (i.e. permanent atrial fibrillation), and **incessant** are characterized by intermittent but repetitive presence.
• **Finally, from an electrocardiographic point of view,** arrhythmias may be divided into either **active or passive** (Table 14.1):
a. **Active arrhythmias**, due to increased automaticity, reentry, or triggered electrical activity (see later and Table 14.2), generate isolated or repetitive premature complexes on the ECG, which occur before the cadence of the regular sinus rhythm. **Premature complexes** may be produced in a parasystolic or extrasystolic ectopic focus that may be supraventricular or ventricular. The extrasystolic mechanism has a fixed coupling interval, whereas the parasystolic has a varied coupling interval. **Premature and repetitive complexes** include all types of supraventricular or ventricular tachyarrhythmias (tachycardias, fibrillation, flutter). In active cardiac arrhythmias, due to classic reen-

Clinical Electrocardiography: A Textbook, Fifth Edition. Antoni Bayés de Luna, Miquel Fiol-Sala, Antoni Bayés-Genís, and Adrián Baranchuk.
© 2022 John Wiley & Sons Ltd. Published 2022 by John Wiley & Sons Ltd.

Table 14.1 Classification of arrhythmias according to their electrocardiographical presentation

Active arrhythmias	Passive arrhythmias
Supraventricular	Escape complex
Premature complexes	Escape rhythm
Tachyarrhythmias	Sinus bradycardia
Different types of tachycardia	Sinoatrial block
Atrial fibrillation	Atrial block
Atrial flutter	Atrioventricular block
Ventricular	Ventricular block
Premature complexes	Aberrant conduction
Different types of tachycardia	Cardiac arrest
Ventricular flutter	
Ventricular fibrillation	

trant mechanisms, a unidirectional block exists in some part of the circuit.

b. **Passive arrhythmias** occur when cardiac stimuli formation and/or conduction are below the range of normality due to a depression of the automatism and/or a stimulus conduction block in the atria, the AV junction, or the specific intraventricular conduction systems (ICS).

From an electrocardiographic point of view, many passive cardiac arrhythmias show a slower than expected heart rate (**bradyarrhythmia**). However, some type of conduction delay or block in some place of the specific conduction systems (SCS) may exist without slow rate, for example, first-degree or some second-degree sinoatrial or AV blocks. Thus, the electrocardiographic diagnosis of passive cardiac arrhythmia can be made because it may be demonstrated that the ECG changes are due to a depression of automatism and/or conduction in some part of the SCS, without this manifesting in the ECG as a premature complex, as it does in reentry. Therefore, atrial or ventricular blocks may be considered arrhythmias. In this book, we have discussed them as a separate entity in Chapters 9 and 10.

Clinical significance and symptoms

The incidence of the majority of arrhythmias increases progressively with age, and arrhythmias are less frequent in children (some exceptions apply like arrhythmias associated to congenital heart diseases and channelopathies

Table 14.2 Mechanisms involved in the main supraventricular and ventricular tachyarrhythmias

Arrhythmia	Main mechanism	Heart rate (bpm)
Sinus tachycardia	↑ automaticity	>90
	Sinoatrial reentry	100–180
Monomorphic atrial tachycardia (Tables 15.4–15.6)	Focus origin (micro-reentry, ↑ automaticity or triggered activity)	90–40 (incessant tachycardia)Till 200–220 (macro-reentrant paroxysmal tachycardia)
	Macro-reentry	If >220, it is considered an atypical flutter
Junctional ectopic tachycardia	Abnormal generation of stimuli	100–180
Junctional reentrant tachycardia		140–200 (paroxysmal tachycardia)
• Reentry only through AV junctional circuit	Reentry in circuit exclusively comprising the AV junction	
• Reentry circuit with anomalous pathway involvement	Reentry in circuit involving also an anomalous pathway (may be paroxysmal or incessant)	Generally <140 (incessant tachycardia)
Chaotic atrial tachycardia	Multiple atrial foci	100–200
Atrial fibrillation	Micro-reentry	350–700 (atrial waves)
	Automatic focus with fibrillatory conduction	
	Rotors with fibrillatory conduction	
Atrial flutter	Macro-reentry	Generally, 240–300 with AV conduction mainly 2 × 1
Classic VT with structural heart disease	Reentry with anatomical or functional circuit (rotors)	From 110 to >200
VT/VF in channelopathies	In most of the cases (long and short QT, and Brugada syndrome) due to differences in the duration and/or the morphology of AP at different myocardial areas	From 140 to >200
Idioventricular rhythm	Increase of automaticity	60–100
VT with narrow QRS	Usually reentry (verapamil-sensitive)	120–160
Parasystolic VT	Protected automatic focus	Generally <140
Torsades de pointes VT	Post-potentials and/or rotors	160–250
VT with no evident heart disease	Triggered activity, reentry or automaticity increase	110–200
Ventricular flutter	Macro-reentry	250–350
Ventricular fibrillation	Micro-reentry with fibrillatory conduction	>400
	Automatic focus with fibrillatory conduction	
	Rotors with fibrillatory conduction	

TAP: transmembrane action potential; VT: ventricular tachyarrhythmia.

(see Brugada syndrome). Data from Holter ECG recordings (see Chapter 25, Holter electrocardiographic monitoring and related techniques) have demonstrated that some isolated premature ventricular complexes (PVC) are present in about 10–20% of young people in 24-hour recordings, and their presence is nearly a rule in the 80+ age group. Similarly, sustained chronic arrhythmias, such as atrial fibrillation, are exceptional in children but are present in about 10% of subjects over 80 years of age. However, **there are arrhythmias that arise particularly in children**, such as some paroxysmal AV junctional reentrant tachycardias using accessory pathways (AVRT), some ectopic junctional tachycardias, as well as some monomorphic ventricular tachycardias (idiopathic), and polymorphic ventricular tachycardias (catecholaminergic). Finally, there are also some cases of congenital AV block.

The most important clinical significance of arrhythmias is related to an **association with sudden cardiac death** (Bayés de Luna and Baranchuk, 2017; Goldstein *et al.* 1994). It is also important to remember that frequently arrhythmias, especially atrial fibrillation, may lead to embolism, including cerebral embolism, sometimes with severe consequences. Also, fast arrhythmias may trigger or worsen heart failure. For further information, consult general references on *Recommended Reading*.

ECG diagnosis of arrhythmias: preliminary considerations

To make a valid ECG interpretation of an arrhythmia and understand the electrophysiologic mechanism that may explain its presence, it may be useful to consider the following tips and recommendations.

• **It is advisable to have a magnifying glass** and a pair of compasses. They may be used to accurately measure the wave duration, the distance between P waves or QRS complexes, the differences in the coupling interval (distance between a premature P wave or QRS complex and the P wave or QRS complex of the preceding basal rhythm), etc. In the modern digital era, amplification of images is simply done using electronic tools. Semiautomatic calipers are also available and measurements are considered more reproducible.

• **It is helpful to take long strips of the ECG tracing** (this is especially important in the case of possible parasystole) **and to record 12-lead ECGs**. This will help to perform the differential diagnosis of ventricular versus supraventricular tachycardias with aberrancy, and it will also help to determine the site of origin and mechanisms of supraventricular and ventricular arrhythmias.

• **In the case of paroxysmal tachycardias, a long strip should be recorded during carotid sinus massage**, and some maneuvers (deep inspiration and Valsalva, as well as other vagal maneuvers) performed for diagnostic and therapeutic purposes (Figure 14.1).

• It is necessary **to obtain ECG recordings during exercise testing**, both in patients with premature complexes, in order to verify if they increase or decrease, and in patients with bradyarrhythmias, to identify an abrupt or gradual acceleration. If acceleration is abrupt, and the heart rate is doubled or even more, this indicates a 2:1 sinoatrial block. If acceleration is gradual, this indicates a bradycardia due to depression or automatism.

• It is useful **to have an overall patient history and previous ECGs**, especially in patients with potential pre-excitation syndrome or in patients with wide QRS complex tachycardias.

• **The "secret" to making a correct diagnosis of arrhythmia is to properly detect and analyze the atrial and ventricular activity and to look at the AV relationship.** For this purpose, over 80 years ago Lewis created some diagrams that are still considered very useful today (Johnson and Denes 2008; Antiperovitch *et al.* 2019). In most cases, only three areas are required to explain the site of onset and the stimulus pathway: atria, AV junction, and ventricles (Figures 14.2–14.4).

• It is convenient **to determine the sensitivity, specificity, and predictive value of the different signs and diagnostic criteria**. This is especially important when performing differential diagnosis in the case of wide QRS tachycardia, between ventricular tachycardia and supraventricular tachycardia with aberrancy (see Chapter 25).

• As previously stated, **it is often necessary to perform special techniques**, such as exercise testing, Holter ECG recording, amplified waves, EPS, imaging techniques, etc., to better understand the prevalence of arrhythmias, the electrophysiologic mechanisms that may explain them, and the correct diagnosis, as well as for prognostic evaluation and the prescription of a particular treatment (see Chapter 25 and Bayés de Luna and Baranchuk, 2017).

Mechanisms responsible for active cardiac arrhythmias

Frequently, active arrhythmias **are triggered by one mechanism and perpetuated by another.** In addition, there are **modulating factors** (unbalanced ANS, ischemia, ionic and metabolic alterations, stress, alcohol and coffee consumption, etc.) that favor the appearance and maintenance of arrhythmias.

When analyzing **tachyarrhythmias**, we can use the analogy of a burning forest (see Table 14.1). The fire may be triggered by a match (premature impulse), but for the fire **to perpetuate,** the bushes and trees (i.e. substrate) must be dry enough. There are many **modulating** factors having an impact on whether the fire (arrhythmia) starts sooner and is perpetuated, such as

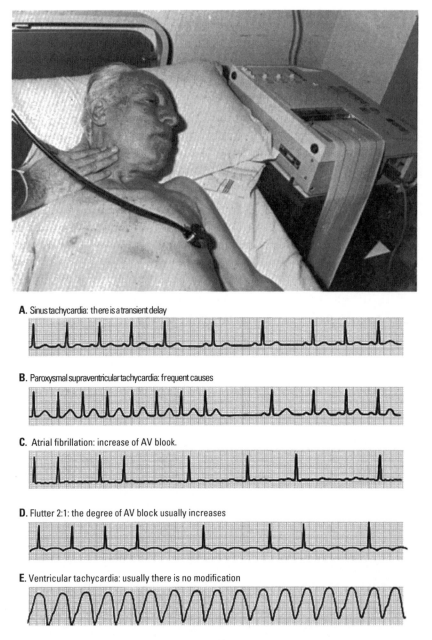

A. Sinus tachycardia: there is a transient delay

B. Paroxysmal supraventricular tachycardia: frequent causes

C. Atrial fibrillation: increase of AV blook.

D. Flutter 2:1: the degree of AV block usually increases

E. Ventricular tachycardia: usually there is no modification

Figure 14.1 Note the correct procedure for carotid sinus massage (CSM). The force applied with the fingers should be similar to that required to squeeze a tennis ball, during a short time period (10–15seconds), and the procedure should be repeated four to five times on either side, starting on the right side. Never perform this procedure on both sides at the same time. It is advisable to auscultate the neck before proceeding with CSM. Caution should be taken in older people and in patients with a history of carotid sinus syndrome. The procedure must include continuous ECG recording and auscultation. A–E: examples of how different arrhythmias react to CSM.

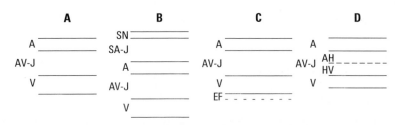

Figure 14.2 Several examples of Lewis (ladder) diagrams including: (A) the atrioventricular (AV) junction, (B) the AV and sinoatrial (SA) junctions, (C) a ventricular arrhythmogenic focus, and (D) a division of the AV junction in two parts (AH–HV).

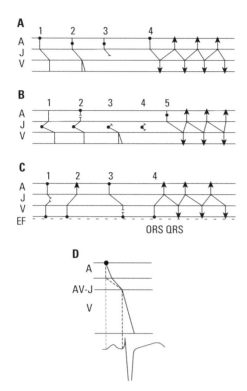

Figure 14.3 (A) (1) Normal atrioventricular (AV) conduction, (2) premature atrial impulse (complex) with aberrant conduction; (3) premature atrial impulse blocked at the AV junction; (4) sinus impulse with slow AV conduction that initiates an AV junctional reentrant tachycardia. (B) (1) Premature junctional impulse with an anterograde conduction slower than the retrograde; (2) premature junctional impulse sharing atrial depolarization with a sinus impulse (atrial fusion complex); (3) premature junctional impulse with exclusive anterograde conduction and, in this case, with aberrancy (see the two lines in the ventricular space); (4) premature junctional impulse concealed anterogradely and retrogradely; (5) premature atrial impulse leading to AV junctional reentrant tachycardia. (C) (1) Sinus impulse and premature ventricular impulse that cancel mutually at the AV junction; (2) premature ventricular impulse with retrograde conduction to the atria; (3) sinus impulse sharing ventricular depolarization with a premature ventricular impulse (ventricular fusion beat); (4) premature ventricular impulse triggering an AV junctional reentrant tachycardia. (D) Shows the way of the stimulus through the AV junction as per the diagram shown in Figure 14.2 A. The solid line shows the real way of the stimulus across the heart. In general, the dashed line is used instead, because it is the place at which the atrial and ventricular activity starts. Thus, the time that the stimulus spends to cross the AV junction, the most important information, is more visible. EF: ectopic focus.

wind or heat (equivalent to tachycardia, instability of the ANS, ischemia, etc.), or is extinguished early, such as rain or cold (equivalent to the stability of the ANS, sympathetic nervous system integrity, etc.).

We will now look at the specific mechanisms that initiate and perpetuate different arrhythmias. We will further discuss the triggering and/or modulating factors when

we examine each particular arrhythmia in the following chapters.

Active arrhythmias may be related to the basal rhythm or occur independently. In the first case, the premature isolated P′ or QRS complex, or the first P′ wave or QRS complex in rapid rhythms, displays a **fixed or nearly fixed coupling interval** in the ECG. This is because the arrhythmia is initiated by a mechanism that depends on the previous basal rhythm. The coupling interval is defined as the time from the onset of the preceding QRS complex (if the active arrhythmia is a ventricular arrhythmia), or the P′ wave (if it is an atrial arrhythmia), to the beginning of the ectopic P′ or QRS complex (Figure 14.5A,B).

The active arrhythmias independent of the baseline rhythm are much less frequent. Usually they are isolated complexes of parasystolic origin and nearly always have a **remarkable variable coupling interval** (Figure 14.5C,D). These arrhythmias rarely occur as sustained tachycardias (see Chapter 16). We will now discuss the ECG features of these two types of active arrhythmias.

The different mechanisms of active arrhythmias are shown in Table 14.2.

Active arrhythmias with fixed coupling interval

Active arrhythmias appearing as isolated complexes or repetitive runs of several complexes (non-sustained tachycardia) usually show a fixed coupling interval of the first complex (Figure 14.5A,B). Parasystolic active arrhythmias have a variable coupling interval of the first complex (see Active arrhythmias with variable coupling interval: the parasystole, below) (Figure 14.5C,D).

Abnormal generation of stimulus

Increased automaticity

Automaticity is the capacity of some cardiac cells (the automatic slow response cells present in the sinus node and to a lesser degree in the AV node) to not only excite themselves but also to produce stimuli that can propagate (Figure 14.6). Therefore, automatic cells excite themselves and produce stimuli that may propagate, whereas contractile cells are only excited by a stimulus from a neighboring cell, transmitting it to the nearest cell (domino effect theory) (see Figure 5.26). Under normal conditions, contractile cells are not automatic cells because they do not excite themselves.

Certain electrophysiologic characteristics of the automatic cells derive from the ionic currents responsible for the ascending slope of transmembrane diastolic potential (DP) (phase 4). In particular, the rapid inactivation

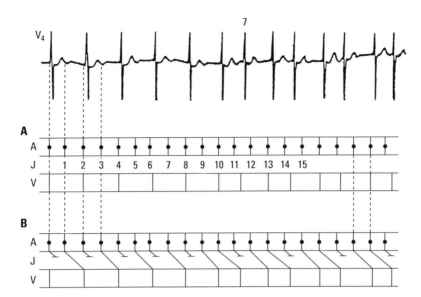

Figure 14.4 Placement of atrial and ventricular waves within the atrial and ventricular spaces, as seen at first glance (A). Although at first glance we do not see two atrial P waves for each QRS, we presume that atrial waves are ectopic (negative in V4 and very fast) (see arrows), and double than the QRS complexes, one visible and the other hidden within the QRS. This is confirmed when we carefully check the bigeminal rhythm. Later on we joined the atrial and ventricular waves through the AV junction (B). These data come from a patient with cardiomyopathy and digitalis intoxication, showing an atrial rate of 150 bpm and a first ventricular rate of 75 bpm. Later on, they are shown as coupled bigeminal complexes. This is an example of ectopic atrial tachycardia with 2×1 AV block and later Wenckebach 3×2 AV block. The atrial waves are ectopic because their morphology differs from sinus P waves seen in previous ECG, and because there are very narrow (50 ms) and negative in V4. The digitalis intoxication explains the presence of AV block. The first, third, fifth, seventh, and ninth P′ waves conduct with long PR interval. The seventh QRS complex (7) is premature and starts a series of coupled complexes (bigeminal rhythm). This complex is probably not caused by the eleventh atrial wave, as the corresponding P′R lasts only 180 ms, whereas the other conducted atrial waves (P′), with the same coupling interval, show a P′R of 400 ms. Instead, the tenth atrial wave (P′) may be conducted with a P′R of 0,56; and therefore the eleventh P′ is not conducted. The sequence: P′R = 400 ms, P′R = 560 ms, P′ not conducted is afterward repeated, perpetuating the Wenckebach sequence where the twelfth and thirteenth P′ waves are conducted, whereas the fourteenth is not, etc.

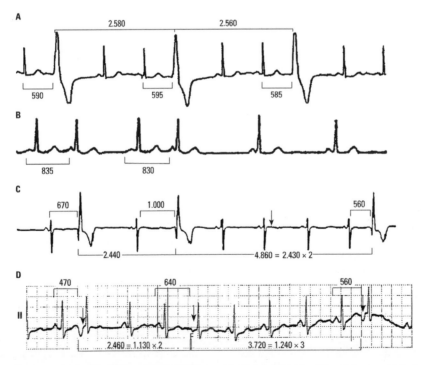

Figure 14.5 (A) Ventricular extrasystole; (B) atrial extrasystole; (C) ventricular parasystole; (D) atrial parasystole (see text). All numbers are expressed in milliseconds.

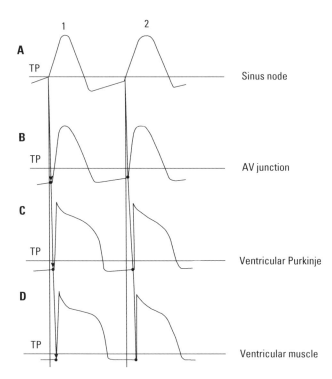

Figure 14.6 Sinus node transmembrane action potential (TAP) (A) transmitted to the atrioventricular (AV) junction (B), the ventricular Purkinje (C), and ventricular muscle (D).

during diastole of the outward K (I_p) current by the inward diastolic current I_f has an impact on heart rate (see Chapter 5). The **most important characteristics are as follows**:

• **The rate of rise of DP (phase 4)**: the faster the rise, the faster the heart rate and vice versa (Figure 14.7A).

• **The level or threshold potential (TP)**: the lower heart (further from 0), the faster the heart rate and vice versa (Figure 14.7B).

• **The baseline level of the previous DP**: the more negative (further from 0), the lower the heart rate and vice versa (Figure 14.7C).

The modifications of these three factors account, in general, for the increase or decrease of the heart automaticity (Figure 14.8). Under normal conditions, the sinus automaticity is transmitted to the AV node and then to the ventricle (see arrows in Figure 14.8), immediately after which these two structures depolarize.

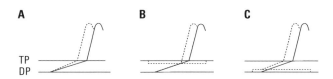

Figure 14.7 Factors influencing the increase of automaticity (broken lines). (A) Faster diastolic depolarization. (B) Threshold potential (TP) decrease. (C) Transmembrane diastolic potential (DP) less negative than normal.

The top part of Figure 14.8 shows how the normal sinus automaticity (1 and 2) produces a transmembrane action potential (AP) capable of propagating itself (B1 and C1). If for any of the reasons previously mentioned, such as reduced rate of the DP rise (b and b′), a lower baseline DP level (c), or a TP level nearer 0 (d), the normal sinus automaticity (a) decreases, the AP curve will not form in time (Figure 14.8: continuous line 2) but later, decreasing the sinus automaticity (A: broken line 2b). On the other hand, through an opposite mechanism, the sinus automaticity will increase and AP generation will take less time. This happens in the case of increase of the phase 4 slope of the AV node or ventricular cells (Figure 14.8 Bh and Ci). The decrease of level of TP or an increase in baseline level of the previous DP, explains the occurrence of active arrhythmias due to an increased automaticity (Figures 14.7 and 14.8). The effect of all these phenomena on the ECG becomes evident with the presence of heart rate variations under sinus rhythm (sinus bradycardia and tachycardia) and the presence of premature or late supraventricular and ventricular QRS complexes (see right side of Figure 14.8, and legend).

At least 10% of paroxysmal supraventricular tachycardias, as well as some ventricular tachycardias and supraventricular and ventricular premature complexes (extrasystoles) with fixed or nearly fixed coupling intervals, **are caused by increased automaticity.** It has been found (Haïssaguerre *et al.* 1998) that premature atrial impulses arising around the pulmonary veins trigger most paroxysmal atrial fibrillations in the absence of significant heart disease.

Triggered electrical activity

Another mechanism that can produce active arrhythmias with fixed or nearly fixed coupling intervals due to an abnormal generation of stimulus is the triggered electrical activity (Antoons *et al.* 2007; Wit and Boyden 2007). This is due to the presence of **early or late post-potentials** significant enough that their oscillatory vibrations initiate a response that can be propagated (Figure 14.9).

Reentry

Reentry is the mechanism that explains many active arrhythmias, the majority of premature complexes, and tachyarrhythmias.

Classical concept

The classical concept of reentry (Moe and Méndez 1966) involves an active wave front propagating around an anatomic circuit in such a way that the wave front loops back on itself (reentry). For this phenomenon to exist, **three conditions** are necessary: **(i) the presence of a circuit, (ii) a unidirectional block in part of the circuit,**

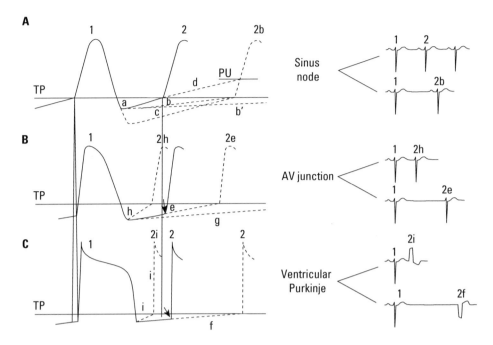

Figure 14.8 (A) Sinus node transmembrane action potential (AP) curve. (B) Atrioventricular (AV) junction TAP curve. (C) Ventricular Purkinje AP curve. It is observed how under normal conditions the stimulus is propagated from the sinus node to the AV junction and to the ventricular Purkinje system, before these structures reach the threshold potential (TP) by means of their own automaticity. **Left:** See the lines joining the APs of the sinus node, the AV junction, and the ventricular Purkinje system. This figure shows the generation of active and passive arrhythmias due to disturbances of automaticity: (a) normal diastolic depolarization curve of the sinus node; (b) diminished diastolic depolarization curve; (c) diastolic depolarization curve of sinus node with normal rate of rise but starting at a lower level; (d) normal diastolic depolarization curve with a less negative TP; (e) normal diastolic depolarization curve of the AV junction; note that before this curve is complete (i.e. before it reaches the TP), the sinus stimulus (arrow) initiates a new AP (end of the continuous line in "e"); (f) normal diastolic depolarization curve of a ventricular Purkinje fiber (the same as in "e" applies); (g) marked decrease of the automaticity of the AV junction; (h) increase of automaticity of the AV junction; (i) increased automaticity in ventricular Purkinje fibers. Therefore, under pathologic conditions, the increased automaticity of the AV junction (h) and the ventricular Purkinje system (i) may be greater than that of the sinus node (active rhythms). Alternatively, the normal automaticity of the AV junction (broken lines in "e" and "g") or the ventricle (broken line in "f") may substitute the sinus depressed automaticity (b and b') (passive rhythms). Right: ECG examples of the different electrophysiologic situations commented on (normal sinus rhythm: 1–2; sinus bradycardia: 1–2b; junctional extrasystole: 1–2h; junctional escape complex 1–2e; ventricular extrasystole: 1–2i and ventricular escape complex: 1–2f).

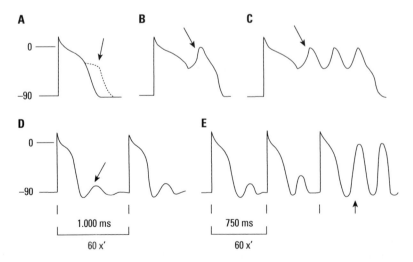

Figure 14.9 The presence of early (A–C) and late (D and E) post-potentials is the mechanism that explains the occurrence of early stimuli (complexes) caused by triggered activity.

and (iii) an appropriate conduction velocity (Bayés de Luna and Baranchuk, 2017; Zipes and Jalife 2004; Enriquez *et al.* 2017) (p. XII).

A. The presence of anatomic circuit through which the stimuli may circulate (reentry). To make this phenomenon occur, there must be somewhere in the circuit a zone with an unidirectional block and an adequate conduction velocity.

1. The reentrant circuit may **be initiated in a small area (micro-reentry) of the Purkinje network or the Purkinje-muscular junction,** in the atrial or ventricular muscle (Figure 14.10). This mechanism explains the majority of premature atrial and ventricular complexes. Traditionally, it was believed that most cases of atrial fibrillations were caused by multiple micro-reentries. It has been shown that the "rotor theory" (Jalife *et al.* 2000) and the increase in automaticity, especially at the pulmonary veins level (Haïssaguerre *et al.* 1998) (see above) may account for many cases of atrial fibrillation, in particular paroxysmal atrial fibrillation (see Figure 14.11).

2. The reentrant circuit may **be located in more extensive areas of the ventricle** (i.e. an area surrounding a post-infarction scar) or through the specific intraventricular conduction system (branch–branch reentry) (Figure 14.10) (see Chapter 16).

3. The reentrant circuit consists of **macro-circuits localized preferably in the right atrium** causing typical or common flutter (counterclockwise rotation) and reverse flutter (clockwise rotation) (Figure 14.12A,B). The atypical flutter and the macro-reentrant atrial tachycardia usually originate in the left atrium and, less frequently, in the right atrium (Figure 14.12C). We use the term atrial tachycardia if the heart rate is <200–220 bpm and atypical flutter if the heart rate is > 220 bpm.

4. A reentrant circuit may **involve the AV junction,** either alone or with the involvement of the AV junction and an accessory pathway (macro-reentry).

In the case of a circuit comprising only the AV junction (Figure 14.13), it was previously believed that this

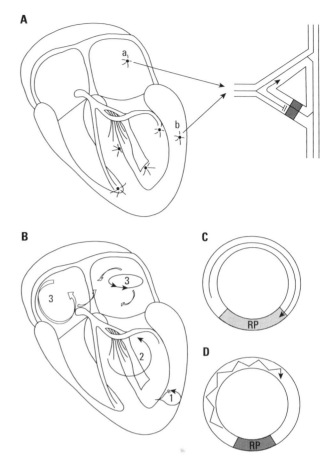

Figure 14.10 Examples of circuits involved in classical reentrant atrial and ventricular arrhythmias. (A) The circuit is usually located in the Purkinje–atrial muscle junction (a) or Purkinje–ventricular muscle junction (b) (micro-reentry). (B) It may also be located in a necrotic area of the ventricle (1) or in a circuit involving the left specific intraventricular system (2), or in the atria (3) (flutter or macro-reentrant tachycardia) (see Figure 3.7). (C and D) Perpetuation of a reentry depends on the refractory period (RP) duration and the conduction velocity (CV). If the RP is long and the CV is fast, reentry is not perpetuated (C), while it is perpetuated (D) if the RP is short and the CV slow (= area of unidirectional block).

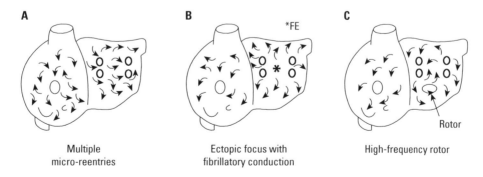

Figure 14.11 The three mechanisms dealing with the onset and perpetuation of atrial fibrillation. (A) Micro-reentry located in an ectopic focus induces multiple reentries (classical concepts). (B) Ectopic focus (EF) with increased automaticity (pulmonary veins) (asterisk) and fibrillatory conduction. (C) Atrial extrasystole located in an ectopic focus initiates a high-frequency rotor that perpetuates the arrhythmia with fibrillatory conduction.

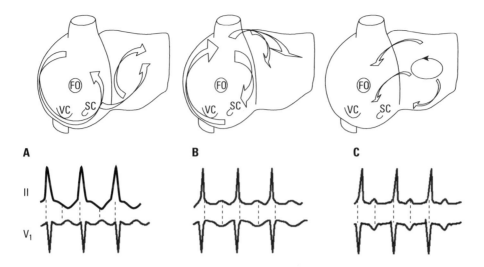

Figure 14.12 (A and B) Circuits explaining the presence of common flutter with counterclockwise rotation and non-common (reverse) flutter with clockwise rotation. (C) Possible macro-reentrant circuit in case of an atypical flutter, as well as macro-reentrant atrial tachycardia.

circuit was functional and located within the AV node (intranodal). It was presumed that the AV node had a longitudinal dissociation, with a slow conduction tract (α) and fast conduction tract (β) (Figure 14.13A). Now it is known (Wu and Yeh 1994; Katritsis and Becker 2007) that these circuits have an anatomic basis in which tissue of the lower atrium is also involved (AV junction) (see Figure 4.10).

The tachycardias originating in these circuits are of slow–fast type. **Slow–fast type tachycardias** are paroxysmal AV nodal reentrant tachycardias (**AVNRT**) in which a premature stimulus (atrial premature impulse) is blocked in the fast pathway (β) still in the absolute refractory period (ARP). It may go through the α pathway with a shorter refractory period, albeit with a lower conduction velocity. As a result, this stimulus is conducted to the ventricles (1 in Figure 14.13A) with a longer P'R than the baseline PR interval. At some point, because the fast pathway (β) is out of the refractory period, the premature stimulus retrogradely invades this pathway and rapidly reaches the atrium (P'), while at the same time entering again into the slow pathway (α), and is conducted to the ventricles to generate the QRS-2 complex (2 in Figure 14.13B). Conduction to the atrium is very fast, and the ectopic P' is concealed in the QRS complex or stuck at the end of it, simulating an "S" or "r" wave.

In the case of a **reentrant circuit with the involvement of the AV junction and an accessory pathway (macro-reentry)**, two types of tachycardias may be observed: with **retrograde conduction** over the accessory pathway or with **anterograde conduction** over the accessory pathway.

In the case of tachycardias with retrograde conduction over the accessory pathway (orthodromic), the QRS is narrow. These can also be slow–fast tachycardias, as in the case of reentrant tachycardia, with a circuit that exclusively involves the AV junction. **Slow–fast-type tachycardias** are paroxysmal AV reentrant tachycardias with the participation of an accessory pathway (**AVRT**). As in AVNRT, the onset of AVRT also occurs with an atrial premature impulse (atrial extrasystole). The P'R interval of this atrial extrasystole present in both cases a long interval, but it is usually longer in AVNRT (see Figure 14.13A,B). This occurs because in paroxysmal AVNRT, the atrial extrasystole is conducted only by the α pathway as it is blocked in the β pathway used as a retrograde arm of the tachycardia (Figure 14.13A). In the case of paroxysmal AVRT, the atrial extrasystole is not completely blocked in the β pathway and this explains why the PR interval is not lengthened too much. Elsewhere, retrograde conduction to the atria through the accessory pathway lasts longer than in the reciprocating (reentrant) tachycardia with exclusive involvement of the AV junction (AVNRT), and for this reason, the P' is close but clearly located after the QRS, but with a RP' < P'R (Figure 14.13A,B).

In the case of **fast–slow tachycardia**, which is infrequent (<5%), the tachycardia is incessant (atypical AVNRT). The circuit consists of a fast anterograde arm through the normal SCS (β pathway) and a slow retrograde arm that was first thought to be formed by slow retrograde conduction over a pathway (Coumel *et al.* 1974) (Figure 14.14). This explains the P'R < RP' relationship.

Tachycardias with anterograde conduction over one accessory pathway and retrograde conduction through the SCS, or, in some cases, over another accessory pathway (antidromic tachycardias) show a wide QRS and may

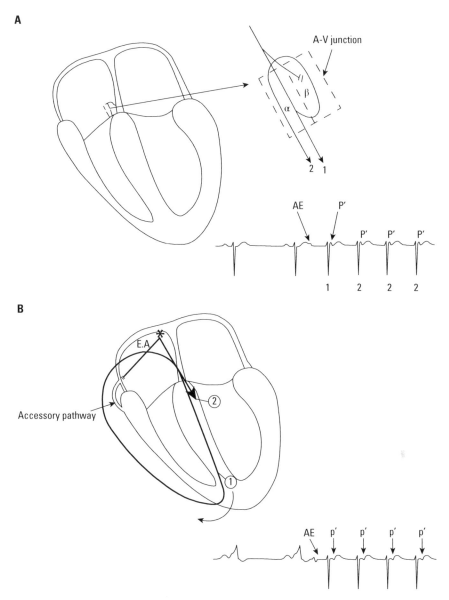

Figure 14.13 (A) Example of reentrant arrhythmias with circuit involving the AV junction exclusively, (A) or also involving an accessory pathway (B). In the first case (A), the premature atrial extrasystole (AE), which does not undergo anterograde conduction on the β pathway is conducted through the α pathway. This facilitates a reentry through the β pathway, with fast atrial retrograde activation (P′), which may be concealed within or at the end of the QRS complex (it may mimic an r′ or S wave). In the second case (B), the circuit has the following composition: His-Purkinje system—ventricular muscle—accessory pathway—atrial muscle—His-Purkinje system. An atrial extrasystole (AE) is blocked in the accessory pathway that shows a unidirectional block, thus being conducted through the normal pathway. Consequently, the resulting complex (1) does not show a delta wave. This impulse reenters retrogradely over the accessory pathway, activates the atria, and initiates a reentrant tachycardia with narrow QRS complexes (2) (without delta wave). In this case, due to longer retrograde conduction over the accessory pathway, the P′ is recorded close but at a short distance from the QRS (RP′ < P′R).

be included in the differential diagnosis of all wide QRS tachycardias (see Chapter 16 and Figure 16.18).

B. The **presence of unidirectional block in a zone of the circuit** is necessary to complete the reentry (see Figure 14.10).

C. The conduction velocity through the circuit has to be **appropriate**: not too quick (the stimulus would find part of the circuit still in the refractory period) and not too slow (the next sinus complex would penetrate the circuit).

Other types of reentry

There are other types of reentry with a functional, rather than anatomic, basis. Some are related to a circular movement, such as:

• Allessie's leading circle reentry (Allessie *et al*. 1977) (Figure 14.15B);

• reentry by one or double spiral waves (rotors) (El-Sherif *et al*. 1997; Jalife *et al*. 2000; Vaquero *et al*. 2008) (Figure 14.15C,D);

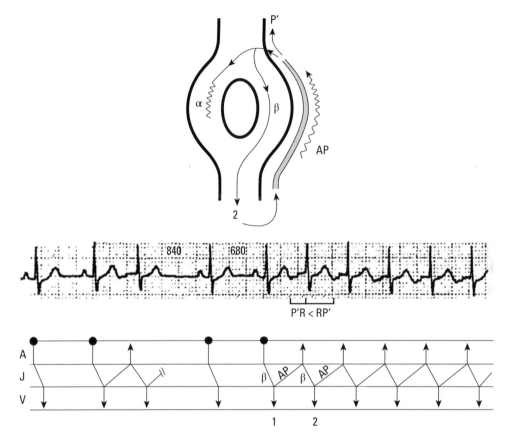

Figure 14.14 Above: Example of fast–slow tachycardia with the involvement of an anomalous pathway (AP) with slow retrograde conduction (P'R < RP'). Middle and below: Onset and end of an episode. β: β pathway.

• reentries related to the dispersion of repolarization between two areas of the myocardium (phase 2 reentry) (Figure 14.15E). These two areas may lie between different layers of the left ventricle (intramural dispersion) (Yan and Anzelevitch 1998) (TAP longer in the endocardium/M cells than in the epicardium) or between different areas of myocardium (transregional dispersion) (Noble 1979; Opthof *et al.* 2007).

Other mechanisms

Unexpected conduction: Supernormal excitability and conduction

In some circumstances, premature stimuli are blocked even when earlier stimuli are conducted. This interesting phenomenon, classically known as supernormal conduction, is believed to occur when the earliest stimulus is conducted because it falls in the supernormal excitability phase (Childers 1984) (Figure 14.16). This supernormal conduction of a stimulus may be explained by the gap phenomenon (Gallagher *et al.* 1973, Elizari *et al.* 2014) (Figure 14.17) or by concealed conduction (see later and Figures 14.29 and 14.30).

Active arrhythmias with variable coupling interval: the parasystole

These are premature impulses not related to the basic rhythm, which therefore have a variable coupling interval. This is caused by an ectopic focus that is prevented from being depolarized by the impulses from the basic rhythm, usually because of a unidirectional entrance block (Figure 14.18). However, when the surrounding tissue is out of the refractory period, the ectopic stimuli produced in this so-called parasystolic focus may come out, resulting in variable premature complexes (independent of the basal rhythm—parasystolic complexes) (Koulizakis *et al.* 1990; Steffens and Gettes 1974, McIntyre 2011, Coronel *et al.* 2014).

From an ECG point of view, these not only have a variable coupling interval, but also interectopic intervals that are multiples of each other, giving rise to **fusion complexes** if the sinus and parasystolic complexes occur simultaneously. A fusion complex is produced when both the sinus and the ectopic ventricular stimuli each partially activate the ventricle (see Figure 14.18).

In a very few cases, for example, when the parasystolic focus is a multiple of the basal rhythm, the parasystolic

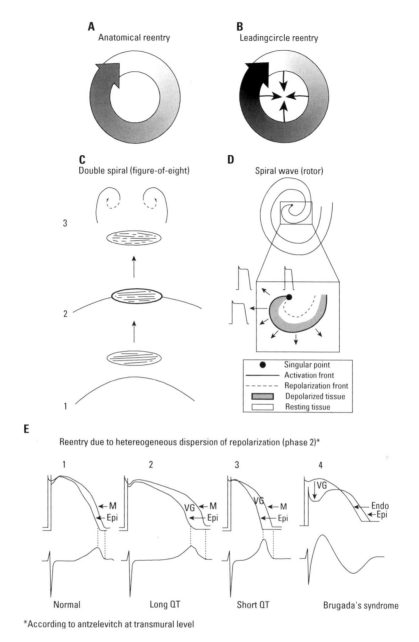

Figure 14.15 (A) Classical reentry (anatomical obstacle) (see Figure 14.10). (B) Allessie's model—leading circle (functional obstacle). In the classical circuit, the tip of the activation wave is far away from the refractory tail (A), while in Allessie's model, it is very close to the refractory tail (B). This justifies how in (B) the excitability zone is narrow and, in most cases, incomplete. In (A), the presence of an anatomical obstacle prevents the activation wave to enter into the circuit, while in (B) the wave can penetrate the circuit, at least partially. (C) Double spiral (rotors): figure-of-eight model: (1) an activation front approaches an obstacle (either anatomical or functional) in its refractory period, reaches it (2) and under the appropriate conditions, it splits into two fixed fronts resembling a figure-of-eight (continuous line: activation front; broken line: circular movement of singular points) (3). (D) Single spiral wave (rotor) theory. The activation front of the rotor (continuous black line) adopts a spiral shape and its curvature bends toward the rotation center. A voltage gradient (VG) exists between the rotation center (singular point), which is in passive status (short AP), and the neighboring areas (activation front), which are active and show a longer AP. The depolarized area (gray) and the resting area (white) are shown. The AP is shortened as it approaches the singular point due to the hyperfunction of K currents. Although the AP shortening is necessary to establish a high-frequency rotor, if it becomes too short, the areas more distal to singular point (with a longer AP) cannot conduct at the speed of the rotor, with a high discharge rate. This may lead to the disruption of the spiral wave that may initiate fibrillatory conduction. (E) Example of phase 2 reentry due to heterogeneous dispersion of repolarization (HDR). According to Anzelevitch, dispersion takes place at a transmural level and the AP of M cells is the longest compared with the AP of the rest of the wall areas. This HDR produces a ventricular gradient (VG) between the areas with longer AP and the area with shortest AP (epicardium) and accounts for the possible occurrence of VT/VF in patients with long QT syndrome (2) and short QT syndrome (3). In the Brugada syndrome (4), the HDR takes places between the endocardium and the epicardium of the RV at the beginning of phase 2 (VG), because of the transient predominance of outward I_{to} current. Epi: Epicardium; M: M cells.

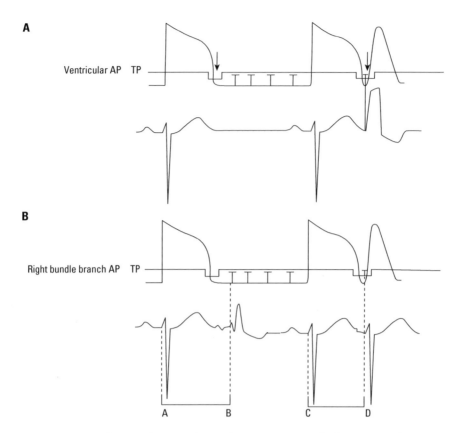

Figure 14.16 Apart from the reentrant mechanisms, there are other mechanisms accounting for the existence of early stimuli triggered by a preceding stimulus (extrasystole). In this figure, it can be seen how the subthreshold stimuli (T) originating in an ectopic focus may generate an AP and turn into a premature complex (supernormal conduction) only when they fall into the supernormal phase of ventricular excitability (arrow) (A). On the other hand, an atrial extrasystole (which is usually conducted with a right bundle branch block morphology) may be normally conducted when it occurs earlier, when the right bundle branch is in a supernormal phase of excitability (AB>CD, in part B of the figure).

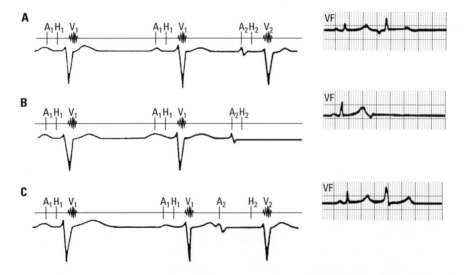

Figure 14.17 **Left**: (A, B and C) Diagrams showing the gap phenomenon. (A) The extra stimulus A2 is normally conducted. (B) The extra stimulus A2 is not conducted to the ventricles, and it is blocked in the area below the His fascicle (normal A2–H2 conduction). (C) If the extrastimulus A2 occurs earlier, it may be conducted with some delay through the AV node (long A2–H2), getting to the His fascicle later than in the previous case (B), and therefore being possibly conducted through the His-Purkinje system (V2). **Right**: Three examples of VF lead in the same patient featuring different atrial impulses with variable coupling intervals [increasingly premature from top to bottom (500, 400, and 320 ms)] and different impulse conductions. (A) The atrial extrasystole is normally conducted; (B) the atrial extrasystole is not conducted; (C) the atrial extrasystole is conducted with aberrancy. If no histogram is performed, there is no objective data supporting whether a phenomenon like this is a gap phenomenon or explained by supernormal conduction.

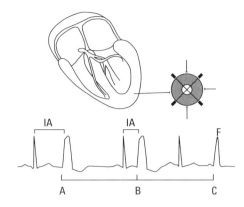

Figure 14.18 The parasystolic mechanism is generally explained by an entry block in the ectopic focus. The central point represents the parasystolic focus, surrounded by an area with an entry block (shaded area). Parasystolic stimuli may be conducted out of this zone but external stimuli cannot get into it. Usually, some degree of exit block also exists (see Figure 16.24). Bottom: Scheme of parasystolic ventricular premature complexes with the characteristic three electrocardiographic features: variable coupling interval, multiple interectopic intervals, and fusion complexes (Figure 14.5).

rhythm may have a fixed or nearly fixed coupling interval (Oreto *et al.* 1988).

Mechanism responsible for passive arrhythmias

Depression of automaticity

When the sinus automaticity is depressed, an ectopic subsidiary rhythm from the AV junction or ventricles takes over control of the heart rhythm at the natural discharge rate (e and f in Figure 14.8). This discharge rate is lower when the pacemaker is in the ventricular Purkinje fibers, because the junctional AV pacemaker is also depressed. The ventricular or AV junctional complexes appearing as a result are called QRS escape complexes, if isolated, and escape rhythms, if repetitive.

Depression of conduction

Conduction alterations that may explain many passive arrhythmias include: (i) heart block, (ii) aberrant conduction, and (iii) concealed conduction.

Heart block

The slowing down of the stimulus conduction can take place at the sinoatrial junction and the AV junction (see Chapter 17), the atria (see Chapter 9), and the ventricles (see Chapter 11).

In general, we refer to block as an anterograde stimulus block, although it is evident that blocks may be unidirectional (anterograde or retrograde) or bidirectional.

According to their degree of delayed conduction, three degrees of block may be distinguished: (i) **first-degree block**, when there is a delay in the stimulus conduction but no stimuli are blocked, (ii) **second-degree block**, when only some stimuli are blocked; this is classified as type I (Mobitz I) or Wenckebach type if a progressive conduction delay occurs before the block is complete and type II or Mobitz II if the block appears suddenly; and (iii) **third-degree block**, when all stimuli are blocked.

In second-degree type I block at sinoatrial and AV level, the conduction delay increases but the increase of the delay is progressively smaller (see Figures 14.19B and 14.20B). This explains, both at the AV junction and at the sinoatrial junction, how the RR intervals are increasingly shorter (AB > BC) after the pause initiated as a result of the total block of stimuli, until a complete conduction block occurs and another pause is observed. This phenomenon, which implies progressively shorter RR intervals due to the increasingly small increases in the block delay, is known as the Wenckebach phenomenon.

In the AV junction, apart from the previously mentioned phenomenon related to the RR intervals, which is the only diagnostic clue to determine a second-degree sinoatrial Wenckebach-type block, the increasing delay of conduction is observed by measuring the PR interval, which progressively lengthens, although the increases are smaller each time ($x + 60, x + 80$ ms). These rules frequently do not apply in blocks at AV level, where the increases are greater or smaller than expected (**atypical Wenckebach phenomenon**). Figure 14.20E shows two examples, one caused by concealed conduction and the other by a reciprocal complex.

In rare cases, the Wenckebach phenomenon in the AV junction occurs in the presence of a 2:1 fixed AV block. In this case, the blocked P wave of the 2:1 fixed AV block remains unchanged, whereas the conducted P wave presents the characteristics of the Wenckebach phenomenon with the PR interval increasing until the P wave is blocked (**alternating Wenckebach phenomenon**) (Figure 14.20F). This probably occurs because the two block types appear at two different levels of the AV junction: the 2:1 fixed block at a proximal level and the Wenckebach-type AV block at a more distal level (Halpern *et al.* 1973; Amat y Leon *et al.* 1975; Chacko *et al.* 2018).

In second-degree Mobitz II-type block, the non-conducted stimulus is preceded by a fixed or nearly fixed conduction (Figures 14.19 and 14.20C). At the AV junction, this is shown by a blocked P wave without previous PR lengthening, which leads to a pause equaling approximately twice the baseline RR. This unexpected pause, which approximately doubles the baseline RR interval, is the only diagnostic evidence of this block at a sinoatrial junction level.

In third-degree block at sinoatrial or AV junction, the pacemaker of the heart is located below the blocked zone (see Figures 14.19 and 14.20, and Chapter 17).

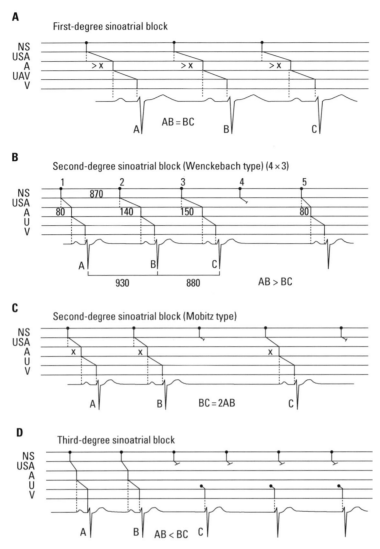

Figure 14.19 (A) First-degree sinoatrial block. The sinoatrial conduction is consistently slowed down (>*x*), but this does not translate onto the surface ECG (*x* =normal sinoatrial conduction time). (B) Second-degree sinoatrial block (Wenckebach type, 4:3). The sinoatrial conduction time progressively increases from normal (80 ms) to absolute block (80 = *x*, *x* +60, *x* +70) and block. The distance between the first two RR (930 ms) is greater than that between the second and the third RR (880 ms). The sinoatrial conduction cannot be determined. However, considering that distances 1–2, 2–3, 3–4, and 4–5 are the same and assuming that the sinus rhythm cadence is 870 ms, 1, 2, 3, 4, and 5 theoretically represent the origin of the sinus impulses. Therefore, as we have assumed that the first sinoatrial conduction time of the sequence is 80 ms, the successive increases in the sinoatrial conduction which explain the shortening of RR duration and the subsequent pause should be 80 + 60 (140) and 140 + 10 (150). Thus, it is explained that in Wenckebach sinoatrial block the greatest increase occurs in the first cycle of each sequence, after each pause (AB > BC). The PR intervals are constant. The second RR interval is 50 ms shorter, since this is the difference between the increases of sinoatrial conduction between the first and the second RR cycles. Actually, the first RR cycle equals 870 + 60 = 930 ms, while in the second cycle it equals 930–50 (50 is the difference between the first increment 60 and the second one 10) = 880 ms. (C) Second-degree sinoatrial block (Mobitz type). Sinoatrial conduction (normal or slowed down) is constant (*x*) before the stimulus is completely blocked (BC = 2AB). (D) Third-degree sinoatrial block. An escape rhythm appears (in this case, in the AV junction) with no visible P waves in the ECG (AB < BC). The escape rhythm may retrogradely activate the atria (not seen in the scheme).

Aberrant conduction

Aberrant conduction is an abnormal and transient distribution of an impulse through the atria, or more frequently through the ventricles, resulting in a change in the P wave (**atrial aberrancy**) (Chung 1972; Julia *et al.* 1978) (Figure 9.28 and Chapter 9) or in the QRS complex morphology (**ven-tricular aberrancy**) (Singer and Ten Eick 1971; Rosenbaum *et al.* 1973) (see Figure 11.14 and Chapter 11). When a ventricular aberrancy occurs in a healthy heart, given that the right bundle branch usually constitutes the structure of the specific system of ventricular conduction with the longest refractory period, the most frequent ECG pattern found is an advanced right bundle branch block.

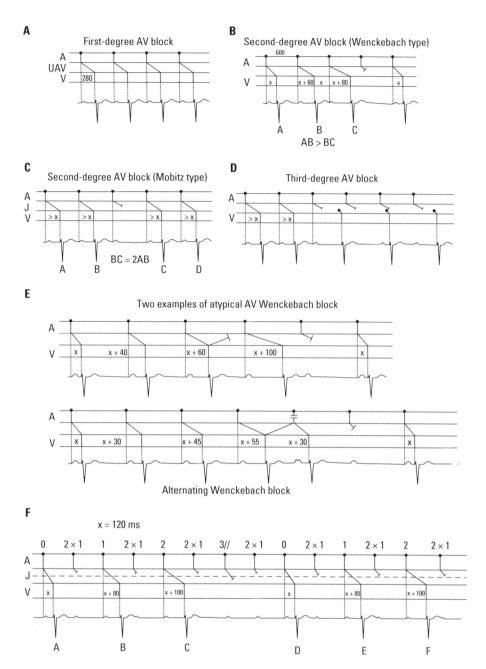

Figure 14.20 (A) First-degree AV block. The PR interval is always prolonged (>200 ms); (B) second-degree AV block 4 × 3 (Wenckebach type). The criterion AB>BC also applies in this case (see text and Figure 14.19B); (C) second-degree AV block (Mobitz type) (BC = 2AB); (D) third-degree AV block. A clear AV dissociation may be seen. After two QRS complexes have been conducted, there is a pause, followed by QRS (at slow frequencies) dissociated from P waves. In this case, the QRS complexes are junctional; (E) atypical Wenckebach blocks. Top: With abnormal lengthening of the increase preceding the pause (PR = $x + 100$) due to a concealed retrograde conduction of the preceding complex in the AV junction. Bottom: The abnormal PR shortening is due to the existence of a reciprocal complex in the AV junction; (F) example of an alternating Wenckebach block (see text).

Phase 3 aberrancy

The aberrant ventricular conduction pattern is, by definition, a transient pattern (**second-degree ventricular block**) and is generally related to a shortening of the RR interval (phase 3 Rosenbaum aberrancy).

A premature supraventricular complex may or may not have aberrant conduction depending, basically, on the ratio between the preceding diastole length and the coupling interval (Figures 14.21 and 14.22).

If the coupling interval is not changed, aberrancy occurs when the preceding RR cycle is longer, as it implies that the subsequent TAP is wider. Therefore, an impulse with a similar coupling interval may fall in the refractory period of the right bundle branch and may

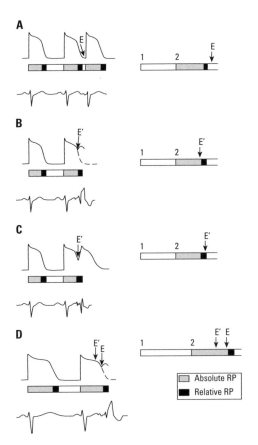

Figure 14.21 (A, B, C, D) Diagrams showing how the combination of a preceding long diastole and a short coupling interval favor the appearance of aberrancy related to a shortened cycle (phase 3 aberrancy). Left: Right bundle branch TAP (top); right bundle branch absolute refractory period (ARP) (bottom, gray); right bundle branch relative refractory period (RRP) (bottom, black) (the sum of both equals the total refractory period of the right bundle). The morphology of lead V1 in different situations depending on the preceding RR interval (cycle length) and the coupling interval is shown; Right: Diagrams (A, B, C, and D) showing a premature stimulus falls in or out of the ARP (gray) or RRP (black) left by the preceding RR cycle (distance 1–2). A premature stimulus is not conducted through the right bundle branch if it falls into its ARP (E′ in B and D). If the preceding RR is longer (D), a premature stimulus (E) (which could be conducted when the preceding RR was shorter) (A), may fall in ARP (D), thus not being conducted (rsR′ in V1) or being slowly conducted showing a partial RBBB morphology (rsr′ in V1) if it falls in the relative refractory period (C) (E′ in C). A premature stimulus falling out of the total refractory period (E in A) is normally conducted, although if the preceding RR interval is longer (D), the same premature stimulus may fall into the total refractory period and thus it may not be conducted (compare E in A and D). **In summary**, a stimulus falling in the final part of phase 3 of a TAP of the right bundle (E′ in C, in the relative refractory period of right bundle) is conducted with a partial right bundle branch block morphology, and an stimulus falling in phase 2 or an initial part of phase 3 of a TAP of the right bundle (absolute refractory period–ARP-of such branch, E′ in B and D) is conducted with a morphology of advanced right bundle branch block. Rosenbaum called this type of aberrancy "phase 3 aberrancy," which means that a stimulus that falls in phase 3 of TAP of the right or left bundle branch is not conducted through such bundle branches, and will have a right or left bundle branch block morphology.

not be conducted (Figure 14.21D), and the other may be normally conducted (Figure 14.21A) if the previous RR is shorter.

In the presence of a shorter coupling interval, aberrancy occurs with the same previous RR (compare E and E′ in Figure 14.21A,B).

Obviously, there is a greater chance of aberrancy if both phenomena occur at the same time, for example, if the preceding diastole is prolonged and the coupling interval becomes shorter.

Premature supraventricular impulses in the sinus rhythm follow this rule consistently (prolonged preceding RR interval + short coupling interval = aberrancy; Gouaux–Ashman criteria) (Figure 14.22). The subsequent complexes of a supraventricular tachycardia with a preceding short RR interval show an aberrant morphology less frequently, unless the refractory period of some SCS parts (right or left bundle branch) is pathologically prolonged. Occasionally, aberrancy may persist for several complexes when the refractory periods of some SCS parts are not able to adapt to sudden changes in the heart rate (Figure 14.23).

Exceptions to the explained above can be observed in premature atrial fibrillation complexes. Complexes that should be aberrant are not, whereas other complexes not following Gouaux–Ashman criteria are indeed aberrant. This may be explained by the different degrees of concealed "f" wave conduction in the AV junction, as well as in the branches. Isolated or maintained aberrant morphologies secondary to concealed retrograde conduction in the branches may also occur (Figure 15.29).

From a clinical viewpoint, it should be noted that **in the presence of atrial fibrillation, most wide QRS complexes are ectopic, especially if they do not have the typical right bundle branch block (RBBB) morphology**. Therefore, the presence of a typical RBBB morphology in lead V1 (rsR′) favors the occurrence of aberrancy, and not the presence of an R morphology with a notch in the descending limb of the R wave (compare Figures 14.24 and 14.25). However, if the wide complex beat is preceded by a short–long–short sequence, aberrancy should be considered. In the presence of atrial fibrillation, the irregular ventricular rhythm of fibrillation is also present when there are aberrant QRS complexes. When the wide QRS complexes have the same morphology but the RR intervals are regular, the atrial fibrillation is considered to have turned into an atrial flutter. If a regular rhythm but a different wide QRS morphology exists, the presence of ventricular tachycardia should be considered.

Phase 4 aberrancy

In some cases, the aberrant morphology is associated with a lengthening of the RR cycle (Rosenbaum phase 4 aberrancy). This may be explained by the presence of a

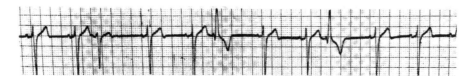

Figure 14.22 The first atrial extrasystole is conducted with minimal aberrancy, even without rsr' morphology, while the following extrasystoles are conducted with a morphology corresponding to an advanced right bundle branch block. By means of the compass, it is observed how the Gouaux–Ashman criteria are met. Therefore, the 6th and 9th complexes, clearly aberrant, show a slightly shorter coupling interval and/or a slightly longer preceding diastole than the 3rd complex. This is enough to fall in an absolute (6th and 9th complexes) or relative (3rd complex) refractory period of the right bundle.

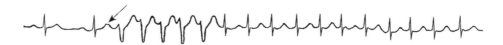

Figure 14.23 Sustained aberrancy during different complexes at the beginning of a supraventricular paroxysmal tachycardia. The first complex of the tachycardia shows classical aberrancy phase 3, the others due to the lack of adaptation to sudden change of heart rate, during a short period, of refractory periods of part of the intraventricular conduction system.

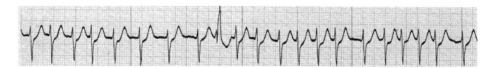

Figure 14.24 Atrial fibrillation (AF) patient with one wide premature QRS complex with a distinct morphology in V1. In general, the Gouaux–Ashman criteria in the presence of wide QRS complexes during AF are not as useful to distinguish between aberrancy and ectopy as in sinus rhythm. Nevertheless, the rsR' morphology in V1, as seen in this case, suggests that the aberrancy is more probable.

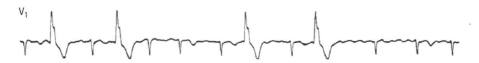

Figure 14.25 A patient with atrial fibrillation (AF) showing wide QRS complexes with a single R in V1. The notch in the descending arm of the QRS and the fixed coupling interval definitely point to an ectopic origin, ruling out aberrant conduction.

spontaneous diastolic depolarization increasing the right bundle branch up to the level observed in a phase 3 aberrancy (Figures 14.26B and 14.27).

Aberrancy without RR changes

Sometimes different mechanisms result in aberrant QRS complexes without changes in the RR intervals (Figure 14.28). On occasions, the aberrant QRS complexes may appear in alternans beats (Shinde *et al.* 2011).

Concealed conduction

Sometimes a structure may be partially depolarized by a stimulus that does not cross it completely. This partial depolarization is not directly observed on the surface ECG. However, it may be seen by its effect on the conduction of successive complexes (concealed conduction). An example of this is seen in **interpolated premature ventricular complexes**. The PR interval of the complex following the premature ventricular impulse is usually longer, as it partially depolarizes the AV junction. As a consequence, the atrial stimulus (P wave) finds the AV junction in the relative refractory period, and thus is conducted more slowly (Figure 14.29).

Concealed conduction explains other phenomena in the field of arrhythmology, including: (i) **the irregular rhythm of the QRS complex in the presence of atrial fibrillation** as a result of the "f" waves depolarizing the

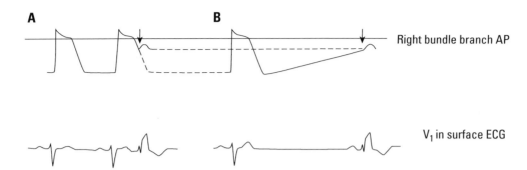

Figure 14.26 Comparison between the aberrancy related with cycle shortening (phase 3) (A) and that related with cycle lengthening (less frequent) (phase 4) (B). In this case, due to an important diastolic depolarization during the long cycle, the right bundle gets to a point, as in phase 3 aberrancy, where it is not excitable, and thus not able to generate a TAP to be conducted (arrow in B at the same level as A). As in phase 3, in the surface ECG an aberrant QRS complex with right bundle branch block morphology (rsR′) is recorded.

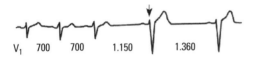

Figure 14.27 Example of a phase 4 left bundle branch block. Note the left bundle branch block pattern appearing after a significant lengthening of the previous RR cycle. The presence of the same PR interval in all complexes favors phase 4 aberrancy instead of an idioventricular escape rhythm.

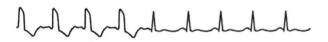

Figure 14.28 Intermittent aberrancy without apparent changes in heart rate.

AV junction to a lesser or greater extent, leading to an irregular conduction (Figure 14.30), and (ii) the presence of a wide aberrant QRS in patients with atrial fibrillation

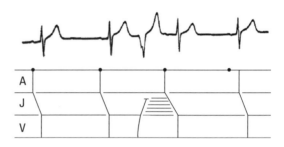

Figure 14.29 Interpolated ventricular extrasystole. The following P wave is conducted with a longer PR due to the concealed conduction of the ventricular extrasystole at the AV junction.

who do not follow the Gouaux–Ashman rule (Longo and Baranchuk 2017). This is explained by concealed conduction of "f" waves in the right or left bundle branch (see Figure 14.31 and Chapter 15).

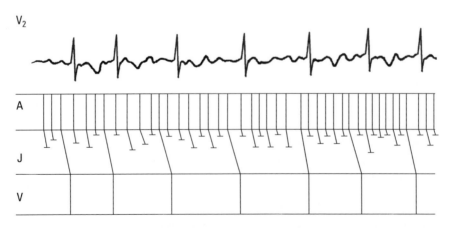

Figure 14.30 V2 recording showing the different morphologies of "f" waves (atrial fibrillation) and the variability of RR due to different degrees of conduction of the "f" waves in the atrioventricular node (concealed conduction).

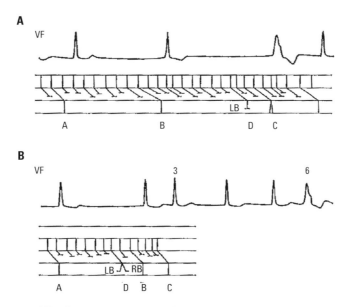

Figure 14.31 (A) Taken from an atrial fibrillation (AF) patient with generally narrow QRS and eventual wide QRS complexes with previous variable RR interval, which is very long in this case. It is probably not a ventricular escape because it is identical to other previous wide QRSs with shorter coupling intervals; it may be explained by the concealed conduction of a previous "f" wave in the left bundle branch (LBB) that has changed its sequence from AB–BC, which should not show left bundle branch block (LBBB) aberrancy, to BD–DC, which may show this aberrancy. (B) An opposite example to that the one shown in part A: the QRS complex (number 3) that appears early with a long previous RR cycle does not show aberrancy, whereas other less premature complexes with a shorter preceding RR cycle show aberrancy (6). An explanation for this may be that an "f" wave located in the preceding diastole has penetrated into both branches, changing the sequence from AB–BC (aberrant) to DB–BC (not aberrant).

References

Allessie MA, Bonke FI, Schopman FJ. Circus movement in rabbit atrial muscle as a mechanism of tachycardia. III. The "leading circle" concept: a new model of circus movement in cardiac tissue without the involvement of an anatomical obstacle. *Circ Res* 1977;41:9.

Amat y Leon F, Chuquimia R, Wu D, *et al.* Alternating Wenckebach periodicity: a common electrophysiologic response. *Am J Cardiol* 1975;36:757.

Antiperovitch P, Bayés de Luna A, Nunes de Alencar J, et al. Old teaching tools should not be forgotten: the value of the lewis' ladder diagram in understanding bigeminal rhythms. *Ann Noninv Electrocardiol* 2019;24:e12685.

Antoons G, Oros A, Bito V, *et al.* Cellular basis for triggered ventricular arrhythmias that occur in the setting of compensated hypertrophy and heart failure: considerations for diagnosis and treatment. *J Electrocardiol* 2007;40(suppl 6):8.

Bayés de Luna A, Baranchuk A. *Clinical Arrhythmology*. 2nd edn. Wiley-Blackwell, 2017.

Chacko S, Glover B, Baranchuk A. Wenckebach periods of alternate beats: an unusual phenomenon. Section conduction disorders. In Shenasa M, Josephson ME, Estes III NAM, Amsterdam EA, Scheinman M (eds) *ECG Master's Collection: Favorite ECGs from Master Teachers Around the World II*. CARDIOTEXT, Minn, USA; 2018, Case 2.6

Childers RW. Supernormality: recent developments. *PACE* 1984;7:1115.

Chung EK. Aberrant atrial conduction. Unrecognized electrocardiographic entity. *Br Heart J* 1972;34:341.

Coronel A, Cibalerio M, Stambuli G, et al. Unusual modulated ventricular parasystole due to premature beats. *J Inn Card Rhythm Manag* 2014;5:1636–1637

Coumel P, Fidelle J, Attuel P, *et al.* Les tachycardies réciproques à évolution prolongée chez l'enfant. *Arch Mal Cœur* 1974;1:23.

Elizari MV, Schmidberg J, Atienza A et al. Clinical and Experimental Evidence of Supernormal Excitability and Conduction. *Current Cardiology Reviews*, 2014,**10**,202–221

El-Sherif N, Chinushi M, Caref EB, Restivo M. Electrophysiological mechanisms of the characteristic electrocardiographic morphology of torsade de pointes tachyarrhythmias in the long QT syndrome-detailed analysis of ventricular tridimensional activation patterns. *Circulation* 1997;96:4392.

Enriquez A, Frankel DS, Baranchuk A. Pathophysiology of ventricular tachyarrhythmias. From automaticity to reentry. *Herzschrittmacherther Elektrophysiol* 2017; **28(2)**:149–156

Gallagher JJ, Damato AN, Varghese PJ, *et al.* Manifest and concealed reentry: a mechanism of A–V nodal Wenckebach in man. *Circulation* 1973;47(4):752–757.

Goldstein S, Bayés-de-Luna A, Guindo Soldevila J. *Sudden Cardiac Death*. Futura Publishing Company, 1994.

Haïssaguerre M, Jaïs P, Shah DC, *et al.* Spontaneous initiation of atrial fibrillation by ectopic beats originating in the pulmonary veins. *N Engl J Med* 1998;339:659.

Halpern MS, Elizari MV, Rosenbaum MB, *et al.* Wenckebach periods of alternate beats. Clinical and experimental observations. *Circulation* 1973;48:41.

Jalife J, Berenfeld D, Mansour M. Mother rotors and fibrillation conduction: a mechanism of atrial fibrillation. *Circ Res* 2000;54:204.

Johnson NP, Denes P. The ladder diagram (A 100+year history). *Am J Cardiol* 2008;101:1801.

Julia J, Bayés De Luna A, Candell J. Auricular aberration: apropos of 21 cases. *Rev Esp Cardiol* 1978;31:207.

Katritsis D, Becker A. The AV nodal reentrant circuit. *A Proposal Heart Rhythm* 2007;4:1354.

Koulizakis NG, Kappos KG, Toutouzas PK. Parasystolic ventricular tachycardia with exit block. *J Electrocardiol* 1990;23:89.

Longo D, Baranchuk A. Ashman Phenomenon Dynamicity during Atrial Fibrillation: The critical role of the Long Cycles. *J Atr Fibrillation* 2017;10(3):1656

McIntyre WF, Baranchuk A. Left ventricular outflow tract parasystole. *Arch Cardiovasc Dis* 2011;104:359–360

Moe GM, Méndez C. Physiological basis of reciprocal rhythm. *Prog Cardiovasc Dis* 1966;8:561.

Noble D. *The Initiation of the Heartbeat.* Oxford University Press, 1979.

Opthof T, Coronel R, Wilms-Schopman FJ, *et al.* Dispersion of repolarization in canine ventricle and the ECG T wave: T interval does not reflect transmural dispersion. *Heart Rhythm* 2007;4:341.

Oreto G., Satullo G, Luzza F, *et al.* Irregular ventricular parasystole: The influence of sinus rhythm on a parasystolic focus. *Am Heart J* 1988;115:121.

Rosenbaum MB, Elizari M, Lazzari JO, *et al.* The mechanism of intermittent bundle branch block. Relationship to prolonged recovery, hipopolarization and spontaneous diastolic depolarization. *Chest* 1973;63:666.

Shinde RS, Carbone V, Oreto G., *et al.* Right bundle branch block on alternate beats during acute pulmonary embolism. *Ann Noninvasive Electrocardiol* 2011;16:311.

Singer D, Ten Eick, R. Aberrancy: Electrophysiological aspects. *Am J Cardiol* 1971;28:381.

Steffens T, Gettes L. Parasystole. In: Fisch Ch (ed). *Complex Electrocardiography 2.* FA Davis, Philadelphia 1974. pp. 99–110.

Vaquero M, Calvo D, Jalife J. Cardiac fibrillation: from ion channels to rotors in the human heart. *Heart Rhythm* 2008;5:872.

Wit AL, Boyden PA. Triggered activity and atrial fibrillation. *Heart Rhythm* 2007;4(3 suppl):S17.

Wu D, Yeh S. Double loop figure of eight reentry as a mechanism of multiple AV reentry. *Am Heart J* 1994;127:83.

Yan GX, Anzelevitch C. Cellular basis for the normal T wave and the electrocardiographic manifestations of the long-QT syndrome. *Circulation* 1998;98:1928.

Zipes D, Jalife J. *Cardiac Electrophysiology: From cell to bedside,* 4th edn. WB Saunders, 2004.

Chapter 15
Active Supraventricular Arrhythmias

Premature supraventricular complexes

Concept and mechanisms

Premature supraventricular complexes are premature complexes of supraventricular origin. These include those of atrial (A-PSVC) and atrioventricular junctional origin (J-PSVC).

Most PSVCs have a fixed or nearly fixed coupling interval (distance from the beginning of the previous sinus P wave to the beginning of the premature ectopic P'), because their origin is dependent on the baseline heart rhythm. They are commonly called extrasystoles. The most frequent mechanism causing PSVC is micro-reentry in the atrial muscle.

Premature supraventricular complexes that have an extremely variable coupling interval are called parasystoles, and the most common mechanism is increased automatism. The automatic focus is protected from the basic rhythm (entry and exit block), and is therefore independent of it.

ECG findings
Morphology

In the ECG, a premature ectopic P (P') wave is observed, which is followed, if not blocked in the atrioventricular (AV) junction, by a QRS complex, which is also premature. The P' wave is usually hidden in the previous T wave, which is usually modified by the P' wave, resulting in a masked P' morphology (Figure 15.1).

If the origin of a PSVC is the AV junction (J-PSVC), then the premature P wave is always negative in II, III, and aVF due to retrograde activation of the atrium from the junction region.

PSVCs may be isolated or occur in runs (Figure 15.2). They rarely comply with the ECG criteria for atrial parasystole (see Figure 14.5D).

Conduction to the ventricles

PSVCs may be conducted to the ventricles in three different ways: normal conduction, aberrant conduction, or blocking in the AV junction (non-conducting), leading to a pause (Figure 15.1).

When supraventricular tachyarrhythmia runs occur, sometimes the first complex of the run shows an aberrant morphology which is a result of the Gouaux–Ashman phenomenon (Figure 15.3B) (Longo and Baranchuk 2017).

The differential diagnosis between aberrant PSVCs and ventricular complexes is shown in Table 15.1.

Clinical implications

From a clinical point of view, PSVCs are generally benign. It is important to determine: (i) their frequency; (ii) if they are associated with paroxysmal arrhythmias, (iii) if they disappear with exercise; and (iv) any etiological factors.

PSVCs may be associated with heart disease (i.e. ischemic heart disease (IHD), cor pulmonale, thyroid dysfunction, pericardial diseases, psychologic factors, drugs, digitalis intoxication, etc.) or may be due to functional disturbances. In healthy individuals, they are usually related to digestive problems (aerophagia, etc.), coffee consumption, alcohol, and stress. More recently, the number (burden) of PSVCs in 24 hours has been associated with an increased risk of atrial fibrillation (Prasitlumkum et al. 2018).

Sinus tachycardia (Tables 15.2 and 15.3)

Concept

Sinus tachycardia is defined as sinus rhythm with a rate greater than 100 bpm.

Clinical Electrocardiography: A Textbook, Fifth Edition. Antoni Bayés de Luna, Miquel Fiol-Sala, Antoni Bayés-Genís, and Adrián Baranchuk.
© 2022 John Wiley & Sons Ltd. Published 2022 by John Wiley & Sons Ltd.

Mechanisms

Most cases of sinus tachycardia are caused by an increase of sinus automaticity as a response to different physiologic sympathetic stimuli (exercise, emotions, etc.) (Figure 15.4), or other specific causes such as fever, hyperthyroidism, pulmonary embolism, acute myocardial infarction, heart failure, etc.

Occasionally, orthostatism leads to an exaggerated sinus tachycardia (postural orthostatic tachycardia syndrome (POTS)).

There have been cases caused by an inappropriate increase of sinus automaticity, probably due to a lack of autonomic modulation of the sinus node or a sinoatrial reentrant tachycardia (Gomes *et al.* 1985; Femenía et al. 2012) (Figure 15.5).

ECG findings

In the ECG, sinus tachycardia presents as an increase in heart rate that occurs progressively in the majority of cases, and persists over a certain amount of time, with certain changes, until the triggering stimulus disappears. Heart rate during exercise, especially in young people with sympathetic overdrive, may reach 180–200 bpm. If the P wave falls in the refractory period of the AV junction, it may conduct with a long PR interval, resulting in a PR > RP. In such cases, in order to better visualize the P wave, some maneuvers (Figure 15.5) or an amplifying technique, a filtering T wave technique, or special leads (Lewis leads) are useful.

In patients with sinus tachycardia due to physiologic sympathetic overdrive (exercise, emotions, etc.), it is frequently observed that the PR and ST segments form part

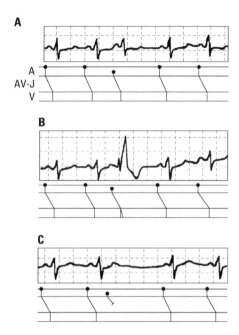

Figure 15.1 Sinus rhythm alternating with paroxysmal atrial fibrillation (AF) episodes and frequent premature supraventricular complexes (PSVCs). (A) A PSVC is conducted normally. (B) A PSVC is conducted with aberrancy because it occurs earlier. (C) A PSVC is blocked, because it occurs earlier in the cycle and the preceding diastole is a little longer. The pause is due to an active, not to a passive arrhythmia.

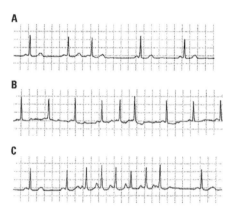

Figure 15.2 Examples of supraventricular premature complexes: (A) isolated; (B) in pairs; (C) in runs.

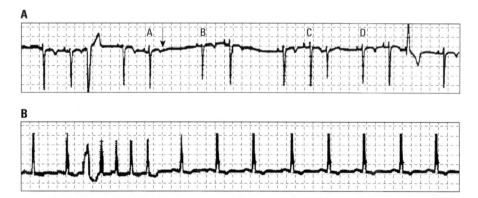

Figure 15.3 (A) A healthy 8-year-old girl with atrial trigeminy, at times normally conducted and at other times blocked (see change in T wave morphology in the AV-pause, arrow (compare AB = CD)). Sometimes, it was conducted with right bundle branch (RBB) and other times with left bundle branch (LBB) morphology. (B) A short run of supraventricular tachycardia. Only the first complex of the run is aberrant due to the Gouax–Ashman phenomenon.

Table 15.1 ECG evidence indicative of the presence of ectopy or aberrancy when early wide isolated QRS complexes are observed in the presence of sinus rhythm[a]

Indicative of ectopy: ventricular extrasystoles

- Wide QRS complex not preceded by a P′ wave (premature ectopic P) (it should be confirmed it is not concealed within the previous T wave)
- QRS morphology in V1: and QRS morphology in V6:
- Presence of complete compensatory pause.

Indicative of aberrancy: supraventricular extrasystoles

- P′ wave preceding a wide QRS complex (slight changes in the previous T wave should be identified)
- QRS morphology in V1: , particularly if QRS morphology in V6 is
- In the presence of wide and narrow premature QRS complexes, it should be checked that only wide QRS complexes meet Gouaux–Ashman criteria (see text).

---

[a] Specificity ≥90%.

of a circumference, as the PR segment descends whereas the ST segment ascends (Figure 15.4).

The appearance of abrupt sinus tachycardia suggests sino-reentrant mechanisms (Figure 15.6).

Clinical implications

Sinus tachycardia caused by a large sympathetic over-drive decreases at night or at rest because of vagal prevalence. This helps to distinguish it from sinus tachycardia due to pathologic causes such as pulmonary embolism, hyperthyroidism, or heart failure, in which sinus tachycardia is more persistent.

Treatment for sinus tachycardia consists of suppression of the underlying triggering cause, if feasible (i.e. stimulant intake), or treating the underlying disease (heart failure, hyperthyroidism, fever, etc.) and usually prescribing beta blockers and/or ivabradine (Femenía *et al.* 2012). Physiologic tachycardia will disappear when the triggering factor is removed, as previously discussed.

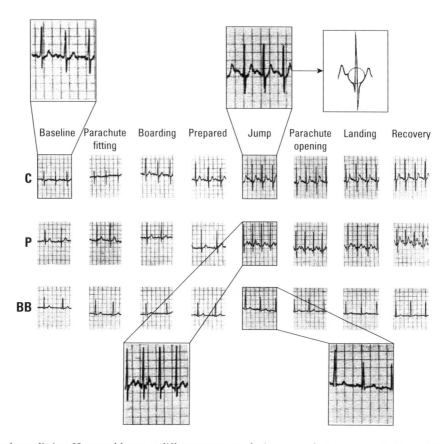

Figure 15.4 Sinus tachycardia in a 32-year-old man at different moments during a parachute jump: control jump (C), with placebo (P), and after taking a beta blocker (BB). Beta blocker (propanolol) administration leads to a less accelerated heart rate. During the control and placebo jumps, a typical ECG sympathetic overdrive pattern is observed (140 bpm), where PR and ST are part of an arch circumference (drawing).

Table 15.2 Supraventricular active rhythms

- Premature supraventricular complexes
- Supraventricular tachyarrhythmias
  - Sinus tachycardia
  - Monomorphic atrial tachycardia (MAT)
  - Atrioventricular (AV) junctional reentrant tachycardia (JRT)
  - AV junctional tachycardia due to an ectopic focus (JT-EF)
  - Chaotic atrial tachycardia
  - Atrial fibrillation
  - Atrial flutter

Table 15.3 Classification of supraventricular tachyarrhythmias according to RR (regular or irregular)

Regular RR (Figure 15.20)
- Sinus tachycardia with fixed AV ratio (almost always 1 × 1) (including sinus node-dependent reentry) (Figures 15.4–15.6)
- Monomorphic atrial tachycardia due to an ectopic focus (MAT-EF), with fixed AV ratio (generally 1 × 1) (Figures 15.7–15.10)
- Junctional reentrant tachycardia (JRT) (Figures 15.11–15.13)
- Junctional tachycardia due to an ectopic focus, with fixed AV conduction to ventricles (JT-EF) (Figures 15.17 and 15.18)
- Atrial flutter with fixed AV conduction, generally 2 × 1 (Figure 15.32)

Irregular RR
- Atrial fibrillation (Figure 15.25)
- Atrial flutter with variable AV conduction (Figures 15.38)
- Multimorphic or chaotic atrial tachycardia (Figure 15.21)
- Monomorphic atrial tachycardia with variable AV conduction (Figure 15.9)
- Junctional tachycardia due to an ectopic focus, with variable AV conductiobn to the ventricles (see Figure 18.10H)

Monomorphic atrial tachycardia (Tables 15.4–15.7)

Concept

Monomorphic atrial tachycardia includes all types of atrial tachycardias that display non-sinus monomorphic P waves (P′) on the surface ECG. Both the initial P′ waves, which initiate the tachycardia, and the subsequent waves have the same morphology (Figure 15.7). The high atrial tachycardias close to the sinus node (parasinus origin) usually produce a P′ wave that may be identical to a sinus P wave.

Mechanisms

There are two well-defined types of monomorphic atrial tachycardia (MAT):

- **Tachycardia originating in a small localized zone (ectopic focus) (MAT-EF).** This may be due to increased automaticity, triggered activity, or micro-reentry. Its clinical presentation could be paroxysmal or incessant. Generally, the different mechanisms cannot be differentiated with a conventional surface ECG, especially when the tachycardia is already established. The most important and useful differences, from a clinical point of view, are shown in Table 15.4 (Chen *et al.* 1994; Wharton 1995).
- **Tachycardia due to an atrial macro-reentry (MAT-MR).** This is usually paroxysmal and is observed in patients with atrial postsurgical incisions, generally following operations for congenital heart disease or atrial ablation procedures. Tachycardia due to an atrial macro-reentry may produce morphologies of different types of

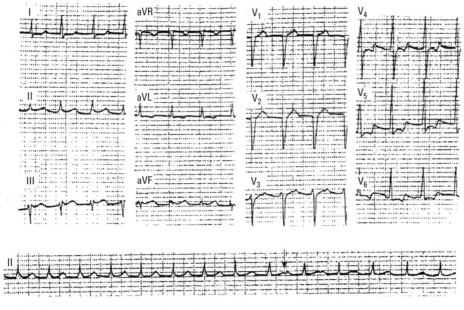

Figure 15.5 Above: Tachycardia at 110 bpm with barely visible atrial activity (a notch following the QRS complex is observed in V3). Breathing (II, continuous trace) results in a slowed down tachycardia, allowing us to see the atrial wave, which is close to the end of the T wave and shows sinus polarity (arrow).

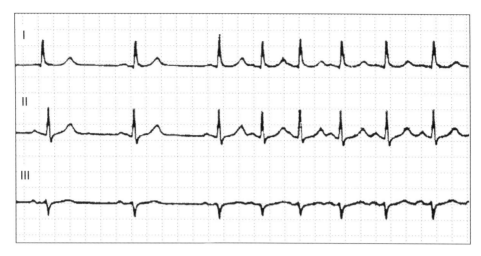

Figure 15.6 Sudden onset of supraventricular tachycardia at a rate of 110bpm with P wave identical to the sinus wave. This may correspond to reentrant sinoatrial tachycardia.

Table 15.4 Clinical, electrophysiological, and pharmacological differences between the different types of monomorphic atrial tachycardia with ectopic focus (MAT-EF), depending on their triggering mechanism (micro-reentry, increase of automatism, or triggered activity)

	Micro-reentry[a]	Increase of automatism	Triggered activity
• Progressive acceleration and desacceleration of tachycardia, both at the beginning (warming-up) and at the end (cooling-down)	No	Yes	Sometimes
• Initiation due to premature systole or programmed stimulation (PS)	Yes	No	Yes
• Termination due to premature systole or programmed stimulation	Yes	No	No
• Vagal maneuvers (carotid sinus massage)	Generally, they have no effect, although it may cause an AV block	Transient suppression	Termination
• Beta blockers	No effect	Transient suppression	Termination
• Adenosine	Contradictory results. Most of the times, it has no effect	Transient suppression	Termination
• Clinical presentation	Paroxysmal form is more frequently observed	Generally incessant type	Paroxysmal or incessant

[a] This group includes the micro-reentry originating in an ectopic focus and also the macro-reentry originating in the area surrounding an atrial postsurgical scar.

flutter, and even of MAT due to an ectopic focus (MAT-EF), by surface ECG (see later).

ECG findings (Tables 15.5 and 15.6)
Paroxysmal monomorphic atrial tachycardia due to an ectopic focus
P wave morphology in sinus rhythm
The P wave usually shows, in the case of MAT-EF of the left atrium, the majority originating from the pulmonary veins, a prolongation of P wave that is often notched.

The ECG during the tachycardia (Figures 15.7–15.10)
• **Heart rate and rhythm:** The MAT-EF initiated in the right atrium presents with a low heart rate (usually ≤150bpm), which is lower than the MAT-EF from the left atrium (Bazán *et al.* 2010).

• **The morphology of the ectopic atrial wave (P').** The P' wave voltage is usually low and the P'R interval is characteristically shorter than the RP' interval, except when the P' wave falls on the AV junctional refractory period and then is conducted with some delay. If the ectopic P' wave is clear we have to consider the following: **(i) negative or +–P wave in lead V1** suggests that the tachycardia originates in the right atrium (100% specificity); **(ii) positive or –+ in lead V1** suggests a left atrium origin (100% sensitivity).

Figure 15.10 summarizes the sites of origin and an algorithm allowing their identification by ECG (Kistler *et al.* 2006).

Table 15.5 Characteristics of atrial activity in monomorphic supraventricular tachyarrhythmias[a]

ECG diagnosis	Atrial activation	Morphology (II, III, aVF)	Morphology V1	Atrial activity frequency	AV block
Sinus tachycardia (Figures 15.4–15.6)	Sinus	Generally, positive or ± in III. It rarely may be ± in II, III, and aVF	Positive or ±	100–180 bpm Sometimes, (mainly in young people) it may even be >200 bpm	Rarely present, even in the fastest types
Monomorphic atrial tachycardia (Figures 15.7–15.10)	Focal origin (MAT-EF) or due to an atrial macro-reentry[a] (MAT-MR)	Depends on the focus location in case of ectopic origin (Figure 15.10) macro-reentrant tachyarrhythmias may feature different morphologies	Depends on the focus location. Macro-reentrant tachyarrhythmias may feature different morphologies (see text)	Generally <150 bpm. It may reach 240 bpm (see text).	Sometimes, in the fastest types
Common flutter (Figures 15.32 and 15.33)	Permanently counterclockwise. This explains the lack of isoelectric baseline in some derivations	Sawtooth F predominantly negative waves. No isoelectric baseline	Generally positive and not very narrow F waves, except in the presence of significant atrial disease	200–300 bpm'	Generally present
Reverse flutter (Figure 15.34)	Clockwise. Generally permanent	Positive F waves in II, III, and aVF generally without isoelectric baseline	F waves generally wide and negative in V1, with no isoelectric baseline	200–300 bpm	Generally present
Atypical flutter[b] (Figure 15.35)	Probably a left atrial macro-reentry. Often unknown	Generally positive waves in II, III, and aVF Frequently a slight undulation is observed	Usually positive	220–280 bpm	Very frequently
Junctional reciprocant tachycardia (JRT) (Figures 15.11 and 15.12)	Retrograde, either in the AV junction or in an anomalous pathway	Concealed in the QRS complex or stuck at its end (AVNRT) or following the QRS complex (AVRT)	If the circuit exclusively comprises only the AV junction, it frequently simulates an r'	Generally 130–200 bpm	Not present
Junctional tachycardia due to an ectopic focus (Figure 15.17)	Retrograde, except in the case of AV dissociation	A negative retrograde activation is observed	Variable	100–200 bpm	AV dissociation due to interference is frequently observed (Figure 15.17)

[a] Monomorphic atrial tachycardias generated in the areas surrounding a postsurgical scar in patients operated for congenital heart disease or subjected to atrial ablation procedures (atrial macro-reentry) may feature different ECG morphologies: the most characteristic ones are identical to those observed in the reverse flutter, although sometimes they may show the same morphologies as the common or atypical flutter (see Atypical flutter), or even MAT-EF.

[b] It is usually considered that its morphology cannot be distinguished from that of fast macro-reentrant atrial tachycardias, and that both mechanisms are the same (generally left atrial macro-reentry). An atypical flutter is named when the arrhythmia rate >220 bpm, and MAT-MR when the arrhythmia rate is lower.

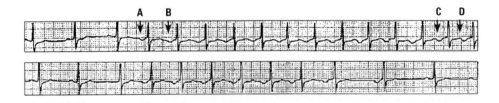

Figure 15.7 Upper tracing: A 20-year-old patient with dilated cardiomyopathy and incessant atrial tachycardia due to an ectopic focus (AB = 0.64 sec and CD = 0.52 sec). Lower tracing: After amiodarone administration, the focus activity is slowed down, with a progressive reduction of rate discharge. All of this suggests that the cause is increased automaticity (see Table 15.4).

Table 15.6 ECG characteristics of the different types of paroxysmal supraventricular tachyarrhythmias with regular RR and narrow QRS complexes[a] (onset during tachycardia)

	Atrial flutter	Junctional reciprocant tachycardia[a]		Sinus tachycardia	Monomorphic atrial tachycardia[b]	Junctional tachycardia due to an ectopic focus
		AVNRT[c]	AVRT[c]			
Beginning of tachycardia	Usually initiated with a premature supraventricular impulse	P′ wave initiating the tachycardia shows a different morphology, compared with the subsequent P′ waves	P′ initiating the tachycardia is generally different to subsequent P′ waves	Progressive initiation. P wave does not feature significant changes	Initial P′ wave is identical to the subsequent P′ waves	Initiation and termination may be either abrupt or gradual. Initial P′ wave is identical to the following P′ waves
Status of the atrial activity wave (P, P′, or F) during tachyarrhythmia	Flutter waves, generally two waves per each QRS complex. Almost never 1 × 1	P′ within the QRS complex = 65%. P′ following the QRS complex = 30% (very close to it). P′ preceding the QRS complex = 5% (Figure 15.13)	P′ following the QRS complex in 100% of the cases, but with RP′ < P′R	P preceding the QRS complex shows a sinus polarity. Almost always P-QRS < QRS-P	P′ wave precedes the QRS complex, usually with P′-QRS < QRS-P′	It is generally concealed in the QRS complex or, more frequently, an AV dissociation is observed
Presence of ventricular block	Depends on the underlying disease and the heart rate	Rarely seen. Almost always features a RBBB morphology	Sometimes observed	Depends on the underlying disease and the heart rate	Depends on the underlying disease and the heart rate	Depends on the underlying disease and the heart rate
QRS alternans (voltage difference >1 mm)	No	No	20% of the cases	No	No	No
AV dissociation	Usually a 2 × 1 AV block is present	Never, unlike what is observed in JT-EF[d]	Never. If AV dissociation is observed, Kent bundle involvement in the circuit is excluded	Generally not present	2 × 1 AV block may be present	Frequently AV dissociation due to interference is observed (ventricular rhythm faster than atrial rhythm, if this is of sinus origin)
Mechanism and clinical presentation	Atrial macro-reentry, usually in heart disease patients. It may be a paroxysmal or chronic flutter	Reentry exclusively in the junction. Almost always in healthy patients. The incessant type rarely occurs	Reentry through an anomalous pathway. Almost always in healthy patients. The incessant type rarely occurs	Generally, it is due to a physiological increase of automatism. On some rare occasions, sinus reentry may be involved	It may be to an ectopic focus (EF) or because of an atrial macro-reentry (AM). Those due to an EF may be paroxysmal or incessant. Those due to a macro-reentry are paroxysmal tachycardias	In many cases, it is observed in heart disease patients. Initiation and termination sometimes are not abrupt. Incessant types may be observed

[a] Basal ECG with or without WPW-type pre-excitation.
[b] MAT may be due to an ectopic focus (MAT-EF) or an atrial macro-reentry (MAT-MR).
[c] AVNRT: tachycardia exclusively involving the AV junction; AVRT: tachycardia with a circuit also involving an anomalous pathway.
[d] JT-EF: junctional tachycardia due to an ectopic focus; MAT: monomorphic atrial tachycardia.

The AV conduction

The AV conduction is often 1 : 1. When the rate of tachycardia is high, sometimes due to the effect of different drugs (digitalis), various degrees of AV block and even AV dissociation may be seen (Figure 15.9). The P′R usually is less than the RP′ (P″R < RP′) (Figures 15.7 and 15.13D). However, in cases of first-degree AV block, it may be P′R ≥ RP′. In this case, it may be difficult to make the differential diagnosis with other paroxysmal tachycardias, especially atrioventricular reentrant tachycardias (AVNR) with accessory pathway (see Tables 15.5, 15.6, and 12.1) once the tachycardia is established.

Table 15.7 Differential diagnosis between incessant AV junctional reentrant tachycardia (I-JRT) and incessant tachycardia due to an atrial ectopic focus (I-MAT-EF)

	Heart rate is increased previously to tachycardia initiation	Polarity of the P waves following the P–P′ triggering the tachycardia	Presence of fusion complexes at the beginning or at the end	Progressive acceleration and desacceleration, both at the beginning (warming-up) and at the end (cooling-down) of the tachycardia
Incessant tachycardia due to an atrial ectopic focus	Heart rate is not accelerated prior to tachycardia initiation	Polarity of the P′ wave triggering the tachycardia is the same as that from the successive waves	They may be present	Yes
Incessant AV junctional reentrant tachycardia	Heart rate is accelerated prior to tachycardia initiation	Polarity of the P–P′ wave triggering the tachycardia is not the same as that from the successive P′ waves	Not present	No

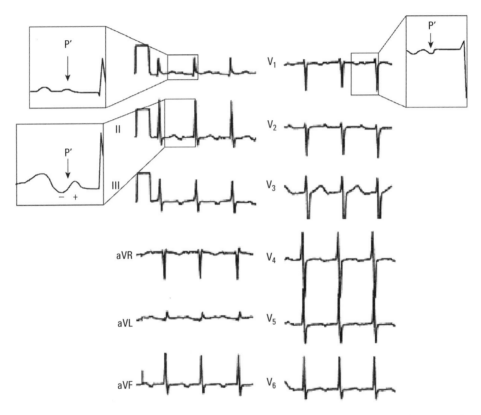

Figure 15.8 The P wave polarity is clearly indicative of the ectopic origin in the low right atrium around the tricuspid ring (negative P′ wave in V1, III, aVF and −+ in II). Therefore, this is a clear case of monomorphic atrial tachycardia at a low rate (110 bpm) misdiagnosed as a sinus tachycardia by the computerized interpretation as a result of the erroneous assessment of the polarity in lead II (−+), which cannot be a sinus polarity. A stress test showed that the tachycardia disappeared when the sinus rhythm accelerated to a higher rate.

The QRS complex

The QRS complex is usually equal to the baseline rhythm. Occasionally, it is wide due to an aberrant ventricular conduction.

The carotid sinus massage

This has a variable effect (Table 15.4).

Monomorphic atrial tachycardia due to macro-reentry

MAT-MR is not characterized by a specific ECG morphology.

The atrial wave morphology varies from the typical to the reverse or atypical atrial flutter. It may even be similar to MAT-EF morphology.

Incessant monomorphic atrial tachycardia due to an ectopic focus

In incessant monomorphic atrial tachycardia due to an ectopic focus (I-MAT-EF), the heart rate typically varies between 90 and 150 and P′R < RP′ (Figure 15.7). All the aspects related to the morphology of ectopic P′ have been previously explained.

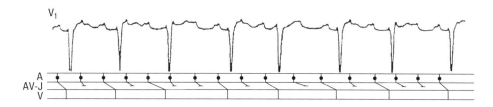

Figure 15.9 A digitalis-intoxicated patient with atrial tachycardia due to an ectopic focus at 175 bpm, with P waves that are different from the preceding sinus waves but not narrow. The atrial waves have some variable cadence and different degrees of AV block.

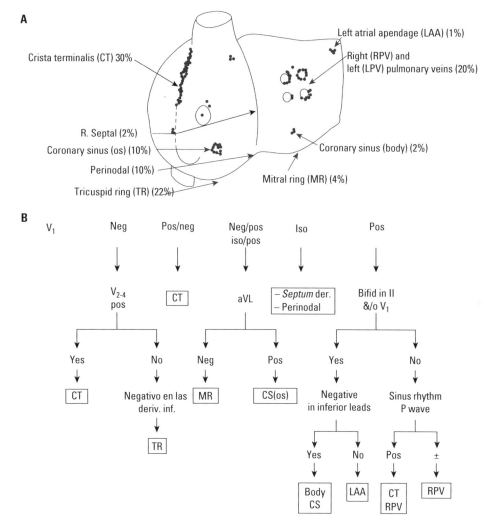

Figure 15.10 (A) Most frequent locations of atrial tachycardias of focal origin. (B) Algorithm to localize the most frequent sites of origin of tachycardias based on P′ wave morphology in V1 (see location inside the figure) (Adapted from Kistler *et al.* 2006).

The main differential diagnosis of I-MAT-EF is with incessant junctional reentrant tachycardia (I-JRT), which once established, also features a P′R<RP′ interval (Figure 15.15) (see Table 15.7).

Clinical implications

The prognosis depends on the heart rate, the underlying pathology, and the impact over LV function and whether the tachycardias are paroxysmal or incessant. The prognosis and treatment depend particularly on the tachycardia rate and the patient's clinical condition. In the case of a stable patient, a paroxysmal episode may be treated, if vagal maneuvers fail, with adenosine, beta blockers, or amiodarone (class I aC). However, pharmacologic treatment is often not useful.

If the tachycardia rate is high and not well-tolerated, electrical cardioversion (CV) may be required (class IB). Later, ablation techniques should be considered to resolve the arrhythmia (class IB), usually with a high success rate.

Junctional reentrant (reciprocating) tachycardia

Concept

No consensus has been reached with regard to the most appropriate name for tachycardias due to a reentrant mechanism, whose circuits are exclusively located in the AV junction or involve an accessory pathway (see Chapter 14). However, the most accepted names according to the guidelines are junctional AV reentrant (reciprocating) tachycardia with a circuit exclusively involving the AV junction (AV node) (**AVNRT**) and junctional reentrant (reciprocating) tachycardia with circuits involving an accessory pathway (**AVRT**).

The tachycardias may be **paroxysmal (slow–fast type)** (Figures 15.11 and 15.12), which are much more frequent and often have characteristic clinical features (sudden onset, polyuria, etc.) (Josephson 1978; Wu *et al.* 1978; Bar *et al.* 1984; Inoue and Becker 1998; Katritsis and Becker 2007), or incessant (**fast–slow type**) (Figure 15.15), which are much less frequent and often seen in the pediatric population (Coumel *et al.* 1974).

Mechanism

Paroxysmal tachycardias (slow–fast circuit)

The circuit may be located just in the AV junction (AVNRT) or may include an accessory pathway in the circuit (AVRT) (see Chapter 14). In all cases, tachycardia is initiated when there is a unidirectional block (anterograde) in some part of the circuit.

When the circuit exclusively involves the AV junction (AVNRT tachycardia) (Figure 15.11), the block takes place in the AV junction where the β pathway is located (see Figure 4.10). The same β pathway is used by the stimulus to reenter. This slow–fast tachycardia is thus characterized by a long AH (atrial–His) interval and a short HA interval (His–atrial) as shown in Figure 15.11C.

When a Kent bundle-type accessory pathway is involved in the circuit (Figure 15.12A), the block generally occurs antregradely in the accessory pathway and the stimulus reaches the ventricles through the normal AV conduction. The stimulus reenters retrogradely over an accessory pathway (see Figure 14.11). The retrograde atrial activation shows a longer HA interval than when the circuit exclusively involves the AV junction, as the circuit is larger (compare Figures 15.11C and 15.12B). Because the anterograde conduction is through the normal AV junction, paroxysmal tachycardias with the involvement of an accessory pathway have a narrow QRS complex, although very often a pre-excitation delta wave is observed in the ECG without tachycardia (Wolff–Parkinson–White (WPW) syndrome). In just a very few cases showing anterograde conduction through the accessory pathway, a wide QRS tachycardia can be seen (differential diagnosis with ventricular tachycardia)

(see Figure 16.18) (Nadeau-Routhier and Baranchuk 2016).

The onset of paroxysmal junctional reentrant tachycardia (Figures 14.13 and 15.11D) is triggered by a premature impulse. The termination of the tachycardia also helps in establishing the mechanism, thus, the differential diagnosis (Chiale *et al.* 2015).

Incessant tachycardias (fast–slow circuit)

Incessant tachycardias usually start as a result of a critical shortening of the sinus RR interval (Figure 15.15).

In incessant or permanent tachycardias, the anterograde block occurs in the AV junction (α pathway). The stimulus reaches the ventricles by the β pathway and reentry occurs over an anomalous bundle with a slow retrograde conduction (Figures 14.14 and 15.15).

ECG findings

Paroxysmal junctional reentrant tachycardia (slow–fast type circuit)

Sinus rhythm

The baseline ECG of patients with AVNRT and AVRT are usually normal. In nearly 40% of cases, a usually non-ischemic negative T wave is present at the end of the episode (Paparella *et al.* 2000). In AVRT the WPW pattern could be present if there is anterograde pre-excitation in sinus rhythm; however, in cases of accessory pathway with retrograde conduction only (concealed pre-excitation), the short PR and delta wave will not be seen (see Table 12.1).

During tachycardia

The **heart rate** generally varies between 130 and 200 bpm. The QRS complex morphology is the same as or very similar (see later) to the baseline rhythm when the circuit exclusively involves the AV junction (AVNRT). If the baseline ECG shows WPW-type pre-excitation (AVRT), this pattern disappears during the tachycardia (narrow QRS complex).

To determine which type of circuit is involved in the paroxysmal junctional reentrant tachycardia, it is essential to determine the relationship between the P' wave and the QRS complex (Figure 15.13).

If the circuit includes the AV junction exclusively (AVNRT), then the P' wave will be within the QRS in 60% of cases, or will appear immediately afterward (30–40%). It simulates an "r" in lead V1, a slurred "s" in inferior leads, or a notch in aVL (Di Toro *et al.* 2009; Nadeau-Routhier and Baranchuk 2016) (Figures 15.11 and 15.13A,B).

If an accessory pathway is involved in the circuit that forms its retrograde arm, the path from the ventricles to the atria is longer, resulting in a P' wave that is always slightly behind the QRS complex (Figures 15.13C and 15.12B). If the accessory pathway is found on the left

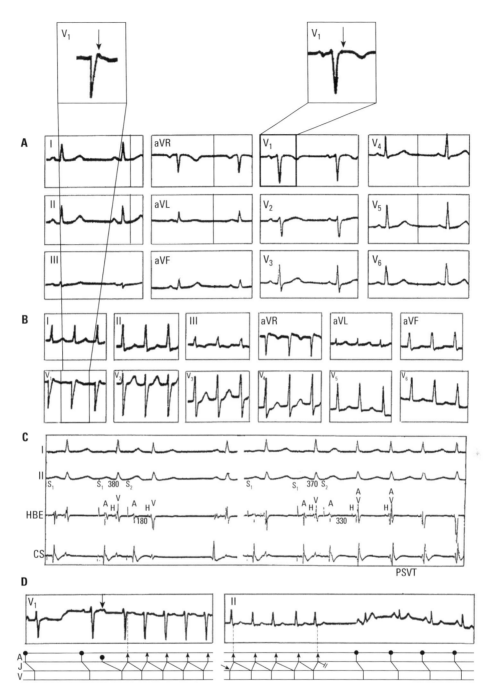

Figure 15.11 (A) ECG of a patient with no heart disease and episodes of paroxysmal supraventricular tachycardia (AVNRT). The tracing is normal. (B) ECG during one episode: "s" wave appears in II and aVF, whereas a minimal r' is observed in V1. Apart from this, no other modifications are observed in the ECG. (C) The same patient with extra stimulation (S1 S2 at 380 ms): a significant AH lengthening is reported (180 ms) but no paroxysmal tachycardia (PT) is initiated. When extra stimulation is coupled at 370 ms, a critical AH lengthening (330 ms) is reached, initiating the junctional reentrant tachycardia with synchronic atrial and ventricular activation (AV junctional exclusive circuit). HB: His bundle; CS: coronary sinus. (D) Onset and termination of a AVNRT episode. We can observe the initial P'R lengthening and the small QRS changes during the episode due to the P' overlapping (r' in V1 and s in II and aVF (compare with A and B).

side, the P' wave is frequently negative in lead I, because the atrial activation occurs from left to right.

Relatively often (≈40% of cases) during tachycardia, ST segment depression appears, but this does not necessarily represent ischemia.

If during the tachycardia, the AV conduction is over one accessory pathway (Kent bundle) or a long atriofascicular tract (see Chapter 12), the QRS is wide (**antidromic tachycardia**) (Figure 15.16). In this case, the retrograde arm of the circuit may be the His–Purkinje system or another accessory pathways. These types of tachycardias must be included in the differential diagnosis of wide QRS tachycardias, along with supraventricular tachycardias with bundle branch block (aberrancy) and ventricular tachycardias (see Chapter 16).

When bundle branch block morphology appears during paroxysmal AVRT reentrant tachycardia, the RR lengthens if the accessory pathway is on the same side as the blocked branch. This happens because the stimulus descending through SCS will have to cross the septum (a longer distance) to complete the reentry circuit.

Junctional reentrant tachycardias usually have a narrow QRS complex, either when the circuit exclusively involves the AV junction (AVNRT) (Figure 15.11), or when it also involves an accessory pathway (AVRT) (Figure 15.12), because the stimulus reaches the ventricles through the AV junction usually with a normal intraventricular conduction.

Incessant junctional reentrant tachycardia (fast–slow type of circuit)

The ECG characteristics of I-JRT are the following (Figure 15.15) (Table 15.7):

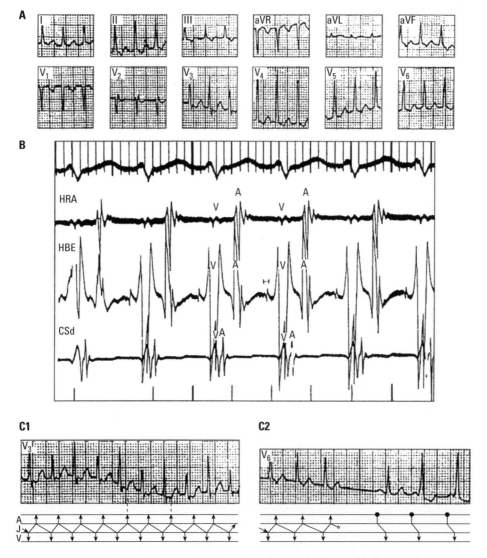

Figure 15.12 (A) Example of junctional paroxysmal tachycardia with left accessory pathway (Kent bundle) in the reentrant circuit (AVRT type). The QRS complex is narrow and the ectopic P is negative in I, II, III, aVF, and V6 (after QRS), with RP′ < P′R. In V3 a QRS complex alternans is presumed (see C left). (B) Electrophysiologic study showing an atrial retrograde activation in which the left atrium is the area first depolarized. As seen in the CS lead (distal), this is where the retrograde atrial activation (A) is first recorded. This may be suggested by surface ECG because in I and V6, the retrograde p′ is clearly negative (leads I and V6 are facing the tail of the atrial activation vector). HRA: high right atrium; HB: His bundle; CS: coronary sinus. (C) AVRT. **Left**: V3, where alternans of QRS complexes are observed. **Right**: V6, where the termination of the episode with anterograde block in the AV junction is observed, with an onset of pre-excitation in the second sinus complex.

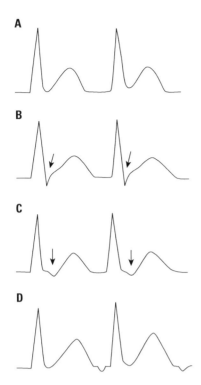

Figure 15.13 Location of P′ waves in paroxysmal supraventricular tachycardias. (A) Non-visible P′ wave, hidden within the QRS (circuit exclusively involving the AV junction). (B) P′ wave that distorts the end of the QRS (simulating that it ends with an S wave) (circuit exclusively involving the junction as well). (C) P′ wave separated from the QRS, but with RP′ < P′R (reentrant) (circuit involving an accessory pathway). (D) P′ wave preceding the QRS with P′R < RP′ (atrial circuit or atrial ectopic focus).

- The heart rate is usually lower (120–150 bpm) than in paroxysmal junctional reentrant tachycardias.
- The P′ wave is located before the QRS complex and, therefore, the RP′ interval is >P′R interval.
- The beginning of the tachycardia is associated with a critical shortening of the baseline RR interval (Figure 15.15). The triggering atrial wave is generally of sinus origin, although it may also be due to an atrial extrasystole or a programmed early atrial stimulation.
- The polarity of the initial atrial wave (usually sinus) is different from the remaining atrial waves (P′), which, as previously discussed, have caudocranial polarity.
- Generally tachycardias occur in runs, which are usually short and separated by a few sinus impulses (incessant). When the tachycardia is always present, it is considered a permanent tachycardia.

Differential diagnosis

The differential diagnosis of **paroxysmal** AV reentrant tachycardias is shown in Tables 15.5 and 15.6 and has already been discussed. Regarding the **incessant** reentrant AV tachycardias, it is important to differentiate I-JRT

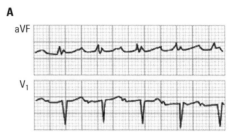

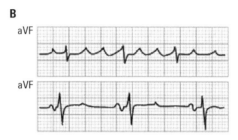

Figure 15.14 (A) aVF and V1 in a patient with heart failure and fixed ventricular rate throughout a 24 h examination. This led us to suspect that the rhythm was not sinus, although a possible sinus P wave around 120 bpm might be inferred in V1. The compression of the carotid sinus blocked the AV node temporarily, which allowed for the identification of "f" waves from an atypical flutter (aVF, B top). The cardioversion successfully restored sinus rhythm. Note the P ± waves in II, III, and aVF corresponding to an advanced interatrial block with retrograde conduction to the left atrium (VF, B bottom).

from I-MAT-EF. The most relevant data have also already been mentioned (see Table 15.7).

Clinical implications

The diagnosis of paroxysmal reentrant tachycardias has to be suspected by history taking, especially when the onset and offset are sudden, and because polyuria is observed especially in long-lasting episodes. Diagnosis of AVNRT-type is supported by the presence of pounding in the neck, and is more common in female patients whose first episode appears after childhood (González-Torrecilla *et al.* 2009).

In general, paroxysmal AV reentrant tachycardias are not life threatening, although they can be very troublesome, because of fast heart rate, the duration of the tachycardia, and the underlying illness, if present. Cases with an accessory pathway involved in the circuit (AVRT) may be potentially dangerous because in rare cases, a rapid atrial fibrillation may be triggered (see later).

To terminate an episode due to a paroxysmal junctional reentrant tachycardia immediately after it starts, it is important to block the circuit at any level, usually at the AV junction. This may be achieved by: (i) hard coughing; (ii) performing a carotid sinus massage (CSM), if feasible; and (iii) administering drugs immediately, if the episode persists, to terminate it as soon as possible. A treatment,

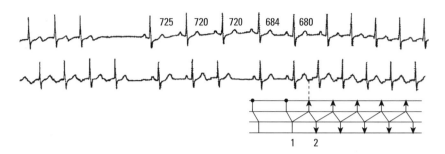

Figure 15.15 Holter continuous recording. Incessant junctional reentrant tachycardia with the fast–slow circuit type AVRT. The accessory bundle with slow conduction constitutes the retrograde arm of the circuit (see Figure 14.13). Bottom: Lewis diagram corresponding to the onset of one episode.

known as the "pill-in-the-pocket" approach (recommendation class IIa), was proposed by Lown more than 30 years ago (Alboni *et al.* 2004).

If the crisis does not cease, after some time (from minutes to hours depending on the tolerance), the patient should be hospitalized, and if the tachycardia is of AVNRT-type (this diagnosis may be suggested by ECG non-visible P′ or a slight change at the end of QRS (Figure 15.11), intravenous adenosine (treatment of choice) or other antiarrhythmic drug such as amiodarone should be administered. Ablation of the slow pathway (AVNRT) or accessory pathway (AVRT) is now considered first line of treatment.

In cases of WPW pattern, even without crisis of AVRT, after discussing the situation with the patient, especially in the case of young people practicing sports, we advise ablation in a well-experienced center after examining the results of the exercise testing, Holter monitoring, and electrophysiologic studies (Bayés de Luna and Baranchuk 2017). This is based on the infrequent but real risk that the first episode could lead to a fast atrial fibrillation that, in very rare cases, may trigger ventricular fibrillation. Exercise testing has limitations to determine the risk of sudden death in patients with anterograde conduction over a pathway, and ablation can be curative (Jastrzębski *et al.* 2017)

In the majority of cases of repetitive crisis, ablation techniques solve the problem. Therefore, ablation is the best solution for patients who do not tolerate junctional reentrant tachycardias or experience them frequently.

Tables 15.5 and 15.6 and Figures 15.11 and 15.12 show the most important ECG characteristics of these two types of tachycardias, as well as the differential diagnosis with other types of supraventricular paroxysmal tachycardias with narrow QRS and regular RR. The location of the P′ wave is a key point (for differential diagnosis see Figure 15.13).

Atrioventricular junctional tachycardia due to ectopic focus

Concept, mechanism, and clinical presentation

Junctional tachycardia due to ectopic focus (JT-EF) is a rare tachycardia, which originates in an ectopic focus of the AV junction, as a result of increased automaticity or triggered activity (Ruder *et al.* 1986).

JT-EFs are observed in patients with severe heart disease, for example, acute myocardial infarction and electrolyte disorders. They are also found in children, and in some cases it is considered congenital (Dubin *et al.* 2005; Collins *et al.* 2009).

ECG findings

This arrhythmia is **usually characterized by a fast rhythm (>150 bpm), a sudden onset and offset, and often presents with AV dissociation.** The atrial rhythm may be of sinus origin (Figure 15.17), ectopic atrial rhythm, atrial fibrillation or flutter (Figure 15.18). Conduction into the ventricles is usually fixed.

The JT-EFs that present with progressive onset and termination (**non-paroxysmal**) usually have a slower heart rate (<130 bpm).

Bidirectional tachycardias of supraventricular origin are atrial, or more often atrioventricular junctional tachycardias due to ectopic focus with alternant ventricular aberrancy (right bundle branch block + superoanterior hemiblock, alternating with right bundle branch block + inferoposterior hemiblock) (see Chapter 16).

When the rate is low (≤100 bpm) but above the normal rhythm of the AV junction, it is considered an accelerated AV junctional rhythm. Occasionally, the accelerated idionodal rhythm competes with the sinus rhythm, producing numerous atrial fusion complexes (Figure 15.19). The rhythms of the AV junction observed in heart rates below 50 bpm are called "escape rhythms" and are discussed in Chapter 17.

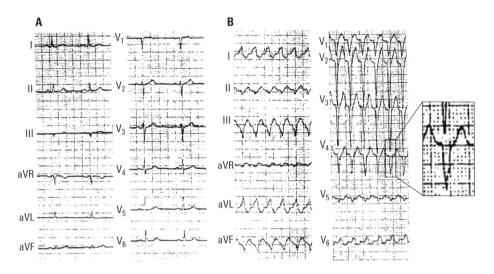

Figure 15.16 A 28-year-old patient without heart disease and a normal ECG (A), who presented with episodes of paroxysmal tachycardia with wide QRS (B). This is an antidromic tachycardia through a long right atriofascicular tract (see Chapter 18, Atypical pre-excitation) that shows a morphology similar to that of an advanced left bundle branch block (LBBB), with wide QRS complexes and an rS morphology in V2–V4, as opposed to the relevant R wave in V3–V4 that is observed in antidromic supraventricular tachycardias over a right accessory atrioventricular pathway (Kent bundle) (see Figure 16.19 and Table 18.1).

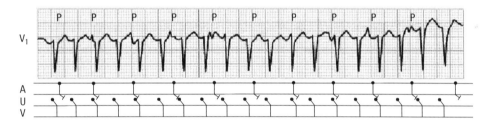

Figure 15.17 Example of a fast junctional ectopic focus tachycardia (180 per minute) with complete atrioventricular dissociation. Atrial rhythm is sinus rhythm.

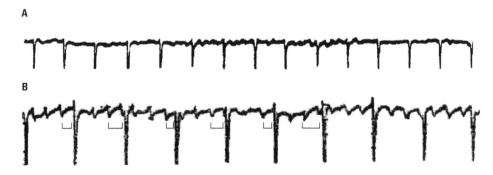

Figure 15.18 (A) Atrial fibrillation with regular RR. The ECG is from a patient with a junctional tachycardia and digitalis intoxication who showed atrial fibrillation as an atrial rhythm. (B) F flutter waves of variable morphology and changing FR intervals coinciding with fixed QRS intervals. This supports the existence of a junctional ectopic focus that is dissociated from the atrial rhythm (atrial flutter).

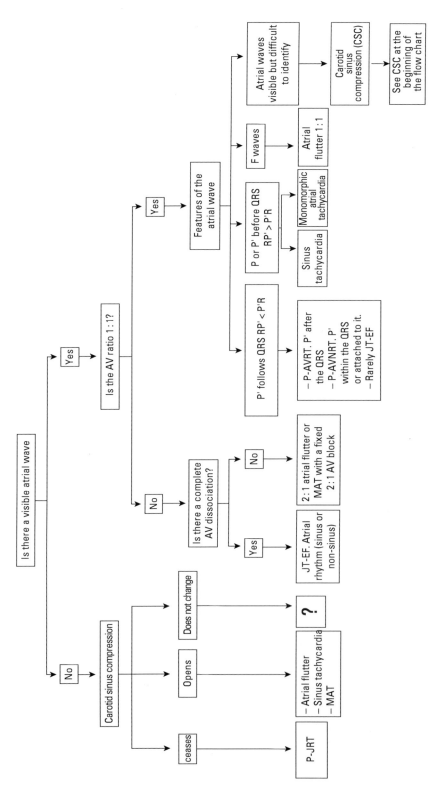

Figure 15.19 Algorithm for the diagnosis of active supraventricular arrhythmias with regular RR intervals and narrow QRS.

Figure 15.20 shows how we can perform diagnosis of this type of tachycardia in a surface ECG using a **step-by-step diagnosis of supraventricular tachyarrhythmias with regular RR and narrow QRS complexes.** In addition, Tables 15.5 and 15.6 show some of the most important aspects of differential diagnosis. A similar diagnostic algorithm was recently published in a free-access i-Book (Nadeau-Gouthier and Baranchuk 2016)

Clinical implications

The prognosis depends on the clinical context (digitalis intoxication, electrolyte imbalance, etc.) and the heart rate. Tachycardia that occurs in childhood, especially in newborns, may be serious and may need urgent treatment including ablation. However, sudden death that sometimes occurs may be due to associated congenital advanced AV block.

Chaotic atrial tachycardia

Concept, mechanism, and clinical presentation

This is an arrhythmia with a variable heart rate (between 100 and 200 bpm) due to the presence of three or more atrial ectopic focuses.

From a clinical point of view, this is a very infrequent arrhythmia. It usually occurs in patients with cor pulmonale (and enlarged right atrium) and is associated with hypoxia episodes.

ECG findings

ECG diagnosis may be made (Figure 15.21) when the following ECG criteria are met: (i) three or more different P wave morphologies in the same lead; (ii) isoelectric baselines in between P waves; (iii) absence of a dominating atrial pacemaker; and (iv) variable PP and PR intervals, which cause an irregular heart rate.

At first glance, an incorrect diagnosis of atrial fibrillation may be made. It is important to avoid confusion with ectopic P waves and atrial "f" waves (see Atrial fibrillation, below).

Clinical implications

The best treatment for this arrhythmia is to treat the underlying condition and improve oxygenation parameters.

Atrial fibrillation

Concept, mechanisms, and clinical presentation

The incidence of atrial fibrillation increases with age. It is presumed that 10% of octogenarians suffer from atrial fibrillation. Although chronic (permanent) atrial fibrillation may be an isolated finding, it often occurs in patients with heart disease, especially mitral valve disease, ischemic heart disease, hypertensive heart disease, and cardiomyopathies, and may also be present in some specific situations (hyperthyroidism, alcoholism, etc.).

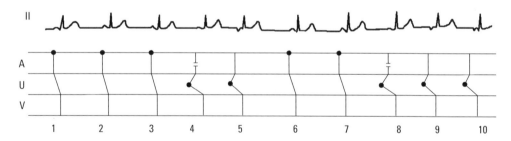

Figure 15.20 The sinus node and atrioventricular junction both compete to be the pacemaker. The heart is at times commanded by the sinus node (complexes 1, 2, 3, 6, and 7), and sometimes by the junction (complexes 5, 9, and 10). On occasion, an intermediate P morphology is observed (complexes 4 and 8, atrial fusion beats). In the fifth and tenth complexes, the junctional focus is accelerated, exceeding 60 bpm, showing a discrete increase of atrioventricular (AV) junction automaticity.

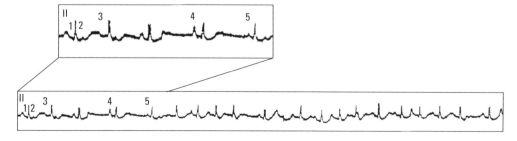

Figure 15.21 A patient with decompensated chronic obstructive pulmonary disease showing all the features of multimorphic or chaotic atrial tachycardia. Note the five different types of P waves in the first five QRS complexes.

Furthermore, it has been demonstrated that higher birth weight is associated with an increased risk of atrial fibrillation during adulthood. Atrial fibrillation may appear as an isolated finding, especially in the elderly or only in presence of some risk factors. In cases of lone atrial fibrillation in young people, it seems possible that some genetic predisposition may play a role (Roberts and Gollob 2010).

Figure 15.22 summarizes the pathophysiological mechanisms involved in the initiation and perpetuating atrial fibrillation (Bayés de Luna and Baranchuk 2017).

Atrial fibrillation has to be considered a progressive disease, starting usually with episodes that are self-controlled (**paroxysmal**), and it is difficult to predict when these will repeat, but in at least in 10% of cases there will be recurrences at 1 year (Figure 15.23). Finally, in the majority of cases, within more or less time (sometimes several decades), the disease becomes **persistent** usually (needs drugs or electrical CV to restore sinus rhythm) or **permanent** (no attempt to restore sinus rhythm) (Figure 15.24). Patients with atrial fibrillation may present with symptoms that are sometimes clinically relevant (angina, dyspnea, and even heart failure in cases of very fast heart rate). However, on some occasions, it is unnoticed by the patient or mildly symptomatic by some palpitations. Unfortunately, especially in the presence of some risk factors, the incidence of cerebral embolism is high and will need preventive anticoagulation treatment (see later).

ECG findings

Diagnosis of atrial fibrillation, although it may be suspected during history taking and physical examination, is confirmed by the ECG. It is based on observation of the fibrillation "f" waves and the ventricular response, which is completely irregular. It is also desirable, if possible, to check the ECG morphology at onset and at the end of the episode, in order to make the differential diagnosis. In the current era, self-detected devices (smart watches, patches, etc.) are part of the diagnostic armamentarium of clinicians. Intracardiac devices are also useful to detect "subclinical AF" which could also lead to an increased risk of embolism (Steinberg *et al.* 2017; Li *et al.* 2019).

During sinus rhythm
Predictor markers

In **sinus rhythm,** there are some ECG changes in the P wave that have been considered "predictor markers" for future atrial fibrillation/atrial flutter episodes. This encompasses: (i) longer duration of P wave with an important negative part of the P wave in V1 (criteria of left atrium enlargement), the presence of left atrium

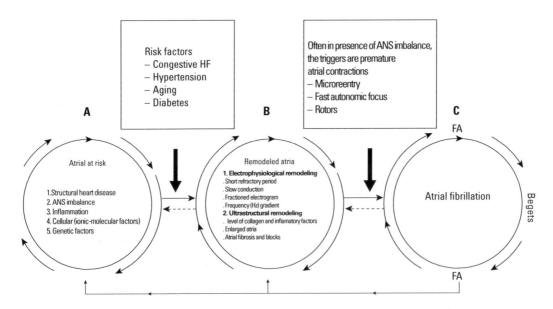

Figure 15.22 Summary of the pathophysiologic mechanisms involved in the initiation and perpetuation of atrial fibrillation (see text).

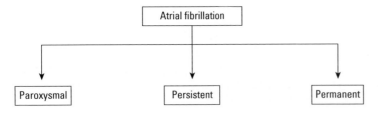

Figure 15.23 Types of atrial fibrillation according to clinical presentation.

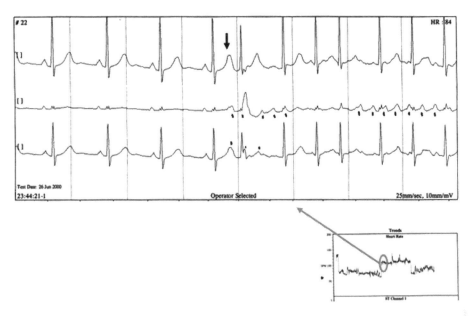

Figure 15.24 A 37-year-old patient who showed frequent paroxysmal atrial fibrillation (AF) episodes despite drug therapy and who was a good candidate for ablation. We see the onset of an episode of paroxysmal AF after a very premature atrial systole that distorts the preceding T wave and is conducted with an aberrant QRS (arrow). Bottom: Onset and end of the episode in the heart rate trend of a Holter recording.

enlargement (P ± V1 with duration ≥120 ms) and signs of right atrial overload (tall initial part of P wave in V1), which may be critical for susceptibility to atrial fibrillation; (ii) the presence of ECG signs of interatrial block (P wave > 120 ms) (Holmqvist *et al.* 2009), especially advanced with ± morphology in II, III, and VF (Bayés de Luna *et al.* 1988) (Figures 9.20 and 15.14). In the last 5 years, the presence of interatrial block in the surface ECG emerged as the most powerful ECG marker of increased risk of AF (currently known as Bayes' syndrome) (Baranchuk and Yeung 2018).

The ECG is often normal in paroxysmal atrial fibrillation and has other various ECG signs according to the underlying heart disease in case of permanent atrial fibrillation.

Atrial waves: "f" waves (Figures 15.25 and 15.26)

The ECG shows small waves (named fibrillatory "f") with a rate between 350 and 700 per minute. Lead V1 is generally the most appropriate lead for observing the fibrillation waves. In some leads and in the presence of atrial fibrosis, the "f" waves are often not well seen. Fibrillatory waves measuring ≥1 mm (coarse "f" waves) are considered to be present more frequently in patients with left atrial enlargement (see Chapter 9). Patients with heart failure and low atrial fibrillatory rate have lower survival (Platonov *et al.* 2012).

The majority of "f" waves are blocked somewhere in the AV junction with different degrees of concealed conduction, producing an irregular ventricular response.

Onset and offset of episodes

Paroxysmal atrial fibrillation is initiated by early premature atrial contractions (short coupling interval) falling in the atrial vulnerable period (AVP) and often with repeated short runs of supraventricular tachyarrhythmias (Figure 15.24).

Persistent atrial fibrillation is initiated by a premature atrial complex that is frequently isolated and usually with longer coupling interval than in paroxysmal episodes.

The end of the episode is usually followed by a short pause. However, often the pause is more or less prolonged. When the pause is very long, it may be indicative of bradycardia–tachycardia syndrome (see Figure 15.27), a form of sick sinus syndrome.

Ventricular response and QRS complex morphology

In normal conditions, it is usually fast (from 130 to 160 bpm) and completely irregular due to the different degrees of concealed conduction of the "f" waves.

In the presence of atrial fibrillation, a regular and slow ventricular rhythm is explained by the presence of an escape rhythm of the AV junction (narrow QRS complex), or ventricular (wide QRS complex) or pacemaker rhythm. If the ventricular rhythm is regular and fast, it is due to an AV junctional tachycardia with narrow QRS (Figure 15.18A), or wide QRS in the case of aberrant conduction, or due to ventricular tachycardia. In both situations, there is a complete AV dissociation due to interference of the high ectopic rhythm, or AV block, if the ventricular rate is slow.

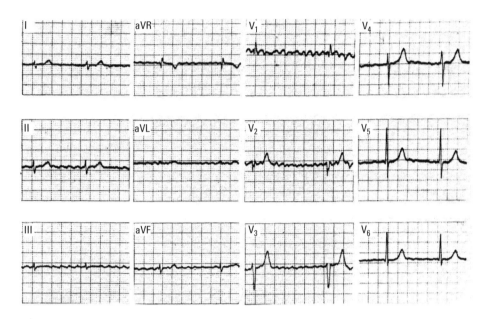

Figure 15.25 A 45-year-old patient with a tight mitral stenosis and mild aortic regurgitation. Note the typical atrial fibrillation (AF) medium-sized waves, which are especially visible in V1.

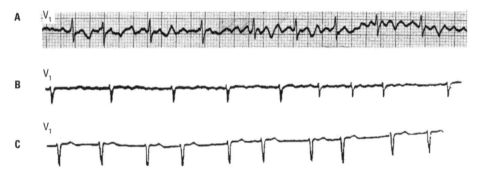

Figure 15.26 (A) Atrial fibrillation (AF) with "f" waves with prominent voltage. (B and C) "f" waves with lower voltage.

Figure 15.27 A long pause frequently occurs after an episode in brady-tachyarrhythmia syndrome, which in this case finishes with a sinus P wave (spontaneous conversion).

The presence of wide QRS complex may be due to aberrancy or ectopy (see later).

Differential diagnosis
With other irregular tachycarrhythmias
Diagnosis of atrial fibrillation is made by surface ECG, or by self-detected devices or intracardiac recordings. In general, this is easy to diagnose. However, it can be confused with the following irregular rhythms:

- **Chaotic atrial tachycardia.** The characteristics of this infrequent tachyarrhythmia are discussed in the section on Chaotic atrial tachycardia, above (Figure 15.21).
- **Atrial flutter with variable AV conduction.**
- **Sinus rhythm with low-voltage P waves and** frequent and irregularly located **atrial extrasystoles.**

Aberrancy versus ectopy in wide QRS complexes
This differential diagnosis has prognostic and therapeutic implications. To explain the wide QRS morphology, the following considerations must be taken into account:

• The presence of runs with irregular wide QRS and typical right bundle branch block (RBBB) morphology rsR′ in V1 (and/or qRs in V6) favors aberrancy (Figure 15.28), mainly if the irregularity of the rhythm during the runs with the RBBB pattern is similar to that observed in the basic rhythm with narrow QRS. The maintained aberrancy with RBBB morphology may be explained by retrograde concealed conduction in the right bundle (Figure 15.28) (Longo and Baranchuk 2017).

• A wide QRS that does not follow the Gouaux–Ashman rule may be explained by different concealed conductions of "f" waves in the intraventricular conduction system (see Figure 15.29) (see legends and Figure 14.31).

The other morphologies are observed to a greater extent when the complexes are ectopic, including the R morphology in V1 with a notch in the descending arm of the R wave and the QS morphology in V6 (Figures 14.25 and 15.29).

Atrial fibrillation in WPW syndrome versus ventricular tachycardia

In WPW syndrome with atrial fibrillation, QRS complexes with different degrees of pre-excitation may be observed, the occurrence of which are not related to the length of the preceding RR interval (Figure 15.30).

The accessory pathway has a faster conduction than the specific conduction system, and therefore atrial fibrillation in the presence of WPW syndrome frequently shows QRS complex morphology with significant pre-excitation and fast heart rate. The refractory period of accessory pathway is also longer. Therefore, an atrial premature beat blocked in the accessory pathway may trigger paroxysmal reentrant AVRT (see Figures 14.13 and 15.12).

Atrial fibrillation in the presence of pre-excitation requires a differential diagnosis with fast ventricular tachycardia runs. The following criteria are indicative of atrial fibrillation in the presence of WPW syndrome (Figure 15.30): (i) the presence of QRS complexes with different degrees of pre-excitation; (ii) the irregularity of the RR intervals; (iii) in ventricular tachycardia, the presence of narrow QRS complexes, if they exist, are sinus captures (premature complexes), whereas in atrial fibrillation with WPW syndrome, the narrow QRS complexes are usually characterized by random occurrence and may be early or late.

Clinical and prognostic implications

Atrial fibrillation is the most prevalent tachyarrhythmia seen in outpatient departments as well as in hospitals. However, the total burden of atrial fibrillation extends

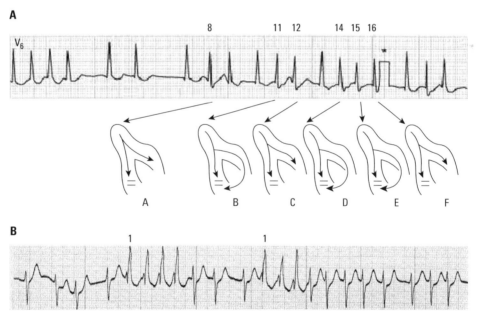

Figure 15.28 (A) Sustained aberrancy. Several wide complexes with right bundle branch block (RBBB) morphology (wide S) are shown in the V6 lead. The eighth wide complex is probably aberrant and may be explained by a phase 3 mechanism (long preceding diastole, short coupling interval). Afterward, there is a couple (complexes 11 and 12), as well as a run (complexes 14, 15, and 16), of aberrant complexes. Complexes 11 and 14 may be aberrant because of the aforementioned classical mechanism (short coupling interval, relatively long preceding diastole). In contrast, the aberrant complexes 12, 15, and 16 without these characteristics may be explained because the preceding ones (11, 14, and 15) may initiate a concealed retrograde conduction over the right bundle branch (RBB), preventing the subsequent stimuli 12, 15, and 16 from crossing this branch in an anterograde fashion (*millivolt). (B) Two runs of QRS with sustained aberrancy are shown. The first complex in each run (1) would be explained by phase 3 aberrancy but not the others. The first aberrant complex of each run, and also the second and third of the first run, and the second of the second run probably retrogradely invade the RBB and the subsequent QRS is aberrant because it cannot be conducted over the RBB as it is in its refractory period due to concealed conduction in the right branch of the preceding QRS complex (see diagram in A). The typical right bundle branch block (RBBB) morphology (rsR′ in V1), and also the irregular RR cadence, similar to narrow subsequent QRS, strongly suggests aberrancy.

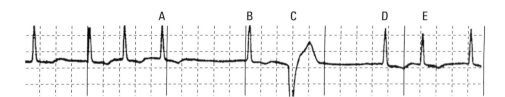

Figure 15.29 Strip of a patient with atrial fibrillation and some wide QRS complexes. The QS morphology of the wide complex in V6 definitely indicates an ectopic origin despite the previous diastole being very long (AB). Note that even with a longer preceding diastole (CD), the following QRS (E) shows a normal morphology, probably because of the concealed conduction of some "f" waves in the branches (see Figure 14.31).

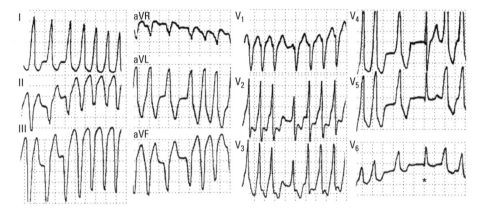

Figure 15.30 Twelve-lead ECG of a Wolff–Parkinson–White (WPW) syndrome in atrial fibrillation. Note the great degree of aberrancy of the complexes, complicating the differential diagnosis with ventricular tachycardia, especially in the presence of a regular ventricular conduction (atrial flutter). This arrhythmia should always be taken into account, because it may easily be mistaken for a very serious ventricular tachycardia. In this case, the diagnosis of WPW syndrome with atrial fibrillation is supported by: (i) the presence of delta waves in some leads (V2, V3) and the presence of different morphologies of QRS, with more or less degrees of aberrancy, as the expression of different degrees of conduction over the accessory pathway; (ii) irregular RR; (iii) narrow QRS, which may or may not be premature (see asterisk) (in ventricular tachycardia, narrow QRS complexes are always premature (captures)); and (iv) awareness of the existence of this arrhythmia.

beyond its symptoms because around **50% of atrial fibrillation episodes are asymptomatic.** These asymptomatic episodes may impact quality of life and cardiac function (Savelieva and Camm 2000). Therefore, in patients at risk, especially those who suffer from valvular heart disease or have had a stroke, it is convenient to use Holter monitoring (or other extended cardiac monitoring strategies) to rule out the possibility of silent atrial fibrillation episodes (Steinberg *et al.* 2017).

Mortality for any reason in patients with atrial fibrillation virtually **doubles the mortality observed in patients with similar clinical status in sinus rhythm.** Isolated atrial fibrillation has a better prognosis. In the remaining cases, it depends on the underlying disease.

In general, **the main dangers of atrial fibrillation are:** (i) fast ventricular rates that are difficult to control with drugs and (ii) the risk of developing systemic embolism, especially cerebral embolism. Fast ventricular rates may lead to hemodynamic deterioration, left ventricle dysfunction, and even to heart failure (tachycardiomyopathy), especially in cases with previous heart disease. In

addition, in rare cases, WPW syndrome may induce serious ventricular arrhythmias, including ventricular fibrillation (see above).

Therapeutic approach

A therapeutic approach comprises four objectives: (i) prevention of the first episode, (ii) conversion to sinus rhythm and prevention of recurrences, (iii) if neither of these are possible, control of ventricular rate, and (iv) prevention of thromboembolism (Fuster *et al.* 2006; Kirchhof and Breithardt 2009; Camm 2011).

Figure 15.31 summarizes when it is necessary to use the different therapeutic approaches (antiarrhythmic agents, anticoagulation, electrical CV, and ablation) along the evolution of the disease. Note that prevention of cerebral embolism is a priority in patients with atrial fibrillation and that the current success rate for ablation in paroxysmal cases is ~70% with relatively lower number of recurrences and a very small number of important complications. No doubt this result will improve in the future, especially if ablation is performed at an appropriate time—"not too

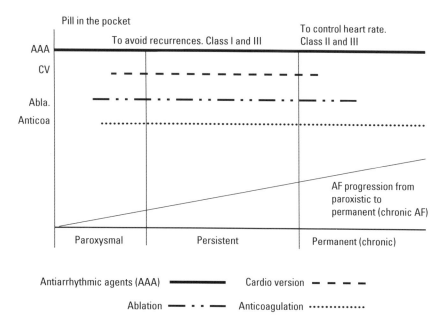

Figure 15.31 Atrial fibrillation is a progressive disease from paroxysmal to persistent and permanent (chronic). The figure shows the time schedule of prescription of different treatments given during the follow-up for this disease. Note that anticoagulation may already have been started if paroxysmal crises are frequent and must be taken during the entire follow-up if there are no contraindications.

early, not too late" and if it includes more cases of persistent atrial fibrillation. For further discussion on all these important aspects, see Bayés de Luna and Baranchuk, 2017.

Atrial flutter

Concept
Atrial flutter is a fast atrial rhythm (240–300 bpm). The cases with a slower rate, even <200 bpm, are explained by the effect of pharmacologic therapy and/or the presence of important conduction delay in the atria. The rhythm is organized and regular, and initiates atrial waves that do not have (at least in some leads, especially the inferior leads) an isoelectric baseline between them (flutter "F" waves).

From a clinical point of view, the etiological characteristics, clinical presentation, and prognosis of atrial flutter are similar to those of atrial fibrillation. Therefore, it may have paroxysmal (sporadic and repetitive) and chronic (persistent and/or permanent) forms. However, atrial flutter is a more "**transient arrhythmia**" that frequently changes to sinus rhythm or atrial fibrillation.

Electrophysiologic mechanism
Although **atrial flutter has some morphological aspects very similar to atrial fibrillation, it is really a very different arrhythmia** because the maintenance mechanism is different. Typical atrial flutter is an arrhythmia of the right atrium, the maintenance mechanism of which is a macro-reentry, and atrial fibrillation is predominantly a

left atrium arrhythmia, the mechanisms of which are never a macro-reentry. However, the triggering and modulating factors (PSVC, autonomic nervous system imbalance, inflammatory markers, etc.) are similar to those of atrial fibrillation.

It is possible that all types of flutter start with a very premature atrial extrasystole, which, when it finds some zone of the atria with unidirectional block, initiates a circular movement (reentry). The slower the conduction of the stimulus or the longer the circuit, the easier it is to perpetuate the arrhythmia.

The depolarization in **common (typical) flutter** is counterclockwise, going down through the anterior and lateral walls of the right atrium and up through the septum and the posterior wall of the right atrium, with a zone of slow conduction in the lower right atrium. Thus, when depolarization reaches the lower part of the septum, another "F" wave is already in development (Figure 14.12A). This explains the lack of isoelectric baseline between "F" waves, and why "F" waves are predominantly negative in leads II, III, and aVF. From leads such as aVF, the positive (craniocaudal) part of the wave lasts longer and is smoother (less visible) than the negative part (caudocranial) (Figures 15.32 and 15.33). Because of this, in leads II, III, and aVF, the negative morphology part predominates over the positive one, especially in the absence of large atria.

In a small number of cases, flutter activation uses the same circuit but follows a clockwise rotation, ascending through the anterior and lateral wall and descending through the posterior and septal wall, so that the circuit is the same, but the rotation is different (**inverse or reverse flutter**) (Figures 14.12B and 15.34). Usually, the ECG shows a different morphology (wide positive waves in leads II, III, and aVF, and wide negative in V1).

It is also possible to find other morphologies that require electrophysiologic study to identify the circuit. They are probably related to a reentry in the left atrium, and correspond to an uncommon type of flutter (**atypical flutter**) (Figures 14.12C and 15.35). These cases are equivalent to macro-reentrant atrial tachycardia but with a higher rate (>220 bpm). In the ablation era (pulmonary vein isolation for atrial fibrillation), the presence of atypical atrial flutters using "old" lines created during prior ablations became more frequent in the EP labs. Learning how to break these flutters and prevent future arrhythmias is paramount in modern EP.

ECG findings
Sinus rhythm
The considerations discussed in the atrial fibrillation section are also valid for atrial flutter (Figure 15.14). The presence of interatrial block during sinus rhythm, after a successful ablation for typical atrial flutter, is a good risk marker for further development of atrial fibrillation (Enriquez *et al.* 2015)

Flutter "F" waves
Common or typical flutter: counterclockwise activation (Figures 15.32 and 15.33)
This comprises predominantly negative "F" waves in leads II, III, and aVF. These are "F" waves with a small voltage in the absence of large atria, and are without an isoelectric baseline, giving them a saw tooth morphology. They are predominantly negative in leads II, III, and aVF, and positive in V1, where the "F" wave is usually narrow and often shows an isoelectric baseline.

Non-common flutter
• **Reverse or inverse flutter**: Clockwise activation (Figure 15.34). Generally, it initiates wide and positive "F" waves in leads II, III, and aVF, without isoelectric baselines between them and with predominantly negative and wide waves in lead V1.
• **Atypical flutter** (Figure 15.35): This term includes positive atrial wave in leads II, III, aVF, and V1 with high rates (>220 bpm) and sometimes with some undulating waves

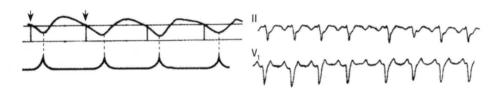

Figure 15.32 Morphology correlation between II and V1 in a common 2 × 1 flutter, with an eventual 3 × 1 conduction.

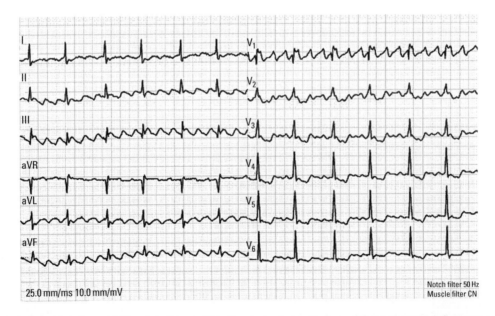

25.0 mm/ms 10.0 mm/mV

Notch filter 50 Hz
Muscle filter CN

Figure 15.33 A 15-year-old patient with Ebstein's disease. Note the sawtooth morphology of the common 3 × 1 flutter waves, which show a voltage greater than usual because of the large size of the atria.

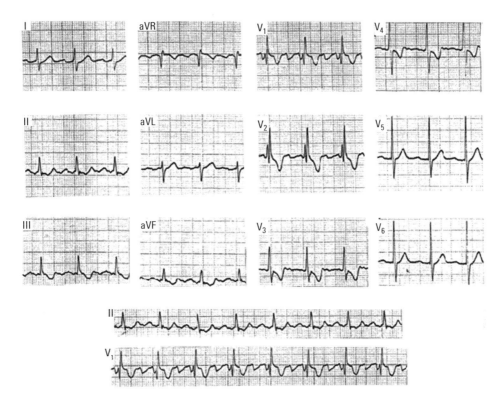

Figure 15.34 Example of reverse atrial flutter (positive "F" waves in I, II, III, and aVF, and wide negative in V1) that appeared after surgery for anomalous drainage of pulmonary veins.

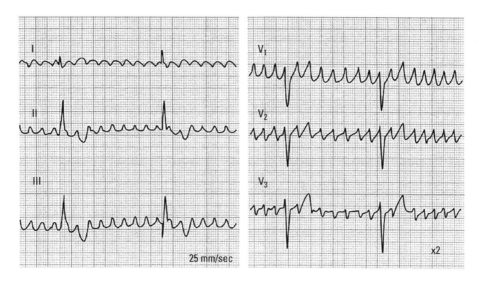

Figure 15.35 Example of atypical flutter with fast atrial waves (~280 x′) and predominantly negative waves in I and positive waves in II, III, aVF, and V1. This type of flutter is very often recorded in patients with advanced interatrial block with retrograde activation of the left atrium.

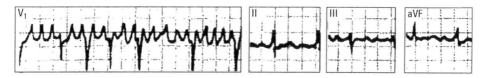

Figure 15.36 Typical fibrillo-flutter morphology. The atrial waves show a fairly regular, slightly faster rate in V1 (as in the flutter), and do not show a saw tooth morphology in II, III, or aVF (as in atrial fibrillation).

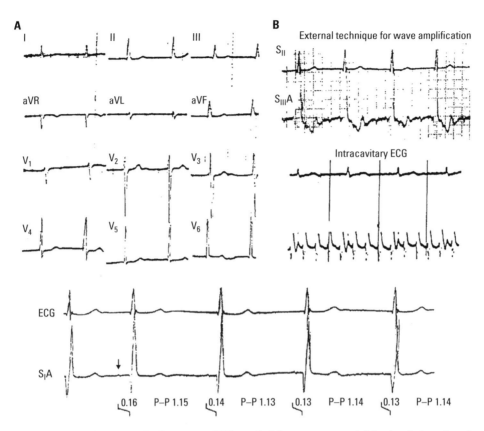

Figure 15.37 (A) ECG of a 66-year-old man with a heart rate of 55 bpm. Atrial waves are not visible, simulating a junctional escape rhythm. (B) With the use of external wave amplification and intracavitary ECG, the concealed flutter waves were exposed. (C) A successful cardioversion was performed, showing afterward, thanks to external amplification of waves (SI A), that it was a small but visible sinus P wave (see arrow).

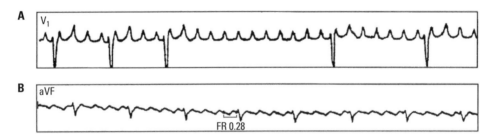

Figure 15.38 (A) Atrial flutter ("F" waves in V1 at 280 bpm) with a significant atrioventricular (AV) block. (B) Typical flutter with a fixed 4 × 1 AV conduction. Note the fixed and long FR interval.

in at least some leads that do not show characteristics of typical or inverse flutter.

Other types of atrial activity

• **Fibrillo-flutter**: In some leads, the atrial waves are typical of fibrillation and in others like flutter waves (Figure 15.36).

• On rare occasions, especially when patients are taking cardioactive drugs (i.e. digitalis), the morphology of the flutter wave varies (Figure 15.18B).

• At other times, when there is significant atrial fibrosis, the flutter "F" waves may not be visible (Figure 15.37).

Ventricular response and QRS morphology

In typical flutter with a rate between 250 and 300 bpm, one of every two "F" waves is blocked in the AV junction, as a rule, and therefore the ventricular response is between 125 and 150 bpm. The FR interval, starting from the beginning of the negative "F" wave, has a duration ≥0.20 sec (Figure 15.38B). However, a higher degree block (3 : 1, rare, 4 : 1, 6 : 1, or more) is found, especially with certain drugs that have depressor effects on the atrioventricular conduction (Figure 15.38A). Sometimes, in the same patient the degree of conduction is variable and can be inclusively 1 : 1 in the same patient (Figure 15.39). If the

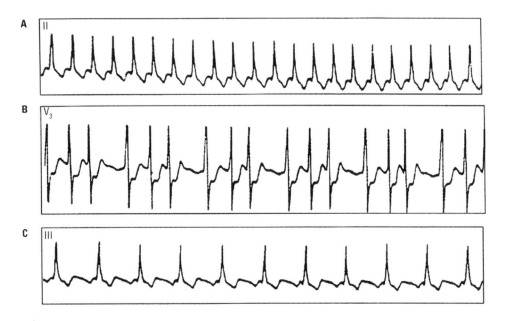

Figure 15.39 A patient with tight mitral stenosis taking antiarrhythmic agents who presented with a 1 × 1 flutter that turned into a Wenckebach-type 4 × 3 conduction (B) and finally a 2 × 1 flutter (C).

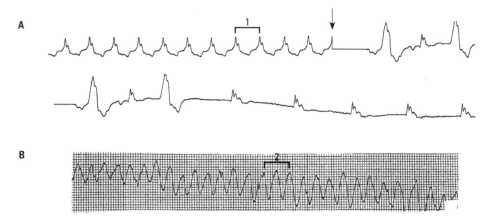

Figure 15.40 (A) A 52-year-old patient with Ebstein's disease and rapid rhythm at 160 bpm suggestive of a 2 : 1 flutter (QRS morphology similar to that under sinus rhythm), which ceased after cardioversion (arrow), turning into a slow escape rhythm with retrograde conduction toward the atria. (B) Afterward, this patient showed a short (monitor strip) run of tachycardia with a heart rate doubled from the previous one (~320 bpm) (1 = 2), which was very badly tolerated, probably indicating a 1 : 1 flutter, which fortunately ceased spontaneously after a few seconds. This tracing, seen isolated, may be taken as a ventricular flutter.

basal QRS complex is wide because of a bundle branch block or pre-excitation, the presence of atrial flutter with 1 : 1 conduction mimics a ventricular flutter aspect (Figure 15.40). Flutter with 1 : 1 is very badly tolerated and represents a real risk of sudden death as a result of its high ventricular rate (usually > 220 bpm).

The presence of variable FR intervals and fixed RR intervals means that AV dissociation exists (Figures 15.18B and 17.4).

The wide QRS morphology may be caused by aberrant conduction (bundle branch block pattern) (Figure 15.40) or conduction along an accessory pathway (Figure 15.41). In cases of 2 : 1 flutter and primarily 1 : 1 conduction, an accessory pathway must be considered when the aberrant QRS complex morphology does not correspond with a bundle branch block pattern and especially if a delta wave is suspected. If the flutter is 1 : 1, the morphology can look like ventricular flutter (compare Figures 15.40B and 15.41B).

Diagnostic difficulties and differential diagnoses

These have already been discussed. They include: (i) diagnostic difficulties due to "F" wave morphology; (ii) diagnostic difficulties due to the "F" wave rate; (iii) diagnostic difficulties due to the width of the QRS complex;

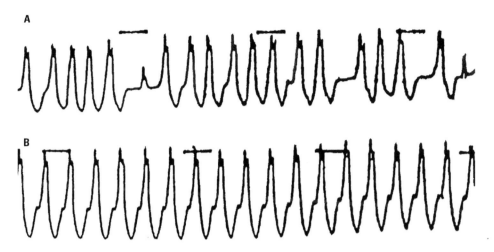

Figure 15.41 A 50-year-old patient with type IV Wolff–Parkinson–White (WPW) atrial fibrillation (top) and atrial flutter (bottom) episodes simulating a ventricular tachycardia. (A) The isolated, wide R morphology, with a notch in the descending arm does not correspond to a right bundle branch block (RBBB)-type conduction aberrancy. The following facts are in favor of a WPW syndrome with atrial fibrillation (in addition to other clinical features and the prior awareness of the WPW syndrome diagnosis): (i) The wide complexes show a very irregular rate and morphology (varying wideness) because of the presence of different degrees of pre-excitation. (ii) The two narrow complexes—6 and the last one in A—are late and premature, respectively. In sustained ventricular tachycardia, QRSs are more regular and if captures occur (narrow complexes), they are always premature (see Figures 15.30 and 16.15). (B) In the WPW syndrome with atrial flutter (in this case 2 : 1, 150 bpm), differential diagnosis with sustained ventricular tachycardia through the ECG is even more difficult.

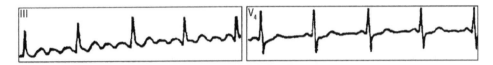

Figure 15.42 A patient with Parkinson's disease who simulates an atrial flutter in some leads (III), although the P wave is clearly visible in other leads (V4).

and (iv) diagnostic difficulties due to artifacts. This has been seen with diaphragm contractions (hiccups) and also as a result of recording problems, for example, when a patient is trembling (Parkinson's tremor disease) (Figure 15.42) (Osman *et al.* 2019).

Clinical implications

In comparison with atrial fibrillation, it is more difficult to control the heart rate in atrial flutter, but the risk of embolism may be lower, but still requiring full oral anticoagulation. However, atrial fibrillation frequently alternates with flutter episodes in the same patient. Thus, the prognosis is similar to that for atrial fibrillation.

There are various options (drugs, electrical CV, atrial pacing, and ablation) for treatment of rapid atrial flutter episodes in hospital. The aim of treatment is to restore sinus rhythm. The success of ablation is higher than in atrial fibrillation with less than 3% recurrence rate and very low intra-procedural complication rate.

References

Alboni P, Botto GL, Baldi N, *et al.* Outpatient treatment of recent-onset atrial fibrillation with the "pill-in-the-pocket" approach. N Engl J Med 2004;351:2384.

Bar FW, Brugada P, Dassen WR, *et al.* Differential diagnosis of tachycardia withnarrow QRS complex (shorter than 0.12 second). Am J Cardiol 1984;54:555.

Baranchuk A, Yeung C. Advanced interatrial block predicts atrial fibrillation recurrence across different populations: learning Bayés syndrome. Int J Cardiol 2018;272:221–222

Bayés de Luna A, Baranchuk A. *Clinical Arrhythmology*, 2nd edn. Wiley-Blackwell, 2017

Bayés de Luna A, Cladellas M, Oter R, *et al.* Interatrial conduction block and retrograde activation of the left atrium and paroxysmal supraventricular arrhythmias. Eur Heart J 1988;9:1112.

Bazán V, Rodríguez-Font E, Viñolas X, *et al.* Atrial tachycardia originating from the pulmonary vein: clinical, electrocardiographic, and differential electrophysiologic characteristics. Rev Esp Cardiol 2010;63:149.

Camm J. Chairman: Guidelines for the management of atrial fibrillation. European Society of Cardiology 2010 (222.escardio/guidelines2010). Eur Heart J 2011.

Chen SA, Chiang CE, Yang CJ, *et al.* Sustained atrial tachycardia in adult patients. Electrophysiological characteristics, pharmacological response, possible mechanisms, and effects of radiofrequency ablation. Circulation 1994;90:1262.

Chiale PA, Baranchuk A, González MD et al. The mechanisms of spontaneous termination of reentrant supraventricular tachycardias. Int J Cardiol 2015;191:151–158.

Collins K, Van Hare G, Kertesz N, *et al.* Pediatric non-postoperative junctional ectopic tachycardia. J Am Coll Cardiol 2009;53:690.

Coumel Ph, Fidelle J, Cloup M, *et al.* Les tachycardies réciproques à évolution prolongée chez l'enfant. Arch Mal Cœur 1974;67:23.

Di Toro D, Hadid C, López C, *et al.* Utility of the aVL lead in the electrocardiographic diagnosis of atrioventricular node reentrant tachycardia. Europace 2009;11:944.

Dubin A, Cuneo B, Strasburger J, *et al.* Congenital junctional ectopic tachycardia and congenital AV block: a shared etiology? Heart Rhythm 2005;2:313.

Enriquez A, Sarrias A, Villuendas R, *et al.* New-onset atrial fibrillation after cavotricuspid isthmus ablation: identification of advanced interatrial block is key. Europace 2015;17(8):1289–93.

Femenía F, Baranchuk A, Morillo CA. Inappropriate sinus tachycardia: current therapeutic options. Cardiol Rev 2012;20(1):8–14

Fuster V, Rydén LE, Cannom DS, *et al.* ACC/AHA/ESC2006 Guidelines for the management of patients with atrial fibrillation: developed in collaboration with the European Heart Rhythm Association and the Heart Rhythm Society. Circulation 2006;15:114:e257.

Gomes JA, Hariman RJ, Kang PS, *et al.* Sustained symptomatic sinus node reentrant tachycardia: incidence, clinical significance, electrophysiologic observations and the effects of antiarrhythmic agents. J Am Coll Cardiol 1985;5:45.

González-Torrecilla E, Almendral J, Arenal A, *et al.* Combined evaluation of bedside clinical variables and the electrocardiogram for the differential diagnosis of paroxysmal atrioventricular reciprocating tachycardias in patients without pre-excitation. J Am Coll Cardiol 2009;53:2353.

Holmqvist F, Platonov PG, Carlson J, *et al.* Altered interatrial conduction detected in MADIT II patients bound to develop atrial fibrillation. Ann Noninvasive Electrocardiol 2009;14:268.

Inoue S, Becker A. Posterior extension of human AV node. Circulation 1998;97:188.

Jastrzębski M, Kukla P, Pitak M, Rudziński A, Baranchuk A, Czarnecka D. Intermittent preexcitation indicates "a low-risk" accessory pathway: time for a paradigm shift? Ann Noninvasive Electrocardiol. 2017;22(6):e12464.

Josephson, ME. Paroxysmal supraventricular tachycardia: an electrophysiological approach. Am J Cardiol 1978;41:1123.

Katritsis D, Becker A. The AV nodal re-entrant circuit. A proposal. Heart Rhythm 2007;4:1354.

Kirchhof P, Breithardt G (LAFNET/EHRA consensus conference on AF). Early and comprehensive management of atrial fibrillation. Europace 2009;11:860.

Kistler PM, Robert-Thomson KC, Haqqani HM, *et al.* P wave morphology in focal atrial tachycardia: an algorythm to predict the anatomic site of origin. J Am Coll Cardiol 2006;48:1010.

Li KHC, White FA, Tipoe T, *et al.* The current state of mobile phone apps for monitoring heart rate, heart rate variability, and atrial fibrillation: narrative review. JMIR Mhealth Uhealth 2019;7(2):e11606

Longo D, Baranchuk A. Ashman phenomenon dynamicity during atrial fibrillation: the critical role of the long cycles. J Atr Fibrillation 2017;10(3):1656.

Nadeau-Routhier C, Baranchuk A. In Nadeau-Routhier C, Baranchuk A (eds) Electrocardiography in Practice: What to Do?. 2016, p. 123–140. Accessed June 2019: https://itunes.apple.com/us/book/electrocardiography-in-practice/id1120119530?mt=13

Osman W, Hanson M, Baranchuk A. Pseudo-ventricular tachycardia, pseudo-atrial fibrillation, and pseudo-atrial flutter in a patient with Parkinson disease: two's company, Three's a Crowd. JAMA Intern Med 2019;179(6):824–826.

Paparella N, Duyang F, Fuca G, *et al.* Significance of newly acquired negative T wave after interruption of paroxysmal supraventricular tachycardia with narrow QRS. Am JCard 2000;85:261.

Platonov P, Cygankiewicz I, Stridh M, *et al.* Low atrial fibrillatory rate is associated with poor outcome in patients with mild to moderate heart failure. Circ Arrhythm Electrophysiol 2012;5(1):77–83.

Prasitlumkum N, Rattanawong P, Limpruttidham N, *et al.* Frequent premature atrial complexes as a predictor of atrial fibrillation: systematic review and meta-analysis. J Electrocardiol 2018;51(5):760–767.

Roberts J, Gollob M. Impact of genetic discoveries on the classification of lone atrial fibrillation. Am J Coll Cardiol 2010;55:705.

Ruder MA, Davis JC, Eldar M, *et al.* Clinical and electrophysiologic characterization of automatic junctional tachycardia in adults. Circulation 1986;73:930.

Savelieva I, Camm AJ. Clinical relevance of silent atrial fibrillation: prevalence, prognosis, quality of life, and management. J Interv Card Electrophysiol 2000;4:369.

Steinberg JS, Varma N, Cygankiewicz I, *et al.* 2017 ISHNE-HRS expert consensus statement on ambulatory ECG and external cardiac monitoring/telemetry. Heart Rhythm 2017;14(7):e55–e96.

Wharton M. Atrial tachycardia: advancesin diagnosis and treatment. Cardiol Rev 1995;3:332.

Wu D, Denes P, Amat-y-Leon F, *et al.* Clinical, electrocardiographic and electrophysiologic observations in patients with paroxysmal supraventricular tachycardia. Am J Cardiol 1978;41:1045.

Chapter 16
Active Ventricular Arrhythmias

In this chapter, we will discuss premature ventricular complexes and various types of ventricular tachycardia as well as ventricular fibrillation and ventricular flutter (Table 16.1).

Premature ventricular complexes

Concept and mechanisms
Premature ventricular complexes (PVCs) are premature impulses (complexes) that originate in the ventricles. Therefore, they have a different morphology from that of the baseline rhythm.

PVCs may be caused by extrasystolic or parasystolic mechanisms (Figures 16.1 and 16.2):

• **Extrasystoles** are much more frequent than parasystoles and are induced by a mechanism related to the preceding QRS complex. For this reason, they feature a fixed or nearly fixed coupling interval (Figure 16.1). This is generally a reentrant mechanism (usually micro-reentry), but also branch to branch, or around a necrotic or fibrotic area (see Figure 14.10). They may also be induced by post-potentials (triggered activity) (see Figure 14.16) or other mechanisms (see Bayés de Luna and Baranchuk 2017; Enriquez *et al.* 2017).

• **Parasystoles** are much less frequent (Figure 16.2). They are impulses that are independent of the baseline rhythm. The electrophysiologic mechanism is an ectopic focus protected from depolarization by the impulses of the baseline rhythm. In general, this is due to the presence of a unidirectional entrance block in the parasystolic focus (see Figure 14.18).

ECG findings
ECG forms of presentation
In the ECG, the PVCs are represented as premature wide QRS complexes with a different morphology from that of the basal QRS.

PVCs usually show a complete compensatory pause (the distance between the QRS complex preceding the PVC and the following QRS complex double the sinus cadence) (Figure 16.3A). This happens because the PVC usually fails to discharge the sinus node. In consequence, the distance BC doubles the distance AB, appearing as two sinus cycles.

If the PVC discharges the sinus node, a non-complete compensatory pause may be observed (BC < 2AB) (Figure 16.3B).

When the sinus heart rate is slow, a PVC, although it may enter the atrioventricular (AV) junction, leaving it in a refractory period (RP), will not prevent the following sinus stimulus from being conducted toward the ventricles, usually with a longer PR interval. This is because of the concealed PVC conduction over the AV junction, leaving it in the relative refractory period (RRP) that slows, but does not prevent, the conduction of the following P wave. Thus, the PVC occurs between two sinus conducted P waves and does not feature a compensatory pause (Figure 16.3C). This type of PVC is known as an **interpolated PVC** (Figures 14.29 and 16.3C).

An isolated PVC may occur sporadically or with a specific cadence. In this case, they may produce a bigeminy (a sinus QRS complex and an extrasystolic QRS

Table 16.1 Lown's classification of premature ventricular complexes (PVCs) according to their prognostic significance (Holter ECG)

Grade 0	No PVC
Grade 1	<30/h
Grade 2	≥30/h
Grade 3	Polymorphic PVCs
Grade 4a	On pairs
Grade 4b	Runs of monomorphic ventricular tachycardia
Grade 5	R/T Phenomenon (PVC falls on the preceding T wave)

Modified from Lown and Wolf (1971).

Clinical Electrocardiography: A Textbook, Fifth Edition. Antoni Bayés de Luna, Miquel Fiol-Sala, Antoni Bayés-Genís, and Adrián Baranchuk.
© 2022 John Wiley & Sons Ltd. Published 2022 by John Wiley & Sons Ltd.

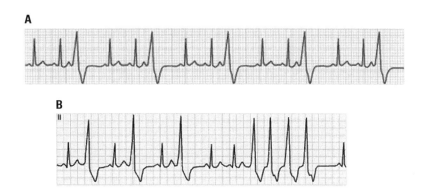

Figure 16.1 (A) Typical example of ventricular extrasystoles in the form of trigeminy. Note similar couple intervals. (B) Another example of ventricular extrasystoles, first bigeminal, then one run of non-sustained ventricular tachycardia (VT) (four complexes).

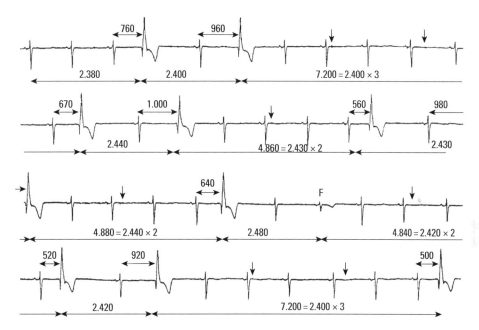

Figure 16.2 An example of parasystole. Note the variable coupling intervals, 760 ms, etc., interectopic intervals are multiple of the baseline interval at 2380, 2400, 2400 × 3, etc., and the presence of a fusion complex (F). The diagnosis of parasystole may be already performed before the appearance of the fusion complex.

complex) (Figure 16.1B) or a trigeminy (two normally conducted QRS complexes and one extrasystolic QRS) (Figure 16.1A). As we have already said, they may also occur in a repetitive form (Figures 16.1B and 16.4D). Short and isolated runs of classical monomorphic ventricular tachycardia with a rather slow rate (Figure 16.4) are considered repetitive forms of PVCs and will be dealt separately within this section.

Lown has classified the PVCs into different types, according to the characteristics shown in Table 16.1 and Figure 16.4 (Lown and Wolf 1971). Ventricular tachycardia (VT) runs correspond to class 4b in Lown's classification (Figure 16.4). If the runs of VT are frequent and repetitive, they are named non-sustained VT (see later). This classification is hierarchical and has prognostic implications (see later).

Characteristics of QRS complexes
Width of the QRS complex

Most PVCs originate in the Purkinje network or in the ventricular muscle. They usually display a QRS complex ≥0.12 sec. Occasionally, if they start in one of the two main branches of the bundle of His or in one of the two divisions of the left bundle branch (LBB), the QRS is <0.12 sec (narrow fascicular PVC), and the morphology, although variable, resembles an intraventricular conduction block with a QRS<0.12 sec. Some of these are parasystolic impulses.

Morphology

QRS morphology varies according to its site of origin (Figure 16.5). If the QRS complex starts in the right ventricle, it may be similar (in lead V1) to that of a left bundle

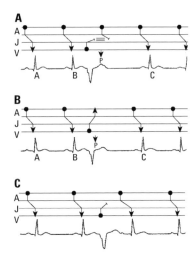

Figure 16.3 (A) Premature ventricular complexes (PVCs) with concealed junctional conduction, which hinders the conduction of the following P wave to the ventricles. (B) PVC with retrograde activation to the atria with depolarization of the sinus node. A change starts in the sinus cadence. (C) PVC with partial atrioventricular (AV) junctional conduction that permits the conduction of the following sinus P wave to the ventricles, albeit with longer PR.

branch block (LBBB) (Figure 16.5B). Those originating in the left ventricle show a variable morphology: when QRS complexes arise mainly from the lateral or inferobasal walls of the heart, they appear positive in all precordial leads (Figure 16.5A); when QRS complexes originate next to the inferoposterior or superoanterior division of the left bundle, they resemble a prominent R wave, sometimes with notches in the descending limb of the R wave, but usually without the rsR morphology that is typical of right bundle branch block (RBBB) in lead V1. The ÂQRS may be extremely deviated to the right or to the left, depending on their origin in the inferoposterior or superoanterior division, etc. The presence of QR morphology suggests associated necrosis (see Monomorphic ventricular tachycardia). Recently, Enriquez *et al.* described an anatomical attitudinal approach to determination of the site of origin (SOO), indicating that some previously considered "right-sided structures" are at the left of the middle line and vice versa. The importance of this preliminary ECG screening of the SOO relies on the ability of guiding the interventionist EP to the proper approach for an ablation (Enriquez *et al.* 2019a).

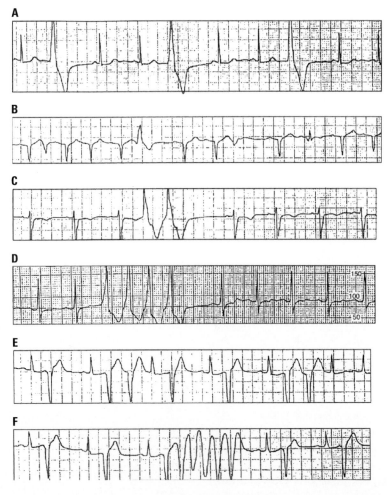

Figure 16.4 Different types of premature ventricular complexes (PVCs) according to Lown's classification: (A) frequent PVCs, (B) polymorphic PVCs, (C) a pair of PVCs, (D) run of ventricular tachycardias (VTs), (E and F) examples of R/T phenomenon with a pair and one run.

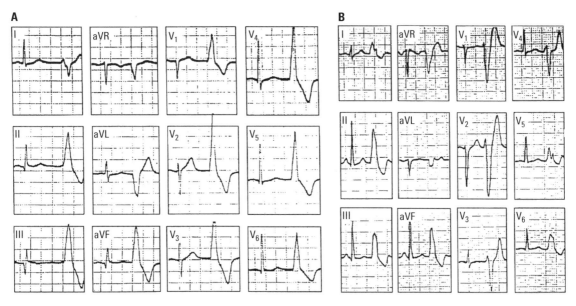

Figure 16.5 (A) Premature ventricular complexes (PVCs) that arise in the lateral wall of the heart (QRS always positive from V1 to V6 and negative in I and aVL). These are frequently observed in heart disease patients. (B) PVCs that arise in the right ventricle. These are frequently observed in healthy individuals, although they may also occur in patients with heart disease.

In general, all QRS of ventricular tachycardias show similar morphologic characteristics to the initial PVC. This is because they usually have the same origin and are caused by the same mechanism. In addition, the intraventricular conduction of the stimulus is usually the same. However, the morphology of QRS complexes may change during an episode of ventricular tachycardia (pleomorphism) (see Polymorphic ventricular tachycardia), or a PVC with a given morphology may produce a polymorphic rather than monomorphic ventricular tachycardia, as is often the case in Brugada's syndrome (see Chapter 21).

In individuals with no evidence of heart disease, PVCs usually show high voltage and non-notched QRS complexes. It is possible for them to have a QS morphology but rarely a notched QR morphology (Enriquez *et al.* 2019a). Repolarization shows an ST segment depression when the QRS is positive, and vice versa, whereas the T wave has asymmetrical branches (Figure 16.6A). This type of PVC may also be observed in patients with heart disease.

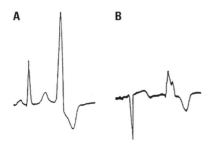

Figure 16.6 Typical ECG morphologies of premature ventricular complexes (PVCs) in healthy individuals (A) and in patients with advanced heart disease (B).

However, the PVCs of patients with significant myocardial impairment show symmetrical T waves more often than healthy subjects, because of the presence of an additional primary disturbance of repolarization. Also, the QRS complexes show notches and slurrings, often with a low-voltage pattern and qR morphology (Moulton *et al.* 1990) (Figure 16.6B).

Extrasystole compared with parasystole (Figures 16.1 and 16.2): The extrasystolic PVC presents a fixed coupling interval. When they are very late (PVCs in the PR interval), they may present fusion complexes (Figure 16.21B). The parasystolic PVCs present usually marked variable coupling interval (>80 ms) and the interectopic intervals are multiples of each other. Lastly, the third key diagnostic point of parasystolic PVCs is the presence of **fusion complexes** that occur when the impulse from baseline and parasystolic foci both activate the ventricle at the same time. The presence of fusion complexes is not necessary for diagnosis of parasystole because they often only appear sporadically and when the diagnosis is already made (Figure 16.2) (consult Bayés de Luna and Baranchuk (2017) for more information, McIntyre and Baranchuk (2011)).

Differential diagnosis

Table 15.1 shows the most relevant data indicative of aberrancy or ectopy in cases of premature complexes with wide QRS. It is very important to determine whether a P wave preceding a wide premature QRS complex is present, because this is crucial for the diagnosis of aberrancy (Figure 16.7). It is also essential to thoroughly observe the PVC morphology, as the presence of patterns consistent

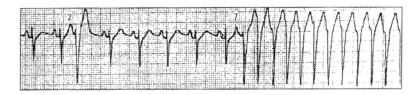

Figure 16.7 Taken from a 51-year-old woman who showed frequent paroxysmal tachycardia episodes. Note how the second and seventh T waves prior to arrhythmia onset are much sharper than the remaining waves, because an atrial extrasystole causes, respectively, an isolated or repetitive aberrant conduction.

with the typical bundle branch block is very much in favor of aberrancy, although we have already stated that fascicular PVC may mimic the pattern of an intraventricular conduction disorder with QRS complexes <0.12 sec.

Clinical implications

If the PVCs are repetitive, they form pairs (two consecutive PVCs) or ventricular tachycardia runs (≥3) (Figures 16.1B and 16.4). Conventionally, a ventricular tachycardia is considered to be sustained when it lasts for more than 30 sec.

PVCs both of extrasystolic and parasystolic origin may be observed in healthy subjects and in heart disease patients. PVCs are more troublesome while resting, particularly when the patient is lying in bed. When frequent, they can cause significant psychologic disturbances. The incidence increases with age, and is more frequent in asymptomatic men after the age of 50 (Hinkle *et al.* 1969). At times, healthy people present with PVCs as a result of consuming foods that cause flatulence, in addition to wine, coffee, ginseng, and some "energy drinks." Emotion, stress, and exercise can also cause PVCs.

The characteristic auscultation finding is interruption of the normal rhythm by a premature beat or beats followed by a pause. If they are very frequent, and especially if they appear in runs, they may end up affecting the left ventricular function, even in patients without previous heart disease (tachycardiomyopathy). Nevertheless, in healthy subjects the prognosis is generally excellent.

The long-term prognosis of healthy subjects with ventricular premature systoles is generally good (Kennedy *et al.* 1985; Kennedy 2002). Nevertheless, the following considerations should be taken into account: (i) if PVCs clearly increase with exercise, this indicates an increasing long-term risk for cardiovascular problems (Jouven *et al.* 2000); (ii) it has been reported that during a stress test, the ST segment depression in the PVC may be a better marker for ischemia than the ST segment depression in the baseline rhythm (Rassouli and Ellestad 2001) (see Figure 20.33); (iii) very frequent PVCs (>10 000–20 000/ day) (Niwano *et al.* 2009) or a PVC burden of >24% (Baman *et al.* 2010) may lead to ventricular function impairment, in which case ablation of the ectopic focus may be advisable (Bogun *et al.* 2008). In the catheter

ablation era, the indications to approach the treatment of PVCs from an invasive perspective have significantly evolved. Today, ablation of PVCs is a common procedure; however, the following rules should be considered before sending a patient for ablation: 1. The PVC "density" should be high (i.e. more than 20 000/day), 2. PVCs should be impacting left ventricular performance (i.e. LVEF < 50%), and 3. symptoms should be debilitating (i.e. patient not able to perform daily activity). If 2/3 of the criteria are present, one should consider treating the PVC (either pharmacologically or by ablation) (Lamba *et al.* 2014; Enriquez *et al.* 2019b).

In addition, it should be noted that Lown's classification is hierarchical (Table 16.1). However, the R/T phenomenon is currently considered to be dangerous, especially in the presence of acute ischemia.

It has been demonstrated (Moss 1983; Bigger *et al.* 1984) that in patients with chronic ischemic heart disease (IHD), especially post-infarction, risk increases after one PVC per hour, especially when complex PVC morphologies and/or heart failure are present. Recently, it has been demonstrated (Haqqani *et al.* 2009) that the characteristics of myocardial infarction scar are more important than the number of PVCs in the triggering of sustained ventricular tachycardia.

In hypertrophic cardiomyopathy, the presence of frequent PVCs, especially the presence of ventricular tachycardia runs, during a Holter ECG recording is an indicator of risk for sudden death (McKenna and Behr 2002).

The severity of PVCs increases in patients with depressed ventricular function and especially in the presence of evident heart failure.

Treatment of PVCs largely depends on the clinical condition of the patient (Bayés de Luna and Baranchuk 2017).

Ventricular tachycardias

Ventricular tachycardias (VTs) may be sustained or non-sustained (runs). They are considered sustained when they last for more than 30 sec. Based on their morphology, ventricular tachycardias are classified as either **monomorphic** or **polymorphic** (Table 16.2). The initial complexes sometimes show certain polymorphisms and may

Table 16.2 Ventricular tachycardias

Monomorphic	Polymorphic
Classical (QRS ≥ 0.12 sec)	Torsades de pointes
Narrow QRS	Bidirectional
Accelerated idioventricular rhythm	Pleomorphism
Non-sustained monomorphic	Catecholaminergic polymorphic
Parasystolic	Other VTs with variable morphology

often feature irregularities of rhythm. Therefore, this classification should be made when the VT is established.

Both monomorphic and polymorphic VT may be sustained or non-sustained (runs). Isolated or infrequent monomorphic ventricular tachycardia runs have been traditionally studied along with PVCs, and are now classified as type IVB in Lown's classification (Figure 16.4). The clinical, prognostic, and therapeutic aspects of frequent monomorphic ventricular tachycardia runs, particularly if they are incessant, may easily trigger a sustained VT in heart disease patients and have a significant hemodynamic impact.

Monomorphic ventricular tachycardia

When monomorphic ventricular tachycardias (VTs) originate in the upper septum/bundle of His branches, they may have a narrow QRS (<0.12 sec). However, if they originate in the Purkinje network, or in any area of the ventricular myocardium, they have wide QRS complexes (≥0.12 sec) (classical VT).

Classical ventricular tachycardia (QRS ≥ 0.12 sec)
Concept
By definition, sustained VTs are those lasting longer than 30 sec. However, from a clinical point of view, most sustained VTs are long enough to develop specific symptoms that may require hospitalization. Most VTs are triggered by extrasystolic PVC. Thus, the initial complex if there are several episodes has the same coupling interval. Parasystolic VTs are very rare and frequently occur at a slow rate. They are generally non-sustained VTs, appearing in runs, and arise from a protected automatic focus, which explains the variable coupling interval (see Figure 16.24).

Classical VT generally originates in the subendocardial area. In a small number of cases in the subepicardium and the majority of these cases in presence of heart disease, especially ischemic and non-ischemic CM. The basal superior region of the LV is the most frequent site of origin of VT of epicardial origin in cases of non-ischemic CM (Valles *et al.* 2010). Localization of the SOO using the ECG has been deeply explored correlating the QRS morphology and sequence of activation with extensive endocardial mapping (Enriquez *et al.* 2019a).

Electrophysiologic mechanism
In subjects with heart disease
In acute myocardial infarction patients without previous scars, sustained VTs are relatively rare, and sudden death generally occurs due to ventricular fibrillation triggered by one isolated or repetitive PVC (Figures 16.31 and 16.32).

Post-infarction VTs in the presence of ischemic CM are usually triggered by alterations in the autonomic nervous system ("modulating factors") assessed by different parameters in the presence of frequent PVCs (Moss 1983; Bigger *et al.* 1984). It has been demonstrated (Haqqani *et al.* 2009) that the characteristics of the scar are more relevant to trigger VTs in chronic IHD patients without residual ischemia than the presence of PVCs (see before). The VT may be perpetuated in post-infarction patients by a reentry mechanism in the area surrounding the infarction scar.

This reentry may be explained by the classical concept of anatomic obstacle or by the functional reentry (rotors).

VTs are also present in patients with non-ischemic CM and in other heart diseases (valvular, congenital) especially in the presence of heart failure.

In some cases, particularly in patients with dilated or ischemic cardiomyopathy, VTs are produced by a reentry where both branches of the specific conduction system (SCS) are involved (Touboul *et al.* 1983).

Channelopathies present VT due to heterogeneous dispersion of repolarization (phase 2 reentry) (Figure 14.15) (Yan and Antzelevitch 1998; Opthof *et al.* 2007) that may induce SD. Also, other inherited heart diseases such as HC and ARVD/C may present VT and SD (see Chapter 21).

In subjects with no evidence of heart disease
The most frequent electrophysiologic mechanisms are as follows (Enriquez *et al.* 2017):
• **A micro-reentry**, usually in the region of the inferoposterior fascicle of the left bundle branch.
• **Triggered electrical activity**: These VTs are sensitive to adenosine.
• **Increased automatism**: These VTs are sensitive to propanolol.
Table 16.3 shows the differences between these three types of idiopathic VTs.

ECG findings
ECG recording in sinus rhythm
If previous ECGs are available, it is useful to compare their morphologies with that of a wide QRS complex tachycardia. For instance, in the case of a tachycardia with a wide QRS complex ≥0.12 sec, the presence of an even wider QRS complex in sinus rhythm due to an advanced LBBB strongly supports the diagnosis of VT. Meanwhile, the presence of an AV block during sinus rhythm favors a wide QRS complex being a VT.

Table 16.3 Idiopathic ventricular tachycardias with QRS >120 ms: ECG morphology[a]

Idiopathic VT with LBBB morphology (generally with "r" in V1). May originate in both ventricles (although usually originates in the RV)[b]	
Inferior (right) ÂQRS Superior (left) ÂQRS	• VT originates in RVOT endocardium. Features a relatively late R transition (V3–V4); R/S in V3 < I) and an isolated unnotched R in V6 (see Figure 16.11). 50% of VT of ARVC show similar morphologies (RVOT) • VT originates near the aortic valve. Features an early R transition (R/S V3 > I) and an isolated notched R in V6. With regard to origin (see Figure 16.9): (i) if QRS morphology in I is rS or QS, the zone close to the left coronary leaflet is involved; (ii) if a notched "r" is observed in V1, the VT originates near the non-coronary valve; and (iii) if qrS pattern is present in V1–V3, the VT originates between the right and left coronary valves • If the VT originates in the area surrounding the mitral ring, a morphology rsr' or RS is observed in V1 • VT originates in the RV free wall and/or near the tricuspid ring. R in I and QS or rS in V1–V2 and late R transition in precordials. ARVC should be ruled out (see Figure 21.7B)
Idiopathic VT with RBBB morphology (generally, R in V1 and "s" in V6; from Rs to rS). Always originates in the LV	
Superior (left) ÂQRS Inferior (right) ÂQRS	• Inferior–posterior fascicular VT: activation similar to RBBB + SAH (Figure 16.10) • Anterior–superior fascicular VT • VT originated in LVOT endocardium near anterior–superior fascicle } Activation similar to the RBBB + IPH

[a] Idiopathic VTs with duration < 120 ms (narrow QRS) present partial RBBB or LBBB morphologies.
[b] Ouyang *et al.* (2002); O'Donnell *et al.* (2003); Yamada (2008).
IPH: inferoposterior hemiblock; LBBB: left bundle branch block; LV: left ventricle; LVOT: left ventricular outflow tract; RBBB: Right bundle branch block; RV: right ventricle; RVOT: right ventricular outflow tract; SAH: superoanterior hemiblock; VT: ventricular tachycardia.

Onset and end

Sustained VT usually starts with a PVC with a morphology similar to the other QRS of the tachycardia, with a relatively short and fixed coupling interval but frequently without R/T phenomena, especially in sustained VT not related to acute ischemia. Sometimes, prior to the establishment of a sustained VT, the number of PVCs and runs increases significantly.

Sustained VT may trigger ventricular fibrillation (Figure 16.34A). This is often the final event in ambulatory patients dying suddenly while wearing a Holter device (Bayés de Luna *et al.* 1989). Tachycardization of sinus rhythm characteristically occurs prior to the sustained ventricular tachycardia, which leads to ventricular fibrillation and sudden death.

Ventricular tachycardia may end by reverting to sinus rhythm or triggering ventricular fibrillation, and, rarely, reverting to asystole (Figure 16.8).

Heart rate

Heart rate usually ranges from 130 to 200 bpm. RR intervals occasionally show some irregularities, especially at tachycardia onset and termination. The rate typically increases before ventricular tachycardia turns into ventricular fibrillation (Figure 16.34A).

QRS morphology

By definition, QRS complexes are monomorphic. The QRS complex patterns depend on the site of origin, the ventricular tachycardia pathways, and the presence of heart disease.

In subjects with no evidence of heart disease: (i) Usually, the QRS morphology does not have many notches, and the T wave is clearly asymmetric. The morphology is similar to that of a LBBB or RBBB. However, the bundle branch block pattern is usually atypical. (ii) Table 16.3 describes the different types of idiopathic VT according to ECG morphology:

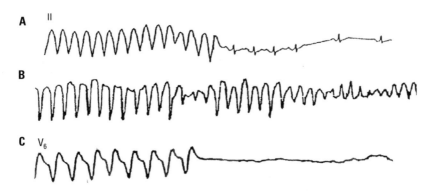

Figure 16.8 Three modes of termination of a sustained ventricular tachycardia (VT). (A) Reverting into sinus rhythm. (B) Initiating a ventricular fibrillation. (C) Turning into asystole (rare).

A

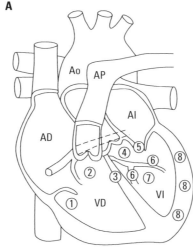

B

Place of origin and incidence	ECG Patent	ÂQRS	Left. If right-handed, the origin is in the superoanterior fascicle. QRS in the frontal plane	It depends on the ÂQRS in V₁	RS transition in precordial leads
(1) Tricuspid ring 5–10%	LBBB	Never right-handed. Between ≃+ 60° and +30°	R in I and VL	QS o rS	Beyond V₃
(2 and 3) RV outflow tract, pulmonary valve and high septum 60–65%	LBBB	Right	R in II, III, and VF	QS or rS	Generally beyond V₃
(4) Below the aortic valve ≈ 5%	LBBB	Right	R in II, III, and VF	– qrS – RS – rS	In V₂–V₃
(5) Mitral ring	Atypical LBBB	Right	R in II, III, and VF	⌇, ⌇	Generally in V₁,V₃
(6) Fascicular. Generally inferoposterior 10–20%	RBBB	Left. If right-handed, the origin is in the superoanterior fascicle.	It depends on the ÂQRS	R	R in V₁

Figure 16.9 (A) Place of origin of idiopathic ventricular tachycardia (VT) (see correlation number location in B). Some, such as the bundle branch (7) and the subepicardial (8) can be observed more often in heart disease cases. (B) ECG features of the most common of these VTs.

RBBB-type with evidence of left or right ÂQRS deviation, or LBBB-type with left or right ÂQRS deviation. (iii) Figure 16.9A,B shows the ECG characteristics of idiopathic VT, depending on their site of origin (Figures 16.10 and 16.11). (iv) Despite having different mechanisms, VTs often originate in areas very close to each other, and therefore have similar morphologies. (v) VTs originating in the left papillary muscles are similar to fascicular VTs; however, they show a wider QRS complex, and there is no Q wave in the frontal plane.

In heart disease patients (Wellens 1978; Josephson *et al.* 1979; Griffith *et al.* 1992; O'Donnell *et al.* 2003), the following characteristics are important: (i) The QRS morphology in heart disease patients compared with the QRS morphology in healthy subjects with VT is usually wider (≥0.16 sec), with more notches and a more symmetrical T wave (Figures 16.12–16.14). (ii) **VTs originating in the left ventricular free wall show wider QRS complexes**, whereas narrower QRS complexes are indicative of VTs originating in the high septum.

Ventricular tachycardias **in heart disease patients may show the following QRS morphologies:**

• a prominent R wave in lead V1 and an "s" wave in lead V6 (**RBBB morphology**) (Figure 16.13);

• an rS in lead V1 with evident R in V6 (**LBBB morphology**) (Figure 16.14);

• **concordance of the QRS complex** patterns in precordial leads (all positive or all negative) (Figure 16.12);

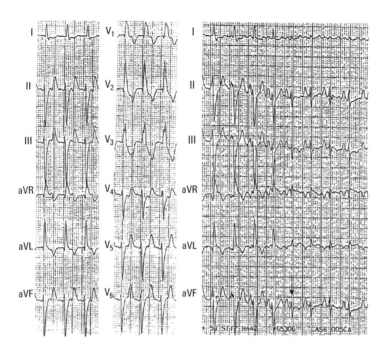

Figure 16.10 An example of verapamil-sensitive ventricular tachycardia (VT). Note the morphology of right bundle branch block + superoanterior hemiblock (RBBB+SAH), but with qR morphology in V1. In the right panel, it can be appreciated how the sinus tachycardia exceeds the VT rate during exercise testing.

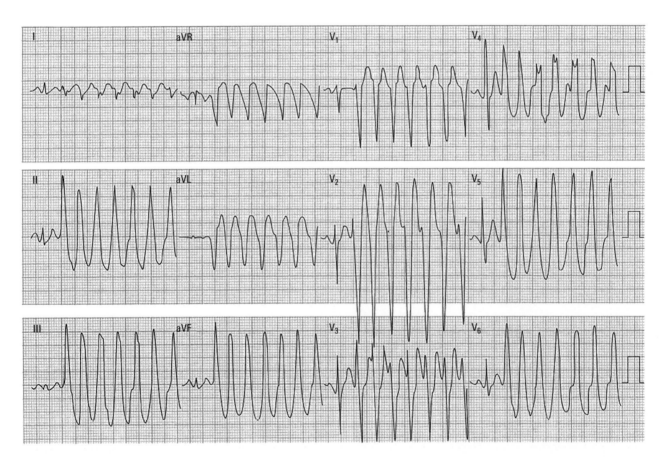

Figure 16.11 An example of left bundle branch block (LBBB)-type ventricular tachycardia (VT) with rightward QRS occurring as repetitive runs during exercise testing in an individual without heart disease.

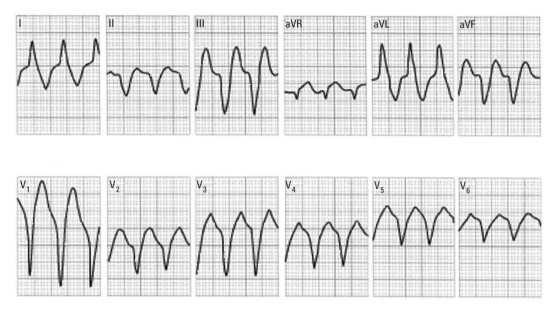

Figure 16.12 The ÂQRS is deviated to the left in the frontal plane, similar to that observed in some cases of left bundle branch block (LBBB). However, all the QRS are negative in the horizontal plane (morphologic concordance in precordial leads), which is not observed in any type of bundle branch block, and this supports diagnosis of ventricular tachycardia (VT).

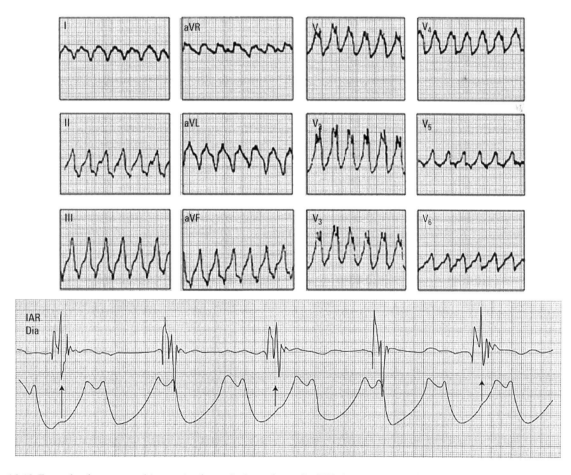

Figure 16.13 Example of monomorphic sustained ventricular tachycardia (VT). An atrioventricular (AV) dissociation is shown with the use of a right intraatrial lead (IAL) and the higher speed of ECG recording, allowing us to better see the presence of small changes in QRS that correspond to atrial activity (arrow). The morphologies of V1 (R) and V6 (rS) also support the ventricular origin.

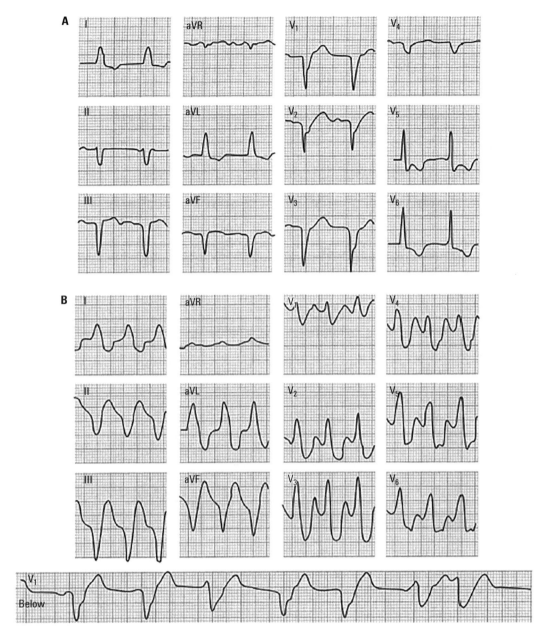

Figure 16.14 A 75-year-old patient with ischemic heart disease. The baseline ECG (A) shows an advanced left bundle branch block (LBBB), with an extremely leftward ÂQRS and poor progression of R wave from V1 to V4, with a notch in the ascending limb of the S wave, suggestive of an associated myocardial infarction. The patient suffered an episode of paroxysmal tachycardia at 135 bpm, with advanced LBBB morphology (B). Despite the fact that the ECG pattern is of LBBB type and the patient presented with baseline LBBB, we diagnose ventricular tachycardia (VT) because of the following: (1) the R wave in V1 was, during the tachycardia, clearly higher than the R wave in V1 during sinus rhythm. Additionally, the bottom panel shows that, in the presence of sinus rhythm, the patient showed premature ventricular complexes (PVCs) with the same morphology as those present during the tachycardia. The first and second PVCs are late (in the PR), and after the second one, a repetitive form is observed; and (2) according to the Brugada algorithm (Figure 16.21), in some precordial leads featuring an RS morphology, this interval, measured from the initiation of the R wave to S wave nadir, is >100 ms.

- **presence of a QR morphology in different leads, seen in post-infarction VT (Wellens** 1978**);**
- Initial slurrings of QRS due to slow conduction delay in the VT of subepicardial origin because less Purkinje fibers are present, explains: (a) pseudo-delta wave pattern; (b) time of intrinsic deflection >85 ms; (c) distance from the

onset of R to the nadir of S >120 ms (Berruezo *et al.* 2004; Bazan *et al.* 2006; Valles *et al.* 2010).
- QS morphology in lead I, less often in inferior leads, is strongly suggestive of non-ischemic CM of an epicardial origin, respectively, in the basal superior or inferior zone of LV (Bazan *et al.* 2006, 2007).

- presence in **lead II of R wave peak time** (distance from the beginning of QRS deflection to the point of first change in polarity, independent of whether the QRS is positive or negative) **≥50 ms** (Pava *et al.* 2010).

With regard to the P wave–QRS complex relationship, there is an AV dissociation in more than 60% of cases.

Occasionally, atrial activity (with or without AV dissociation) (Figure 16.13) may be observed as a notch in the repolarization of isolated PVCs or VTs.

The presence of **AV dissociation** is critical in order to make a diagnosis of wide QRS complex tachycardias of ventricular origin.

Frequently, the sinus impulse cannot depolarize the whole ventricular myocardium, which is only partially depolarized by the tachycardia impulse. In these cases, the ventricular **fusion complex** is non-premature, or only minimally premature, and its width and morphology are half way between the sinus and ectopic impulses (Figure 16.15).

Atrial fibrillation associated to Wolff–Parkinson–White (WPW) syndrome also shows intermediate morphology QRS complexes as a result of different degrees of pre-excitation, or even narrow complexes, such as **capture complexes** (see Figure 15.31) (see Chapter 15 AF in WPW syndrome versus VT).

ECG diagnostic criteria: differential diagnosis of wide QRS tachycardia

ECG criteria with a higher positive predictive value

(PPV) for the diagnosis of VT, as previously discussed are the following:

- The presence of capture and/or fusion complexes (Figure 16.15).
- The demonstration of AV dissociation (Figure 16.13). This occurs in 50–60% of cases.

- Evidence of extremely deviated ÂQRS (between −90° and ±180°).
- A markedly wide QRS complex >140 ms in RBBB tachycardias, and >160 ms in LBBB tachycardias.
- The presence of morphologies that are incompatible with bundle branch block, for example when all QRS complexes are positive or negative in leads V1–V6 (concordance of QRS) (Figure 16.12).
- Determination of QRS complex morphology in leads aVF, aVR, V1, and V6 (Table 16.4) (high PPV).
- Presence of R wave peak time in lead II >50 ms (Pava *et al.* 2010) and presence of ECG criteria of VT of epicardial origin due to initial slurrings of QRS (see ECG findings) (Berruezo *et al.* 2004; Bazan *et al.* 2006; Valles *et al.* 2010).
- Presence of QR or QS pattern in other leads than aVR (see Table 16.4).

Sequential algorithms

In 1991, Brugada described an algorithm incorporating the sequential use of many of the aforementioned criteria, which allows for very specific (>95%) and sensitive (>95%) differential diagnosis. Figure 16.16 shows the steps for applying this algorithm and how to measure the RS interval (AB interval, see Figure 16.16). However, its application is not easy for the emergency physician or the clinical cardiologist because it is necessary to make an effort to learn how to use this algorithm step by step.

The algorithm described by Brugada (1991) is not useful in the case of reentrant bundle branch VT (Figure 16.17) or for differentiating VT from wide QRS complex supraventricular tachycardia (SVT) in WPW syndrome (antidromic tachycardia) (Figure 16.18). In the latter case, Steurer's sequential approach (Steurer *et al.* 1994) is sensitive enough and particularly specific. According to the author, the following features

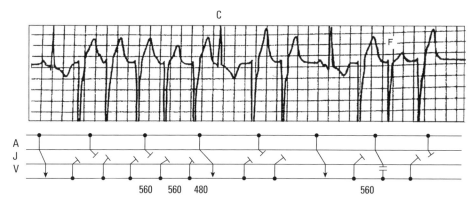

Figure 16.15 After a sinus complex, a ventricular tachycardia (VT) run lasting seven beats occurs. The Lewis diagram represents the complete atrioventricular (AV) dissociation. Between the fifth and sixth complexes of the VT, there is a typical ventricular capture (early QRS with the same morphology as the baseline rhythm). Afterward, after a normal sinus stimulus (not early), there is a short VT run (three QRS complexes). The complex in the middle is a fusion complex, as it has a different morphology from the other two (narrower QRS and a less sharp T wave), and the RR interval is not modified (see Chapter 18: QRS of different morphologies).

Table 16.4 Differential diagnosis between ventricular tachycardia and wide QRS aberrant supraventricular tachycardia with regular RR intervals (morphological criteria)

In favor of ectopy:

V1

V1   especially if in V6

VR

VF:
1) In presence of wide QRS and RBBB pattern
2) In presence of wide QRS and LBBB pattern

In favor of aberrancy:

V1   if in V6

VR

VF:
1) presence of wide QRS and RBBB pattern
2) In presence of wide QRS and LBBB pattern

are suggestive of ventricular tachycardia: (i) negative QRS complex in leads V4–V6, (ii) QR pattern in one of leads V2–V6, (iii) confirmation of AV dissociation, (iv) ÂQRS complex <−60° and >+150°. Figure 16.18 shows an example of antidromic SVT with an accessory AV pathway, which does not meet any of these criteria.

A different algorithm has been described (Vereckei *et al.* 2008) based fundamentally on the information obtained from the aVR lead, which features a slightly higher statistical potential. However, it is not valid for tachycardias with aberrant conduction involving an accessory pathway or for reentrant bundle branch ventricular tachycardia. According to this algorithm, the morphologies of aVR suggestive of aberrancy are usually QS-type complexes with a rapid inscription in the first portion of the QRS complex, which sometimes show an initial "r." The remaining morphologies suggest aVT, in particular the morphologies with or without initial R that has a slow inscription during the first 40 ms of the QRS (Table 16.4 see aVR).

The verification of whether the morphologies of wide QRS tachycardia are consistent with aberrant conduction (Table 16.4) leads to a very high PPV, similar to that obtained through Brugada's algorithm. Because this approach is actually the fourth step of Brugada's algorithm, **we think that the most practical method to make this differential diagnosis is to carefully follow this algorithm step by step, incorporating the ECG pattern of aVR in the fourth step.**

Figure 16.19 shows a typical example of wide QRS tachycardia due to aberrant conduction. The diagnosis is supported by a comparison between the QRS morphologies of a previous ECG in sinus rhythm, and the QRS morphology of wide QRS tachycardia, which does not meet the abovementioned criteria. Figures 16.12–16.14 are clear examples of classical VT.

However, it should be pointed out that the bundle branch reentrant VT (Figure 16.17) generally shows a LBBB morphology often with a QS pattern in V1 that makes the differential diagnosis of SVT with aberrant conduction more difficult. Sometimes, the evidence of AV dissociation, if it is present, allows us to reach the correct diagnosis. Surface ECG recordings at high velocity (Figure 16.13), as well as the potential future implementation of ECG devices with a T wave filter (see Chapter 25), may be helpful.

In cases of diagnostic uncertainty, which rarely occurs following this approach, invasive electrophysiologic study (EPS) should be carried out.

Clinical implications

Sustained VT is a malignant arrhythmia that in many cases, especially in patients with heart diseases with acute ischemia, LV dysfunction or inherited heart diseases, may trigger VF and sudden death. For all information related with this type and the clinical implications and therapeutic approaches of other types of VT, consult Bayés de Luna and Baranchuk (2017).

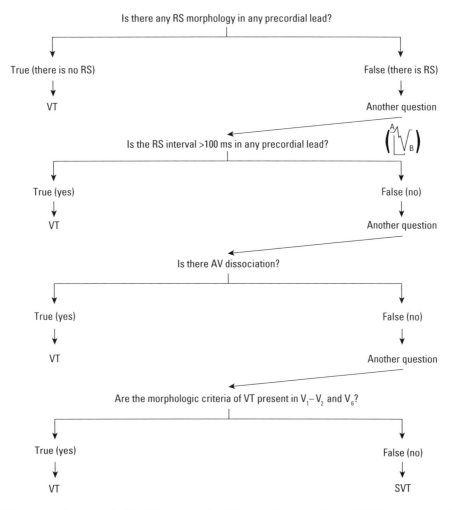

Figure 16.16 Algorithm for the diagnosis of wide QRS tachycardia. When an RS complex is not visible in any precordial lead, we can make a diagnosis of ventricular tachycardia (VT). When an RS complex is present in one or more precordial leads, the longest RS interval should be measured (from start of the R wave to S wave nadir—see inside the figure). If the RS interval is greater than 100 ms, we can make a diagnosis of VT. If the interval is shorter, the next step is to check the presence of atrioventricular (AV) dissociation. If it is present, we can make a diagnosis of VT. If not present, the morphologic criteria for the differential diagnosis of VT should be checked in V1 and V6 leads. According to these, we will diagnose VT or supraventricular tachycardia (Modified from Brugada *et al.* 1991).

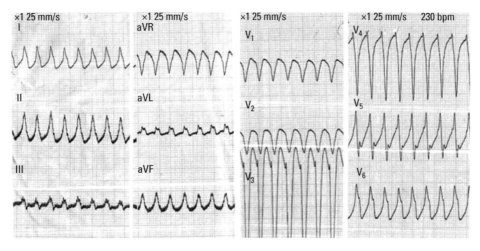

Figure 16.17 An example of a bundle branch ventricular tachycardia (VT) with a typical advanced left bundle branch block (LBBB) morphology (see V1 with a QS pattern).

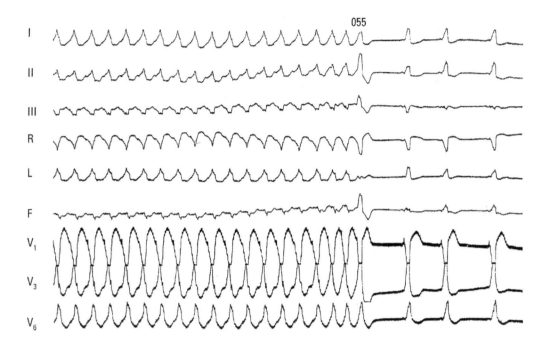

Figure 16.18 A broad QRS tachycardia. This is an antidromic supraventricular tachycardia (SVT) over an accessory atrioventricular (AV) pathway (Kent bundle). The morphology is that of a left bundle branch block (LBBB), although the R wave is clearly visible in V3, which is not usual in antidromic tachycardias through an atriofascicular tract (atypical pre-excitation). Note the persistence of the Wolff–Parkinson–White (WPW) morphology once the tachycardia disappears. None of the criteria in favor of a VT in the differential diagnosis between VT and antidromic tachycardia are met (see Steurer *et al.* 1994 and Differential diagnosis of wide QRS complex tachycardias). All these data suggest that it is a typical antidromic tachycardia (bundle of Kent) with aberrant morphology. Remember that for this differential diagnosis, the algorithm criteria from Figure 16.21 do not apply (Based on Steurer *et al.* 1994).

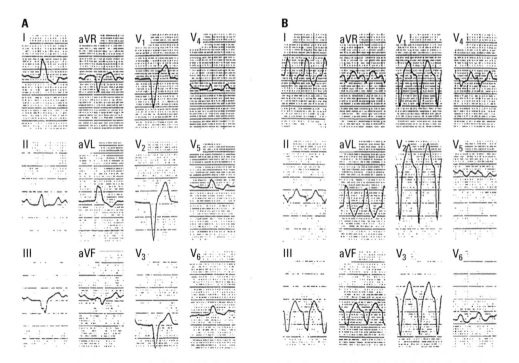

Figure 16.19 Taken from a 48-year-old patient with dilated cardiomyopathy and left bundle branch block (LBBB) morphology in the baseline ECG (A). The patient suffered a paroxysmal tachycardia with a wide QRS very similar to the baseline one (B). The supraventricular origin was suggested by the fact that the QRS morphology in all leads (see especially V1) was identical to that present during sinus rhythm.

Other monomorphic ventricular tachycardias
Narrow QRS complex ventricular tachycardias (fascicular tachycardias) (Hayes *et al*. 1991; Hallan and Scheinman 1996) (Figure 16.20)

Narrow QRS complex VTs are infrequent. They represent fewer than 5% of all VT cases. These tachycardias are characterized by a relatively narrow QRS complex (<0.12 sec), and they originate close to the high septum or the fascicular areas (right bundle branch, left bundle branch trunk, or their two divisions).

The electrical impulse starts in the site of origin, usually by a reentry mechanism, and rapidly spreads through the His–Purkinje system. Narrow QRS complex ventricular tachycardias show partial RBBB morphology, if originated in the left ventricle, with evidence of right or left ÂQRS deviation, depending on the site of origin (close to left superior and anterior division or inferior and posterior division, respectively). The cases of VT with partial RBBB patterns plus evidence of left ÂQRS extreme deviation are verapamil-sensitive. These VTs may have practically the same morphology, but with the QRS complex ≥0.12 sec.

In cases of VT with narrow QRS, it is sometimes difficult to make a differential diagnosis with SVT or atrial flutter with aberrancy when only using a surface ECG. The presence of capture and fusion complexes and the evidence of AV dissociation are suggestive of a tachycardia of ventricular origin (Figure 16.22). However, sometimes intracavitary electrocardiography is often necessary to reach the correct differential diagnosis.

From a therapeutic point of view, the most reasonable and wise option is to treat narrow QRS ventricular tachycardia as a classical wide QRS sustained VT.

Idioventricular accelerated rhythm (IVAR) (Figures 16.21 and 16.22)

This is a ventricular rhythm originating in an automatic ectopic focus with a slightly decreased discharge rate (~80–100 bpm). Unless heart rate is more than 100 bpm, we should not speak of true ventricular tachycardia. The occurrence of an idioventricular accelerated rhythm during reperfusion is particularly due to increased automatism in the His–Purkinje system (Riera *et al.* 2010). The ectopic focus is visible only when the sinus heart rate has a rate below its discharge rate. This explains the frequent fusion beats that appear, especially at the onset and at the end of the runs (Figure 16.21A). In fact, some cases of suspected slow parasystolic ventricular tachycardia correspond to IVAR (see later).

The IVAR is not a true ventricular tachycardia because the rate is below 100 bpm. It appears as an escape but accelerated ventricular rhythm, when the sinus rhythm slows down its rate. Because of this, fusion beats are very frequent (see above) (Figures 16.21 and 16.22).

The impulse that initiates the IVAR features a long coupling interval, which is similar to baseline RR interval. Therefore, there are no different coupling intervals of the first PVCs of the ventricular tachycardia runs, as happens in runs of true parasystolic ventricular tachycardia.

The IVAR usually shows the same ventricular discharge rate. However, occasionally, it may vary in different episodes. Thus, the same focus may, in rare cases, present as a true VT, and in these cases, a treatment

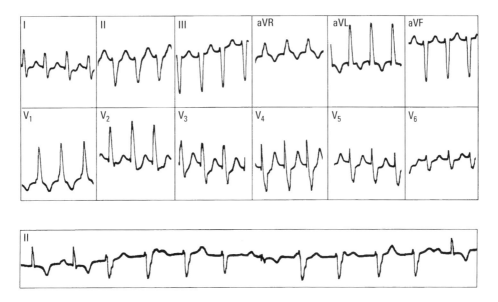

Figure 16.20 The QRS of the tachycardia lasts 110 ms and features a right bundle block and superoanterior hemiblock (RBBB + SAH) morphology. However, the exclusive R wave in V1, and, above all, the presence of captures and fusions (bottom tracing) indicate that this is a narrow fascicular ventricular tachycardia (VT) arising from a zone close to the inferoposterior division.

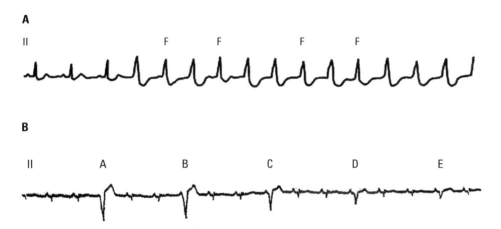

Figure 16.21 (A) Example of different fusion degrees (F) in the presence of an accelerated idioventricular rhythm (about 100 bpm). (B) Late trigeminal PVCs in the PR interval showing progressive fusion degrees from C to E.

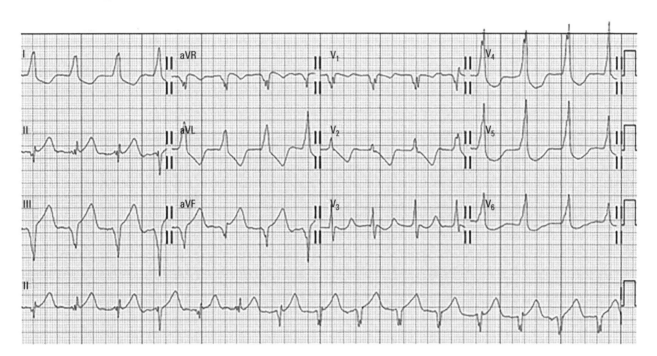

Figure 16.22 45-year-old man with occlusion of the posterior descending coronary artery. During the PCI procedure, intraluminal thrombus and the appearance on the 12-leads ECG of accelerated idioventricular rhythm with frequent fusion beats. Note how in the narrower QRS complexes, there is elevation of ST-T in II, III, aVF and a mirror image in V1–V3.

similar to that applied to classical sustained monomorphic VT may be necessary.

Repeated non-sustained monomorphic ventricular tachycardia

Frequent VT runs and, in particular, the incessant types (repeated non-sustained ventricular tachycardia) may cause significant hemodynamic compromise and alteration of the anatomical substrate (tachymyocardiopathy), particularly when the ventricular rate is high, and finally may trigger sustained ventricular tachycardia (Figure 16.23).

Parasystolic ventricular tachycardia (Chung et al. 1965; Touboul et al. 1967; Roelandt and Schamroth 1971) (Figure 16.24)

Parasystolic VTs are very infrequent arrhythmias that originate in an automatic focus protected from depolarization by a normal impulse (entrance block). Some of published cases correspond to IVAR (see above).

The following ECG findings are suggestive of typical VTs of parasystolic origin:

• The PVC, which initiate the VT runs, show a variable coupling interval and meet all criteria of parasystole.

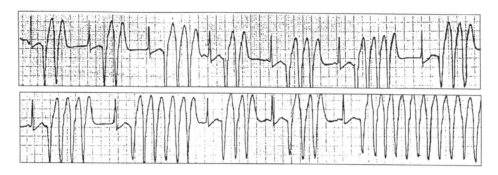

Figure 16.23 Taken from a 66-year-old man with ischemic heart disease. The tracings are successive. Self-limited runs of ventricular tachycardia (VT) with fast rate and incessant rates can be observed, until a sustained VT is initiated.

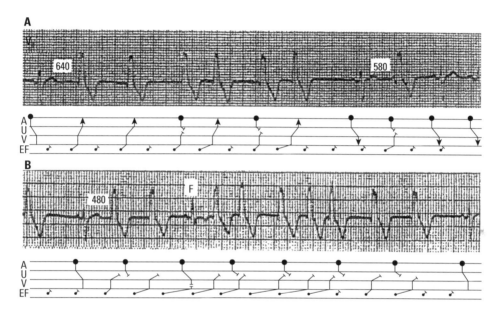

Figure 16.24 (A and B) Two strips from a patient with irregular runs of ventricular tachycardia (VT) of parasystolic origin. The ECG characteristics of parasystolic VT may be seen: (1) different coupling intervals of the first premature ventricular complex (PVC) of each run, (2) the presence of fusion complexes, and (3) the possible explanation of irregular rhythm due to different grades of exit block of the parasystolic ectopic focus (Adapted with permission from Koulizakis *et al*. 1990).

- Although the discharge rate of parasystolic VT is relatively fixed as we have stated before, different degrees of exit block may explain the presence of irregular RR intervals, and also the presence of fusion and capture complexes.

Figure 16.24 shows an example of irregular ventricular tachycardia runs due to parasystolic ectopic focus at 140 bpm with different degrees of exit block that explain the irregularity of ventricular rates. This case meets the criteria of parasystolic VT runs: (i) different coupling intervals of the first PVC and (ii) presence of fusion beats. Irregular RR intervals may be explained by different grades of exit block.

Polymorphic ventricular tachycardia (Table 16.2)

This includes "Torsades des pointes VT," bidirectional VT, and the catecholaminergic polymorphic VT.

Torsades de pointes

There are two different types of torsades de pointes polymorphic VT: the **classical** VT (Dessertene 1966) and the **familiar polymorphic** VT, which features a short coupling interval and lacks a long QT interval (Leenhardt *et al*. 1995).

Classical torsades de pointes ventricular tachycardia (Figure 16.25)

This is the most typical and interesting type due to its prognostic and therapeutic implications. The characteristic torsades de pointes morphology may be related to a counterclockwise rotation of the wave front along the whole ventricular cavity.

Torsades de pointes VT occurs in runs of variable duration (from a few beats to ≥100 beats). The QRS is characteristically non-monomorphic, and cyclical changes

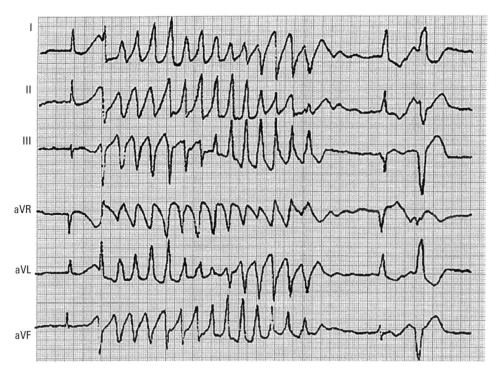

Figure 16.25 A run from a typical torsades de pointes ventricular tachycardia (VT). Taken from a patient with long QT syndrome. Note the typical pattern that is particularly evident in some leads (III, aVF, and aVL).

characterized by a pattern of twisting points (Dessertene 1966) are observed. However, this characteristic twisting morphology is not evident in all ECG leads. The baseline ECG has a long QT interval and the first QRS of the ventricular tachycardia has a long coupling interval, but, due to long QT, the PVCs usually fall close to the peak of the T (or T+U) wave. Figure 16.26 shows the differences between a classical sustained ventricular tachycardia and a torsades de pointes ventricular tachycardia.

The most important **premonitory ECG signs** of a torsades de pointes/VF episode are: (i) QTc interval >500 ms, (ii) T–U wave distortion that becomes more apparent in the QRS-T filter after one pause, (iii) visible macroscopic T wave alternans, and (iv) the presence of evident bradyarrhythmia (sick sinus syndrome or AV block). It is probable that all these ECG signs induce torsades de pointes VF due to genetic predisposition, especially in the presence of ionic imbalance and/or the administration of some drugs (Chevalier *et al*. 2007; Drew *et al*. 2010; Kukla *et al*. 2016).

Pleomorphic VT

Occasionally sustained ventricular tachycardia may alternate morphologies (pleomorphism) such as RBBB and LBBB (Josephson *et al*. 1979). These changes may be gradual or abrupt, and occur over long or short periods of time. They are usually associated with changes in cycle length. Morphologies are considered to be different when they have different patterns (i.e. an advanced RBBB or LBBB), or when the ÂQRS deviation changes ≥45°, even if the bundle branch block pattern is unchanged. These changes in the morphology usually occur after the administration of certain pharmaceutical agents, and coincide with changes in the vT rate (proarrhythmic effect).

Often, in a conventional ECG recording we will probably not see more than one morphology with a regular rhythm. In this case, it would not be possible to differentiate from classical ventricular tachycardia. Therefore, if we rely too much on one ventricular

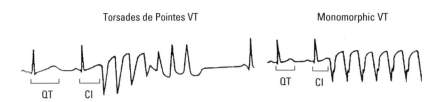

Figure 16.26 Characteristic morphologies of a run of "torsades de pointes" ventricular tachycardia (VT) and of a classic monomorphic VT. CI: coupling interval.

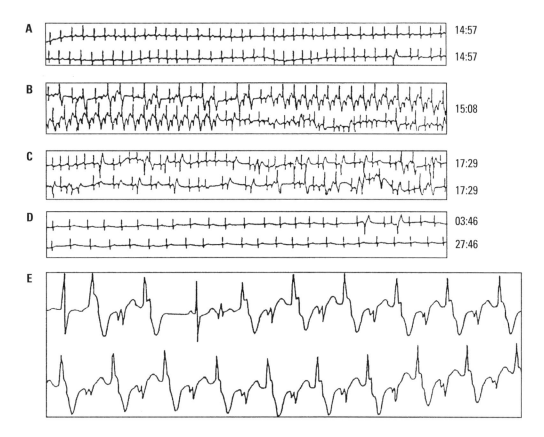

Figure 16.27 Patient with frequent PVCs during psychological stress test. (A) and (D), onset and end of the test. (B) and (C) appearance of different types of polymorphous PVCs with clear evidences of runs of BVT, that is seen enlarged in (E).

tachycardia morphology at a certain time point, we may sometimes misdiagnose the exact place of origin.

Bidirectional ventricular tachycardia (Figure 16.27)

Bidirectional tachycardias are infrequent and may be of supraventricular (BSVT) or ventricular (BVT) origin (Siegal *et al.* 2009; Baranchuk 2010).

The mechanism of BVT is probably delayed afterdepolarization related to excess digitalis intake, ionic imbalance, and catecholamine levels. In a two-dimensional anatomic model of the rabbit ventricles, Baher *et al.* (2011) suggested that the full spectrum of arrhythmias associated with bidirectional VT can be accounted for based on the properties of DAD triggered arrhythmias.

From an ECG point of view (Richter and Brugada 2009), the frontal plane axis (ÂQRS) shows alternative changes of up to approximately 180°, and the RR intervals are usually equal but sometimes show a bigeminal-like pattern (long–short–long).

From the differential diagnosis point of view, the alternans wide QRS morphology compatible with an alternating bifascicular block is very suggestive of supraventricular origin (Rosenbaum *et al.* 1969). In contrast, evidence of AV dissociation supports a diagnosis of ventricular origin (BVT).

Differential diagnosis of bidirectional tachycardias must also be performed with changes of 2 : 1 type QRS morphology, including all cases of true QRS alternans (see Chapter 18) such as: (i) the QRS alternans in AVRT (see Figure 15.12), and (ii) the cyclical changes in the QRS complex voltage in sinus rhythm as observed in cardiac tamponade (see Figure 18.4A).

Other cases in sinus rhythm that have alternatively (2 : 1) different QRS morphologies, such as ventricular bigeminy with late extrasystoles (in the PR interval), alternans pre-excitation in WPW syndrome, and alternans bundle branch block QRS complexes (2 × 1), are considered cases of pseudo-alternans (see Table 18.1).

Catecholaminergic polymorphic ventricular tachycardia (Leenhardt *et al.* 1995) (Figure 16.28)

Catecholaminergic polymorphic ventricular tachycardia is an infrequent form of polymorphic ventricular tachycardia, particularly occurring in young patients with a structurally normal heart. It is usually triggered by exercise, and recent studies have pointed out a genetic origin (Priori *et al.* 2001). It may be associated with different active and passive arrhythmias. As already stated, catecholaminergic polymorphic ventricular tachycardias are preceded by various exercise-induced ventricular

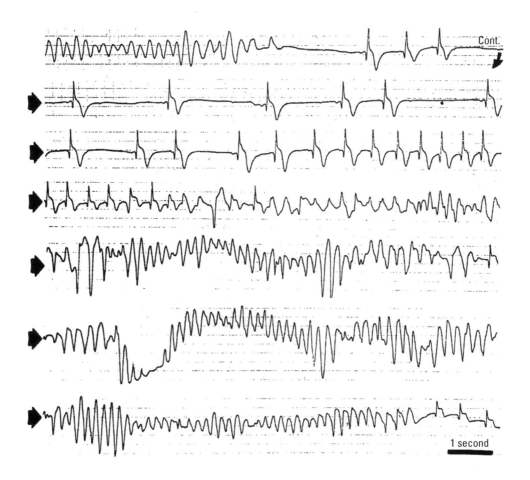

Figure 16.28 Holter recording during a syncope showing a polymorphic ventricular tachycardia, ventricular fibrillation-like, with a spontaneous conversion in transient sinoatrial block with post-critical repolarization changes and then a sinus tachycardia, polymorphic ventricular premature beats, and another episode of polymorphic ventricular tachycardia (30 seconds) (reproduced with permission from Leenhardt *et al.* 1995).

and supraventricular arrhythmias, usually including bidirectional ventricular tachycardias (Femenia *et al.* 2012).

Ventricular flutter

Concept and mechanism

Ventricular rate is very fast (around 300 bpm) and regular (RR variability ≥ 30 ms). It is triggered by a PVC that is usually extrasystolic (exceptionally parasystolic, see Bayés de Luna and Baranchuk 2017), and maintained by a reentry circuit large enough to generate waves, which may trigger very fast yet organized QRS complexes that feature a morphologic pattern. Ventricular flutter is a very fast ventricular tachycardia in which the isoelectric space between the QRS complexes is barely observed. Usually, a very quick ventricular flutter triggers ventricular fibrillation unless it is terminated by cardioversion in CCU or by an implantable cardioverter defibrillator

(ICD) discharge (Figure 16.29). Very infrequently, it is self-limited.

ECG presentation

Ventricular flutter is characterized by the presence of QRS complexes of the same morphology and voltage, with no isoelectric baseline between them and no visible T waves. Therefore, it is no clear separation between the QRS complex and the ST-T segment (Figure 16.29). The ascending limb is the same as the descending limb. For this reason, the ECG looks similar when viewed upside down. The ventricular rate is usually 250–300 bpm.

Frequently, it appears that after a few complexes of fast ventricular tachycardia, they become ventricular flutter complexes.

Occasionally, some ventricular tachycardias show a QRS complex without an evident repolarization wave, at least in some deviations. However, the ventricular rate does not reach 250 bpm.

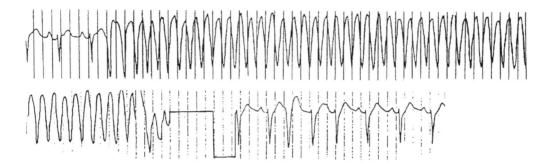

Figure 16.29 Ventricular flutter in a patient with an implantable cardioverter defibrillator (ICD). The discharge from the defibrillator terminates the arrhythmia.

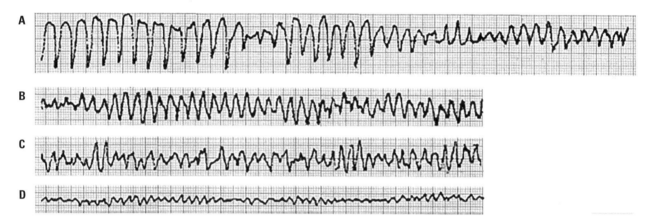

Figure 16.30 (A) Very fast ventricular rhythm of intermediate characteristics between ventricular tachycardia (VT) (it is too fast) and ventricular flutter (typical QRS do not appear in this lead), which quickly turns into ventricular fibrillation (VF). (B, C, and D) Different types of VF waves. (B) A patient with an acute myocardial infarction and frequent, polymorphic, and repetitive PVC, which triggered a ventricular fibrillation (VF) (arrow) that was terminated by cardioversion.

Nevertheless, there are borderline situations between ventricular tachycardia and ventricular flutter, and ventricular flutter and fibrillation, as in the case of atrial fibrillation and atrial flutter (Figure 16.30A).

Ventricular flutter may sometimes be confused with atrial flutter 1×1 with pre-excitation or with bundle branch block aberrancy (Figures 15.40 and 15.41).

Ventricular fibrillation

Concept

Ventricular fibrillation (VF) is a very fast (>300 bpm) and irregular rhythm, which does not generate effective mechanical activity and leads to cardiac arrest and death in a short period of time unless the patient has an ICD implanted or is resuscitated in a few seconds (Figures 12.9C, 16.23, and 16.30). Exceptional cases of self-limiting ventricular fibrillation have been described (Dubner *et al.* 1983; Castro Arias *et al.* 2009). The VF presents significant, cycle

length (RR), morphology, and wave amplitude variability (Figure 16.30).

Ventricular fibrillation is triggered by an isolated or repetitive PVC that is usually extrasystolic (Bayés de Luna and Baranchuk 2017) (Figures 16.31 and 16.32), although exceptionally it may be triggered by a parasystolic PVC (Itoh *et al.* 1996; Bayés de Luna and Baranchuk 2017). It is maintained as a result of repetitive micro-reentries—a mechanism similar to that seen in atrial fibrillation. Recently, it has been suggested that it may be caused by a spiral wave (rotor) that becomes unstable (see Figure 14.15D) and starts chaotic and fibrillatory conduction (Figure 16.33).

ECG presentation (Figure 16.30)

The ECG shows irregular, high-rate (300–500 bpm) QRS complexes of variable morphology and height, where QRS and ST-T are undistinguishable. When the waves of VF are relatively broad, recovery prognosis after electric CV is better than when they are slow and not very high VF.

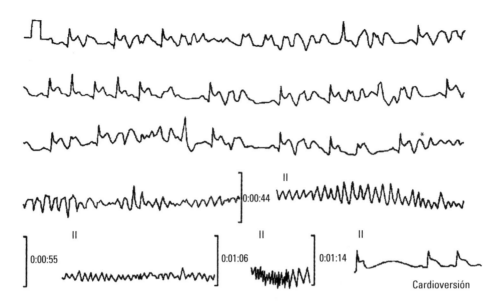

Figure 16.31 A patient with an acute myocardial infarction and frequent, polymorphic, and repetitive PVC, which triggered a ventricular fibrillation (VF) (arrow) that was terminated by cardioversion.

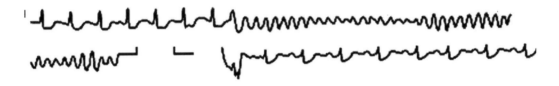

Figure 16.32 Patient with an acute infarction. An isolated premature ventricular complex (PVC) triggers directly a ventricular fibrillation (VF) that ceases after a few seconds (bottom strip) after an electrical cardioversion.

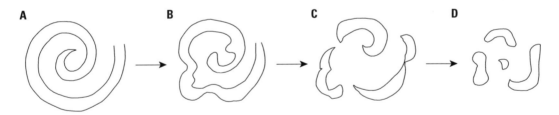

Figure 16.33 Here we see how a spiral wave (rotor) (A) is disrupted and turned into a meandering (B), and later increasingly chaotic conduction until it completely breaks up, resulting in a fibrillatory conduction (C and D).

Clinical implications

The greatest significance of ventricular fibrillation stems from the fact that it is the final arrhythmia that in many cases leads to sudden death. It usually appears in cases of ischemic heart disease and is present in 80–90% of cases of sudden death due to ventricular fibrillation. However, in only around 50% of cases is acute ischemia the trigger of VF, usually with an isolated or repetitive PVC (Figure 16.31 and 16.32). Outside acute ischemia, VF is triggered by a sustained VF (Figure 16.34A) often due to reentry around the myocardial scar (Bayés de

Luna *et al.* 1989). VF outside ischemia usually appears in patients with heart failure or inherited heart diseases (Bayés de Luna and Baranchuk 2017).

Figure 16.35 shows which are the triggering and modulating factors that act on a vulnerable myocardium and trigger primary ventricular fibrillation or ventricular tachycardia leading to ventricular fibrillation. Obviously, given that ventricular fibrillation is the most important mechanism of sudden death in these situations, it is necessary to fight against all these factors.

A

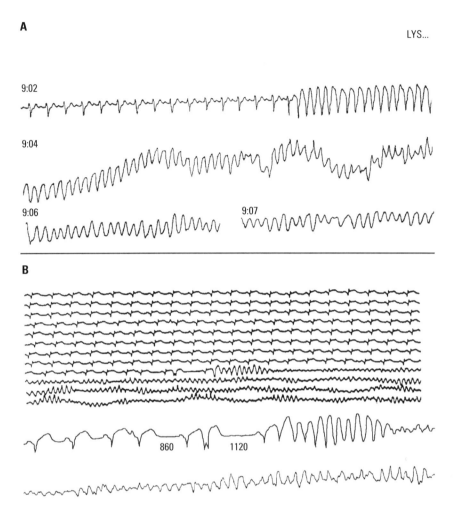

B

Figure 16.34 (A) Ambulatory sudden death due to a ventricular fibrillation (VF) in an ischemic heart disease patient treated with amiodarone for frequent premature ventricular complexes (PVCs). At 9:02 a.m. he presented with a monomorphic sustained ventricular tachycardia (VT), followed by a VF at 9:04 a.m. after an increase in VT rate and width of QRS complex. (B) Ambulatory sudden death due to a primary VF triggered by a PVC with a short coupling interval, after a post-PVC pause (1120 ms) longer than the previous one (860 ms). Note that the sequence of events started with an atrial premature complex, which caused the first shorter pause.

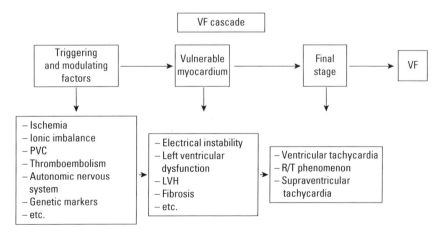

Figure 16.35 Diagram of the precursors of ventricular fibrillation (VF). A triggering factor acts on vulnerable myocardium and provokes the cascade of events leading to VF.

References

Baher AA, Uy M, Xie F et al. Bidirectional ventricular tachycardia: ping pong in the His-Purkinje system. *Heart Rhythm* 2011; 8:599–605

Baman T, Lange D, Ilg K, et al. Relationship between premature ventricular complexes and left ventricular function. *Heart Rhythm* 2010;7:869.

Baranchuk A. Bidirectional ventricular tachycardia or not? That is the question. *Cardiol J* 2010;17(2):214.

Bayés de Luna A, Baranchuk A. *Clinical Arrhythmology*, 2nd edn. Wiley-Blackwell, 2017.

Bayés de Luna A, Coumel P, Leclercq JF. Ambulatory sudden death: mechanisms of production of fatal arrhythmia on the basis of data from 157 cases. *Am Heart J* 1989;117:151.

Bazan V, Baña R, Garcia FC, et al. Twelve-lead ECG features to identify ventricular tachycardia arising from the epicardial right ventricle. *Heart Rhythm* 2006;3:1132.

Bazan V, Gerstenfeld EP, Garcia FC, et al. Site-specific twelve-lead ECG features to identify an epicardial origin for left ventricular tachycardia in the absence of myocardial infarction. *Heart Rhythm* 2007;4:1403.

Berruezo A, Mont L, Nava S, et al. Electrocardiographic recognition of the epicardial origin of ventricular tachycardias. *Circulation* 2004;109:1842.

Bigger JT, Fleiss JL, Kleiger R, et al. The relatinoships among ventricular arrhythmias, left ventricular dysfunction, and mortality in the 2 years after myocardial infarction. *Circulation* 1984;69:250.

Bogun F, Crawford T, Chalfoun N, et al. Relationship of frequent postinfarction premature ventricular complexes to the re-entry circuit of scar-related ventricular tachycardia. *Heart Ruhthm* 2008;5:367.

Brugada P, Brugada J, Mont L, et al. A new approach to the differential diagnosis of a regular tachycardia with a wide QRS complex. *Circulation* 1991;83:1649.

Castro Arias JR, López MA, Sánchez LT. Loop recorder documentation of self-terminating cardiac arrest not receiveing reanimation manoeuvres. *Eur Heart J* 2009;30:1702.

Chevalier P, Bellocq C, Millat G, et al. Torsades de pointes complicating atrioventricular block: evidence for a genetic predisposition. *Heart Rhythm* 2007;4:170.

Chung KY, Walsh TJ, Massie E. Ventricular parasystolic tachycardia. *Br Heart J* 1965;27:392.

Dessertene F. La tachycardie ventriculaire â deux foyers opposés variables. *Arch Mal Cœur* 1966;59:263.

Drew BJ, Ackerman MJ, Funk M, et al. on behalf of the American Heart Association Acute Cardiac Care Committee of the Council on Clinical Cardiology, the Council on Cardiovascular Nursing, and the American College of Cardiology Foundation. Prevention of torsade de pointes in hospital settings: a scientific statement. *Circulation* 2010;121:1047.

Dubner SJ, Gimeno GM, Elencwajg B, et al. Ventricular fibrillation with spontaneous reversion on ambulatory ECG in the absence of heart disease. *Am Heart J* 1983;105:691.

Enriquez A, Frankel DS, Baranchuk A. Pathophysiology of ventricular tachyarrhythmias: from automaticity to reentry. *Herzschrittmacherther Elektrophysiol* 2017; 28(2):149–156.

Enriquez A, Baranchuk A, Briceno D, et al. How to use the 12-lead ECG to predict the site of origin of idiopathic ventricular arrhythmias. *Heart Rhythm* 2019a;16(10):1538–1544pii: S1547-5271(19)30302-9.

Enriquez A, Neira V, Bakker D, et al. Bipolar ablation with half normal saline for deep intramural outflow tract premature ventricular contraction. *HeartRhythm Case Rep* 2019b;5(8):436–439.

Femenia F, Barbosa-Barros R, Sampaio SV, et al. Bidirectional ventricular tachycardia: a hallmark of catecholaminergic polymorphic ventricular tachycardia. *Indian Pacing Electrophysiol J* 2012;12(2):65–68.

Griffith MJ, De Belder MA, Linker NJ, et al. Difficulties in the use of electrocardiographic criteria for the differential diagnosis of left bundle branch block pattern tachycardia in patients with structurally normal heart. *Eur Heart J* 1992;13:478.

Hallan M, Scheinman M. Uncommon forms of ventricular tachycardia. *Cardiol Rev* 1996;4:13.

Haqqani HM, Kalman JM, Roberts-Thomson KC, et al. Fundamental differences in electrophysiologic and electroanatomic substrate between ischemic cardiomyopathy patients with and without clinical ventricular tachycardia. *J Am Coll Cardiol* 2009;54:166.

Hayes JJ., Stewart RB, Green HL, Bardy GH. Narrow QRS ventricular tachycardia. *Ann Intern Med* 1991;114:460.

Hinkle LE Jr, Carver ST, Stevens M. The frequency of asymptomatic disturbances of cardiac rhythm and conduction in middle-aged men. *Am J Cardiol* 1969;24:629.

Itoh E,Aizawa Y, Washizuka T, et al. Two cases of ventricular parasystole associated with ventricular tachycardia. *PACE* 1996;19:370.

Josephson ME, Horowitz LN, Farshidi A, et al. Recurrent sustained ventricular tachycardia. 4. Pleomorphism. *Circulation* 1979;59:459.

Jouven X, Zureik M, Desnos M, et al. Long-term outcome in asymptomatic men with exercise induced premature ventricular depolarizations. *N Engl J Med* 2000;343:826.

Kennedy HL. Ventricular ectopy in athletes: don't worry . . . more good news! *J Am Coll Cardiol* 2002;40:453.

Kennedy HL, Whitlock JA, Sprague MK, et al. Long-term followup of asymptomatic healthy subjects with frequent and complex ventricular ectopy. *N Engl J Med* 1985;24:312.

Koulizakis NG, Kappos KG, Toutouzas PK. Parasystolic ventricular tachycardia with exit block. *J Electrocardiol* 1990;23:89.

Kukla P, Jastrzębski M, Fijorek K, et al. Electrocardiographic parameters indicating worse evolution in patients with acquired long QT syndrome and torsades de pointes. *Ann Noninvasive Electrocardiol* 2016;21:572–579.

Lamba J, Redfearn DP, Michael KA, et al. A. Radiofrequency catheter ablation for the treatment of idiopathic premature ventricular contractions originating from the right ventricular outflow tract: a systematic review and meta-analysis. *Pacing Clin Electrophysiol* 2014; 37:73–78.

Leenhardt A, Lucet V, Denjoy I, et al. Catecholaminergic polymorphic ventricular tachycardia in children. *Circulation* 1995;91:1512.

Lown B, Wolf M. Approaches to sudden death from coronary heart disease. *Circulation* 1971;44:130.

McIntyre WF, Baranchuk A. Left ventricular outflow tract parasystole. *Arch Cardiovasc Dis* 2011; 104(5):359–360.

McKenna WJ, Behr EF. Hypertrophic cardiomyopathy: management, risk stratification, and prevention of sudden death. *Heart* 2002;87:169.

Moss AJ. Prognosis after myocardial infarction. *Am J Cardiol* 1983;52:667.

Moulton KP, Medcalf T, Lazzara R. Premature ventricualr complex morphology: a marker for left ventricular funcion and structure. *Circulation* 1990;81:1245.

Niwano S, Wakisaka Y, Niwano H, *et al.* Prognostic significance of frequent premature ventricular contractions originating from the ventricular outflow tract in patients with normal left ventricular function. *Heart* 2009;95:1230.

O'Donnell D, Cox D, Bourke J. *et al.* Clinical and electrophysiological differences between patients with arrhythmogenic right ventricular dysplasia and right ventricular outflow tract tachycardia. *Eur Heart J* 2003;24:801.

Opthof T, Coronel R, Wilms-Schopman FJ, *et al.* Dispersion of repolarization in canine ventricle and the ECG T wave: T interval does not reflect transmural dispersion. *Heart Rhythm* 2007;4:341.

Ouyang F, Cappato R, Ernst S, *et al.* Electronatomic substrate of idiopathic left ventricular tachycardia: unidirectional block and macroreentry within the purkinje network. *Circulation* 2002;105:462.

Pava L, Perafán P, Badiel M, *et al.* R-wave peak time at DII: a new criterion for differentiating between wide complex QRS tachycardias. *Heart Rhythm* 2010;7:922.

Priori S, Napolitano C, Tiso N, *et al.* Mutations in the cardiac ryanodine receptor gene (hRyR2) underlie catecholaminergic polymorhpic ventricular tachycardia. *Circulation* 2001;103:196.

Rassouli M, Ellestad M. Usefulness of ST depression in ventriuclar premature complexes to predict myocardial ischemia. *Am J Cardiol* 2001;87:891.

Richter S, Brugada P. Bidirecitonal ventricular tachycardia. *Circulation* 2009;54:1189.

Riera AR, Barros RB, de Sousa FD, *et al.* Accelerated idioventricular rhythm: history and chronology of the main discoveries. *Indian Pacing Electrophysiol J* 2010;10(1):40–48.

Roelandt J, Schamroth L. Parasystolic ventricular tachycardia. Observations on differential stimulus threshold as possible mechanism for exit block. *Br Heart J* 1971;33:505.

Rosenbaum MB, Elizari MV, Lazzari JO, *et al.* Intraventricular trifascicular blocks. The syndrome of right bundle branch block with intermittent left anterior andposterior hemiblock. *Am Heart J* 1969;78:306.

Siegal D, Quinlan C, Parfrey B, *et al.* Type II bidirectional ventricular tachycardia as a mechanism of termination of sustained ventricular tachycardia. *J Cardiovasc Electrophysiol* 2009;20(3):345–346.

Steurer G, Gursoy S, Frey B, *et al.* The differential diagnosis on the electrocardiogram between ventricular tachycardia and preexcited tachycardia. *Clin Cardiol* 1994;17:306.

Touboul P, Delaye J, Clement C, *et al.* Tachycardie ventriculaire parasystolique. *Arch Mal Cœur* 1967;63:1414.

Touboul P, Atallah G, Kirkorian G. Bundle branch re-entry: a possible mechanism of ventricular tachycardia. *Circulation* 1983;67:674.

Valles E, Bazan V, Marchlinski FE. ECG criteria to identify epicardial ventricular tachycardia in nonischemic cardiomyopathy. *Circ Arrhythm Electrophysiol* 2010;3:63.

Vereckei A, Duray G, Szénasi G, *et al.* New algorithm using only lead a VR for differential diagnosis of wide QRS complex tachycardia. *Heart Rhythm* 2008;5:89.

Wellens HJ. The value of the electrocardiogram in the differential diagnosis of a tachycardia with a widened QRS complex. *Am J Med* 1978;64:27.

Yamada T, Litovsky SH, Kay GN. The left ventricular ostium: an anatomic concept relevant to idiopathic ventricular arrhythmias. *Circ Arrhyth Electrophysiol* 2008;1:396.

Yan GX, Antzelevitch C. Cellular basis for the normal T wave and the electrocardiographic manifestations of the long-QT syndrome. *Circulation* 1998;98:1928.

Chapter 17
Passive Arrhythmias

This chapter will describe the most important ECG characteristics of the different passive arrhythmias according to the classification in Table 14.1.

Escape complex and escape rhythm

Concept and mechanism

When the heart rate is slow as a result of depressed sinus automaticity, sinoatrial block, or atrioventricular (AV) block, an AV junction pacemaker at a normal discharge rate (40–50 bpm) may pace the electrical activity of the heart by delivering one or more pacing stimuli (escape beat or complex and escape rhythm) (Figures 17.1–17.5). If the AV junction shows depressed automaticity, an idioventricular rhythm at a slower rate (<30 bpm) would command the heart's activity. If the atrial rhythm is atrial fibrillation (AF), the escape rhythm is regular (Figure 17.2) and this is the demonstration of AV dissociation. This never occurs in the presence of atrial fibrillation with normal AV conduction. If the atrial rhythm is atrial flutter, a diagnosis of escape rhythm will be reached based on the slow and regular RR intervals observed, with a variable flutter wave–QRS complex interval (FR interval) (Figure 17.4).

ECG findings

In the ECG, the escape complex is recorded as a wide QRS complex not preceded by a P wave or the preceding P wave has a PR interval <0.12 sec (Figure 17.1A). The escape rhythm is identified as a sequence of dissociated escape QRS complexes (Figures 17.1–17.3), which may be interrupted by sinus captures (Figure 17.1B) that sometimes appear as bigeminal complexes. In this case, a differential diagnosis of bigeminy should be made (Figures 17.1B and 18.6I). The escape rhythm may show retrograde conduction to the atria that is usually slower than the anterograde to the ventricles (Figures 17.1C and 24.1). Sometimes, a progressively slower escape rhythm precedes asystole (Figure 17.5).

The QRS complex is narrow when the escape source is in the AV junction (Figure 17.1). Conversely, when the escape focus originates from the ventricle or from the AV junction but pre-existent bundle branch block or phase 4 aberrancy exists, the resulting QRS complex is wide.

The occurrence of AV junctional escape rhythm or escape complexes at their usual discharge rates should not be necessarily considered pathologic, as this is usually observed in athletes or in subjects with increased vagal tone. In fact, it warrants protection against a slow rhythm. Frequently, if there is no depression of the AV junction automaticity, the implantation of pacemakers would be neither urgent nor most likely necessary. Obviously, pacemaker implantation is urgent if the slow heart rate is due to a depressed AV junctional or ventricular rhythm.

When the AV junction automaticity is very slow or an infrahisian AV block exists, the heart may be controlled by a slow ventricular pacemaker (Figure 17.3).

Sinus bradycardia due to sinus automaticity depression (Figures 17.7 and 17.8)

Concept and mechanism

In this situation, the sinus discharge rate is lower than 60 bpm. The following are the mechanisms explaining sinus automaticity depression (see Figures 14.7 and 14.8): (i) decrease of the slope of phase 4 partly due to the inactivation of the diastolic inward current (I_f); (ii) a threshold potential nearer to zero; and (iii) a more negative transmembrane diastolic potential (TDP).

Exercise, emotions, and adrenergic discharge induce a progressive acceleration of the sinus heart rate, which also shows a progressive deceleration when these physiologic stimuli disappear. The sinus node is considered to be pathologically altered when these physiologic changes do not take place.

Frequently, daytime sinus tachycardia alternates with occasional very slow bradycardia during the night,

Clinical Electrocardiography: A Textbook, Fifth Edition. Antoni Bayés de Luna, Miquel Fiol-Sala, Antoni Bayés-Genís, and Adrián Baranchuk.
© 2022 John Wiley & Sons Ltd. Published 2022 by John Wiley & Sons Ltd.

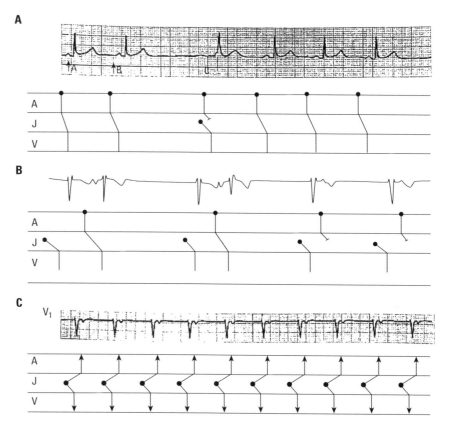

Figure 17.1 (A) A 52-year-old patient with bradycardia–tachycardia syndrome. The AB distance is half the BC distance, indicative of a probable 2 : 1 sinoatrial block. In C, a P wave is initiated, which cannot be conducted because an escape atrioventricular (AV) junctional complex takes place shortly after (third QRS complex). (B) An example of incomplete AV dissociation with slow escape rhythm (first, third, fifth, and sixth complexes) and sinus captures (second and fourth complexes). After the two last QRS complexes, we observe how the P waves are not conducted because they are closer to the QRS complex than the two first P waves, therefore falling in the junctional refractory period. (C) AV junctional rhythm at 64 bpm with retrograde conduction to the atria slower than the anterograde conduction to the ventricles (see the negative P wave following each QRS complex).

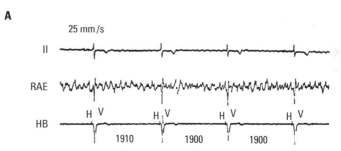

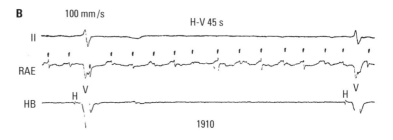

Figure 17.2 (A) Lead II: Regular RR intervals in the presence of underlying atrial fibrillation with narrow QRS complexes. This is indicative of a junctional ectopic rhythm dissociated from the atrial rhythm (atrial fibrillation). See the amplified F waves in the right atrial electrogram (RAE), and how in the His bundle (HB) recording H deflection precedes the narrow ventricular complexes with HV = 45 ms (see B), confirming it is a junctional atrioventricular (AV) block proximal to the bundle of His.

particularly in young athletes, (first-degree or even second-degree AV block may even occur during night) if right vagal (sinus node) and left vagal (AV node) overdrive exist (Figure 17.6) (see later).

ECG findings
Sinus automaticity depression is manifest by a slow sinus rhythm, which in young athletes or in patients with vagal predominance may even be less than 30 bpm (Bjeregaard 1983)

(Figure 17.7). The sinus discharge rate is not fixed, particularly in children. All this is especially evident in the presence of sinus bradycardia. In adults, this variability from one cycle to another is usually less than 10–20%. Sinus arrhythmia may be diagnosed (Figure 17.7B,C) when RR interval variability from one cycle to another is greater than 20%. Sinus arrhythmia is considered to be mild when the change from one cycle to another is <50%, moderate when the change is between 50% and 100%, and severe if it is over 100%.

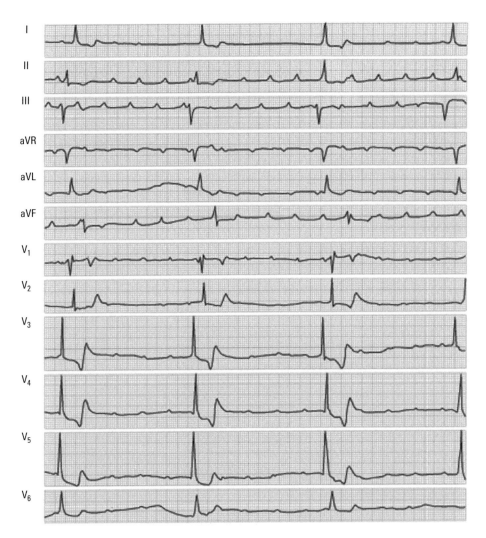

Figure 17.3 Twelve-lead surface ECG in a patient with complete atrioventricular (AV) block (complete dissociated P–QRS relationships), with a somewhat wide (120 ms) QRS complex and a very slow escape rhythm, leading to urgent pacemaker implantation.

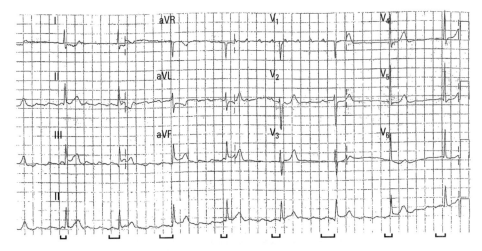

Figure 17.4 Atrial flutter with regular RR at 46 bpm and varying FR distances (see bottom) confirming an atrioventricular (AV) dissociation. This patient suffered from atrial flutter dissociated by AV block of a junctional escape rhythm.

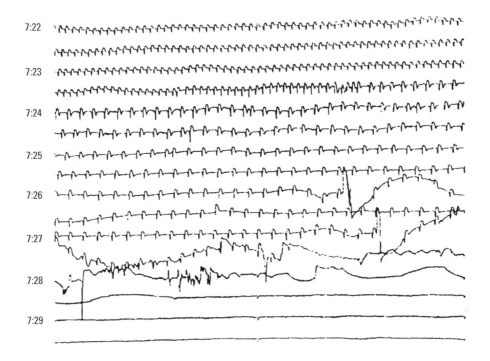

7:22
7:23
7:24
7:25
7:26
7:27
7:28
7:29

Figure 17.5 A 68-year-old patient who presented with sudden death four days after suffering an acute myocardial infarction. In the ECG Holter recording, we observe quick progressive automaticity depression with occurrence of a slow escape rhythm leading to cardiac arrest, probably because of an electromechanical dissociation due to cardiac rupture.

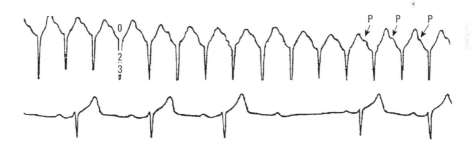

Figure 17.6 A 25-year-old athlete without significant bradycardia with clear ECG signs of sympathetic overdrive during the day (top) and frequent atrioventricular (AV) Wenckebach episodes at night due to the preferential involvement of the left vagus nerve (below).

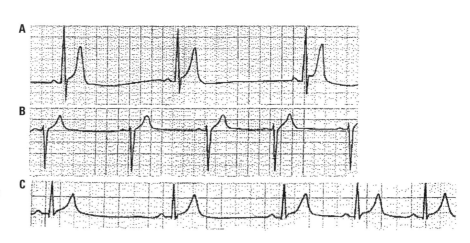

Figure 17.7 (A) Significant sinus automaticity depression. Holter ECG recording (athlete) during sleep showing bradycardia <30 bpm. Note that the PR interval is normal as the left vagus nerve is not involved. (B) A similar example with a heart rate <40 bpm and somewhat irregular, in a healthy young person. (C) Another example of sinus bradycardia in a healthy young person with significant RR irregularity.

Sinus bradycardia is often observed with a normal PR interval (Figure 17.7). Sinus bradycardia and different degrees of AV block are present when a predominant vagal overdrive affects both the right vagus nerve (sinus node) and the left vagus nerve (AV node) (see above) (Figure 17.6).

Finally, it should always be taken into account that a slow sinus rhythm may rarely be explained by the presence of concealed atrial bigeminy (Figures 17.8 and 18.1). It is quite important to consider this possibility and try to identify the small P′ wave deflection at the T wave (Figure 17.8) or close to the end of the T wave, which may be confused with the U wave (Figure 18.1) (arrow), as in these cases the therapeutic approach is quite different to that of a slow rhythm due to a sinus bradycardia.

Sinoatrial block

Concept and mechanism

If the sinus stimulus reaches the atria but with delay, a first-degree sinoatrial block is observed, although the AV relation (P wave–QRS complex) is not altered. This is not the case in third-degree sinoatrial block, where an AV junctional rhythm is the dominant pacemaker. Finally, the second-degree sinoatrial block may be of Mobitz- or Wenckebach-type, similar to the second-degree blocks of the AV junction (see Figures 14.19 and 17.9).

ECG findings
First-degree sinoatrial block
This cannot be detected by surface ECG and may require intracardiac recordings.

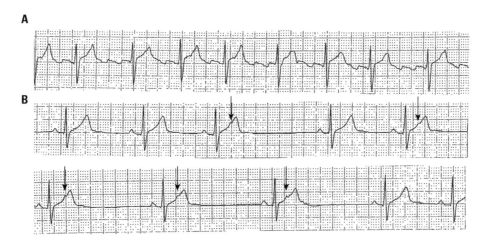

Figure 17.8 (A) Atrial flutter with variable atrioventricular (AV) conduction accounting for the irregular RR and the varying FR. (B) Two continuous strips in sinus rhythm with frequent concealed atrial extrasystoles (notch in T wave ascending limb, see arrow), which give the impression that the basal rhythm, which is already slow, is much more bradycardic.

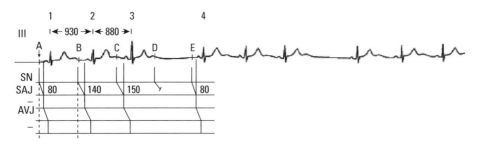

Figure 17.9 Second-degree Wenckebach-type sinoatrial block (4 : 3). The sinoatrial conduction time progressively increases from normality (80 ms) (from A to onset of first P wave) until a complete block occurs (D not followed by a P wave). The distance between the first two RRs (930 ms) is greater than the distance between the second and third RRs (880 ms). Sinoatrial conduction cannot be determined. Theoretically, A, B, C, D, and E represent the origin of the sinus impulses. A–B, B–C, C–D, and D–E distances are the sinus cadence (870 ms). In addition, assuming that the first sinoatrial conduction time in the sequence is 80 ms (distance from the arrow to A), the successive increases observed in the sinoatrial conduction (80 + 60 = 140 and 140 + 10 = 150) account for the shortening of RR and explain the following pause. Therefore, it is confirmed that the more significant increase in the Wenckebach-type block (a sinoatrial block in this case) occurs in the first cycle of each sequence, following a pause (1–2 > 2–3). PR intervals do not change. The second RR interval is 50 ms shorter than the first (930 vs. 880 ms), as this is the difference between the sinoatrial conduction increases of the first and second cycles. In fact, the first RR is 870 + 60 = 930 ms, while the second cycle is 930 – 60 + 10 = 80 ms.

Second-degree sinoatrial block

In the presence of an intermittent-type 2 : 1 second-degree sinoatrial block, the ventricular rate is half the sinus rate (BC = 2 AB in Figure 14.19C). If the 2:1 second-degree block is fixed, the ECG recording will be similar to that of a sinus bradycardia due to automaticity depression. If the 2 : 1 block disappears with exercise, an abrupt increase of the heart rate, usually more than double due to increase in sinus rate, may be observed.

Second-degree sinoatrial block (Wenckebach-type) may also be observed. Usually, this presents as a 3 : 2 (Figure 18.6E) or 4 : 3 block (Figures 14.19B and 17.9). Figure 17.9 explains why in the second-degree sinoatrial block (Wenckebach-type), the RR interval progressively shortens. The block increment is gradually less until the complete block initiates a pause. This type of block does not modify the PR interval because the block is at the sinoatrial level.

From an electrocardiographic point of view, the 3 : 2 sinoatrial Wenckebach block shows a sequence and ECG characteristics similar to those of atrial bigeminy due to premature parasinus atrial impulses (P′ wave is identical or almost identical to the sinus P waves). Figure 17.10

explains the key steps for this differential diagnosis (Bayés de Luna *et al.* 1991).

Third-degree (complete) sinoatrial block

No atrial depolarization due to sinus stimuli is observed. Therefore, the ECG recording shows an AV junctional or ventricular escape rhythm (see Figure 14.19D).

Atrial block

We have discussed all the aspects related to blocks at atrial level in Chapter 9.

Atrioventricular block

Concept and mechanism

Conduction block is observed in the AV junction. As in other types of heart block, we shall refer to first-, second-, and third-degree blocks (see Chapter 14, Heart block). The etiology is due to a degenerative, infection, inflammatory or ischemic process of the AV junction. In rare

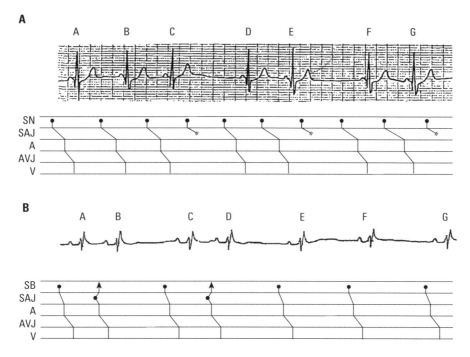

Figure 17.10 Differential diagnosis (Lewis diagrams) between 3 : 2 sinoatrial block and atrial parasinus bigeminy with very similar or identical P′ waves, and a virtually identical ECG pattern. Above (A): After three sinus impulses conducted to the atria, in D a 3 : 2 sinoatrial block sequence starts. Below (B): Two sequences of atrial bigeminy followed by normal rhythm. In the first case (3 : 2 sinoatrial block), AB and BC intervals correspond to the baseline rhythm, which is very similar to the shortest RR interval of coupled bigeminal rhythm (DE and FG distances). Conversely, in cases of atrial parasinus bigeminy, the basal rhythm (EF and FG intervals) is very similar to the longest pause observed in the bigeminal rhythm (BC and DE distances) (below). Therefore, in the presence of a bigeminal rhythm with previous basal RR intervals with the same P, PR, and QRS, the diagnosis of a 3 : 2 sinoatrial block is supported by the fact that the regular RR intervals are very similar to the shortest RR interval corresponding to the bigeminal rhythm. On the other hand, if the regular RR intervals are similar to the longest RR interval of the bigeminal rhythm, it is most likely an atrial parasinus bigeminy.

cases, it may be congenital (see Chapter 24, Advanced AV block). The exact location of the block (suprahisian, hisian, or infrahisian block) is accurately determined only by intracardiac studies (see later; Figure 17.13). However, the presence of a narrow QRS complex escape rhythm and a second-degree Wenckebach-type AV block suggests that the block is located in the AV junction, whereas the presence of a wide QRS complex favors evidence of a block below the bundle of His.

ECG findings

We will discuss below the key diagnostic criteria of the different AV blocks that may be found in the surface ECG.

First-degree atrioventricular block

A first-degree AV block occurs when the PR interval is greater than 0.18 sec in children, 0.20 sec in adults, and 0.22 sec in elderly patients (Figures 14.20A and 17.11).

Second-degree atrioventricular block

One or more P waves are not conducted to the ventricles despite being beyond the physiologic AV junctional refractory period (Figure 14.20B,C). Second-degree AV block may be of a Wenckebach-type (also known as Mobitz I) or of a Mobitz-type block (Mobitz II). In the **Wenckebach-type AV block** (Figure 17.12A), the progressive shortening of the RR interval is due to a progressive reduction of the AV block increment (180 ms–260 ms–300 ms) until a complete AV block is reached.

The mechanism is explained as progressive and decremental prolongation of the PR interval until a P wave fails to conduct to the ventricles. The latter initiates a pause that is longer than any other RR interval. Therefore, a Wenckebach-type AV block is characterized by: (i) a progressive lengthening of the PR interval, starting from the first PR interval after the pause; (ii) the most significant increase being observed in the second PR interval after the pause (Figures 14.20B and 17.12A); (iii) the pause being a longest RR interval; and (iv) the PR interval that initiates each sequence, it is always identical. However, for different reasons, these rules are not always present. Figure 14.21E shows two forms of atypical Wenckebach-type AV block (see legend; Chacko et al. 2017).

In the second-degree A Mobitz II-type, the AV block and consequent pause occur abruptly without previous progressive lengthening of the PR interval. As a result, one or several P waves may be blocked (paroxysmal AV block) (Figures 14.20C and **17.12**B). The second-degree 2 : 1 AV block (one out of two P waves is blocked) may be explained by both Mobitz I or Mobitz II-type blocks (Figure **17.12**C).

On rare occasions, in the presence of a 2 : 1 block in the AV junction (higher portion), the Wenckebach phenomenon may arise from the conducted P waves themselves occurring in the lower part of the AV junction (alternating Wenckebach phenomenon) (Halpern *et al.* 1973; Amat y Leon *et al.* 1975; Baranchuk *et al.* 2009). Figure 14.20F shows an example of this odd electrophysiologic phenomenon.

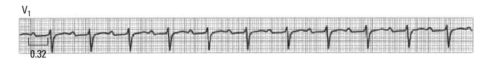

Figure 17.11 First-degree atrioventricular (AV) block (PR 0.32 seconds).

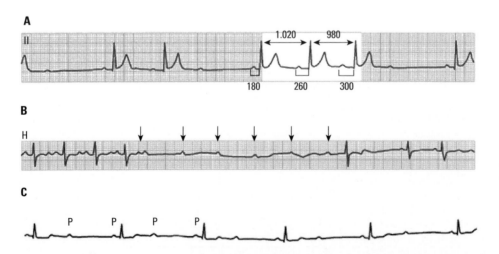

Figure 17.12 (A) Second-degree type I atrioventricular (AV) block (see Wenckebach phenomenon). (B) Paroxysmal second-degree AV block (Mobitz II type). Note the six blocked P waves without a prior increase of the PR interval. The first QRS complex following the pause is an escape QRS complex as it features a very long PR interval. The last two P waves are conducted. (C) Second-degree 2 : 1 AV block.

Third-degree atrioventricular block

In this type of block, a complete dissociation between the P waves and the QRS complexes exists, thus it is frequently named complete AV block (Figures 14.20D, 17.3, and 17.14). The escape rhythm is slow (usually less than 45 bpm), except in some patients with congenital AV block (Figure 17.15), and it is almost always lower than the sinus rate. When the escape ventricular rhythm is greater than the sinus rhythm, we cannot be sure that the AV block is complete, as some P waves may not be conducted as a result of an interference phenomenon (the P waves falls in the AV node's physiologic refractory period).

The width of QRS may be narrow if the AV block is high (suprahisian) or wide if it is infrahisian, or aberrant conduction exists.

The exact location of the block

This can only be determined by intracardiac recordings (see Chapter 25, Intracavitary ECGs and electrophysiologic studies). Figure 17.13 shows examples of first-degree AV block after His level (prolonged HV interval) (A),

second-degree 2 × 1 block before His deflection (B), second-degree AV block after His deflection (C), and second-degree AV block at His level (see two H deflections—H–H′—and the block between the two His deflections H–H′) (D).

Cardiac arrest

A diagnosis of cardiac arrest is reached when the patient carotid pulse is not palpable and no cardiac sounds are heard by auscultation. In continuous ECG recording, it is observed how cardiac arrest may be preceded by a progressive bradyarrhythmia (Figure 17.5) or tachyarrhythmia, usually ventricular fibrillation (see Figures 16.30 and 16.32). Rarely, ventricular tachycardia may directly trigger the cardiac arrest (see Figure 16.8).

Patients in coronary intensive care unit usually are recovered with electrical cardioversion if the cardiac arrest is due to primary ventricular fibrillation (see Figures 16.31 and 16.32).

Hospitalized patients suffering from cardiac arrest should be treated as emergency patients (cardiac arrest protocol).

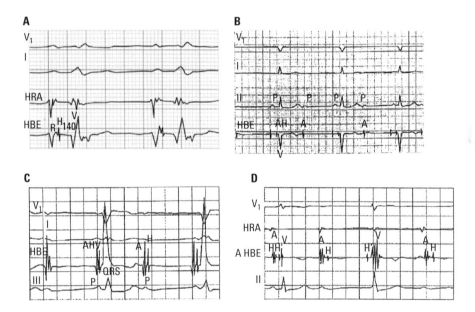

Figure 17.13 (A) Post-hisian first-degree block. In the His lead (EHH), a very long HV is observed (140 ms). The high right atrium (HRA) deflection coincides with the onset of the P wave. (B) Pre-hisian second-degree 2 : 1 atrioventricular (AV) block. The stimulus is blocked after the A deflection and before the H deflection as this is not recorded in the bundle of His lead (EHH). (C) Post-hisian second-degree 2 × 1 block. The P wave is blocked after the deflection of the His bundle. (D) Intrahisian second-degree AV block. Note the split H deflection in the first complex (but with AV conduction), followed by a block after the H deflection. Later, an escape complex is observed, preceded by the second deflection of the His bundle. Finally, there is a block after the first His deflection.

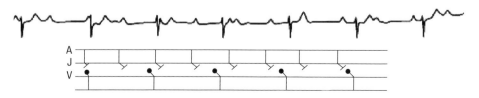

Figure 17.14 Third-degree or advanced atrioventricular (AV) block. A complete AV dissociation is observed.

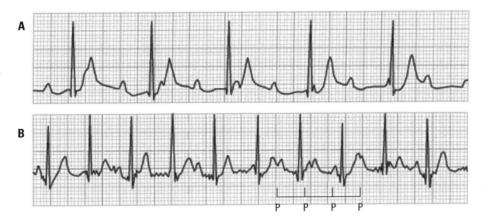

Figure 17.15 (A) Congenital atrioventricular (AV) block with clear AV dissociation in a 20-year-old patient. P waves are independent from QRS complexes, with an escape rate >60bpm. Note the high and sharp T waves. (B) During exercise, there is still AV dissociation, although the sinus heart rate is >130 *x'* (see P–P) and the accelerated escape rhythm is over 100 *x'*. This is a clear example of congenital AV block not yet requiring pacemaker implantation.

The fight against out-of-hospital cardiac arrest is a significant challenge in modern cardiology. Automated external defibrillators (AEDs) are useful at selected locations (airports, sport stadiums, etc.). However the efficiency of this effort, at least in some environments and with current logistics, is limited (Public Access Defibrillation Trial Investigators 2004). Logistic and economic problems make currently universal implementation very challenging. Furthermore, the time elapsed before resuscitation by AED is still too long and many cardiac arrest survivors suffer from neurologic sequels. Finally, it has been suggested that home use of AEDs might offer an opportunity to improve survival for patients at risk (Bardy *et al.* 2008).

The pacemaker electrocardiography (Garson 1990; Kasumoto and Goldschlager 1996; Hesselson 2003; Jastrzebski *et al.* 2014, 2019; ECG University V2 2019) (Figures 17.16–17.28)

Components of the pacemaker ECG

A pacemaker ECG comprises three components: the stimulation spike, the subsequent chamber depolarization, and, finally, the repolarization wave.

Spikes may be either monopolar or bipolar. Monopolar spikes show a higher voltage (currently, only very old pacemakers use unipolar pacing). Bipolar spike voltage may increase due to pacemaker dysfunction. Non-stimulating monopolar spikes may shift the isoelectric line due to their high voltage, mimicking a QRS complex and thus appearing to be normal (Figure 17.23A). Patients with pacemakers may show different types of fusion complexes (Figure 17.25A) due to simultaneous activation of two fronts, the pacemaker stimulus and the intrinsic conduction (ECG University V2 2019).

The QRS complex morphology and the ÂQRS vector direction depend on the pacing site (Figures 17.16–17.18). Stimulation is almost always made from the right ventricle (transvenous-endocardial pacing), and the ECG recording morphology will depend whether the RV lead is placed in the apex, the septum (septal pacing) or the His bundle (Figures 17.16 and 17.17; Courtesy Dr Jastrzebsky).

Resynchronization pacemakers (see below) show a morphology characterized by a narrower QRS complex than that observed at baseline (Figure 17.16 and 17.17). However, different QRS morphologies may be found with resynchronization pacemakers (Steinberg *et al.* 2004; Barold *et al.* 2006a; Jastrzebsky *et al.* 2014).

Figure 17.18 shows the QRS axis in the different types of ventricular stimulation.

Dual-chamber pacemakers (DDD) feature two consecutive spikes, corresponding to atrial and ventricular activation respectively (Figure 17.25C).

Esp-qR morphology observed in I, VL, and V6 usually with "q" ≥0.03 sec is suggestive of old anterior infarction (Figure 17.19) (Barold *et al.* 2006b; Barold 2008).

On the other hand, in patients with intermittent pacing it is observed, as it also happens in intermittent LBBB and right-sided accessory pathway (Wolff–Parkinson–White (WPW) pattern), that the non-pacing complexes have negative T waves that are not due to myocardial ischemia (electrical memory phenomenon) (Figure 17.20). Repolarization disorders are not easily discerned in patients with pacemakers, and thus, in the presence of precordial pain, pacemakers usually hinder the diagnosis. However, when ST changes are significant, they may be clearly observed in the ECG (Figure 17.21).

When patients with pacemakers develop cardiogenic shock, a block between the spike and the paced QRS may occur in the final phase (Figure 17.22). In contrast, a lack

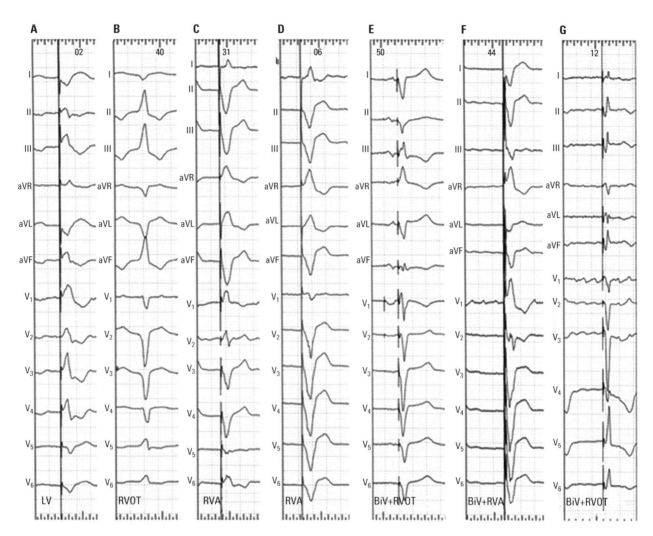

Figure 17.16 *Panel A*: Classic findings during pure left ventricular (LV)-only pacing, shown as a negative lead I, positive lead V1, and negative lead V6. *Panel B*: A negative lead I during pure right ventricular (RV) pacing with outflow tract RV lead position (RVOT) is also a common finding. *Panels C and D*: During RV-only pacing with apical RV lead position (RVA), a positive QRS in lead V1 and/or QS in V6 are not infrequently seen, but lead I remains positive. *Panel E*: Classic biventricular (BiV) pacing pattern in patients with RVOT lead position. Although no dominant R was seen in lead V1, there was QS in lead V6 and lead I was negative. *Panel F*: Classic BiV pattern in patients with RVA lead, showing a dominant R in lead V1, QS in lead V6 and negative lead I. *Panel G*: During BiV pacing in patients with RVOT lead, a very narrow QRS can be achieved, sometimes approaching the morphology of a supraventricular QRS complex, losing most or all three features of LV capture (no negative lead I, no positive lead V1, no QS in lead V6). However, narrow QRS in itself is a potent criterion for LV capture, since such a narrow QRS cannot be achieved during RV-only pacing in a patient with heart failure.

of conduction between the pacemaker spike and the myocardium may also be observed due to pacemaker malfunction (Figure 17.23A) (see below).

Evolution of pacemaker technology (Figures 17.24–17.27)

The first pacemakers were fixed-pace devices, and they could not detect the electrical activity of the heart in the patient (sensing capacity), nor could they be inhibited in the presence of spontaneous electrical activity. Thus, the spontaneous electrical activity of the heart interfered with pacemaker activity. According to the three- and five-letter codes (Parsonnet *et al.* 1981; Bredikis and Stirbys 1985) (Table 17.1),

these pacemakers delivered ventricular (V) pacing, but did not have sensing function (O), and therefore no automatic response (O) to the sensing capacity. **This type of pacemaker (VOO) is no longer used in clinical practice, however; in patients pacemaker-dependent patients (no detectable intrinsic rhythm) requiring thoracic surgery, one may need to program the pre-existent device as VOO to avoid electrical interference from cautery.**

Pacemakers with **sensing capacity to detect spontaneous electrical activity of the heart were designed several decades ago**. The most commonly used pacemaker displays an automatic response to this sensing capacity by inhibiting its discharge. Later, a new response cycle is

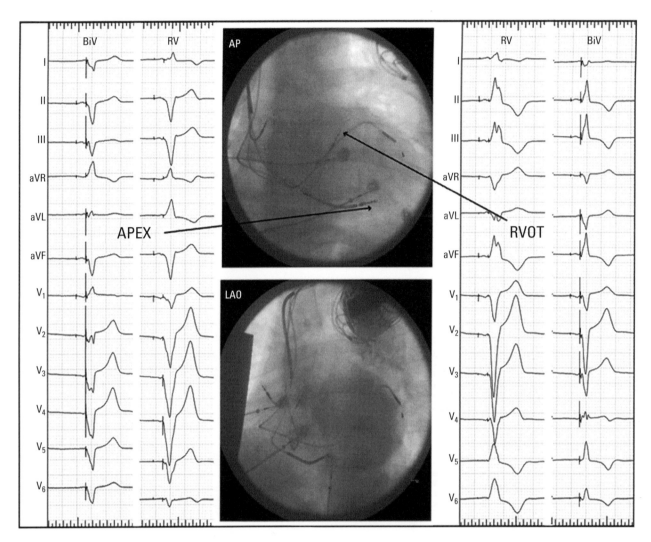

Figure 17.17 Fluoroscopy in anteroposterior (AP) and left anterior oblique (LAO) projections showing a change in the right ventricular pacing site from RVOT (upper arrow) to apex (lower arrow) due to an upgrade from a biventricular pacemaker to a biventricular defibrillator. This case illustrates differences in QRS morphology between BiV with apical and BiV with non-apical RV lead position. Notably, the dominant R wave in lead V1 that was present during BiV pacing with an apical RV lead is absent during BiV pacing with an RVOT lead. The QS complex in leads V5–V6 present during RV-only apical pacing is absent during RV-only RVOT pacing. Note that during both types of BiV pacing, there is an evident change compared to RV-only pacing in both QRS duration and morphology in the final part of the QRS in leads V2–V3. The duration of the QRS from nadir to end in leads V2–V3 is 2–3 times shorter and rises much more steeply than during RV pacing.

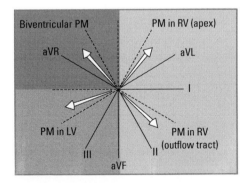

Figure 17.18 ÂQRS in the different types of ventricular stimulation (see Figure 17.16).

initiated, which starts a pacemaker impulse, provided that a spontaneous QRS complex does not occur before. **This type of pacemaker is called VVI pacemaker** (Figure 17.25A) (V: ventricular pacing; V: ventricular sensing; I: demand response (inhibition) if the lead is located in the ventricle). In cases of sinus node disease without AV block, single-chamber pacemakers (**AAI**) (Figure 17.25B) are used (with the lead located in the right atrium). **When the sinus node function is normal but an AV block exists, VDD or DDD pacemakers may be implanted** (Figure 17.25C) (see Choosing the best pacemaker in different clinical settings).

Currently, the most commonly used pacemakers are sequential (dual-chamber) pacemakers, which pace and

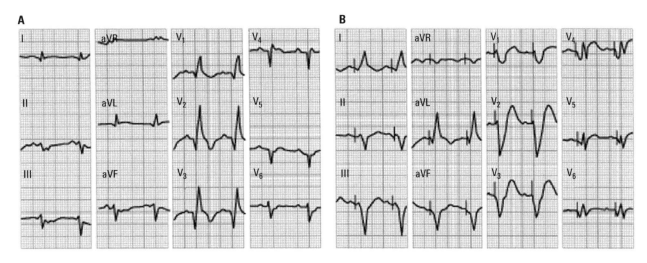

Figure 17.19 (A) Patient with anteroseptal and lateral infarction and advanced right bundle branch block (RBBB) in whom a pacemaker was implanted. (B) Note that Esp-qR morphology is recorded not only in I and aVL, but also in V5–V6, suggestive of necrosis in patients with pacemaker.

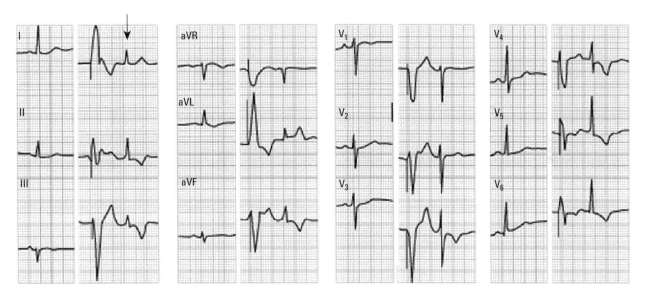

Figure 17.20 Patient with sick sinus in whom a pacemaker was implanted. The left panel of each trace pair shows the basic ECG, whereas the right panel shows the pacemaker ECG, followed in each lead by spontaneous complexes. An alteration in the repolarization of the spontaneous complexes (negative T waves) is observed, which is not due to the presence of ischemia but to the phenomenon of "electrical memory."

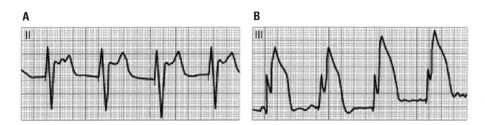

Figure 17.21 Patient with episode of Prinzmetal angina in whom a pacemaker was implanted (A). During an episode (B), a significant ST elevation is observed.

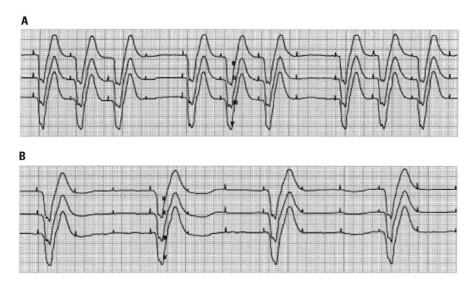

Figure 17.22 (A) A 57-year-old patient with a pacemaker in a cardiogenic shock with spike-myocardium block and some non-stimulating spikes. (B) After a few minutes, agonic rhythm is present (most of the spikes do not stimulate).

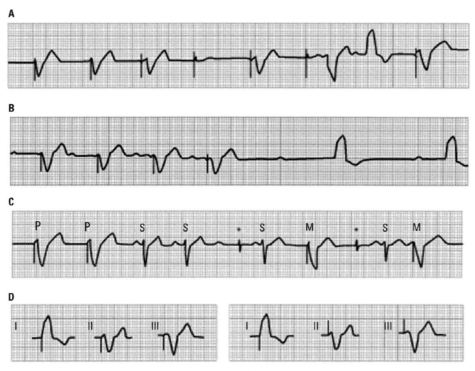

Figure 17.23 (A) Fourth and sixth spikes are not followed by QRS complexes. Note the spike morphology with isoelectric baseline distortion, which may be mistakenly interpreted as a genuine QRS complex. The sixth spike is a ventricular escape and then a sinus capture occurs. (B) After four pacemaker complexes, the spike is not observed and a very slow escape rhythm appears, probably due to cable rupture. (C) Pacemaker complexes (M) alternating with sinus complexes (S). Two different spikes are observed, with a subthreshold stimulation not followed by QRS. (D) Significant changes of spike polarity in many leads. This is an abnormal pattern.

sense both atria and ventricles, and may display inhibition or other types of response. These are DDD pacemakers (Table 17.2 and Figure 17.25C) with two spikes (see above), which initiate atrial and ventricular depolarization in a sequential mode. The addition of a "sensor" allows to determine the metabolic demand of the patient,

to increase (or decrease) the pacing rate according to the perceived metabolic demand ("accelerators").

Many modern pacemakers adapt to normal everyday life because they can increase the heart rate on demand. They sometimes include biosensors, the most commonly used being the P wave. When the P wave rate does not

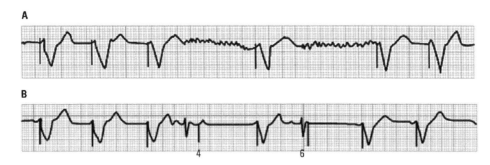

Figure 17.24 (A) Example of oversensing: typical interference by myopotentials. The pacemaker perceives the muscular contraction to be intrinsic activity and becomes inhibited. (B) Example of undersensing. Sensing failure in a patient with a VVI pacemaker. The fourth and sixth spikes fall on the ST of prior complexes and are not followed by new QRS as the myocardium is in refractory period. The reason for the occurrence of these spikes is the failure in the detection of prior QRS because they have a low voltage that is not perceived.

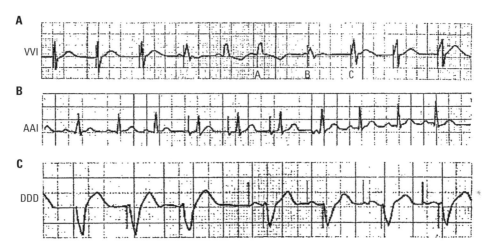

Figure 17.25 (A) VVI pacemaker. Ventricular on-demand pacemaker. The pacemaker is activated when the spontaneous rhythm is slower than its discharge rate. There are fusion impulses (4 and 7). After two sinus impulses (5 and 6), the pacemaker rhythm starts again. The first pacemaker impulse is delayed with regard to the programmed stimulation rate (hysteresis) (AB > BC). (B) AAI pacemaker. The three first complexes and the three final complexes are sinus complexes, start with an atrial spike, followed by an atrial depolarization wave (P wave). From the eighth complex, the sinus activity is again predominant and the pacemaker is inhibited. (C) DDD pacemaker. Example of physiologic (sequential) pacemaker. First, we observe three complexes caused by the pacemaker ventricular stimulation ("atrial sensing"). Next, the sinus rate decreases and starts the pacing by complexes initiated by the physiologic atrioventricular sequential stimulation (two spikes).

increase, due to sinus node disease or atrial fibrillation, other biosensors are used (muscle activity, etc.). Both VVI and DDD pacemakers may have this type of response (**DDDR and VVIR**) (Figures 17.26 and 17.27). External programmers can modify all the pacemaker parameters when necessary. Moreover, advances in the field of multi-programming systems and telemetric interrogation can facilitate the correction of various pacemaker dysfunctions, and allow better pacemaker monitoring. Arrhythmias may also be memorized and diagnosed (**Holter function**). Likewise, implantable defibrillators may be monitored and controlled.

As a result of all these advances, indications for pacemakers have also been changed. Today, they are not only used to prevent sudden death secondary to bradyarrhyth-mias, but also to better treat some tachyarrhythmias or improve ventricular function. Examples of such use include the following:

• **AV node ablation + VVIR pacemaker implantation in** patients with rapid atrial fibrillation in whom the AV node conduction cannot be well controlled with drugs. This approach allows for improvement of the ventricular function and quality of life in atrial fibrillation patients with a very fast ventricular rate. Currently, AV node ablation is combined with biventricular pacing (cardiac resynchronization therapy (CRT)), with acceptable success in cases of advanced heart failure + atrial fibrillation + QRS > 120 ms (Gasparini *et al.* 2006). However, the benefit of CRT is attenuated in cases on permanent AF, due to lack of AV resynchronization.

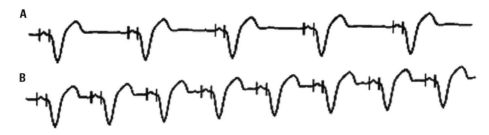

Figure 17.26 (A) DDDR pacemaker in a patient with sick sinus and atrioventricular (AV) block. Note how the pacemaker pacing increases with exercise (B).

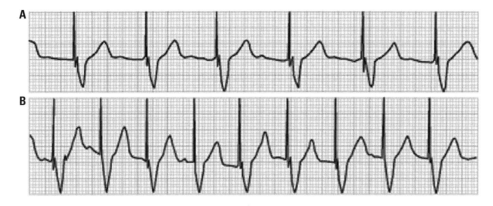

Figure 17.27 (A) VVIR-type pacemaker in a patient with atrial fibrillation (AF) and atrioventricular (AV) block. Note how the pacemaker pacing increases with exercise (B).

• **Ventricular resynchronization pacemakers** (Figures 17.16 and 17.17) are indicated for heart failure patients who present with typical left bundle branch block or for those with right ventricular stimulation inducing dyssynchrony (Cazeau *et al.* 2001; Moss *et al.* 2009). These pacemakers deliver electrical stimulating pulses to both ventricles to coordinate contraction of both chambers. Therefore, these pacemakers correct the dyssynchrony generated by pacemakers located in the right ventricle and/or by the underlying LBBB, improving ventricular contractility and heart failure (CRT). Resynchronization pacemakers are implanted in the left ventricle using a catheter, which is introduced in a coronary vein through the coronary sinus to stimulate the ventricular free wall. Some reviews (Steinberg *et al.* 2004; Barold *et al.* 2006a) have been published commenting on assessment of biventricular pacing, and the diagnostic value of 12-lead ECG during biventricular pacing for cardiac resynchronization. The indications for CRT are discussed elsewhere (see Bayés de Luna and Baranchuk 2017, and ECG University V2).

Stepwise approach to interpretation of an unknown pacemaker ECG: a pacemaker clinic

To interpret the ECG tracing of a patient with a pacemaker, the following stepwise approach should be used: (i) determine the mode of operation of the pacemaker (VVI, DDD, etc.); (ii) measure pacemaker parameters (rate, AV intervals, etc.); and (iii) evaluate the pacemaker function: pacing threshold, sensing threshold, lead impedances and stored events.

Table 17.1 Pacemakers: three- and five-letter identification codes

Types	Category	Letters
I	Chamber(s) paced	V: ventricle A: atrium D: dual (A+V)
II	Chamber(s) sensed	V: ventricle A: atrium D: dual (A+V) O:none
III	Modes of response	T: triggered I: inhibited (on demand) D: dual (triggered/inhibited) O: none (asynchronous) R: reverted
IV	Programmable antiarrhythmic functions	P: single programmable M: multiprogrammable C: communicating R: rate modulation O: none
V	Special functions	B: P = pacing S: shock D. dual (P + 5)

Table 17.2 Characteristics of the main types of pacemakers currently used

Letter position (I II III)	Mode description	Use
VVI	Ventricular on-demand pacemaker (inhibited by R wave) (Figure 17.25) On-demand tachycardization capability (type VVI-R biosensors) (Figure 17.27)	Currently, the most used pacemaker. The spontaneous QRS complex is sensed by the device and the following pacemaker impulse is inhibited. The generator output circuit is recycled and a pacemaker stimulus is generated at a given rate, unless a spontaneous QRS is generated before. It is especially indicated for patients with atrial arrhythmias, particularly atrial fibrillation, slow ventricular rate, advanced age, sedentary lifestyle, infrequent bradycardia episodes and recurrent tachycardia mediated by the pacemaker
AAI	Atrial on-demand pacemaker (inhibited P wave) (Figure 17.25). Capability type AAI-R	Especially indicated for sinus node disease with intact AV conduction, and presumably with no atrial fibrillation in the short-term follow-up
DDD	Universal. Atria and ventricles sensed and paced (Figure 17.25). Different types of programmable parameters may be included. Capability of on-demand tachycardization (DDD-R type) (Figure 17.26)	Sinus node disease and all types of AV block. It does not provide additional benefits over the VVI in case of persistent atrial fibrillation. Pacemaker-mediated tachycardias may occur in the presence of retrograde conduction, which could be prevented by programming the pacemaker without atrial detection

Today's advanced pacemaker technology and increased cost of sophisticated devices require methodological long-term follow-up in order for the patient to receive the optimum pacing benefit and for the treatment to be as cost-effective as possible.

The use of ECG to detect pacemaker complications
Pacemaker complications include those related to implantation, those related to dysfunction of some components of the pacing system, the pacemaker-induced arrhythmias, the pacemaker syndrome, and pacemaker system infection. Complications related to implantation and infection of the system are discussed fully elsewhere (see Bayés de Luna and Baranchuk 2017).

Pacemaker dysfunction
In pacemaker-dependent patients, a dysfunction due to a failure of a component of the pacemaker may induce syncope, hemodynamic deterioration, and even sudden death. Therefore, early detection of possible malfunctions on dependent patients is very important. There are many different reasons for pacemaker dysfunction. We shall briefly look at some ECG clues that may reveal various pacemaker dysfunctions due to stimulation and sensing problems, which are usually caused by dislodged or fractured leads. For further information on the subject, consult Barold *et al.* (2006a), Barold (2008), Hayes and Friedman (2008), Hesselson (2003). A free source of interpretation of ECG of cardiac devices can be found in www.ecguniversity.org.

Pacemaker stimulation problems are generally caused by failure to deliver energy to the myocardium. It is particularly important to check the changes of voltage, as well as the spike duration and transmission. Impedance

measurement also helps to diagnose these problems (this requires the use of a programmer to establish the pacing impedance, which is a reflection of the status of the electrical circuit). The most important stimulation problems occur in the following situations:

- The spike falls outside the myocardial refractory period and therefore has the potential to stimulate. Despite this, it is not followed by a QRS complex, due to an exit block (Figure 17.23A).

- The spike is not permanently or intermittently detected (Figure 17.23B).
- Sometimes, a spike showing a different morphology initiates a subthreshold stimulation (Figure 17.23C).
- In many leads, spike polarity changes are observed (it may be normal if occurring in only one lead), initiating an exit block and occasionally a sensing problem (Figure 17.23D). In the Holter ECG recording, spike polarity changes frequently occur, although generally they are not clinically significant.

Pacemaker sensing problems often manifest as oversensing or undersensing. **Oversensing** occurs when the generator responds to signals different than the QRS complex (or the P wave in the case of atrial pacemakers), which leads to changes in the pacemaker discharge rate because other signals are inappropriately perceived. Oversensing may occur because the **T wave is sensed** or because the pacemaker **wire is partially broken**. It may also be caused by **interference of myopotentials** produced by pectoral muscle contractions (the most common form of oversensing). The pacemaker senses the muscle contraction as an intrinsic cardiac activity and becomes inhibited (Figure 17.24A). In pacemaker-dependent patients, oversensing may result in asystolia. This is consider an urgency and sometimes requires re-programming or the assistance of temporary pacing until final resolution of the sensing problem. **External interference**, such as electromagnetic or radiofrequency interference, can also cause oversensing (McIntyre *et al.* 2010). Oversensing accounts for most of the cases of pauses observed in patients with permanent pacemakers.

In **undersensing**, we observe an inhibited ventricular pacemaker that is unable to sense the QRS complex (or when an inhibited atrial pacemaker cannot sense the P wave). This may be due to a **failure in the pacemaker system** (generator or electrode), or to a **cardiac problem** generally related to a transitory or permanent QRS voltage decrease. In this case, the spike appears regularly, even though there are sinus QRS complexes. These QRS have not been sensed by the VVI system because of their low voltage (Figure 17.24B). Undersensing may also result from **electrode displacement** early after implantation.

Pacemaker-induced arrhythmias (Figure 17.28)

The development of DDD-type dual-chamber pacemakers involves the generation of an artificial reentry circuit. An anterograde arm of the loop comprises the dual-chamber generator with the atrial sensor, whereas the retrograde arm is either the specific conduction system (SCS) or an accessory pathway allowing only retrograde conduction (Figure 17.28).

These circuits may account for the occurrence of pacemaker-mediated supraventricular tachycardias. Figure 17.28 explains how the tachycardia is initiated and perpetuated. During tachycardia, every pacemaker QRS complex is sensed by the atrium, triggering a new pacemaker QRS. This problem may occur in DDD pacemakers if the pacemaker atrial refractory period is shorter than the duration of ventricle–atrial conduction.

Several methods have been designed to prevent pacemaker-mediated tachycardias. Some models automatically prolong the atrial refractory period after sensing the ventricular premature extrasystole, a function which may be programmable. Generators have been designed to interrupt the tachycardia and restore the normal heart rate through a periodic ventricular impulse that transiently interrupts the AV conduction, leading to the reversion of the tachycardia. These tachycardias may be easily terminated by the application of a magnet over the pacemaker, thus inhibiting atrial sensing and producing an asynchronous stimulation. Next, it is necessary to re-program the pacemaker and increase the atrial refractory period (prolongation of the PVARP).

On some occasions, other supraventricular tachyarrhythmias may be triggered (fibrillation, flutter, etc.). Sometimes, an extracardiac cause is involved in the development of these arrhythmias (it may be triggered by myopotentials, magnets, electrocauterization, etc.).

With current lower output pacemakers, the risk of ventricular fibrillation is practically zero, even though the electrical stimulus of the pacemaker may coincide with the patient's T wave (vulnerable ventricular period).

Frequently, ventricular extrasystoles are observed in patients with implantable pacemakers. Although they may disappear when heart rate increases, they may require specific antiarrhythmic treatment. Patients with a doubtful indication for pacemaker implantation are frequently taking antiarrhythmic agents that depress conduction and/or automaticity. This is an important factor when considering pacemaker implantation.

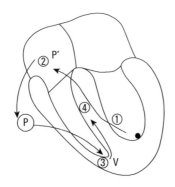

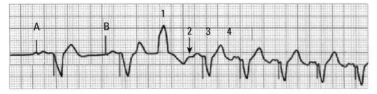

Figure 17.28 Diagram explaining how pacemaker-mediated (DDD) tachycardias are triggered. Note how after two impulses from a sequential pacemaker (A and B), a PVC (!) is conducted retrogradely to the atrium. The retrograde P (2) is sensed by the pacemaker, generating, after a delay in the AV conduction, a new paced QRS complex (3) that may be retrogradely conducted again (4), perpetuating the repetitive phenomenon of the tachycardia. In the case of a VVI pacemaker, no tachycardia would occur, because this type of pacemaker does not sense the atria (Table 17.2), preventing the occurrence of subsequent QRS stimulation.

Pacemaker syndrome

Pacemaker syndrome is caused by a retrograde AV conduction that occurs particularly in VVI pacemakers, causing a "negative atrial kick" that produces a more important hemodynamic impairment than simple loss of AV synchrony (see below).

For a more detailed description of pacemaker ECG, as well as all related main components, goals, logistical needs, and functional aspects of a pacemaker clinic, including the assessment of pacemaker dysfunction, we recommend the interested reader to consult specialized publications (Garson 1990; Hesselson 2003; Barold *et al.* 2006a, 2006b; Barold 2008; Hayes and Friedman 2008), as well as the guidelines of scientific societies and general references. More recently, the International Society of Holter and Non-invasive Electrocardiology (ISHNE) has created a website called ECG University. The ECG University V2 is dedicated to electrocardiology of cardiac implantable devices. Access is free (visit www.ecguniversity.org).

Choosing the best pacemaker in different clinical settings (Figures 17.29 and 17.30)

We must consider: (i) the appropriate pacemaker function for each case and (ii) implantation protocols.

Appropriate pacemaker function for each case

The choice of an appropriate pacemaker function depends on many factors.

Preservation of normal atrial contraction and an appropriate AV conduction synchrony

If an appropriate atrial contraction does not occur in the presence of advanced interatrial block with retrograde left atrial activation (P±leads II, III, and VF), the atrial electrode should be preferentially located in the upper septal region, so that both atria may depolarize at the same time.

Appropriate AV synchrony is very important, as without it atria contract against closed AV valves and venous congestion occurs. The inadequate timing of atrial and ventricular contractions may set off a constellation of signs and symptoms known as **pacemaker syndrome**. This includes decreased cardiac output, hypotension, fatigue, exercise intolerance, dizziness, lightheadedness, and even near-syncope.

Pacemaker syndrome usually occurs when stimulation is VVI with 1×1 retrograde AV conduction. Retrograde VA conduction causes a "negative atrial kick" (see above). Pacemaker syndrome may also occur in the presence of VDD stimulation with retrograde conduction, and also in the case of pacemakers with inappropriate VA synchrony due to incorrect programming. Pacemaker syndrome due

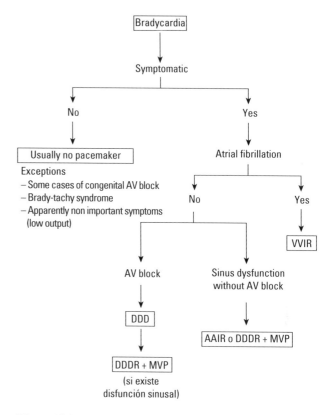

Figure 17.29 Decision tree. Selection of stimulation for all cases of bradycardia, regardless of their origin (see Figure 17.30 and implantation protocols) (*see Nielsen 2010) (Based on Nielsen 2010).

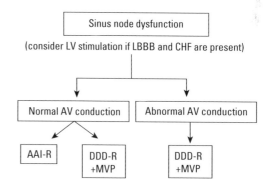

Figure 17.30 Decision tree. Selection of stimulation mode in sinus node dysfunction. AAIR: AAI with rate response; DDD: dual chamber; DDDR: dual chamber with rate response; LVF: left ventricular function; HF: heart failure; MVP: algorithms minimizing ventricular pacing, allowing for maximum stimulation from the specific conduction system (see Implantation protocols and Nielsen (2010)) (Based on Nielsen 2010).

to VVI pacing with VA 1×1 conduction can be eliminated by restoring AV synchrony with atrial pacing, if AV conduction is normal, or with dual-chamber pacing with an appropriate AV delay.

Preservation of the normal ventricular activation sequence

Changes in this sequence produced by pacemaker stimulation in the right ventricular apex or in the case of advanced LBBB may induce hemodynamic alterations and may even trigger heart failure (Stockburger *et al.* 2009; Tops *et al.* 2009). In consequence, when the AV conduction is normal, maintenance of a normal ventricular activation sequence is recommended. Dual-chamber rate-responsive pacing maintains the AV synchrony, but it is not a physiologic pacing modality. It was thought that when the DDDR pacemaker functions more than 40% of the time, the incidence of heart failure and atrial fibrillation increases when compared with patients with an AAI pacing mode. Hence, in patients with sick sinus syndrome requiring DDDR pacing (i.e. AV block), implanting a pacemaker with algorithms allowing maximum pacing through the normal SCS, so that the pacing ventricular stimulation is kept to a minimum, was recommended (i.e. algorithms minimizing ventricular pacing (MVP)) (Figure 17.30). The DDDR pacemaker protects from the small possibility (~2% of annual risk) of future AV block development (see Implantation protocols, and consult Bayés de Luna and Baranchuk 2017).

There is considerable evidence (Zhang *et al.* 2008; Sanna *et al.* 2009) that apical right ventricular pacing (ARVP) produces abnormal heart contractions, and favors left ventricular dysfunction and heart failure. In patients with normal ejection fraction (EF), in a 12-month follow-up, ARVP induces adverse left ventricular remodeling and a decrease in EF when compared with biventricular pacing (Yu *et al.* 2009). Some authors believe that from a hemodynamic point of view, stimulation from the right ventricular outflow tract may be better than that from the right ventricular apex (Cock *et al.* 2003). It has been shown that even survival may improve (Vanerio *et al.* 2008).

The parahisian technique is appropriate to preserve a physiologic AV synchrony and prevent inter- and intraventricular asynchrony (Ochetta *et al.* 2006). Further improvement in the use of appropriate electrodes to stimulate the His region will minimize the current technical limitations. At present, ongoing studies will determine the efficacy of His-pacing, and new strategies (i.e. Left Bundle pacing) are in development.

In patients with LBBB and/or depressed ventricular function requiring pacemaker implantation, biventricular pacing should be recommended. Pacing should reach the left ventricle through the coronary sinus via a cardiac vein contacting the left ventricular lateral wall (Cazeau *et al.* 2001). This leads to resynchronization of the cardiac activation (CRT) and prevents abnormal activation (LBBB-type), occurring with right ventricular activation (Moss *et al.* 2009). Most of the benefit of CRT devices is concentrated in patients with typical LBBB, QRS duration >150 ms, and ejection fraction below 35%.

Maintenance of a normal physiologic chronotropic function

This currently may be achieved with modern technologies (progressive rate-responsive pacemakers) (AAIR, VVIR, and DDDR) (Vardas *et al.* 2007).

Implantation protocols

Various protocols, including guidelines for implantation and selection of the correct cardiac pacemakers, are now available (see guidelines of the scientific societies) (Vardas *et al.* 2007; Epstein *et al.* 2008; Martínez Ferrer *et al.* 2009).

Figures 17.29 and 17.30 show the respective algorithms used to determine the best pacemaker for sick sinus syndrome and bradycardia due to any cause.

In patients with sick sinus syndrome (Figure 17.30), pacemaker is recommended (Chapter 24) and even without AV block, the first pacing choice is probably the DDDR (DANPACE trial) (Nielsen 2010). The AAIR has the inconvenience that an AV block may eventually occur. If AV block is not present at the time of implantation (a progressive atrial stimulation warranting a 1×1 AV conduction up to a rate of 140 bpm should be made), the annual risk of AV block is about 2%.

When symptomatic bradycardia occurs in the presence of slow atrial fibrillation, the VVIR mode pacemakers are the option most widely used (Figure 17.29).

The presence of an acquired AV block requires pacemaker implantation in most cases. However, in cases of congenital AV block, it is a questionable procedure (see Chapter 24).

In patients with advanced AV block and normal sinus function, DDD pacemakers are the first choice. In the presence of sinus node dysfunction, a DDDR pacemaker with (for example) MVP function should be implanted (other algorithms like VIP, were introduced in the market to avoid unnecessary RV pacing) (Figure 17.29).

References

Amat y Leon F, Chuquimia R, Wu D, *et al.* Alternating Wenckebach periodicity: a common electrophysiologic response. Am J Cardiol 1975;36:757.

Baranchuk A, Kang J, Shaw C, *et al.* Electromagnetic interference of communication devices on ECG machines. Clin Cardiol 2009;**32**(10):588–592.

Bardy G, Lee K, Mark D, *et al.* Home use of automated external defibrillators for cardiac arrest. N Engl J Med 2008;358:1793.

Barold SS. *Cardiac Pacemakers and Resynchronization Therapy: Step by Step. An Illustrated Guide*, 2nd edn. Wiley-Blackwell, 2008.

Barold SS, Giudici MC, Herweg B, *et al.* Diagnostic value of the 12-lead electrocardiogram during conventional and biventricular pacing for cardiac resynchronization. Cardiol Clin 2006a;24:471.

Barold SS, Herweg B, Curtis AB. Electrocardiographic diagnosis of myocardial infarction and ischemia during cardiac pacing. Cardiol Clin 2006b;24:387.

Bayés de Luna A. Baranchuk A. *Clinical Arrhythmology*, 2nd edn. Wiley-Blackwell, 2017.

Bayés de Luna A, Guindo J, Homs E, *et al*. Active vs. Passive rhythms as an explanation of bigeminal rhythm with similar P waves. Chest 1991;99:735.

Bjeregaard P. Incidencia y significación clínica de las bradiarritmias en individuos sanos. Rev Latina Cardiol 1983;4:47.

Bredikis JJ, Stirbys P. A suggested code for permanent cardiac pacing leads. Pacing Clin Elecrophysiol 1985;8:320.

Cazeau S, Leclercq C, Lavergne T, *et al*. Effects of multisite biventricular pacing in patients with heart failure and intranventricular conduction delay. N Engl J Med 2001;344:873.

Chacko S, Glover B, Baranchuk A. Wenckebach periods of alternate beats: an unusual phenomenon. Section conduction disorders. In Shenasa M, Josephson ME, Estes III NAM, Amsterdam EA, Scheinman M (eds) *ECG Master's Collection: Favorite ECGs from Master Teachers Around the World II*, CARDIOTEXT, USA, 2017.

Cock CC, Giudici MC, Twisk JW. Comparison of the haemodynamic effects of right ventricular outflow-tract pacing with right ventricular apex pacing: a quantitative review. Europace 2003;5:275.

ECG University V2 (www.ecguniversity.org). Steinberg J, Dubner S, Baranchuk A (Directors), 2019.

Epstein AE, DiMarco JP, Elenboge KA, *et al*. ACC/AHA/HRS 2008 Guidelines for device-based therapy of cardiac rhythm abnormalities: a report of the American College of Cardiology/American Heart Association task force on practice guidelines (writing committee to revise the ACC/AHA/NASPE 2002 Guideline update for implantation of cardiac pacemakers and antiarrhythmia devices): developed in collaboration with the American Association for Thoracic Surgery and Society of Thoracic Surgeons. Circulation 2008;117:350.

Garson A. Stepwise approach to the unknown pacemaker ECG. Am Heart J 1990;118:924.

Gasparini M, Auricchio A, Regoli F, *et al*. Four-year efficacy of cardiac resynchronization therapy on exercise tolerance and disease progression: the importance of performing atrioventricular junction ablation in patients with atrial fibrillation. J Am Coll Cardiol 2006;48:734.

Halpern MS, Nau GJ, Levi RJ, *et al*. Wenckebach periods of alternate beats. Clinical and experimental observations. Circulation 1973;48:41.

Hayes DL, Friedman PA. *Cardiac Pacing, Defibrillation and Resynchronization: A Clinical Approach*, 2nd edn. Wiley-Blackwell, 2008.

Hesselson AB. *Simplified Interpretation of Pacemaker ECGs*. Futura/Blackwell, 2003.

Jastrzebski M, Kukla P, Fijorek K, Czarnecka D. Universal algorithm for diagnosis of biventricular capture in patients with cardiac resynchronization therapy. Pacing Clin Electrophysiol 2014;37(8):986–993.

Jastrzębski M, Moskal P, Bednarek A, Kiełbasa G, Vijayaraman P, Czarnecka D. Programmed his bundle pacing: a novel maneuver for the diagnosis of his bundle capture. Circ Arrhythm Electrophysiol 2019;12(2):e007052.

Kasumoto FM, Goldschlager N. Cardiac pacing. N Engl J Med 1996;334:89.

McIntyre WF, Michael KA, Baranchuk A. Electromagnetic Interference Induced by Magnetic Resonance Imaging. Can J Cardiol 2010;26(2):e64.

Martínez Ferrer J, Fidalgo Andres ML, Barba Pichardo R, *et al*. Novedades en estimulación cardiaca. Rev Esp Cardiol 2009;62:117.

Moss AJ, Hall WJ, Cannom DS, *et al*. Cardiac resynchronization therapy for the prevention of heart failure events. N Engl J Med 2009;361:1329.

Nielsen JC, on behalf of the DANPACE investigators. The Danish multicenter randomized trial on single atrial (AAIR) versus dual chamber pacing in sick sinus syndrome, 2010. http://www.escardio.org/congresses/esc-2010/congress-reports/page798.1DANPACE.aspx.

Ochetta E, Bortnik M, Magnani A, *et al*. Prevention of ventricular desynchronization by permanent parahisian pacing after atrioventricular node ablation in chronic atrial fibrillation. J Am Coll Cardiol 2006;47:1938.

Parsonnet V, Furman S, Smyth NP. A revised code for pacemaker identification. Pacing Clin Electrophysiol 1981;4:400.

Public Access Defibrillation Trial Investigators. Public access defibrillators and survival after out-of-hospital cardiac arrest. N Engl J Med 2004;351:637.

Sanna I, Franceschi F, Pevot S, Basturd E, Dehero JC. Right ventricular apex pacing: it is obsolete? Arch Cardiovasc Dis 2009;102:135.

Steinberg JS, Maniar PB, Higgins SL, *et al*. Noninvasive assessment of the biventricular pacing system. Ann Noninvasive Electrocardiol 2004;9:58.

Stockburger M, Celebi O, Krebs A, *et al*. Right ventricular pacing is associated with impaired overall survival, but not with an increased incidence of a tachyarrhythmias in routine cardioverter/defibrillator recipients with reservedly programmed pacing. Europace 2009;11:924.

Tops LF, Schalij MJ, Bax JJ. The effects of right ventricular apical pacing on ventricular function and dyssynchrony. J Am Coll Cardiol 2009;54:764.

Vanerio G, Vidal JL, Fernandez P, *et al*. Medium-and long-term survival after pacemaker implant: improved survival with right ventricular outflow trac pacing. J Interv Card Electrophysiol 2008;21:195.

Vardas PE, Auricchio A, Blanc JJ, *et al*. Guidelines for cardiac pacing and cardiac resynchronization therapy: The Task Force for cardiac pacing and cardiac resynchronization therapy of the European Society of Cardiology. Developed in collaboration with the European Heart Rhythm Association. Eur Heart J 2007;28:2256.

Yu CM, Chan JY, Zhang Q, *et al*. Biventricular pacing in patients with bradycardia and normal ejection fraction. N Engl J Med 2009;361:2123.

Zhang XH, Chen H, Sin C, *et al*. New-onset heart failure after permanent right ventricular apical pacing in patients with acquired high-grade atrioventricualr block and normal left ventricular function. J Cardiovasc Electrophysiol 2008;18:136.

Chapter 18
Diagnosis of Arrhythmias in Clinical Practice: A Step-by-Step Approach

In this chapter, we will discuss the different steps to properly diagnose an arrhythmia.

Determining the presence of a dominant rhythm

It is generally easy to identify whether the dominant rhythm is of sinus or ectopic origin, and, in this latter case, to know what kind of arrhythmia it is. Occasionally, however, it may be difficult to determine which rhythm is dominant. For instance, in the case of chaotic atrial tachycardia (see Figure 15.21), by definition, there is no dominant rhythm (see Chapter 15, Chaotic atrial tachycardia). At times, it may also be difficult to distinguish between sinus rhythm and flutter with 2 : 1 conduction (see Figure 15.14).

In particular, when the atrial rate is around 200 bpm, it is challenging to distinguish between atypical flutter and tachycardia due to an atrial macro-reentry (MAT-MR). In fact, these two arrhythmias could be considered the same (see Chapter 15, Atrial flutter: ECG findings) from a morphological point of view, but different in terms of definitive treatment with ablation.

When atrial activity is not observed, it may also be quite difficult to determine which the dominant rhythm is. In this case, carotid sinus massage and other vagal maneuvers (see Figure 15.5) could be helpful. The use of T wave filtering techniques, if available (see Chapter 25) can also help to determine the dominant rhythm. Intracavitary studies may also be useful in many cases, even in atrial fibrillation/atrial flutter with small or apparently nonexistent "f" waves (Figures 15.37 and 18.1).

Atrial wave analysis

Be sure that the atrial activity is visible in the ECG

In an ECG tracing with narrow or broad QRS tachycardia, sometimes atrial activity is not observed because the atrial wave is hidden within the QRS complex (see Figure 15.13A). Sometimes, it could be useful to take an ECG during deep breathing (see Figure 15.5) or during carotid sinus compression. If, despite all these measures, the atrial wave is not seen (Bayés de Luna *et al.* 1978), it is useful to use voltage amplification techniques (see Figure 13.24) and, if possible, to apply the T wave filter (Goldwasser *et al.* 2011) (see Figure 25.16). However, the fact that no atrial activity is detected in the surface ECG even in the presence of slow heart rate is not conclusive evidence for atrial paralysis (see Figure 15.37), because the atrial rhythm may be concealed in the QRS complex or undetectable in the surface ECG (Figure 15.37). Atrial paralysis is only confirmed when no atrial activity is observed in intracavitary recordings.

Morphology and polarity

The atrial wave morphology suggests sinus or ectopic origin. In sinus rhythm, it is positive in leads V2–V6 and I, and negative in lead aVR; it is frequently ± in lead V1, whereas in rare cases it is ± in leads II, III, and aVF (Bayés de Luna *et al.* 1985; Bayes de Luna and Baranchuk 2017); finally, it is negative or ± I in aVL.

In the case of monomorphic atrial tachycardia of ectopic focus (MAT-EF), the algorithm shown in Figure 15.10 allows us to localize the atrial origin of the ectopic P′ wave (Kistler *et al.* 2006). On the other hand, a very

Clinical Electrocardiography: A Textbook, Fifth Edition. Antoni Bayés de Luna, Miquel Fiol-Sala, Antoni Bayés-Genís, and Adrián Baranchuk.
© 2022 John Wiley & Sons Ltd. Published 2022 by John Wiley & Sons Ltd.

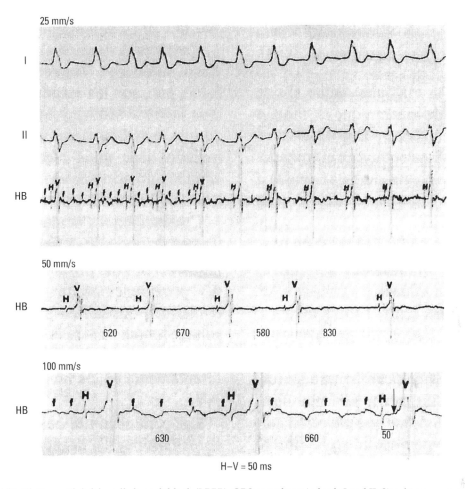

Figure 18.1 Atrial fibrillation with left bundle branch block (LBBB)–QRS complexes in leads I and II, Simultaneous recording of His bundle electrocardiogram (HBE) depicts the "f" waves, which are non-visible on surface ECG, and demonstrates that the H deflection precedes the ventricular complexes, with a normal H–V interval of 50 ms. Tracings taken at higher speeds show better the oscillations in the duration of RR intervals (50 and 100 mm/sec).

narrow P wave (<0.06 sec) is indicative of ectopic origin, although it should be pointed out that many ectopic P′ waves are wide (see Figures 15.7 and 15.9).

F waves of atrial fibrillation show low but variable voltages, being more evident in V1 (see Figures 15.25 and 15.26), whereas the typical common flutter waves display a sawtooth morphology with a predominant negative component in leads II, III, and VF (see Figure 15.33).

Figure 18.2 shows the morphology of atrial activation waves in the different supraventricular tachycardias with regular and monomorphic waves (see also Table 15.5) and Figures 18.3 and 18.4 show the different algorithms that, depending on whether atrial activity is present or not, allow us to determine the type of active supraventricular arrhythmia with narrow QRS and regular (Figure 18.3) or irregular RR (Figure 18.4).

Cadence

The cadence of atrial activity may be regular or irregular. In sinus rhythm, the cadence is regular, although it

usually shows a little variability, especially during respiration (see Chapter 15, Sinus tachycardia). Ectopic atrial waves may show a regular or irregular cadence. The cadence of atrial activity is regular in all ectopic forms or reentrant tachycardias (of atrial or junctional origin) and in atrial flutter, whereas cadence is irregular in chaotic atrial tachycardia and atrial fibrillation (Figures 18.2 and 18.3). Relatively often, ectopic atrial tachycardias show some changes in the heart rate at the onset or end of the crisis (see below), in relation to some stimuli (exercise, etc.) or after some drugs administration (digitalis).

Rate

• Sinus rate during rest is not usually faster than 80–90 bpm, although this rate may be higher in sympathetic overdrive or in different pathologic situations (fever, acute myocardial infarction, hyperthyroidism, heart failure, etc.). Exercise and emotions (see Figure 15.4) lead to a progressive increase of up to 180–200 bpm in young people, whereas a progressive slowing down is

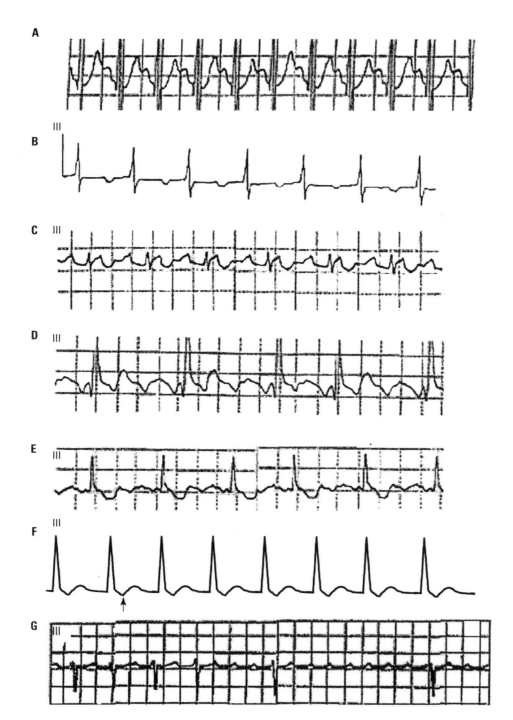

Figure 18.2 Different morphologies of monomorphic atrial waves. (A) Sinus P wave. (B) Monomorphic atrial tachycardia due to ectopic focus (MAT-EF) with 1 : 1 conduction. (C) MAT-EF with 2 : 1 atrioventricular (AV) conduction. (D) "F" waves of common flutter with variable AV conduction. (E) "F" waves of reverse flutter with a 3 : 1 conduction. (F) Retrograde P' in case of AVRT (junctional reciprocating tachycardia–accessory pathway). (G) Atypical flutter waves with variable conduction.

observed when the stimuli disappear. The sinus rate during sleep or rest may be slower than 50 or even 40 bpm (see Chapter 17, Sinus bradycardia due to sinus automaticity depression). The rate is also increased in inappropriate sinus tachycardia and in sinus reentrant tachycardia (see Chapter 15, Sinus tachycardia).

• In MAT-EF, the P' wave ranges between 100 and 200 bpm. In some cases, its rate increases during exercise and at the onset of tachycardia (warming up) (see Figure 15.7).
• In MAT-MR, the atrial rate is usually fast and does not change with exercise. If it reaches ~200 bpm, it may

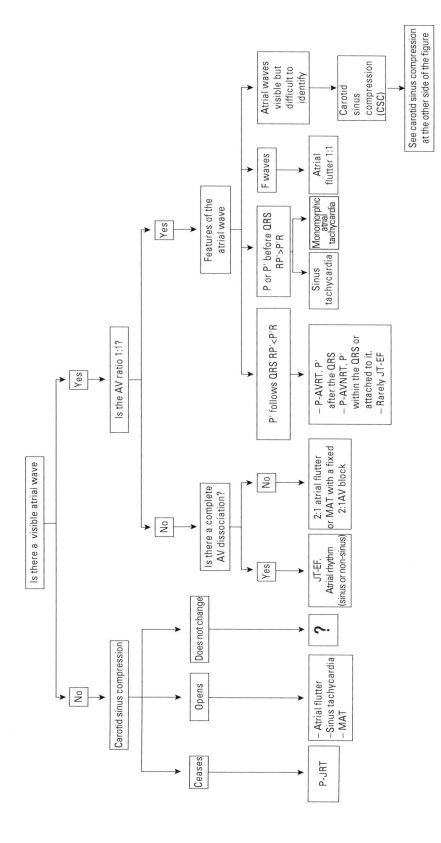

Figure 18.3 Algorithm for detecting active supraventricular arrhythmias with regular RR intervals and narrow QRS complexes.

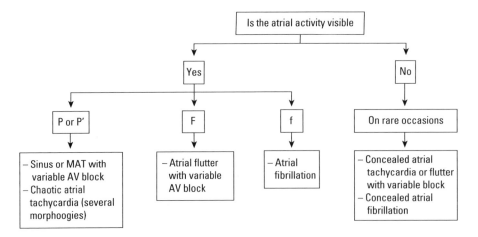

Figure 18.4 Algorithm for detecting active supraventricular arrhythmias with irregular RR and narrow QRS complexes.

resemble an atypical flutter. In fact, both names probably correspond to the same arrhythmia (see Chapter 15, Atrial flutter).

• The rate in the two types of AV junctional tachycardias due to reentrant mechanism (JRT)—exclusively junctional and with accessory pathway—is usually high (~150–180 bpm).

• The rate of atrial rhythm in atrial fibrillation and flutter (A.Fl) and the ventricular rate is usually high (360–700 bpm and irregular in AF, and 200–300 bpm and regular in A.Fl), and the ventricular rate, depends on the grade of concealed AV conduction of f or F waves (see Chapter 15).

• A not very fast but fixed rate (100–130 bpm) both during the day and night supports diagnosis of ectopic rhythm (atrial tachycardia or 2 : 1 flutter instead of sinus rhythm) (see Figure 15.14).

• A slow regular atrial rate (<60 bpm) is indicative of sinus bradycardia, or, in rare cases, of a sinoatrial 2 : 1 block. In the latter case, the heart rate may double with exercise, whereas in sinus bradycardia the heart rate increases progressively.

Location of the atrial wave in the cardiac cycle (RR)

• The sinus P wave and most MAT P′ waves precede the QRS complex, with a PR<RP relationship (see Figure 15.13D).

• In paroxysmal junctional tachycardias, where the reentrant circuit exclusively involves the AV junction (atrioventricular nodal reentry tachycardia (AVNRT)), the P′ wave is located within the QRS complex (and is therefore not visible) or it is attached to its end, resulting in morphology distortion (see Figure 15.13A,B). If the reentry involves an accessory pathway (AVRT), the P′ wave follows the QRS complex closely so that P′R>RP′ (see Figure 15.13C).

• In junctional ectopic tachycardia when there is ventriculoatrial conduction, the P′ may be located before or after, or be hidden within the QRS complex (see Chapter 15, Atrioventricular junctional tachycardia due to ectopic focus).

QRS complex analysis

Width and morphology

The QRS complexes may be narrow (<120 ms) or wide (≥120 ms).

• Narrow QRS complexes are the result of normal ventricular activation due to sinus rhythm if they are preceded by a sinus P wave, or due to different types of supraventricular tachyarrhythmias (see Tables 15.2 and 15.3). Narrow QRS complexes in the case of slow rates not preceded by sinus P waves correspond to junctional escape complexes or rhythm.

• Wide QRS complexes may be the result of intraventricular aberrant conduction, over an accessory pathway, or of ventricular origin (see below).

Cadence

In the presence of narrow QRS complexes, the RR cadence may be regular or irregular (see Table 15.3). Based on this premise, the different types of fast regular or irregular rhythms with narrow QRS complexes may be diagnosed using the algorithms of Figures 18.3 and 18.4. In addition, Tables 15.2 and 15.3 display the most important ECG aspects of paroxysmal regular supraventricular tachyarrhythmias with narrow QRS complexes. The presence of premature atrial or ventricular complexes may convert a regular rhythm into an irregular one.

All the types of slow regular or irregular rhythms, usually with narrow QRS complexes (sinus bradycardia, escape functional rhythm, etc.), are discussed in

Chapter 17. A proposed algorithm for narrow complex tachycardias can be consulted for free at www.ecguniversity.org or by downloading for free a new i-book (Baranchuk and Nadeau-Rauther 2016; Baranchuk *et al.* 2018).

When the QRS is wide and the ventricular rate is fast and regular, a differential diagnosis between ventricular tachycardia (see Figures 16.12–16.14) and supraventricular tachycardia with aberrant intraventricular conduction (see Figure 16.19) or with anterograde conduction over an accessory pathway (see Figure 16.18) has to be performed. In most cases (when the substrate is ischemic), differential diagnosis may be established using the algorithm developed by Brugada *et al.* (1991). For more detailed information on the algorithm, visit www.ecguniersity.org.

The presence of wide QRS complexes and irregular rhythm is seen in the case of atrial fibrillation or atrial flutter with variable conduction and aberrant intraventricular conduction or pre-excitation (see Figures 15.40 and 15.41). The presence of capture or fusion complexes may show if the fast irregular rhythm is due to ventricular tachycardia or atrial fibrillation with aberrant conduction (see Figures 15.31 and 16.15). From a clinical point of view, a wide complex tachycardia in a patient with history of structural heart disease should be treated as ventricular tachycardia until the diagnosis can be properly established by an expert electrocardiologist.

The possible explanations of wide QRS in the presence of slow heart rate include sinus bradycardia with bundle branch block, and ventricular escape rhythm or AV junctional with aberrancy (see Chapter 17).

On occasion, the QRS complexes occur in a repetitive form (alloarrhythmia), for example bigeminal rhythm (see Repetitive arrhythmias analysis: bigeminal rhythm, and Figure 18.10) (Antiperovitch *et al.* 2019).

Rate

The QRS complex may show a fast rate (>90 bpm), normal rate (60–90 bpm), or low rate (<60 bpm).

High ventricular rates correspond to active arrhythmias, but in many cases normal and low ventricular rates may also be seen in active rhythms, as in the case with regular rhythms (particularly flutter with 4 : 1 AV conduction) or irregular rhythms (particularly atrial fibrillation with low ventricular rate due to advanced AV block). In the case of flutter with 4 : 1 AV conduction and heart rate of about 75 bpm, it may be mistakenly considered to be sinus rhythm both through palpation and auscultation. However, with exercise, the heart rate usually shows abrupt increases (due to a decrease of AV block), or remains stable, whereas the sinus rhythm increases the heart rate progressively.

The majority of passive arrhythmias have low ventricular rates. There are exceptions, for example, first-degree sinoatrial block or AV block (see Figures 14.19A and 14.20A).

Atrioventricular relationship analysis

This information is very important to obtain the correct diagnosis of arrhythmia. Evidence of AV anterograde conduction, regardless of the type (sinus P wave–QRS complex, P′ wave-QRS complex, F flutter or f fibrillation waves–QRS complex), as well as the eventual ventriculoatrial (VA) retrograde activation, is often a key parameter to correctly diagnose the different arrhythmias (Figure 18.2).

If no AV or VA relationship is observed, we may state that AV dissociation is present, which may be due to a block or interference (see Chapter 14, Decreased conduction: blocks). In the first case, the ventricular rate is slow, due to an advanced block or a complete block (see Figures 14.20D, 17.3, and 17.14), whereas in the second case the ventricular rate is fast. If the QRS is wide, it is very suggestive for ventricular tachycardia (see Figure 16.13). Less often, it may be due to junctional ectopic tachycardia with aberrant conduction.

Premature complex analysis

Premature complexes may show normal or wide QRS morphology (aberrant or ventricular ectopy). The most frequent causes of premature complexes are **extrasystoles of supraventricular or ventricular origin** (see Figures 15.1 and 16.1). Other possible causes of premature QRS complexes that should be considered include:
- parasystolic complexes (see Figures 15.2 and 16.2);
- reciprocating complexes (if they are repetitive, they are indicative of a reentrant tachycardia) (see Figures 14.10–14.15);
- sinus captures in the presence of ventricular tachycardia (see Figure 16.15) or escape rhythm (see Figure 17.1);
- premature complexes in the case of atrial flutter with variable conduction, even in atrial fibrillation;
- premature complexes due to sinus arrhythmia (see Figure 17.7).

Pause analysis

The presence of a pause is generally a result of a passive rhythm (second-degree or transient advanced sinoatrial or AV block, or sudden depression of the sinus node automatism). In children and athletes, pauses are occasionally caused by a marked physiologic sinus arrhythmia (see Figure 17.7) and excessive vagal tone.

Rarely, pauses are caused by an active rhythm, such as a blocked supraventricular extrasystole (see Figures 17.8 and 18.5), or even a concealed junctional extrasystole that is not conducted to the atria or the ventricles yet precludes the conduction of the next sinus P wave.

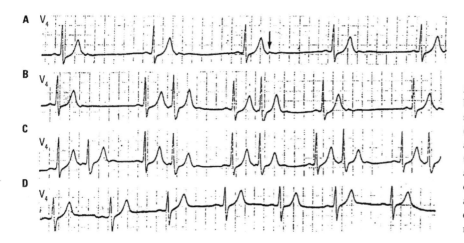

Figure 18.5 (A) Significant sinus bradycardia (30 bpm) featuring small sharp and short waves after the T wave (arrow), corresponding to concealed atrial extrasystoles, very different from the smooth and longer U wave. In (B) and (C), the same extrasystoles are observed after being conducted. After administration of propafenone (D), the extrasystoles disappeared and the heart rate increased.

Delayed complex analysis

Late QRS complexes are usually escape complexes (see Figure 17.1B), which may be narrow or wide (aberrant phase 4 junctional escape complexes or ventricular escape complexes).

They may also be sinus complexes, as a result of a sudden decrease in sinus automatism with delayed normal P wave. Sometimes, delayed sinus complexes occur after a sinoatrial or second- or third-degree AV block (see Figures 17.9 and 17.10), or after a tachyarrhythmia episode that may be followed by a long pause ("brady-tachy" syndrome), after which a sinus P wave or an escape complex occurs (see Figure 15.28). To be sure that the delayed complex is of sinus origin, the preceding P wave should be conducted to the ventricles (PR interval ≥ 120 ms). Often, the sinus P wave occurs simultaneously with the escape complex. This diagnosis is made because the PR interval is ≤ 120 ms, or the QRS complex overlaps the P wave (coincident complex) (see Figure 17.1A).

Analysis of the P wave, the QRS complexes, and the ST-T of variable morphology (Figures 18.6–18.9 and Table 18.1)

Morphology changes in the same tracing frequently affect QRS complexes, although occasionally the P wave and ST/T segment may also display changes.

QRS complexes of variable morphology

• **Fusion QRS complexes** occur when the ventricles are depolarized partially by the sinus (atrial) impulse and partially by the ventricular impulse (see Bayés de Luna and Baranchuk 2017).

• QRS complexes with **different degrees of ventricular fusion** are particularly observed in relatively slow ventricular tachycardia (see Figure 16.15), accelerated idioventricular rhythm (see Figure 16.21), or in ventricular extrasystoles in the PR interval (see Figure 18.6). Different degrees of fusion may also be found in parasystolic rhythms (see Figure 16.2).

• **Capture complexes** may also be considered to have a variable morphology because they are different of basal rhythm (Figure 16.15). They have already been discussed when referring to premature complex analysis (see Premature complex analysis, above).

• Rare cases of **Wenckebach-type bundle branch block** QRS complexes of variable morphology may also appear (see Figure 18.9).

• Sometimes, QRS complexes with variable morphology are observed **in the precordial leads V2–V5 due to respiratory changes**. A clear example of this is when a QS complex **in lead III turns into qR with a deep breath (positional change)** (Figure 18.6), which rules out that the Q wave is due to necrosis.

• QRS complexes with variable morphology also include the various types of **electric alternans of the QRS complex** that may be seen in sinus rhythm and in different arrhythmias (AVRT, bidirectional ventricular tachycardia, and Figure 18.7). Table 18.1 shows the most frequent situations in which alternating QRS/ST-T are seen (Bayés de Luna and Baranchuk 2017).

ST-T with variable morphology

ST-T morphology changes may be irrelevant when associated with QRS complex morphology changes during deep breathing (for instance, in lead III (Figure 18.6)). In this case, changes do not show alternans but a cyclical pattern related to respiration.

When evident ST-T electrical alternans are observed, as in the case of important acute ischemia (Figure 18.7B) in the presence of electrolyte and/or serious metabolic disorders (Figure 18.7D), as well as in the long QT syndrome (Figure 18.7C), they constitute a marker for malignant arrhythmias and sudden death (see Chapter 21, Long QT syndrome).

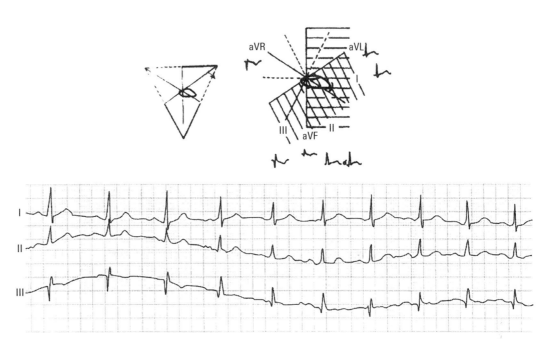

Figure 18.6 QRS–T changes during deep breathing in III (Qr turns into qR).

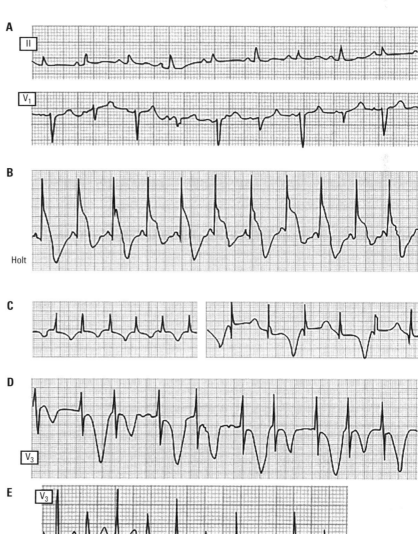

Figure 18.7 Typical examples of electrical alternans (Table 18.1). (A) QRS alternans in a patient with pericardial tamponade. (B) ST/T alternans in Prinzmetal angina. (C) Repolarization alternans in a congenital long QT syndrome. (D) Repolarization alternans in significant electrolytic imbalance in a patient with atrial fibrillation. (E) QRS alternans during a reentrant atrioventricular junctional tachycardia involving an accessory pathway (see also Figure 16.27).

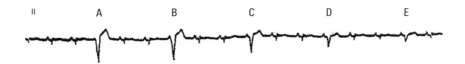

Figure 18.8 Late trigeminal premature ventricular complexes (PVCs) occurring in the PR interval, and showing progressive fusion degrees from C to E.

Table 18.1 Most frequent causes of QRS–T alternans

QRS alternans	ST-T alternans

• Cardiac tamponade
• Presence of AVNRT (Figure 15.12)
• Bidirectional VT (Figure 16.27)
• False alternans:
  • Related to breathing (in precordial leads)
  • Bundle branch block or WPW 2 × 1
  • Late bigeminal PVC. QRS complexes in the PR interval
	• Serious hyperacute ischemia
	• Long QT syndrome
	• Electrolyte imbalance

AVNRT: atrioventricular nodal reentry tachycardia; PVC: premature ventricular complex; WPW: Wolff–Parkinson–White.

P waves with variable morphology

In some instances, P waves with variable morphology may be caused by different degrees of atrial fusion, as in the case of atrial parasystole (see Figure 15.2), or when late junctional extrasystoles are present (see Figure 15.20). If these are bigeminal, they may originate an evident alternans of the P wave.

Various changes in P wave morphology due to other causes may also be found in the same ECG tracing (wandering sinus pacemaker, respiratory movements, artifacts, aberrant atrial conduction, and so on, see Figures 9.28 and 9.32).

Repetitive arrhythmia analysis: bigeminal rhythm

Occasionally, the heart rhythm shows an irregular pattern over time (alloarrhythmia). If short and long RR alternate, we refer to this as bigeminal rhythm. On rare occasions, the sequences of repetitive arrhythmia are due to trigeminal or quadrigeminal rhythms (for instance, two or three normal QRS complexes followed by a third or fourth premature complex). The latter are generally explained by the same mechanisms accounting for bigeminal rhythm, which will be described in the following paragraphs (Antiperovitch *et al.* 2019).

Figure 18.10 shows different examples of bigeminal QRS complex, with repetitive short and long RR intervals. This figure illustrates the more common mechanisms, explaining the different causes of bigeminal rhythm that may be

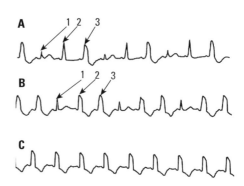

Figure 18.9 Lead I in a patient with different degrees of left bundle branch block. (A) Progressive left bundle branch block—Wenckebach type (1–3). (B) Intermittent left bundle branch block (2 and 3). (C) Fixed left bundle branch block (Modified from Brenes *et al.* 2006).

determined by the surface ECG. We also encourage the reader to make the correct diagnosis in the last tracing (k) marked with a question mark (see legend of the Figure 18.10), and to practice by placing the corresponding Lewis diagram (Chapter 14, Preliminary considerations) for each example.

We will now briefly comment on the key signs used for obtaining the correct diagnosis in the different examples:

A. Atrial bigeminy: the atrial bigeminal wave (P′) is different from the sinus P wave, as is the case when atrial premature systoles are observed.

B. Ventricular bigeminy: the bigeminal QRS complexes are wide and show a fixed coupling interval.

C. Concealed atrial trigeminy: the T wave of the bigeminal complexes are slightly different from the T wave of the sinus rhythm due to the presence of a concealed P′ wave.

D. Escape–ventricular extrasystole sequence. The first QRS complex of the bigeminal rhythm is not preceded by a P wave.

E. 3 : 2 sinoatrial block: This should be differentiated (differential diagnosis) from parasinus atrial bigeminy (see Figure 17.10).

F. 2 : 1 atrial flutter alternating with 4 : 1 atrial flutter.

G. Sinus rhythm with second-degree Wenckebach-type AV block with 3 : 2 AV conduction.

H. AV junctional ectopic rhythm with a 3 : 2 Wenckebach-type AV block. There is no evident atrial activation. The patient also showed an ECG with regular junctional tachycardia with a relatively slow rate (110 bpm).

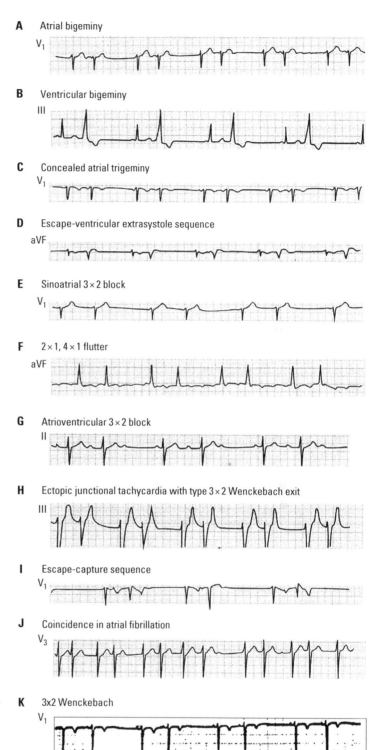

A   Atrial bigeminy

B   Ventricular bigeminy

C   Concealed atrial trigeminy

D   Escape-ventricular extrasystole sequence

E   Sinoatrial 3 × 2 block

F   2 × 1, 4 × 1 flutter

G   Atrioventricular 3 × 2 block

H   Ectopic junctional tachycardia with type 3 × 2 Wenckebach exit

I   Escape-capture sequence

J   Coincidence in atrial fibrillation

K   3x2 Wenckebach

Figure 18.10 Different types of bigeminal QRS complexes. The different mechanisms are shown within the figure, except for the case K, which corresponds to a concealed atrial trigeminy (similar to case C). Note that in K, the second T wave of each QRS bigeminy is less deep, because these is hidden a positive P wave. Other parts of the ECGs tracing show atrial trigeminy. This subtle T wave alteration led us to reach the correct diagnosis.

I. Escape–capture sequence with different degrees of aberrant conduction of sinus complex (captures).

J. Atrial fibrillation may occasionally and randomly show apparently bigeminal complexes.

K. We expect the reader to detect the subtle T wave morphology changes in the bigeminal rhythm, a key factor in determining that it is caused by concealed atrial trigeminy (see C).

The most frequent causes of bigeminal rhythm are supraventricular or ventricular extrasystoles. However, as already discussed, there are many other active and passive arrhythmias that may initiate bigeminal rhythm (Figure 18.10). Obviously, sometimes the diagnosis is uncertain. In this case, it is advisable to review the previous chapters and to use Lewis diagrams to determine the type of arrhythmia. We advocate to maintain alive the use of the Lewis diagram as an easy, inexpensive tool to understand electrophysiological mechanisms of arrhythmias (Antiperovitch *et al.* 2019). If needed, other complementary techniques should be used (complementary leads, Lewis lead (Bakker *et al.* 2009), atrial wave amplification, T wave filtering (Goldwasser *et al.* 2011), intracavitary ECG, etc.).

Differential diagnosis between several arrhythmias in special situations

We present a review of some of the ECG clues in some situations where reaching a correct diagnosis is somewhat difficult.

Sinus rhythm misdiagnosed as ectopic rhythm

The patient may show moderate tachycardia (100–130 bpm) with no visible atrial activity. In this situation, it is useful to perform maneuvers that lead to rhythm changes (for instance, deep breathing) to assess whether the P wave appears, in which case it is probably sinus rhythm (see Figure 15.5). Occasionally, atrial rhythms may feature subtle changes with maneuvers, but the P wave polarity will usually allow for distinction between sinus and ectopic atrial tachycardia.

Very rarely, misdiagnosis is due to the fact that although a sinus rhythm is present, the P wave is not visible (concealed sinus rhythm). This is the result of a significant atrial fibrosis generating low voltages that cannot be measured by surface ECG, although they may be detected through wave amplification techniques (Bayés de Luna *et al.* 1978) (see Figure 15.37).

Sinoventricular conduction is a rare type of cardiac activation where the P wave is sometimes not visible because the sinus rhythm is conducted to the AV node and ventricles with delayed atrial activation that even may be hidden in the QRS complex (Bellet 1969). This type of conduction usually occurs in certain cases of electrolyte disorders, such as hyperkalemia, and accounts for some of the rare cases of sinus rhythm with short PR interval or non-visible P wave (Figure 23.20). This is due (see Figure 7.2) to delayed atrial activation, which may explain a short PR interval, and may be confused with a pre-excitation with short PR interval (see Figure 7.2B), or even within AV junctional rhythm when the delayed P wave is hidden within the QRS (see Figure 7.2C).

Differential diagnosis between 2 : 1 flutter and sinus rhythm

This confusion may occur when the flutter rate is slow (around 200 bpm) and, therefore, the rate of QRS complex is around 100 bpm. In this situation, one "f" wave may be hidden within the QRS complex or it may not be appropriately observed, whereas the other "f" wave may be mistaken for a sinus P wave (see Figure 15.14). For a correct diagnosis to be reached, it is important: (i) to be aware of this possibility (i.e. that flutter waves may be concealed in the QRS complex), and (ii) to assess whether the patient has a fixed heart rate over time, which is not the case in sinus rhythm, and this therefore supports a diagnosis of 2 : 1 flutter.

Meanwhile, as previously discussed, it is often impossible to distinguish between a slow atypical flutter and a fast monomorphic atrial tachycardia (see Chapter 15, Atrial flutter). From a clinical point of view, the latter is not a relevant problem, because both may be considered the same arrhythmia, in contrast with the case where 2 : 1 flutter is misdiagnosed as sinus rhythm, because this mistake may lead to incorrect diagnosis and management.

Aberrant supraventricular tachycardia misdiagnosed as ventricular tachycardia

In this situation, regardless of the diagnostic criteria already discussed (see Chapter 16, Classical monomorphic ventricular tachycardias, Table 16.4 and Figure 16.16), when assessing a wide QRS complex tachycardia it is useful to remember the following:
* In the presence of heart disease, and above all in ischemic heart disease, the arrhythmia is most likely of ventricular origin (Baranchuk and Nadeau-Rauther 2016).
* Ventricular tachycardias may show slightly irregular patterns, especially at onset. However, when a significant rhythm irregularity is observed, and narrow QRS complexes are present and do not meet the criteria for captures (in ventricular tachycardia, the narrow sinus captures are always premature) because they appear early or late, it is most likely atrial fibrillation in a patient with Wolff–Parkinson–White (WPW) syndrome, rather than ventricular tachycardia (see Figure 15.31).

The following supraventricular tachycardias may have wide QRS complexes:
* atrial 2 : 1 flutter in patients with WPW syndrome (see Figure 15.41B);
* reentrant tachycardia with anterograde conduction over an accessory pathway (see Figure 16.18);
* reentrant junctional tachycardia with anterograde conduction through an atypical preexcitation tract (see Figure 15.16);
* typical supraventricular tachycardia or flutter pre-existent with bundle branch block (see Figure 16.19).
* pacemaker-mediated tachycardia.

Fast paroxysmal supraventricular rhythm with QRS complex <0.12 sec and r′ in lead V1

If in an ECG tracing atrial waves are not seen, it is most likely that the QRS pattern in V1 with terminal r′, which is sometimes very tiny, is not due to incomplete right bundle branch block (r′). The cause of terminal QRS complex deflection is a P' wave due to retrograde VA conduction of a junctional reciprocating tachycardia of AVNRT type (see Figures 15.11–15.13).

If an atrial wave is observed preceding the QRS complex, and there is also an r', the latter may be the second F wave of a 2 : 1 flutter that is attached to the end of the QRS complex. The cadence of the atrial waves (F waves) should be assessed with a compass to prove that the apparent r' wave in lead V1 is, in fact, an F wave (Figure 15.33).

Pause due to active arrhythmia

Occasionally, concealed atrial extrasystoles initiate a pause that is not caused by a passive arrhythmia, but rather an active one. In some cases, when concealed bigeminy is present, a slow regular rhythm exists. The key in diagnosis is to demonstrate the presence of the ectopic P wave at the end of the T wave as a short and sharp low-voltage wave (Figure 18.5), or a slurring in the ascendant–descendent slope of the T wave (see Figure 17.8).

If this cannot be suggested by means of a surface ECG, other techniques may be used to assess whether an ectopic P wave is actually concealed in the T wave: wave amplification, faster registration speed (see Figure 15.37), T wave filtering (Chapter 25), and use of special leads (see Chapter 25).

References

Antiperovitch P, Bayés de Luna A, Nunes de Alencar J, *et al.* Old teaching tools should not be forgotten: the value of the Lewis ladder diagram in understanding bigeminal rhythms. *Ann Noninvasive Electrocardiol* 2019;24(5):e12685.

Bakker AL, Nijkerk G, Groenemeijer BE, *et al.* The Lewis lead. Making recognition of P waves easy during wide QRS complex tachycardia. *Circulation* 2009;119:92.

Baranchuk A, Nadeau-Rauther C. Electrocardiography in Practice: What to do. I-Book. https://books.apple.com/ca/book/electrocardiography-in-practice-what-to-do/id1120119530, 2016.

Baranchuk A, Dubner S, Steinberg J. www.ecguniversity.org, 2018 (accessed Nov 2019).

Bayés de Luna A, Baranchuk A. *Clinical Arrhythmology*, 2nd edn. Wiley-Blackwell, 2017.

Bayés de Luna A, Boada FX, Casellas A, *et al.* Concealed atrial electrical activity. *J Electrocardiol* 1978;11:301.

Bayés de Luna A, Fort de Ribot R, Trilla E, *et al.* Electrocardiographic and vectorcardiographic study of interatrial conduction disturbances with left atrial retrograde activation. *J Electrocardiol* 1985;18:1.

Bellet S. *Clinical Disorders of the Heart Beat.* Lea & Febiger, 1969.

Brenes C, Brenes-Pareira C, Castellanos A. Wneckebach phenomenon at the left bundle branch. *Clin Cardiol* 2006;29:226.

Brugada P, Brugada J, Mont L, *et al.* A new approach to the differential diagnosis of a regular tachycardia with a wide QRS complex. *Circulation* 1991;83:1649.

Goldwasser D, Bayés de Luna A, Serra G, *et al.* A new method of filtering T waves to detect hidden P waves in electrocardiogram signals. *Europace* 2011;13:1028.

Kistler PM, Roberts-Thomson KC, Haqqani HM, *et al.* P-wave morphology in focal atrial tachycardia: development of an algorithm to predict the anatomic site of origin. *J Am Coll Cardiol* 2006;48:2010.

Part 5
The Clinical Usefulness
of Electrocardiography

Chapter 19
The Diagnostic Value
of Electrocardiographic Abnormalities

Introduction

The assessment of 12-lead ECGs requires the detection of any abnormalities. If present, the diagnostic value and possible clinical implications of these abnormalities must be determined.

Electrocardiography plays a key role in the diagnosis of arrhythmias, atrial and ventricular conduction abnormalities, pre-excitation, and many inherited heart diseases. In such cases, a diagnosis can be made reliably using the ECG alone. **With regard to other conditions, such as chamber enlargement and the different stages of ischemic heart disease, the ECG is not always sufficient to make the diagnosis** and, on certain occasions, as has already been commented on, its capacity for diagnosis is lower with respect to other techniques (as occurs with echocardiography and chamber enlargement; see Chapter 10). Furthermore, ECG abnormalities used as diagnostic criteria for chamber enlargement (Chapters 9 and 10) or ischemia (Chapters 13 and 20) can occasionally be explained by other causes. Therefore, it is necessary to know the sensitivity, specificity, and predictive value of the different ECG diagnostic criteria in each situation, in order to understand them correctly (Chapter 8).

In the first group of diseases (i.e. those in which electrocardiography represents the main diagnostic technique), the ECG is the "gold standard" for comparisons. When the diagnosis is incorrect, the physician interpreting the ECG tracing is usually to blame because it demonstrates a poor understanding of ECG tracing or a lack of knowledge of the criteria considered necessary to establish such a diagnosis. For example, a delta wave and/or a short PR interval may be overlooked because the physician does not know that it is pivotal for the diagnosis of a pre-excitation. **In the second group of diseases**, the physician interpreting the ECG tracing can suspect the diagnosis or even assure or confirm it on certain occasions, can even assure it, especially when data for clinical

correlation are available. An example of this type of disease is acute myocardial infarction.

It is possible to diagnose certain diseases (e.g. advanced right bundle branch block) just by looking at the ECG. At other times, it may be suspected for certain conditions, such as right ventricular enlargement. Some ECG patterns **may also indicate** a marker for a serious process or a risk of sudden death (e.g. channelopathies and some cardiomyopathies, etc.). Often, **data related to the patient's clinical status are crucial to the interpretation** of the importance of an ECG abnormality. For example, in the case of the rsR' morphology in V1, the importance of the clinical setting (bedside diagnosis) is illustrated by the following examples:

- A pattern of advanced right bundle branch block (QRS≥0.12 sec) together with tachycardia and dyspnea that appear suddenly in a bedridden patient suggest a significant pulmonary embolism. However, a similar ECG pattern with no associated abnormal clinical data in an elderly person is not a marker for poor prognosis.
- An rsR' morphology recorded in V1 in a child or adolescent with a QRS complex duration of less than 0.12 sec and normal repolarization and no change in heart rate during respiration must lead to suggestion of an atrial septal defect. The auscultation of a fixed double second cardiac sound and the presence of increased pulmonary flow in the chest X-ray support the diagnosis, which can be confirmed by echocardiography.

In the following sections, we will explain how a thorough study of the ECG waves and intervals, as well as knowing their normal values, allows not only for the identification of whether an ECG tracing is within a normal range but also for the diagnosis of an ECG abnormality and understanding of its clinical implications. Some of the ECG patterns observed could correspond to normal variants or a pathological condition, and it is generally necessary to have clinical data or other techniques available to clarify this doubt. SI, SII, SIII morphology is a good example of this situation (see Figure 10.13).

Clinical Electrocardiography: A Textbook, Fifth Edition. Antoni Bayés de Luna, Miquel Fiol-Sala, Antoni Bayés-Genís, and Adrián Baranchuk.
© 2022 John Wiley & Sons Ltd. Published 2022 by John Wiley & Sons Ltd.

We would like to emphasize that some aspects of this chapter have already been discussed in Chapter 7, where the normal value of the different parameters is discussed extensively. Here, we describe especially the abnormalities of these parameters.

We will subsequently study the different cardiac intervals (PR and QT) and waves' (P, QRS, ST–T–U) abnormalities. The reader should refer to Chapter 7 in order to review the normal features of all these parameters. We will also list the characteristics of sinus rhythm and the main cardiac rhythm abnormalities.

Abnormal PR interval

Under normal conditions, the PR interval can shorten with sympathetic overdrive and lengthen with vagal overdrive (see Chapter 7). Normal adult values are 0.12–0.20 sec. The upper limit is shorter in children (0.18 sec) and longer in the elderly (0.22 sec).

A **long PR interval** is secondary to a first- or second-degree AV block (see Chapter 17) while a **short PR interval** is observed in various atrial arrhythmias, such as monomorphic atrial tachycardia (see Chapter 15), in the pre-excitation syndromes (see Chapter 12) and, in rare cases of sinoventricular conduction (Bellet and Jedlicka 1969) (see Chapter 18, Figure 7.2). At times, a pre-excitation syndrome presents a borderline PR interval and the delta wave is not very evident. These two facts

may confuse the ECG pattern of pre-excitation with right bundle branch block, right ventricle hypertrophy, or ischemic heart disease (Figure 19.1).

Abnormal QT interval

The clinical usefulness of the abnormal QT intervals (short QT interval and long QT interval) and the existence of abnormal differences in the QT interval assessment in different surface ECG leads (QT interval dispersion) will be examined. Normal QT interval characteristics have been shown in Chapter 7, and how the interval should be measured is also discussed. We will refer here to the heart rate-corrected QT interval (QTc) (see Figures 7.8 and 7.9. and Table 7.3), although an excessively long non-corrected QT interval, > 440–460 ms and, especially when > 500 ms, is always pathological. Occasionally, this measurement is quite difficult because the T wave is flattened and/or it is not absolutely clear whether a U wave is present or not. There are **inherited and acquired causes of short and long QT** that will be discussed in depth in Chapters 21 and 24.

Short QTc interval
Some rare cases of very short QT interval not related to any known etiology and in all different heart rates in families with a history of sudden death have also been described as newly inherited heart disease (**short QT**

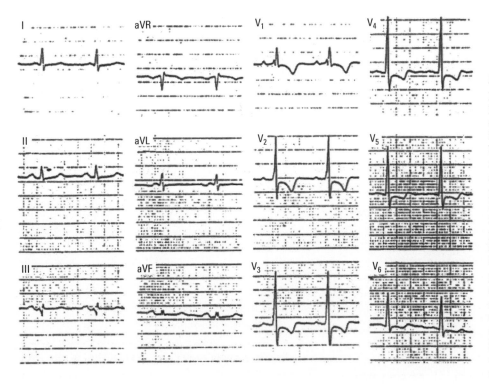

Figure 19.1 A 55-year-old patient with a history of paroxysmal tachycardia episodes and no chest pain. The ECG was interpreted for years as right bundle branch block plus myocardial ischemia (q in lead III and ST depression in several precordial leads). However, the lack of any history suggestive of ischemic heart disease, the presence of ECGs for more than 20 years, and the borderline PR interval raised the suspicion of pre-excitation (see the morphology of V2 with a possible delta wave). A definite diagnosis of Wolff–Parkinson–White was obtained during an atrial fibrillation episode and was confirmed by electrophysiologic studies.

interval syndrome) (Gaita *et al.* 2003). Also, a diagnostic score has been published (Gollob *et al.* 2011) (see Table 21.7 and Figure 21.13).

A somewhat short QT interval can occasionally be seen in cases of **early repolarization (ER)**, a pattern considered benign but that in some cases may have a bad prognostic significance due to the association with idiopathic ventricular fibrillation (Haïsaguerre *et al.* 2008) (see Figure 24.8). In fact, a high prevalence of early repolarization in the presence of short QT syndrome has been recently reported (see Chapter 24).

An acquired short QT interval is found as a consequence of **digitalis** administration; this effect begins during the therapeutic range, but it is clearly more evident in digitalis toxicity (Figures 23.14 and 23.15). In some ionic imbalances such as **hypercalcemia and hyperkalemia,** a short QT interval is observed (Figure 23.22).

A short QT interval in Holter recordings could be, like the long QT interval, a marker of poor prognosis (Algra *et al.* 1993).

Long QTc interval

A long QTc interval occurring in the setting of an inherited long QT syndrome is a marker of sudden death secondary to malignant ventricular arrhythmias (**Jervell and Lange-Nielsen syndrome and Romano–Ward syndrome**) (Zareba *et al.* 1998; Schwartz *et al.* 2001; Moss *et al.* 1995). This is discussed in Chapter 21 (Inherited heart diseases).

Acquired long QT may be seen in **post-infarction patients** (Schwartz and Wolff 1978), and during stroke and **ionic abnormalities**. The latter sometimes occurs in the presence of severe conditions, such as **sepsis, toxic or metabolic shock**, and may trigger ventricular fibrillation (see Figure 24.7). The factors that predispose to prolongation of the QT interval are listed in Table 19.1.

A significant amount of evidence has been reported showing that **repolarization can be lengthened by the action of a variety of drugs**. Table 19.2 shows the different types of drugs associated with lengthening the QT interval and the potential risk of arrhythmias (for more

Table 19.1 Predisposing factors for QT interval prolongation

- Heart disease: Ischemic heart disease, heart failure, etc.
- ECG alterations: baseline prolonged QT, abnormal U wave, T wave alternans, deep and negative T wave, significant bradycardia
- Acute neurological accidents
- Ionic and metabolic alterations: diabetes, anorexia, hypoglycemia, hypothyroidism, obesity
- Septic shock
- Female sex
- Advanced age
- Hypothermia
- Intoxications

Table 19.2 Drugs associated with QT prolongation and potential arrhythmogenic risk (for more details, please consult www. qtdrugs.org)

Antiarrhythmic drugs:	Generally, types I and III. Also, recently studied drugs (azimilide, ibutilide). Propafenone is probably less risky, in the absence of heart failure. A drug with less antiarrhythmic effect, despite the fact it significantly prolongs the QT interval, is amiodarone and dronadorone (see text) Type II and IV drugs are safe
Macrolide antibiotics:	Azithromycin, clarithromycin, erythromycin
Fluoroquinolones:	Ciprofloxacin, levofloxacin, etc.
Antidepressants:	Amitriptyline, disopyramide, fluoxetine, imipramine, paroxetine, etc.
Antipsychotics:	Haloperidol, risperidone
Antihistaminics:	Terfenadine (withdrawn)
Gastrointestinal tract:	Cisapride (withdrawn)

information consult www.qtdrugs.org). Recently, health agencies (FDA, EMEA) have imposed strict control of new drugs affecting repolarization because even a relatively slight lengthening of the QT interval due to the use of these drugs **can be related to the development of torsades de pointes and sudden death** (Sarapa *et al.* 2004). Among these drugs, class I antiarrhythmic drugs as well as several drugs with different therapeutic properties, such as terfenadine and cisapride, are included (see Chapter 24). On the other hand, the long QTc interval that is observed following the administration of amiodarone **can be associated with a beneficial antiarrhythmic effect** (Surawicz *et al.* 1984). This is most likely explained by the fact that, even when repolarization is lengthened, this lengthening is homogeneous, producing less refractory period dispersion and a lower risk for reentry arrhythmias.

QT interval dispersion

QT dispersion represents the difference in QT measurement in different leads. In general, there is not much difference in healthy individuals (<50 ms) (**low QT dispersion**). Significant differences in length have been reported in patients with congenital long QT interval (>80–100 ms) and, to a lesser extent, in post-infarction patients and those with other heart diseases (Day *et al.* 1990).

Certain doubts still remain regarding the **electrophysiological explanation of QT interval dispersion.** The authors who demonstrated in experimental studies that differences in the QT interval length could be explained by a **local effect**, meaning differences in the duration of repolarization in different areas in the heart (Zabel *et al.* 1995), have not found QT interval length to be useful in clinical practice, even when using the best parameters to measure QT dispersion (Zabel *et al.* 1998). Meanwhile, the Rotterdam group considers that the QT interval dispersion is not secondary to repolarization duration heterogeneity, but rather a **projection effect**, which refers to the impossibility of measuring the end of repolarization in some leads because the final part of the T wave loop, especially when round, does not generate measurable vectors since its projection on such leads is null (Kors *et al.* 1999). The group has found that the QT interval and the QT interval dispersion measurement are good clinical parameters to stratify prognosis (De Bruyne *et al.* 1999).

These discrepancies regarding the mechanism accounting for QT interval dispersion are an added disadvantage in assessing its usefulness. Certainly, the latter is limited since the methodological problems inherent in the way that QT dispersion is measured, the type of equipment that should be used (for greater accuracy, all 12 leads should be assessed), and the normal limits are not still not known.

To summarize, QT interval dispersion is clearly found in some heart diseases, such as inherited long QT syndrome, where differences in measurements >80–100 ms are often seen. However, some doubts still remain due to the methodological limitations regarding clinical usefulness when measurements are just slightly above the normal values, as frequently occurs in postinfarction patients and in those with heart failure. Consequently, the **measurement of the QT interval dispersion has not been systematically accepted in acquired heart disease for clinical practice.** Exceptionally, it is sometimes used in clinical pharmacology to assess the potential proarrhythmic effect of some drugs that alter repolarization.

Abnormal P wave

In Chapter 7, we have described the different parameters of P wave, named P wave indices by Magnani (duration, morphology, axis, voltage and area, see Figure 7.3), and in Chapter 9 we have commented all types of P wave abnormalities, especially all related with atrial enlargement and atrial blocks.

Now, we will make some comments in different aspects of abnormal P wave, especially abnormal P wave axis and P wave morphology.

Abnormal P wave axis (ÂP)

With regard to the ÂP, verticalization of the heart shifts the ÂP to the right, no more than +90° (flattened P wave in I), while horizontalization shifts it to the left. Under pathological conditions, such as right atrial enlargement in adults (cor pulmonale, valvular heart diseases with right-side compromise), ÂP is usually deviated to the right (**P pulmonale**), although no further than +90° (see Chapter 9). In addition, it is relatively common in patients with congenital heart diseases with right-sided involvement that the ÂP is somewhat deviated to the left, just as it is in cases with left atrial enlargement (**P congenitale**).

ÂP abnormal is a very good parameter (P wave indices), jointly P wave duration and advanced interatrial block to study the risk of future atrial fibrillation and stroke (P wave score) (Alexander *et al.* 2019) (see Chapter 9).

Abnormalities of the morphology and voltage of the P wave

With regard to P wave morphology and voltage, the following must be highlighted:

• A P wave taller than 2.5 mm or wider than 0.10 sec must be considered pathological (see Figure 7.5). However, P wave height can increase in normal individuals with sympathetic overdrive and hypoxia, or can even be modified clinically with respiration. It can be hidden or at least masked within the ST segment during exercise.

• The sinus node P wave should never be negative in lead I. If present, it can be explained by three mechanisms: artifacts (electrodes interchange in the arms); congenital heart disease with atrial inversion, with the right atrium on the left side, such as in dextrocardia; or an ectopic rhythm, the most frequent explanation.

• A positive or ± but predominantly positive P wave is seen in V1 under normal conditions. In Chapters 7 and 9, we have discussed all related with the P terminal force in V1 (PtfV1), and there we explain the doubts about the value of this pattern to diagnose LAE. Only insist in the need that to evaluate the PtfV1 we have to be sure that the electrode in V1 is well located in 4th ICS. Finally, just to say that the P wave may be transiently pathological in V1 (predominance of the negative component) in the presence of acute pulmonary edema (see Figure 9.13).

• A ± P wave in II, III, and aVF is always pathological. An advanced interatrial conduction block with left atrial retrograde activation is the underlying explanation (Bayés de Luna *et al.* 1985, 1988) (see Figure 9.18). We have demonstrated that the presence of this type of interatrial block is quite frequently a marker of future supraventricular arrhythmias, especially atrial fibrillation and non-common atrial flutter (Bayés de Luna *et al.* 1988), and thus is considered a new arrhythmic syndrome (Braunwald 2012) (Daubert *et al.* 1996) that after Conde and Baranchuk (2014), and Bacharova and Wagner (2015) has been named Bayés syndrome (Baranchuk 2017). The Bayés syndrome has been also associated to stroke, dementia, and increased mortality (Bayés de Luna *et al.* 2020) (see more information in Chapter 9, about that and all the aspects related with P wave indices).

• It should be remembered that the atrial repolarization wave (Ta) is usually masked by the QRS complex. However, it can be visualized both in normal (sympathetic) and pathological (e.g. atrial infarction, pericarditis, long PR interval) situations (see Chapter 9).

Abnormal QRS complex

Characteristics of the normal QRS complex in terms of voltage and morphology, as well as the QRS complex normal spatial orientation (ÂQRS) have been described in Chapter 7. The clinical usefulness of some of these QRS complex abnormalities will be discussed.

Abnormal ÂQRS

In most cases, normal ÂQRS ranges between 0° and +90°, but it can be found anywhere between –30° and +100° in quite horizontalized or verticalized hearts, respectively (see Chapter 7).

Right-deviated ÂQRS

An ÂQRS very deviated to the right in patients with no heart disease or with no vertical heart could be explained by the presence of fewer than normal Purkinje fibers in the left ventricular apical (anteroseptal) area. This would cause a depolarization delay in this area, with the subsequent ÂQRS deviation to the right. This hypothesis cannot be easily demonstrated. For that, it would be necessary to perform necropsy studies in healthy subjects without the vertical heart dying accidentally, and in patients, in whom a previous ECG recording with an ÂQRS very deviated to the right was available.

The pathological situations in which an ÂQRS evidently deviated to the right is found are the following:
• right ventricular enlargement either isolated (see Figure 10.3) or associated with right or left bundle branch block (see Chapters 10 and 11);
• inferoposterior hemiblock either isolated (Figure 11.42) or associated with right bundle branch block (RBBB) (see Chapter 11);
• some types of Wolff–Parkinson–White (WPW) syndrome (see Figure 12.8);
• some infarctions usually of the anterior and/or lateral wall (see Figures 13.70 and 13.94);
• a pacemaker located in the left ventricle (see Chapter 17).

Left-deviated ÂQRS

ÂQRS hyperdeviation to the left can reach –30° due to a simple position change (cardiac horizontalization) or left ventricular enlargement. In theory, this could also occur in a healthy subject due to a mechanism similar to that used to explain ÂQRS deviation to the right in the absence of heart disease or cardiac verticalization (i.e. fewer Purkinje fibers in the left ventricle anterolateral area). In this case, in the absence of heart disease, a depolarization delay in this area would be generated, thereby shifting the QRS axis to the left.

The pathological situations that could present with a left ÂQRS deviation greater than –30° are the following:
• superoanterior hemiblock (SAH) either isolated (see Figure 11.35) or associated with RBBB (see Chapter 11);

• some inferior infarctions, with or without associated superoanterior hemiblock (see Figure 13.99);
• some cases of type III WPW syndrome (see Figures 12.4 and 12.5);
• a pacemaker located in the right ventricular apex (see Chapter 17);
• advanced left bundle branch block with delayed transeptal depolarization in the superoanterior area (due to associated right peripheral block or SAH) (see Figure 11.29).

The most difficult challenge is to differentiate between a normal variant and a pathological situation in cases with a "borderline" ÂQRS deviation to the left (close to –30°). These cases can be explained both by a partial superoanterior hemiblock or left ventricular enlargement, as well as a normal variant. The evolution from a normal ÂQRS close to –30° to an ÂQRS very deviated to the left (–60°) would confirm that a "borderline" ÂQRS is the expression of a partial SAH (see Figure 11.38).

Indeterminated ÂQRS

The ÂQRS cannot be measured on certain occasions. This occurs in the presence of an SI, SII, SIII morphology, in which an evident S wave with S≥R in all three frontal plane bipolar leads is observed (see Figures 11.19). Although the overall ÂQRS cannot be measured, the direction of the electrical forces in the first and second parts of the QRS complex can be obtained. This type of recording can be found in three situations:
• normal variant with the cardiac apex of the heart directed backward or with fewer Purkinje fibers in the basal area of the right ventricle (Bayés de Luna *et al.* 1987) (see Figure 7.27);
• right ventricular enlargement (see Figure 10.13);
• peripheral block of the right bundle branch (see Figure 11.19).

Absolute differentiations between these three possibilities using a surface ECG recording alone are sometimes impossible (see Chapters 10 and 11). The presence of a pathological P wave and, of course, auscultation, physical examination, other complementary ECG techniques, and especially an echocardiogram along with other imaging techniques that allow us to detect an associated right-side pathology, may be useful (Bayés de Luna *et al.* 1987).

The utility of the ÂQRS–ÂT spatial angle

At the early days of ECG utilization, great importance was given to the angle between the depolarization (QRS complex) and repolarization (T wave) spatial orientation, the so-called "ventricular gradient" (Wilson *et al.* 1934). Recently, this concept has been revisited and the usefulness of the ÂQRS–ÂT spatial angle measurement (angle between ÂQRS and ÂT) and the analysis of T wave morphology loop as a prognosis predictor has been demonstrated both in the post-infarction setting (Zabel *et al.* 2000) and in the general population (Kardys *et al.* 2003) (see Chapter 3, Improving the capacity of the ECG).

Abnormal QRS complex duration and voltage
QRS voltage
Normal QRS voltage varies significantly, according to age and sex (see Tables 7.3–7.5). The normal upper range in different leads is difficult to determine, but QRS complexes ≥20 mm in I and II or ≥11 mm in aVL are rarely seen. However, QRS complexes of up to 25–30 mm or more can be seen in left precordial leads, especially in adolescents, with no left ventricular enlargement. It is also seen in some elderly subjects, mainly in very thin women. ECG criteria for ventricular enlargement according to the QRS complex voltage and its limitations are discussed in Chapter 10 (Tables 10.1–10.8).

Low QRS complex voltage
Abnormal low QRS voltage exists when the sum of QRS voltage in leads I, II, III of the frontal plane is lower than 15 mm, and in precordial leads if the amplitude of the largest QRS deflection is 8 mm or less.

Low voltage can be found in the absence of heart disease when a frontier factor (obesity, pleural effusion, pericarditis, emphysema, or myxedema, etc.) exists. It is frequently seen in patients with dilated cardiomyopathy in the frontal plane, but not in the horizontal plane and also in some cases of ischemic heart disease (see Chapters 13, 20, and 22).

In dilated cardiomyopathy, the QRS voltage in V3 is much higher in cases of idiopathic etiology than in cases of ischemic etiology (Bayés-Genís *et al.* 2003).

The QRS complex voltage is usually high in hypertrophic cardiomyopathy. However, the presence of a relatively low voltage has been described as a marker of heart failure in the long term (Ikeda *et al.* 1999) (see Figure 21.4).

High QRS voltage
QRS complex voltage is higher than the range considered normal in various heart diseases, especially in different types of ventricular enlargement (see Chapter 10). However, there are many factors that modify the QRS voltage, interfering with the diagnosis of left ventricular enlargement (see Chapter 10).

In addition, QRS complex voltages above the normal range are sometimes seen in apparently healthy individuals, especially in very lean individuals (see Chapter 10).

The following parameters may be considered probably abnormal:
• initial or terminal R wave in aVR greater than 3–4 mm;
• an R wave in aVL >11 mm;
• an R wave in aVF >20 mm.

The ECG criteria for high QRS voltage in frontal and horizontal plane leads are discussed in Chapter 10.

QRS duration
QRS complex duration in right precordial leads is usually, under normal conditions, slightly longer (0.01–0.02 s) than that of frontal plane leads. A ÂQRS complex duration ≥0.12 sec is always abnormal and is explained by significant intraventricular conduction blocks or pre-excitation. Ventricular enlargement may reach 0.12 sec if parietal or fascicular blocks are associated (see Chapters 10 and 11).

The intrinsicoid deflection time (IDT) (time from the beginning of QRS to the peak of R) is increased in some cases of ventricular enlargement and in ventricular blocks (see Chapters 10 and 11). However, some athletes and individuals presenting with vagal overdrive with a normal heart may exhibit an IDT in V5–V6 that is above normal.

Abnormal QRS complex morphology
Pathological Q wave
The characteristics of the normal "Q" wave in each lead are described in Chapter 7 (see QRS complex), and the identification of a pathological "Q" wave is explained in Chapter 13 (Table 13.7). Any pathological "Q" wave should be assessed taking into account the clinical setting. The first possibility to consider is a pathological Q wave secondary to ischemic heart disease. A lack of coronary symptoms does not imply the absence of ischemic heart disease; it should therefore be ruled out by the history taking and complementary techniques.

In the absence of ischemic heart disease, the presence of a pathological Q wave can be explained by one of the following causes (see Table 13.9):
• normal variants (thoracic anomalies, position changing, etc.); it is especially important to bear in mind that a deep "Q" wave can be recorded in lead III that even disappear with deep inspiration (see Figure 18.6) and that a QS morphology can often exist, especially in the elderly in V1 and even in V2 in the absence of evidence of underlying heart disease (see later and Chapter 7, Elderly people);
• right or left ventricular enlargement (hypertrophic cardiomyopathy (see Figure 10.24) or dilated or restrictive cardiomyopathy (see Figure 22.3)) and many other diseases with myocardial involvement (see Table 13.9);
• advanced or even partial left bundle branch block (QS in V1–V2) (see Chapter 11);
• WPW syndrome, etc. (see Chapter 12).

Morphologies with a significant or predominant R wave in V1 (R, R ≥ S, rsR′ (r′))
Normal and pathological conditions that can exhibit a predominant R wave or a r′ (R′) wave in V1 are shown in Table 10.3.

Pathological conditions include:
• right ventricular enlargement and biventricular enlargement (see Chapter 10);

- septal hypertrophy in cardiomyopathies (see Chapters 21 and 22);
- typical or atypical partial and advanced RBBB (see Chapter 11);
- some types of WPW syndrome (see Chapter 12);
- some type of Brugada pattern (see Chapter 21);
- lateral myocardial infarction with a predominant R wave in V1 (see Chapters 13 and 20);
- block of the middle fibers of the left bundle branch could probably explain some cases of RS morphology in V1–V2 especially if is transient (Chapter 11) (Pérez Riera *et al.* 2011). However, it may be possible that the same pattern may be explained by transient incomplete RBBB (Peñaloza *et al.* 1961) (see Chapter 11).

A rsr′ (R) or even predominant R wave in V1 could also be a normal variant.

An rSr′ morphology found in normal children usually exhibits the following characteristics: (i) a low-voltage initial r′ wave (exceptionally ≥8 mm), (ii) an r′ wave of <6 mm, and (iii) an rSr′ morphology modified with deep breathing (see Figure 7.40). In contrast, in most congenital heart diseases and in over half the cases with acquired heart disease, an rSr′ morphology is usually above the mentioned values. Also supporting the possibility that the rSr′ morphology is abnormal is the lack of an evident S wave in leads I and V6 and the presence of a pathological P wave or QRS complex.

An rsr′ morphology can be secondary to **a V1 electrode located too high** in terms of cardiac position (second or third right intercostal space) in very lean individuals with a longilineal thorax. The P and T waves are usually negative in these cases, because the electrode located above the normal position records the tail negativity of the vectors corresponding to the P and T waves, while the initial r wave could be minimal, if present, when the initial ventricular depolarization forces are directed downward. When the V1 electrode is located in the correct position (fourth intercostal space), the rSr′ pattern disappears (see Figure 11.18).

Frequently, an rSr′ morphology is found in individuals with **thoracic abnormalities** (pectus excavatus and straight back syndrome) in the absence of underlying heart disease. It is attributed to the change in heart position in these cases, caused by a reduction in the thoracic anteroposterior diameter. Usually, the P wave in V1 is negative. Some of these patterns occur with a slight upward deviation of the ST segment that is convex to the isoelectric baseline ("saddle-back" pattern) (see Figure 7.16).

Similar patterns with rSr′ may be also seen in **athletes**. Figure 7.16 shows the more important ECG characteristics used to differentiate rSr′ in athletes from a similar ECG pattern seen in patients with pectus excavatum and type II Brugada pattern. It is important to remember that the r′ wave seen in patients with thoracic deformities (pectus excavatum) and athletes or when electrodes are incorrectly placed is narrow, while the r′ observed in the Brugada's syndrome is usually wide (see Chapter 21).

Taller-than-normal R waves (R≥S) in V1 with low-voltage R could correspond to a normal variant in adults who were **born post-term**. In addition, the presence of prominent R in V1–V2 may theoretically be caused by the presence of fewer than normal Purkinje fibers in the apical (anteroseptal) area, producing a delayed depolarization at that level. Finally, an extreme levorotation can also favor the occurrence of RS morphology in V2 and, possibly, even in V1 (see Table 10.3).

In 2015, Baranchuk published a paper explaining differential ECG characteristics of patients that presented rSr′ in V1 (Figure 19.2).

Absence of a q wave in I, aVL, and V6, and absence of an r′ wave in V1 (V1–V2) in patients with a QRS complex < 0.12 sec

The presence of an old septal infarction can explain the QS morphology in V1–V2, especially in the presence of symmetrical negative T waves. This may be further suggested in the ECG by the presence of qrS or fragmented QRS in V1–V2.

A slight delay in the stimulus conduction through the left bundle branch due to a partial left bundle branch block (LBBB) can explain the lack of a "q" wave in leads I, aVL, V5, and V6, and the lack of an "r" in V1. This causes the left septal area to be depolarized late and, therefore, the initial forces of the ventricular depolarization, which are generated in the left heart, are thus counteracted by the forces arising from the right side (bundle). Naturally, this can also explain why a QS and unique R wave pattern are the morphologies found in V1 and V6 in the presence of an advanced LBBB.

QS morphology in V1 and sometimes V2 and absence of "q" in V6 with R pattern may also be explained, as an isolated abnormality, simply by septal fibrosis, which can generate a similar pattern of partial LBBB because of the lack of the septal vectors. However, the lack of septal "q" wave is not considered a strong criterion for block of middle fibers as was suggested by MacAlpin (2004) (see Chapter 11) (Bayés de Luna *et al.* 1983). Occasionally, a small "r" wave can exist in V1 as the expression of the depolarization forces corresponding to the right ventricle.

Furthermore, a poor progression of the "r" wave from V1 to V3 can occasionally be seen in elderly individuals in the absence of any underlying heart disease, which may also be related to septal fibrosis or partial LBBB (see Figure 7.45).

QRS complex alternans

In Chapter 18 (see also Figure 18.7 and Table 18.1), the P wave, QRS–T complexes, and waves with variable morphology including all types of electrical alternans are described.

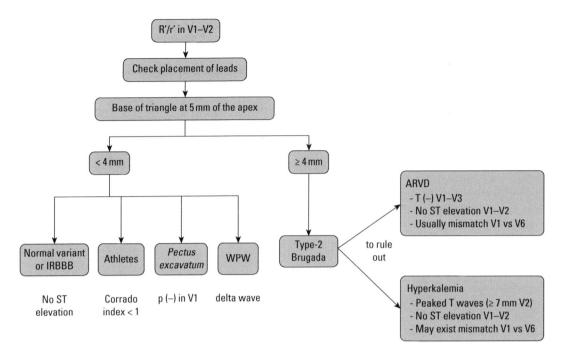

Figure 19.2 Proposed diagnostic algorithm in patients with r′ in leads V1–V2. Baranchuk *et al.* 2015.

Repolarization abnormalities: from innocent to very serious findings

Any change in the normal repolarization parameters (see Chapter 7) can be considered a repolarization abnormality. Therefore, repolarization abnormalities encompass not only any change of ST segment and T and U waves that are not considered normal, but also the changes of QT duration and dispersion previously described.

For many years, repolarization abnormalities have been divided into minor and major or evident categories. The first are considered small deviations of the ST segment (ups and downs of ST < 1 mm) and the T wave (small changes in morphology with more symmetric T wave and/or subtle changes in voltage) and minor changes in the U wave. Major changes are considered to be evident ST changes (ups and downs of ST) and an evident negative T wave.

Currently, any change of repolarization may or may not represent one of the following:
- an ECG sign of ongoing acute cardiac ischemia;
- a marker of post-ischemic change;
- evidence of other heart diseases (pericarditis, ventricular enlargement, ventricular blocks) or other pathologies, or various circumstances (drugs, alcohol, etc.) (see Chapter 23);
- some variant of normal pattern.

With this in mind, ECG change must be assessed not only in relation to the morphological importance of the change, but specially in the light of clinical context. In fact, a large ST elevation or depression is always an alarming finding, but a strikingly negative T wave is not usually a marker of emergent problems. However, any small ST shifts or even the presence of minor T wave abnormalities may be considered dangerous in the context of possible acute coronary syndrome (ACS). In this context, we will now comment on the presence of repolarization changes in various clinical settings.

ST-T changes in a patient presenting with acute chest pain or the equivalent: diagnostic approach

It is important to consider every possibility to explain acute chest pain or equivalent (e.g. tenderness, oppression, or sudden dyspnea). Figure 19.3 shows how to rule out non-ischemic patients arriving at the Emergency Department with chest pain. Sometimes, it is easy to conclude that the pain is non-ischemic, or to diagnose ischemic origin, but in approximately 25–30% of cases the pain is dubious and we need to perform complementary explorations to reach a definitive conclusion.

We will now discuss the importance of history taking, blood tests, and especially the surface ECG, bedside diagnostic methods that may be used in any medical center and usually are sufficient to arrive at a diagnosis.

The following possibilities should be considered in a patient with acute chest pain (Figure 19.3 and Table 19.3).

Chest pain of ischemic origin

From the ECG point of view, in Chapter 13 we explained all the ECG changes related to acute ischemia and its differential diagnosis. Now, we would just like to stress that

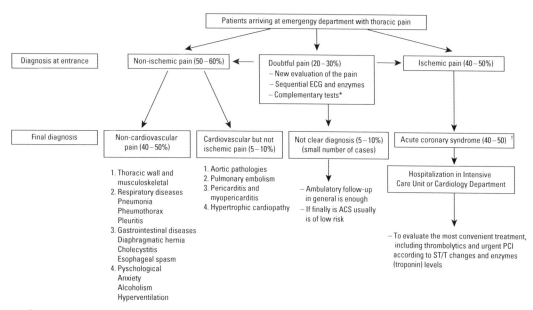

Patients arriving at emergengy department with thoracic pain

Diagnosis at entrance

Non-ischemic pain (50 – 60%)

Doubtful pain (20 – 30%)
– New evaluation of the pain
– Sequential ECG and enzymes
– Complementary tests*

Ischemic pain (40 – 50%)

Final diagnosis

Non-cardiovascular pain (40 – 50%)

Cardiovascular but not ischemic pain (5 – 10%)

Not clear diagnosis (5 – 10%) (small number of cases)

Acute coronary syndrome (40 – 50) [†]

1. Thoracic wall and musculoskeletal
2. Respiratory diseases
   Pneumonia
   Pheumothorax
   Pleuritis
3. Gastrointestinal diseases
   Diaphragmatic hernia
   Cholecystitis
   Esophageal spasm
4. Pyschological
   Anxiety
   Alcoholism
   Hyperventilation

1. Aortic pathologies
2. Pulmonary embolism
3. Pericarditis and myopericarditis
4. Hypertrophic cardiopathy

– Ambulatory follow-up in general is enough
– If finally is ACS usually is of low risk

Hospitalization in Intensive Care Unit or Cardiology Department

– To evaluate the most convenient treatment, including thrombolytics and urgent PCI according to ST/T changes and enzymes (troponin) levels

*X Ray, exercise testing, and if necessary, echocardiography, other imaging techniques and coronary angiography
[†]Clinical, ECG, enzymatic characteristics

Figure 19.3 How to rule out non-ischemic pain in patients who present at the Emergency Department with thoracic pain: types of thoracic pains, diagnosis at arrival, and how to proceed to reach a final diagnosis (see text) (Fiol-Sala *et al.* 2020).

sometimes it is very easy to diagnose because the patient presents with clear changes in the ST segment (ST elevation myocardial infarction (STEMI) or non-STEMI) that may suggest acute coronary syndrome, although other pathologies, such as pericarditis, myocarditis, dissecting aneurysm, and even normal variant (early repolarization), should be ruled out. Table 19.3 shows the most important data taken from clinical history, ECG, and blood tests to perform this differential diagnosis.

The first ECG manifestation of a possible STEMI is often a tall and wide T wave that is usually a very transient pattern evolving into STEMI. Sometimes, this pattern is persistent. According to Birnbaum *et al.* (1993), these patients present with grade I of ischemia, but in other series (De Winter *et al.* 2008) it seems that the grade of ischemia is at least moderate and often also presents with an upsloping ST depression (see Figure 20.9). A complete occlusion of LAD is frequently found in these cases but the presence of collateral circulation/preconditioning diminishes the impact of the occlusion and explains the ECG pattern having not only tall T wave but also some grade of ST depression. The upsloping ST depression plus tall T wave is a result of the presence of very important subendocardial involvement that includes zones with more subendocardial ischemia patterns (ST depression– ECG pattern of injury) or less subendocardial ischemia (tall T waves). If the patient is left untreated, usually clear transmural homogeneous involvement will appear accompanied by ST elevation evolving into myocardial infarction (see Figures 20.6 and 20.7).

A patient may appear in the Emergency Department or Medical Outpatient Department because he or she has had chest pain of dubious origin in the past 24–48 hours, although sometimes the patient is more anxious because of the location rather than because of the intensity of the pain. The ECG is usually normal, or in any case only small changes appear that have to be considered together with any previous ECGs if they exist. This comparison may help to evaluate any small changes of repolarization that may be misinterpreted with only one ECG (see Figure 20.15). These small changes may be dangerous in the clinical context of recent past chest pain. It is necessary to start medical treatment, but in the absence of chest pain, the practice of percutaneous coronary intervention (PCI) may be considered urgent.

Sometimes, patients will come to the Emergency Department because of acute chest pain but upon arrival the pain temporally disappears and the ECG shows an ST elevation evolving to a deep negative T wave, or the negative T wave is the only ECG change recorded during the stay in the Emergency Department. This pattern, usually seen in V1–V2 to V4–V5 in cases of LAD compromise, is a sign of an at least partially open artery and therefore it is not necessary to perform an emergency PCI; on the other hand, when there is a persistent ST elevation this represents acute ischemia and myocardial muscle in danger: "time is muscle," and an emergency PCI is needed.

A deep and negative T wave that appears in the evaluative phase of a STEMI before evolving into a Q wave myocardial infarction means that the artery is totally or

Table 19.3 Differential diagnosis between pericarditis, early repolarization, acute coronary syndrome, and dissecting aneurysm

	Pericarditis	Early repolarization	Acute coronary syndrome	Dissecting aneurysm
Medical history Age	Any age	Any age. Often in young people with vagal overdrive/ or sportsmen	Exceptional before the age of 30	Adults and elderly
Risk factors for ischemic heart disease/sudden death	No	Sometimes ventricular fibrillation (see Chapter 24)	Often	Often. Frequent in patients with hypertension
Previous respiratory infections	Frequent. Sometimes fever	No (occasional)	No (occasional)	No (occasional)
Pain characteristics	Visceral pain often with: • Pain increase during respiration. It may seem that pain increases with the exercise because the latter increases respiration frequency • Typical radiation toward the left shoulder • Sometimes recurrent	Can coexist with osteo-articular pain or pain of any other origin (see Figure 19.2)	• Ischemic pain often with typical irradiation (see text) • During rest or light exercise Can be present in any part of the thorax, and even any pain above the navel is suspicious	Intensive, visceral pain, mainly located in the back of the thorax. If this occurs, it is always important to rule out a dissecting aneurysm or an MI of the lateral wall
ECG	ST elevation in the early phase. Often, but not always convex with respect to the isoelectric line; presented mainly in the precordial leads • Sometimes typical evolutive changes (see Figure 22.9) • Often PR segment elevation in VR and depression in II (see Figures 9.3 and 22.10) • There is no change during an exercise stress test	• ST elevation, convex with respect to the isoelectric line. In general not >2–3 mm, mainly in precordial leads from V2–V3 to V4–V5 • Sometimes in the inferior wall slurrings at the end of QRS • Elevation of PR segment not evident The ST elevation disappears during a stress test (Figure 19.5)	• ST elevation, which in its most typical form is concave with respect to the isoelectric line, usually evident • PR elevation in VR is not frequent. It can be present in atrial MI, but then there are clear signs of Q-wave MI	• No typical pattern. In general is related to the associated diseases (HBP previous ischemic heart disease) • ST elevation as a mirror pattern (Figure 19.4).
Blood tests	Mild-moderate elevation of the troponin (perimyocarditis)	Within the normal range	Can be within the normal range (unstable angina) or elevated, very often with important increase	• In general, no increase troponin • Increase D-dimer (high SE, low SP)
Evolution	In general, good clinical evolution Sometimes evolutive ECG changes, but not always typical (see Figures 22.9 and 22.10) Q wave is missing	• Usually no change • Occasionally related to sudden death (Chapter 24)	Often evolution into Q wave and non-Q wave MI	Often bad evolution/ prognosis

Reproduced with permission from Fiol-Sala *et al.* 2020.
MI: myocardial infarction; HBP: high blood pressure.

partially open, and this is a marker of post-ischemic change. However, this does not mean that the problem is over. If the artery is re-occluded again (new thrombus or coronary spasm), this post-ischemic pattern may show a pseudonormalization of the T wave and if occlusion persists, a new ST segment elevation may soon appear (Figure 20.4B). At other times, the clinical state stabilizes and the ECG stays the same with negative and deep T waves in V1–V4 for months. These cases usually have an open artery or at least the flow of blood is correct at this time, thanks to a very good collateral circulation/preconditioning. Nevertheless, the normalization of this negative T wave with time is a sign of a better prognosis (Tamura *et al.* 1999) (Chapter 20).

We always have to remember that in a few cases the ECG remains normal or unmodified during an ACS (see Chapters 13 and 20).

Cardiovascular non-ischemic pain

It is essential to perform differential diagnosis with pericarditis, myocarditis, and some other processes. As already mentioned, Table 19.1 shows the most important

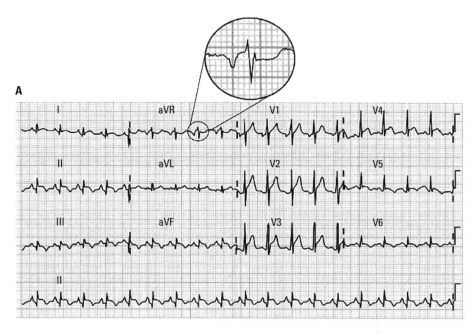

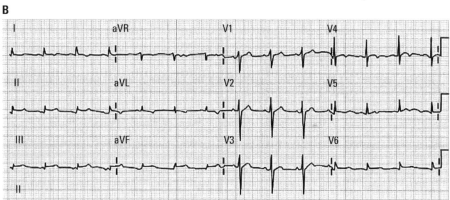

Figure 19.4 (A) A 39-year-old patient with long-standing precordial pain without ischemic characteristics. There is an ST segment elevation in many leads and in someone with final negative T wave but without Q waves and with PR elevation in aVR with depression in II (myopericarditis). The clinical history ECG and the follow-up (B) with an ECG that shows an evolution compatible with pericarditis (negative T wave without Q wave) suggests this diagnosis.

clinical, blood test, and ECG characteristics that help to differentiate ACS with ST elevation from acute pericarditis, dissecting aneurysm, and early repolarization.

In pericarditis, the ST segment elevation is not usually very striking although there are exceptions. It is not followed by a Q wave and the negative T waves are not very deep and do not usually have evident mirror images. However, sometimes differential diagnosis is difficult (see Chapter 13; Figure 19.4) (Spodick 1982; Gintzon and Laks 1982). Occasionally, when myopericarditis exists, both the ST segment elevation and T wave may be more evident and difficult to distinguish only with the ECG from ACS (Figure 13.18). Furthermore, a mild increase in troponin levels sometimes makes the diagnosis more difficult.

It would be a mistake to interpret the ST elevation in V1–V2 as a primary pattern and not to recognize that it is a mirror pattern of left ventricular strain pattern in V5–V6. In the case of left ventricular hypertrophy in hypertensive patients with chest pain, this may be due to

dissecting aneurysm, especially if the pain is in the back (Figure 19.5). In this case, it is important to measure D-dimer, which is a very sensitive blood test, although the specificity is low.

As has already been mentioned, it is also important to make a differential diagnosis, especially in the acute stage of pericarditis when only a slightly convex ST segment elevation exists, with the normal variant known as **early repolarization**. In the case of early repolarization pattern, there is a clear ST elevation resolution with exercise (Figure 19.6).

In cases of **pulmonary embolism and acute decompensation of cor pulmonale,** an ST elevation may appear (see Figure 10.16). Other ECG patterns may also appear (deep negative T waves in right precordial leads—see Figures 10.14 and 10.15, new RBBB—see Figure 10.16, etc.) that have to be considered in the differential diagnosis of patients with acute chest pain or equivalents and ECG changes (see Figures 10.14–10.16).

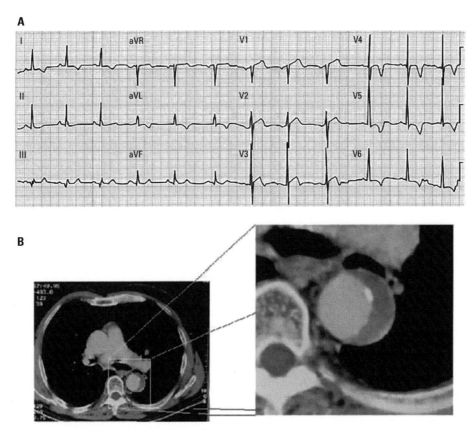

Figure 19.5 (A) A patient with thoracic pain due to a dissecting aortic aneurysm. An ST segment elevation in V1–V3 can be explained by the mirror pattern of an evident left ventricular enlargement (V6) due to hypertension. This ST segment elevation has been erroneously interpreted as due to an acute coronary syndrome. As a consequence, fibrinolytic treatment was administered, which was not only unnecessary but even harmful. (B) The CAT scan imaging shows the dissecting aneurysm of the aorta. This case demonstrates that before accepting a diagnosis of STE-ACS, other diseases that may cause ST segment elevation should be ruled out.

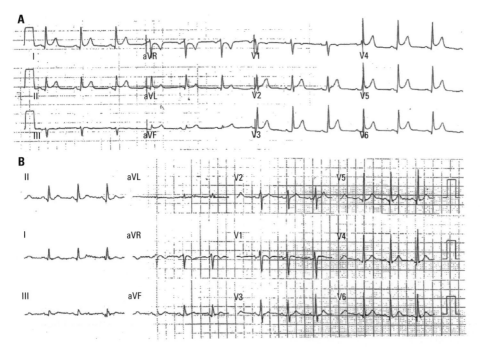

Figure 19.6 (A) A patient with thoracic pain and mild ST segment elevation in many leads. ECG was considered by automatic interpretation as pericarditis. (B) The ST segment elevation disappears with exercise, which favors the diagnosis of early repolarization pattern. This is an example of misdiagnosis of automatic interpretation.

The differential diagnosis should also include the **chronic pattern of ischemic heart disease with ST elevation** such as the presence of **ventricular aneurysm**, the newly described **Tako-Tsubo syndrome**, and the evanescent ST elevation pattern of **coronary spasm** (see Figures 20.44 and 20.46).

Finally, ST depression may appear in patients without ischemia during exercise test (see color Plate 3), and also in the course of **fast supraventricular tachycardia** (Figure 19.7). Usually the ST depression is upsloping but it may show a downsloping ST depression pattern. In the latter case, it is especially necessary to rule out the presence of ischemia (see Figure 19.7).

Pain of non-cardiovascular origin (Figure 19.3)

Pain of non-cardiovascular origin may be caused by: (i) problems in the thoracic wall and thoracic/neck muscles; (ii) lung disease; (iii) problems in the gastrointestinal tract; (iv) problems of psychiatric origin.

ECG is not changed in these cases. Using history taking, physical examination, blood tests (biomarkers), and complementary techniques, we are usually able to reach a correct diagnosis in the majority of cases.

Acute dyspnea

May be the most important manifestation of LV failure and pulmonary edema (see Figure 9.13). We have to rule out severe heart disease (acute myocarditis, acute MI, etc.).

In acute cor pulmonale secondary to pulmonary embolism (see Figure 10.16) or worsening of a chronic cor pulmonale produced by a sudden right chamber overload—usually related to a respiratory infection (see Figure 10.14)—negative T waves may be observed in the right precordial leads and/or in II, III, and aVF. In addition, ST changes in the frontal and/or horizontal plane may be confused with those seen in ischemic heart disease.

Other lung diseases such as pneumothorax (see Chapter 23) may present with acute dyspnea and ECG changes (see Figure 23.5). Also bronquial asthma has to be considered.

On some occasions, dyspnea may be the equivalent of pain in cases of acute ischemic attack.

Presence of rapid palpitations or syncope (near-syncope)

Various tachyarrhythmias, especially atrial fibrillation, but also supraventricular reentrant tachycardia, even in young individuals, and obviously ventricular tachycardia may present as chest pain probably of hemodynamic origin. In any case, this possibility has to be considered in the history taking. The ST changes are often striking and the coronary perfusion is usually normal (see above). This opens the possibility that tachycardization may explain some types of repolarization change (Birnbaum *et al.* 2011).

We will not discuss the differential diagnosis of all the causes that may induce syncope or near-syncope (see Bayés de Luna and Baranchuk 2017). We just want to say that the causes may be benign (vasovagal syncope) or malignant (tachyarrhythmias especially VT–VF). It is necessary to rule out acute ischemia, pulmonary embolism, and inherited heart disease. The surface ECG may give many crucial information and the history taking is also very important.

ST-T alternans

This topic is discussed in Chapter 18 (see Figure 18.7 and Table 18.1) and in Chapter 20.

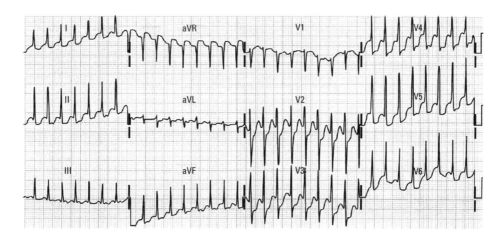

Figure 19.7 This is a case of young man with a very rapid reentrant tachycardia with a circuit exclusive of the atrioventricular junction (AVNRT). The patient presents with chest discomfort and shows evident ST depression as may be seen in the absence of ischemic heart disease in the case of fast heart rate (see Chapter 15).

ECG changes in repolarization found in patients with no precordial pain and in the absence of current or past symptoms suggestive of ischemic or pericardial disease

Differential diagnosis of all causes of T wave abnormalities (T wave taller and wider (Table 13.2) or flat/negative (Table 13.3)) and ST shifts (ST elevation (Table 13.4) and ST depression (Table 13.5)) should be performed. It is also important to bear in mind the clinical context of the patient. In a recent publication (Jayroe *et al.* 2009), it has been demonstrated that even experts in ECG diagnosis make several mistakes when faced with an ECG with ST elevation without clinical context. However, by applying all the information explained in this book, especially in Chapters 10–13, this chapter, and Chapters 20–22, the possibility of performing the correct diagnosis is very high.

In the presence of moderate/important right and left ventricular enlargement, repolarization abnormalities are secondary to depolarization abnormalities. In more advanced cases, the most striking pattern is the so-called "strain pattern": (see Figures 10.21 and 10.26). The negative T wave in these cases is typically asymmetric. Therefore, if a pattern with somewhat symmetric T wave is found, some type of primary factor (ischemia, drugs) may be influencing the ECG pattern (mixed pattern—see Figure 10.28).

Undoubtedly, advanced bundle branch blocks, especially LBBB, and significant enlargement of both ventricles are often accompanied by marked secondary repolarization abnormalities.

Various heart diseases, such as mitral valve prolapse and myocarditis, can generate repolarization abnormalities that are occasionally even more striking than those observed in ischemic heart disease.

In general, cardiomyopathies frequently exhibit T waves that are quite pathological. This is especially true in apical hypertrophic cardiomyopathy (see Figure 10.25). Sometimes, the only abnormality seen in right ventricular arrhythmogenic dysplasia—bearing in mind that 20% of those cases exhibit a normal ECG—is a negative T wave that is generally not very deep but sometimes symmetric in the right precordial leads (see Figure 21.7).

ST segment and especially T wave abnormalities are seen in congenital long QT syndrome, including T wave alternans (see Figure 21.10). Brugada's syndrome may also exhibit repolarization abnormalities. An upsloping ST segment elevation concave with respect to the isoelectric baseline is the most characteristic feature, often without evidence of an RBBB morphology (without final r' wave in V1 and aVR and S wave in V6) (see Chapter 21).

Striking repolarization abnormalities (evident negative T wave, ST segment depression ≥ 1 mm) may be seen in the absence of ischemic or other type of heart disease. This is sometimes seen in athletes (Serra-Grima *et al.* 2000)

(see Chapter 23; see also Figures 7.16 and 23.11), in the presence of ionic disturbances (see Figures 23.19–23.21), in neurological disease (see Figures 13.15D, 13.16H and 23.1), when secondary to drug effects (see Figures 23.13 and 23.15), or due to so-called "cardiac memory" when the activation is normal, in patients with a baseline anomalous ventricular activation (right ventricular pacemakers, advanced LBBB, intermittent WPW syndrome with right ventricular pre-excitation) (see Figure 17.20).

Negative T waves may be seen not only in V1 but also in V2 or even V3 in some women and Black people. Normally, the T wave is symmetrical and not deep. The differential diagnosis between a sudden right chamber overload and acute ischemic attack may be difficult using only the ECG, since these morphologies are sometimes quite similar. However, the history taking and the evolving nature of this morphology should make the diagnosis easier.

It should be remembered that fleeting repolarization abnormalities can often be seen (e.g. flattened bimodal T wave or even slightly negative, slight ST segment depression deviation) after alcohol or carbohydrate intake, with a change of position (standing) and with hyperventilation (see Figure 7.47). Persistent repolarization abnormalities can also be detected with intake of certain drugs (e.g. amiodarone (Figure 23.13) and digitalis (Figure 23.15)), in chronic alcoholism (see Figure 23.16) and in some ionic disturbances, particularly hyperkalemia (tall and peaked T wave) and with hypokalemia (ST segment downward deviation) (see Figures 23.19–23.21) (Surawicz 1967).

However, sometimes no apparent reason is found to explain repolarization abnormalities. In such cases, it is advisable to rule out hidden WPW syndrome, mitral valve prolapse, and hypertrophic cardiomyopathy, and obviously silent ischemic heart disease or silent pericarditis/myocarditis. A complete clinical history should be taken and the required explorations, including, if necessary, a coronary artery angiogram (Figure 19.7) carried out in order to ensure that such abnormalities are not due to ischemic heart disease.

Repolarization abnormalities observed in the ECG recording should be assessed within the patient's clinical context. However, sometimes even in presence of abnormal repolarization the coronarography is completely normal and the ECG remains unchanged for years (Figure 19.8)

Heart rate and cardiac rhythm abnormalities in a surface ECG

The step-by-step requirements that have to be taken for the sequential diagnosis of various arrhythmias are described in Chapter 18.

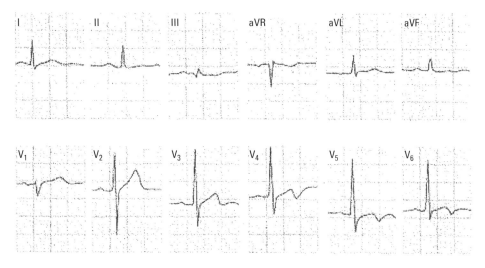

Figure 19.8 This is a case of a 56-year-old man without any past or present clinical symptoms suggestive of ischemic heart disease or other cause that may explain this evident repolarization abnormality. The ECG was recorded during a check-up. All the complementary tests, including coronarography, were normal, and the ECG has remained practically the same for over 10 years.

References

Alexander B, Milden J, Hazim B, *et al*. New electrocardiographic score for the prediction of atrial fibrillation: The MVP ECG risk score (morphology-voltage-P wave duration). Ann Noninvasive Electrocardiol 2019;00:e12669.

Algra A, Tijssen JG, Roelandt JR, Pool J, Lubsen J. QT interval variables from 24 hour electrocardiography and the two year risk of sudden death. Br Heart J 1993;70:43.

Bacharova L, Wagner GS. The time for naming the interatrial block syndrome: Bayes syndrome. J Electrocardiol 2015;48:133–134.

Baranchuk A. *Interatrial block and supraventricular arrhythmias. Clinical implications of Bayés' Syndrome.* Cardiotext Publishing, Minneapolis, Minnesota, USA, 2017.

Baranchuk A, Enriquez A, García-Niebla J, *et al*. Differential diagnosis of rSr' pattern in leads V1-V2. Comprehensive review and proposed algorithm. Ann Noninvasive Electrocardiol 2015;20(1):7–17.

Bayés de Luna A, Baranchuk A. *Clinical Arrhythmology*. 2nd edn. Wiley-Blackwell, 2017.

Bayés de Luna A, Serra-Genís C, Guix M *et al*. Septal fibrosis as determinant of Q wave in patients with aortic valve disease. Eur Heart J 1983;4(suppl E):86.

Bayés de Luna A, Fort de Ribot R, Trilla E, *et al*. Electrocardiographic and vectorcardiographic study of interatrial conduction disturbances with left atrial retrograde activation. J Electrocardiol 1985;18:1.

Bayés de Luna A, Carrió I, Subirana MT, *et al*. Electrophysiological mechanisms of the SI SII SIII electrocardiographic morphology. J Electrocardiol 1987;20:38.

Bayés de Luna, A., Cladellas, M., Oter, R. *et al*. Interatrial conduction block and retrograde activation of the left atrium and paroxysmal supraventricular arrhythmias. Eur Heart J 1988;9:1112.

Bayés de Luna A, Martínez-Sellés M, Bayés-Genís A, *et al*. Síndrome de Bayés. Lo que todo clínico debe conocer. What every clinician should know about Bayés Syndrome. Rev Esp Cardiol (Engl Ed) 2020;73:758–762.

Bayés-Genís A, Lopez L, Viñolas X, *et al*. Distinct left bundle branch block pattern in ischemic and non-ischemic dilated cardiomyopathy. Eur J Heart Failure 2003;5:165.

Bellet S, Jedlicka J. Sinoventricular conduction and its relation to sinoatrial conduction. Am J Cardiol 1969;24:831.

Birnbaum Y, Sclarovsky S, Blum A, Mager A, Gabbay U. Prognostic significance of the initial electrocardiographic pattern in a first acute anterior wall myocardial infarction. Chest 1993;103:1681.

Birnbaum Y, Zhu S, Wagner G. New considerations of ST "elevation" and "depression" and accompanying T wave configuration in acute coronary syndromes. J Electrocardiol 2011;44:1.

Braunwald E. Foreword. *Clinical electrocardiography: a textbook*, 4th edn. Ed. A. Bayés de Luna. Wiley-Blackwell, Londres, 2012.

Conde D, Baranchuk A. Bloqueo interauricular como sustrato anatómico-eléctrico de arritmias supraventriculares: Sindrome de Bayés. Arch Cardiol Mex 2014;84(1):32–40.

Daubert JC, Mabo P, Berder V, Gras D. Atrial flutter and interatrial conduction block: preventive role of biatrial synchronous pacing? In Waldo AL, Touboul P (eds). *Atrial Flutter: Advances in mechanisms and management*. Futura Publishing Company, 1996.

Day CP, McComb JM, Campbell R. QT dispersion: an indication of arrhythmia risk in patients with long QT intervals. Br Heart J 1990;63:342.

De Bruyne MC, Hoes JA, Kors JA, *et al*. Prolonged QT interval predicts cardiac and all-cause mortality in the elderly. Eur Heart J 1999;20:278.

De Winter RJ, Verouden NJ, Wellens HJ, Wilde AA. Interventional Cardiology Group of the Academic Medical Center: a new ECG sign of proximal LAD occlusion. N Engl J Med 2008;359:2071.

Fiol-Sala M, Birnbaum Y, Nikus K, Bayés de Luna A. *Electrocardiography in Ischemic Heart Disease. Clinical and Imaging Correlations and Prognostic Implications*. 2nd edn. Willey-Blackwell, 2020.

Gaita F, Giustetto C, Bianchi F, *et al*. Short QT syndrome: a familial cause of sudden death. Circulation 2003;108:965.

Gintzon LE, Laks MM. The differential diagnosis of acute pericarditis from the normal variant: new electrocardiographic criteria. Circulation 1982;65:1004.

Gollob MH, Redpath CJ, Roberts JD. The short QT syndrome: proposed diagnostic criteria. J Am Coll Cardiol 2011;57:802.

Haïsaguerre M, Derval N, Sacher F, *et al*. Sudden cardiac arrest associated with early repolarization. N Engl J Med 2008;358:2016.

Ikeda H, Maki S, Yoshida N, *et al*. Predictors of death from congestive heart failure in hypertrophic cardiomyopathy. Am J Cardiol 1999;83:1280.

Jayroe BJ, Spodick DH, Nikus K, *et al*. Differentiating ST elevation myocardialinfarction and non ischemic causes of ST elevation by analyzing the presenting ECG. Am J Cardiol 2009;103:301.

Kardys I, Kors JA, van der Meer IM, *et al*. Spatial QRS-T angle predicts cardiac death in a general population. Eur Heart J 2003;24:1357.

Kors JA, van Herpen G, van Bemmel JH. QT dispersion as an attribute of T-loop morphology. Circulation 1999;99:1458.

MacAlpin RN. Clinical significance of QS complexes in V1 and V2 without other electrocardiographic abnormality. Ann Noninvasive Electrocardiol 2004;9:39.

Moss AJ, Zareba W, Benhorin J, *et al*. ECG T-wave patterns in genetically distinct forms of the hereditary long QT syndrome. Circulation 1995;92:2929.

Peñaloza D, Gamboa R, Sime F. Experimental right bundle branch block in the normal human heart. Am J Cardiol 1961;8:767.

Pérez Riera A, Ferreira C, Ferriera Filho C, *et al*. Electro-vectorcardiographic diagnosis of left septal fascicular block: anatomic and clinical considerations. Ann Noninvasive Electrocardiol 2011;16:196.

Sarapa N, Morganroth J, Couderc JP, *et al*. Electrocardiographic identification of drug-induced QT prolongation: assessment by different recording and measurement methods. Ann Noninvasive Electrocardiol 2004;9:48.

Schwartz P, Wolff S. QT interval prolongation as a predictor of sudden death in patients with myocardial infarction. Circulation 1978;57:1074.

Schwartz PJ, Priori SG, Spazzolini C, *et al*. Genotype-phenotype correlation in the long QT syndrome: gene-specific triggers for life-threatening arrhythmias. Circulation 2001;103:89.

Serra-Grima JR, Estorch M, Carrio I. Marked ventricular repolarization abnormalities in highly trained athletes' electrocardiograms: Clinical and prognostic implications. J Am Coll Cardiol 2000;36:1310.

Spodick DH. Acute pericarditis: ECG changes. Primary Cardiol 1982;8:78.

Surawicz B. Relationship between electrocardiogram and electrolytes. Am Heart J 1967;73:814.

Surawicz B, Knoebel SB, Long QT. Good, bad or indifferent? J Am Coll Cardiol 1984;4:398.

Tamura A, Nagasi KM, Kriya Y, *et al*. Significance of spontaneous normalization of negative T wave during healing of anterior myocardila infarction. Am J Cardiol 1999;84:1341.

Wilson FN, Macloed AG, Barker PS, Johnston FD. Determination of the significance of the areas of the ventricular deflections of the electrocardiogram. Am Heart J 1934;10:46.

Zabel M, Portnoy S, Franz MR. Electrocardiographic indexes of dispersion of ventricular repolarization: an isolated heart validation study. J Am Coll Cardiol 1995;25:746.

Zabel M, Klingenheben T, Franz MR, Hohnloser SH. Assessment of QT dispersion for prediction of mortality or arrhythmic events after myocardial infarction: results of a prospective long-term follow-up study. Circulation 1998;97:2543.

Zabel M, Acar B, Klingenheben T, *et al*. Analysis of 12-lead T-wave morphology for risk stratification after myocardial infarction. Circulation 2000;102:1252.

Zareba W, Moss AJ, Schwartz PJ, *et al*. Influence of genotype on the clinical course of the long-QT syndrome. International Long-QT Syndrome Registry Research Group. N Engl J Med 1998;339:960.

Chapter 20
The ECG in Different Clinical Set of Ischemic Heart Disease

Introduction

From exercise angina to acute coronary syndrome, and myocardial infarction

Myocardial ischemia can occur through two different pathophysiological mechanisms, **in the majority of cases related to the presence of atherothrombosis**. These mechanisms are:

• an **abrupt decrease in blood flow** that constitute the clinical syndrome of ACS–evolving MI, and

• **increased myocardial demand**, the prototype of which is exercise angina.

Other types of ACS–MI will be discussed later in the section on ECG changes due to decreased blood flow not related to atherothrombosis (Table 20.1).

Abrupt decrease in blood flow: acute coronary syndrome–myocardial infarction (Table 20.2)

There are two types (Myocardial Infarction Type I, Thygesen *et al*. 2019):

• **ACS with decreased flow due to occlusive thrombosis** that is usually total or nearly total (≥90%) with reduced perfusion (TIMI flow 0/1) and transmural involvement (ST elevation ACS). This type is called ST elevation myocardial infarction (STEMI) because in the majority of cases, some degree of necrosis and increase of biomarkers exist. The culprit artery in case of a single occluded artery is more frequently (From *et al*. 2010) the left anterior descending coronary artery (LAD) (≈45%) followed by the right coronary artery (RCA) (≈35%), and left circumflex artery (LCX) (≈20%). The culprit artery is rarely the left main trunk (LMT), the intermediate, first septal, or first diagonal branches.

• **ACS due to a decreased flow usually involving a patent artery often with non-occlusive thrombus** (usually TIMI flow 2/3) and non-completely transmural involvement (non-ST elevation ACS) (NSTE-ACS or NSTEMI). Throughout this book, we use STEMI and NSTEMI rather than STE-ACS and NSTE-ACS (Jacobs 2011).

• **STEMI represent ≈30% of cases of ACS** arriving in the Emergency Department in our hospital and NSTEMI ≈50%. The rest (20%) are cases of ACS with confounding factors (left ventricular hypertrophy, wide QRS) that often may also be classified into these two types, although the diagnosis especially in case of NSTEMI is more difficult (see later). Now, we will comment the cases of ACS with narrow QRS.

• In spite of this clear differentiation of NSTEMI and STEMI types, ACS is a dynamic process (Figure 20.28) and sometimes, with or even without treatment, a patient with a STEMI pattern evolves to a NSTEMI pattern and vice versa. This has management implications (see changes from NSTEMI to STEMI and vice versa).

Acute coronary syndrome due to total or near total occlusive thrombosis and with complete transmural involvement: STEMI (Table 20.2)
Pathophysiology and clinical setting

Coronarography shows complete or nearly complete thrombotic occlusion in the patient with a ruptured plaque and reduced blood flow (TIMI 0/1). The presence of total or near total occlusion may be intermittent and associated with coronary spasm and/or new thrombosis. However, sometimes after removal of the thrombus, the coronary stenosis is not very significant (<50%). There is **complete transmural involvement** of at least part of one left ventricular wall, often in myocardium previously relatively unaffected by the ischemia.

In general, very little collateral circulation or preconditioning (mechanism of adaptation to ischemia mediated by ATP-sensitive potassium channels and adenosine) is present (Tomai *et al*. 1999). The biomarkers are positive, and usually evolve to Q wave MI.

According to the guidelines, if the patient presents with angina that has started within the last 12 hours, treatment to open the artery (fibrinolysis or percutaneous coronary intervention (PCI) if possible) should be started immediately in order to avoid or minimize development of Q wave MI ("time is muscle").

Clinical Electrocardiography: A Textbook, Fifth Edition. Antoni Bayés de Luna, Miquel Fiol-Sala, Antoni Bayés-Genís, and Adrián Baranchuk.
© 2022 John Wiley & Sons Ltd. Published 2022 by John Wiley & Sons Ltd.

Table 20.1 Classification of ECG changes in clinical settings due to myocardial ischemia

1. DECREASED BLOOD FLOW
   A. Acute coronary syndrome–myocardial infarction (ACS–MI)
      a. Due to atherothrombosis
         - ACS with narrow QRS
         - ACS with confounding factors
         - Chronic MI with narrow QRS
         - Chronic MI with confounding factors
      b. Other ECGT changes usually ACS not due to atherothrombosis
         - Hypercoagulability
         - Tachyarrhythmia
         - Coronary dissection
         - Tako–Tsubo syndrome
         - Congenital abnormalities
         - PCI and bypass surgery
         - Coronary spasm
         - X syndrome
         - Myocardial bridging
         - Miscellaneous
2. INCREASED DEMAND
   A. Exercise angina due to atherothrombosis
   B. Others: Pulmonary hypertension, chronic anemia, tachyarrhythmia, etc.

Summary of ECG changes (see later)

The ECG shows ST segment elevation usually occurring after a transient period of a peaked, tall, and positive T wave (see Figures 13.5B and 20.4B) (see later and Table 13.1). Although the ST elevation is the most striking ECG manifestation, some leads with ST depression as a mirror pattern are also observed. Correlating the ups and downs of ST is crucial to identifying the culprit artery, the location of the obstruction, and the area at risk in the case of STEMI (see Chapter 13 and Figures 13.38–13.52), and later: ECG changes in ACS due to decreased blood flow (STEMI).

Acute coronary syndrome usually with patent artery and non-complete transmural involvement: NSTEMI (Table 20.2)

Pathophysiology and clinical setting

These cases occur due to ulcerated plaque often with rupture and, in around 40% of cases, thrombus but with patent artery (non-complete occlusion). Patients with NSTEMI may present with either elevated biomarkers (non-Q wave MI or true NSTEMI) or not increased biomarkers (unstable angina). The average diameter of stenosis is slightly larger than in STEMI but the thrombus usually does not occlude the artery completely. However, if the artery is occluded—which occurs in around 20–25% of cases (Dixon 2008; Pride *et al.* 2010)—**there is no complete homogeneous transmural involvement** because of the presence of collateral circulation and/or preconditioning. The involvement of left ventricular walls by the ischemia is not completely transmural and occurs usually in the presence of already previous evident impairment of subendocardial flow and increased left ventricular

Table 20.2 Summary of ECG, clinical, angiographic, and pathologic findings in ST elevation myocardial infarction (STEMI) and non-ST elevation myocardial infarction (NSTEMI)

ECG	Clinical	Angiographic	Pathology	Treatment
ACS with narrow QRS STEMI (30% of total) - Tall T wave - ST elevation - Evolving MI - Atypical patterns (Table 20.3)	Rest pain or equivalents	- Total or nearly occluded artery by fresh thrombus - TIMI 0/I flow	- Usually ruptured plaque. After some time of subendocardial involvement there is a transmural homogeneous involvement	- Emergency PCI - Medical treatment (see guidelines scientific societies) - Fibrinolysis if PCI is not feasible
NSTEMI (50% of total)[a] (During pain) - ST depression (70%) - Flat/negative T wave (≈15%) - U changes (<1%) - Normal or unchanged (≈15%) - Sometimes in the absence of pain the ECG is normal/nearly normal	With or without permanent rest pain	- Patent artery in >70% cases. - Non-occluded thrombus (≈50%) - Acute total occlusion in 10–20% case but with collaterals/ preconditioning	- Usually ulcerated plaque - Predominant subendocardial involvement - Usually non-transmural homogeneous involvement or, if exists (10–0% cases) is in general in the "mute" (basal) areas	- Antithrombotic and antiplatelet agents - Non-emergency PCI except in a high-risk group. However, often PCI is urgent

[a] The rest (20%) are cases of ACS with confounding factors (see text).

ACS: acute coronary syndrome; MI: myocardial infarction; NSTEMI: non-ST elevation myocardial infarction; PCI: percutaneous coronary intervention; STEMI: ST elevation myocardial infarction.

telediastolic pressure. The coronary flow is decreased (TIMI flow 2 or sometimes 3).

Angiographic studies of NSTEMI have demonstrated that compared with STEMI, they are more likely to present with a more spontaneous patent artery, better flow (TIMI >1), and less median stenosis (Abbas *et al.* 2004).

The culprit artery may be LMT or any of three coronary arteries or their main branches at all levels. Frequently, there is two- or three-vessel disease but usually only one culprit artery.

The patient may present with pain upon arrival at the Emergency Department. This depends on whether the coronary flow is sufficiently open (spontaneously or with treatment) for blood to reach the ischemic zone. However, antithrombotic treatment must be urgently applied to stop the progression of the disease. The **decision to perform PCI is usually not emergent**, especially if pain ceases, but often an urgent, as soon as possible, PCI is recommended if feasible.

Summary of ECG changes

The ECG changes include ST depression and/or postischemic flat/negative T wave, or even unmodified or normal ECG.

Hence, the name non-ST elevation acute coronary syndrome (non-STEMI) (Thygesen *et al.* 2019). However, ST elevation is often present in some leads, especially in aVR and V1 (mirror pattern) (see further discussion about all the ECG changes found in NSTEMI).

In the following sections, ECG changes in various clinical settings will be fully discussed. We know that some aspects have already been mentioned, but we consider that it is convenient to reinforce its importance.

ECG patterns in acute coronary syndrome with ST segment elevation (STEMI) (Table 20.3, Figure 20.1) with narrow QRS

In the past, many cases of STEMI evolved to an MI, which was usually of Q wave type (Figures 20.1A). If modern treatments to open the artery are available, more Q wave MIs can now be aborted (see Figure 20.1B).

Typical ECG patterns (Chapter 13, ST segment in ACS, and Figures 20.1–20.4 and 13.38–13.52)

The typical ECG pattern is ST segment elevation. Other patterns may also be seen (see later).

The ST segment elevation criteria for ischemia according to the new universal definition of MI (Thygesen *et al.* 2019) includes New ST elevation at the J-point in two contiguous leads with the cut-point: ≥1 mm in all leads other than leads V2–V3 where the following cut-points apply: ≥2 mm in men ≥40 years; ≥2.5 mm in men <40 years, or ≥1.5 mm in women regardless of age. This type of ST segment elevation of these characteristics is considered abnormal and evidence of acute ischemia in the clinical

Table 20.3 ECG patterns in ST elevation myocardial infarction (occluded/nearly occluded artery with homogeneous transmural involvement) (see text)

Typical pattern	ST elevation with mirror pattern (≈ 30% of all ACS)[a]
Equivalent pattern	Mirror pattern in V1–V3–V4 with ST depression (LCX occlusion) (≈5%). Often, some ST elevation in inferior/lateral leads (Figure 20.4A)
Patterns that may be seen during the acute process	At early phase: Tall and usually very transient T wave (Figure 20.4 B1) (<2%). Sometimes the tall T wave is persistent (hours) and may present ST depression (Figures 20.4B2 and B3) (<2%) After resolution of ST elevation without evolution to Q wave MI: deep negative T wave, especially in LAD occlusion (V1–V2 to V4–V5) (≈5%) (Figure 20.4C)

[a] Based on our experience (Sant Pau Hospital, Barcelona) with the ECG at arrival to Emergency Department (≈30% STEMI, 50% NSTEMI—see Table 20.4—and the rest ≈20% ECG with confounding factors (Fiol-Sala *et al.* 2020).
ACS: acute coronary syndrome; MI: myocardial infarction.

setting of ACS (presence of precordial pain or the equivalents). Whenever possible, it is important to compare this pattern with previous ECGs (Table 13.1).

The morphology of the ST segment elevation may show a concave or convex shape with respect to the isoelectric line or just a rectified line. Often, the shape of the morphology changes at follow-up with a greater concave shape after a hyperacute period. In this phase, the height of the ST elevation may be considered, causing the S waves to be pulled up (Figure 20.2C). This decreases during the subacute phase (Figures 13.32 and 13.34).

The evolution of ST segment elevation, if the MI is not treated, leads to Q wave MI with a progressive resolution of ST elevation. It is considered MI if the ST remains elevated after 20 m. The degree of ST elevation rapidly reaches a peak elevation that usually occurs at 1 hour after the onset of pain. The plateau last up 12 hours. Afterward, a progressive decline takes place that lasts a few days. In the pre-fibrinolytic era, complete resolution was found in 95% of cases of inferior MI and in 40% of cases in anterior MI after two weeks (Mills *et al.* 1975). Currently, the course is very different and the resolution of ST elevation is often very rapid with fibrinolysis and especially PCI (see Figure 20.1).

The ST resolution is accompanied by the progressive appearance of Q wave and T wave inversion indicating transmural involvement, or at least involvement of some layers of left ventricular wall outside the subendocardium (see Figures 13.32 and 13.61). In fact, the appearance of a negative T in the evolving process of Q wave MI is due to the LV intraventricular pattern (window phenomenon of

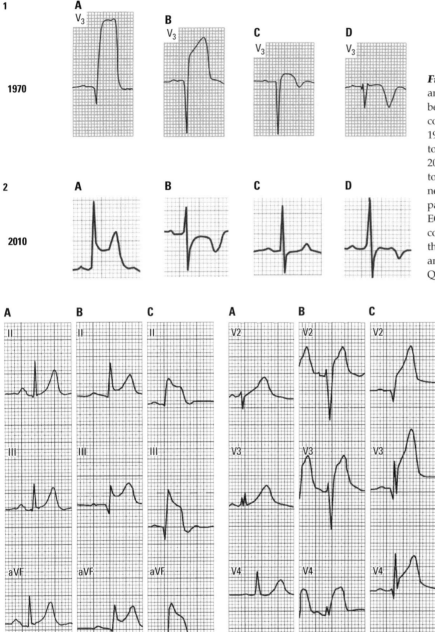

Figure 20.1 Comparison of the evolution of an STEMI of the anteroapical zone in 1970 before thrombolysis and percutaneous coronary intervention (PCI) and currently. In 1970, from A to D, we may see the evolution to a large Q wave myocardial infarction. In 2010, the patient with STEMI (A) is submitted to successful PCI (B), and a post-ischemic negative T wave appears. Later on, (C) the patient presented with pain again and the ECG pseudonormalizes. A new coronarography demonstrates thrombosis of the stent and new PCI solves the problem, and again a negative T wave appears (D). The Q-wave infarction was aborted.

Figure 20.2 (1): The three types of repolarization abnormalities that may be seen in an acute phase of myocardial infarction involving the inferolateral zone: (A) tall and/or wide T waves in inferior leads; (B) abnormal ST segment elevation, with no changes of the final part of QRS; (C) important ST segment elevation and distortion of the final part of QRS. (2): The three types of repolarization abnormalities that may be seen in an acute phase of myocardial infarction involving the anteroseptal zone: (A) tall and/or wide T waves especially seen in right precordial leads; (B) abnormal ST segment elevation, with no changes of the final part of QRS; (C) important ST segment elevation and distortion of the final part of QRS (see text).

Wilson) (Figures 13.6E and 13.61). The ST may remain slightly elevated even in the chronic phase. Sometimes this ECG pattern of Q wave MI diminishes or even disappears (see Figures 13.32 and 20.35).

ST elevation prevails in the leads facing the affected zone, producing a **direct ECG pattern**. In some opposing leads, the ST segment depression is seen as an **indirect mirror ECG pattern** (see Figures 13.35–13.37). These same features also occur in the chronic phase, with a Q wave producing the direct pattern and an R wave in V1–V2 as the mirror pattern (see Figure 13.73). In STEMI, the global evaluation of direct and reciprocal changes (ups and downs of ST) is important for detecting which artery is

the culprit (the RCA or the LCX in case of ST elevation in II, III, and aVF) (see Figure 13.39), as well as to find the location of the LAD occlusion in cases of ST elevation in the precordial leads (Figure 13.38).

An **ST segment elevation may be observed as a normal variant in V1–V2**, especially in males including 1–2 mm of ST elevation with an slightly convex shape with respect to isoelectric line, an ascending ST slope, and asymmetric T waves (Figure 7.13H). ST elevation may also be seen in many other normal situations such as in athletes or thoracic abnormalities (pectus excavatum) (see Figure 7.16).

Abnormal ST elevation due to other causes may be seen in Table 13.4 and Figure 13.59.

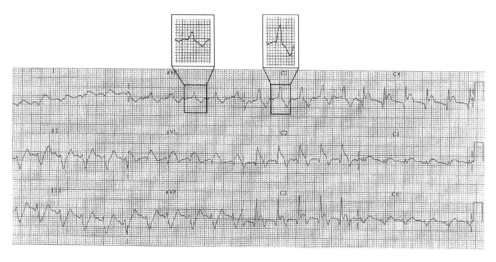

Figures 20.3 Patient with STEMI and very bad hemodynamic status in cardiogenic shock, due to complete occlusion of the left main trunk (LMT). Observe the right bundle branch block (RBBB) with superoanterior hemiblock (SAH) and the ST shifts with ST elevation in I, aVL, and from V2 to V6, and ST depression in II, III, aVF. V1 and aVR are isoelectric due to the influence of LCX involvement that counteracts the ST elevation in V1 and aVR that usually is seen in case of proximal to S1 LAD occlusion (except in case of great conal artery—see text).

Atypical ECG patterns (Figure 20.4, Table 20.3)

The following ECG patterns without ST elevation may be noted as the most striking ECG change in patients with the clinical ECG angiographic syndrome of STEMI (occluded or near occluded coronary artery with transmural involvement).

• **Presence of ST depression in V1–V3, V4.** When the ST depression is evident already in V1 without a final tall positive T wave (see before), this pattern is usually the **mirror pattern of** transmural lateral ischemia, due to LCX occlusion or rarely distal occlusion of long RCA. Therefore, it is a **true STEMI** with transmural involvement by a totally occluded artery, usually LCX, that usually presents with ST elevation in opposing leads. Unfortunately, these patients are often misdiagnosed as NSTEMI. In general, ST elevation in inferior or lateral leads is seen but sometimes the ST shift is very slight (Figures 20.4A and 20.5).

We have discussed previously the great importance of recognizing this pattern as a case of STEMI (see mistakes in the interpretation of ACS).

• We should remember, however, that **ST depression in V1–V4 more often corresponds to NSTEMI.** Usually, in these cases there is little if any ST depression in V1 and the final T wave is, in general, positive and tall. Therefore, it seems that NSTEMI are much more frequent when the culprit artery is the LCX, although there is no logical hypothesis to explain that. The only explanation is that LCX STEMI are misdiagnosed as NSTEMI because ST depression in V1–V4, with mild or even no ST elevation in other leads is often present as the most relevant ECG change, in the hiperacute phase of ACS (Figure 20.5). Therefore, it is very important to recognize these changes, which probably can be done with 12-lead ECG if we observe some subtle changes

(Figure 20.5), because these cases need emergency PCI. Furthermore, the ST depression in V1–V2 to V3–V4 in the case of LCX occlusion (mirror pattern) usually presents in the hiperacute phase-evident ST depression in V1 without final positive T wave. In contrast, the ST depression in V1–V2 to V4–V5 in the case of LAD subocclusion never/nearly never presents with evident ST depression in V1 (compare Figures 20.5 with 20.6B, and with 20.20). Furthermore, in cases of LAD subocclusion, the T wave in V2–V3 is more positive. Some hours after the onset of ACS, cases with LCX occlusion may present final positive T wave (ST depressed T positive) as a mirror pattern of evolving lateral MI. Figure 20.22 shows the various culprit coronary arteries found in cases of isolated ST depression in V1–V4 in the Triton 38 TIMI trial (Pride *et al.* 2010) (see below).

In some phases of STEMI, ECG patterns other than ST elevation may be seen, including the following:
• In general, only **for a very brief period, the first recorded ECG change during hyperacute ischemia is a change in the T wave morphology (wider and peaked and often taller)** accompanied by an increase in the QT interval (Kenigsberg *et al.* 2007) (Figures 20.4B-1 and 20.12). This is because the first area of left ventricle to be affected by the ischemia is the subendocardium, and often the tall T wave is the ECG pattern of subendocardial ischemia (see Figures 13.6B, 13.7B, and 13.10). Sometimes, an ST depression usually mild may also be seen. This pattern is not frequently seen in the Emergency Department because it is very transient and quickly followed by an ST segment elevation (Figure 20.4B-1). The same occurs in case of abrupt occlusion in human beings not due to classical ACS (coronary spasm, Figure 20.45) or PCI (Figure 20.14).

Atypical patterns of STE-ACS (STEMI)

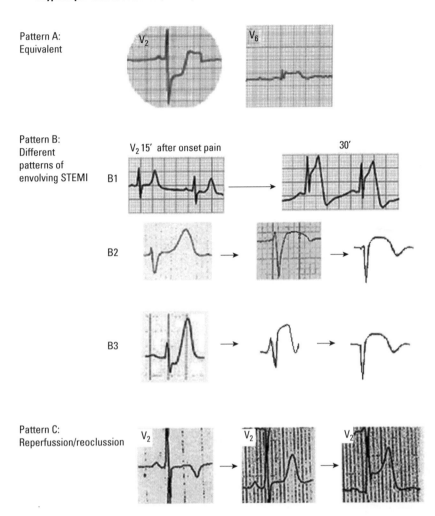

Pattern A:
Equivalent

Pattern B:
Different
patterns of
envolving STEMI

B1

B2

B3

Pattern C:
Reperfussion/reoclussion

Figure 20.4 Atypical patterns of STE-ACS: Pattern A: STEMI equivalent. In the case of LCX occlusion (involvement of LCX). Pattern B: Three patterns of tall and wide T wave as a first sign of ischemia. B-1: Transient pattern followed by ST elevation (STEMI) after a few minutes. B-2 and B-3: Examples of persistent tall T wave (several hours), before complete occlusion and transmural involvement evolving to Q wave MI (see text). Pattern C: deep negative T wave when the pain disappears in case of STEMI (post-ischemic change). However, the pain may appear again (new occlusion due to new thrombus or coronary spasm), and the T wave first pseudonormalizes and later evolves to ST elevation.

• **The presence of this tall and symmetrical T wave**, sometimes with slight ST segment depression or elevation may persist for hours (Figures 20.6 and 20.7) (Sagie *et al*. 1989). According to Birnbaum *et al*. (1993), it corresponds to a grade I of ischemia and in general occurs in patients with an occluded artery but good collaterals (Figures 20.2A and 20.4B-2). A similar pattern in general with mild or even moderate ST depression followed by a tall and wide T wave in V2 to V4–V6 has been recently reported in 2% of patients with LAD occlusion (De Winter *et al*. 2008). In these cases, there are not too many collaterals and the grade of ischemia was probably greater (moderate increase of biomarkers) (Figure 20.4B-3). The most logical explanation for tall T waves and mild ST depression is that there is a delay in the repolarization in the subendocardial area, when only a tall T wave is present (Sagie *et al*. 1989), in addition to small change in the shape of the transmembrane action potential (TAP) of this area when there is also mild ST depression. The sum of this slightly changed TAP (small area with slow ascent and longer duration) with the normal TAP of the subepicardium

explains both the ST depression and the peaked and tall T waves in the ECG tracing. This situation of predominant subendocardial ischemia without transmural involvement may also exist in cases of total occlusion of the LAD if important collateral circulation/preconditioning is present (De Winter *et al*. 2008; Gorgels 2009) (see Figures 13.6 and 20.6).

• **During the evolution of a STEMI due to a LAD proximal occlusion**, when the artery has been opened either spontaneously or after treatment (drugs) (fibrinolysis or PCI) without the pattern evolving to Q wave MI (Figure 20.4C), and once the pain has vanished, **a striking negative T wave** (>3–5 mm) may appear. This indicates an open artery or, at least, in the case of an occluded artery, a sign that a very good collateral circulation/preconditioning exists. However, it is not a guarantee that the problem is resolved. In fact, it was considered in the past a pattern of impending MI (De Zwan *et al*. 1982) because in the past, the artery often reoccludes spontaneously (see Figure 20.4C). In this case, if the patient presents again angina the ECG changes, first presents pseudonormaliza-

A

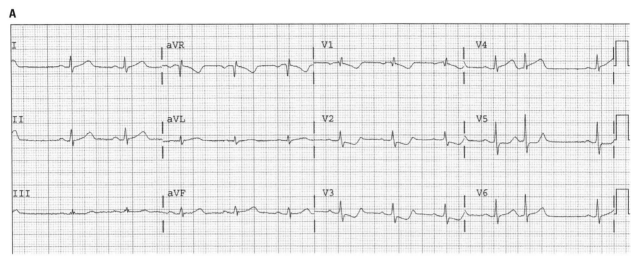

B

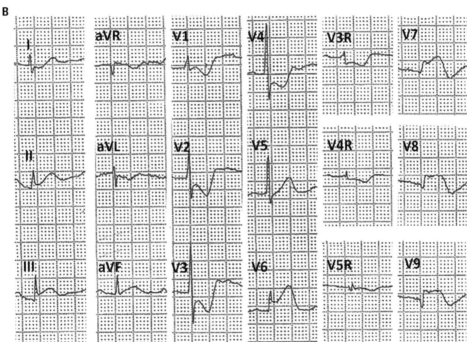

Figure 20.5 (A) ECG recorded during chest pain in a patient with acute occlusion of the LCX coronary artery. No significant lesions were present in the other coronary arteries. The ECG shows ST depression in leads V1–V4 and only minor ST elevation, not fulfilling (STEMI) criteria, in leads I, aVL, and V6. (B) A similar case in which ST depression in many precordial leads is seen (V1–V5) with mild ST elevation in II, III, aVF. The recording of V7–V9 visualizes the STEMI better. However, it may be diagnosed already by 12-lead ECG and corresponds to true STEMI equivalent.

tion of the T wave sometimes with the presence of negative U wave (Figure 20.26) and later reappearance of ST segment elevation.

Therefore, patients with deep negative T waves in the right precordial leads who have had anginal pain in the hours previously should be submitted to coronarography as soon as possible. This situation is not, however, considered an emergency, unlike the case of a clear ST elevation, because the presence of a deep negative T wave indicates

that the myocardial tissue is at this moment more or less perfused (open artery).

Furthermore, once the acute phase has passed, this pattern may remain for a long time, even years, without requiring urgent study. The resolution of the patterns to a normal positive T wave, however, is a sign of good prognosis (Tamura *et al.* 1999).

Recently, it has been demonstrated in a few cases by correlation with cardiovascular magnetic resonance

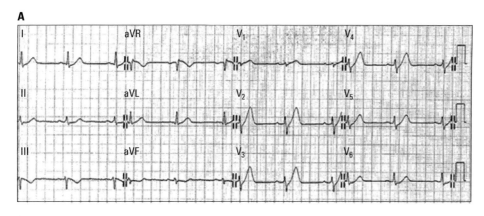

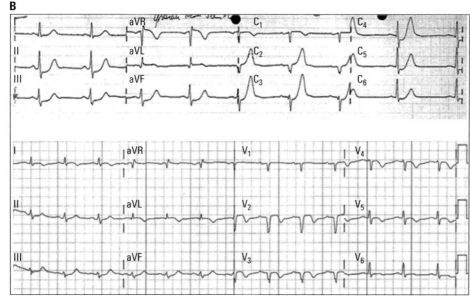

Figure 20.6 Two cases of STE-ACS with persistent pattern of tall T wave in V1 to V3–V4 in (A) without evident ST shifts (as cases of Sagie *et al.* 1989), and in (B) with some ST depression in many precordials (as cases of Dressler and Roesler 1947 and De Winter *et al.* 2008). Both present with proximal occlusion of the LAD without important collateral circulation and non-important involvement in RC and LCX. The implantation of one stent in LAD proximal solves the problem in both cases but the patient of case B finally presented with a QS pattern of myocardial infarction in right precordials (see below).

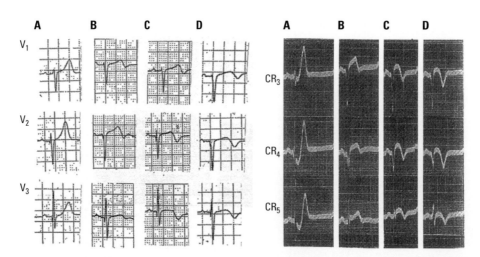

Figure 20.7 Left: Patient with acute chest pain and evolving anterior wall myocardial infarction. (A) During prolonged chest pain showing positive peaked T waves without ST segment elevation. (B and C) ECG recorded 12 hours (ST elevation) and 24 hours (negative T wave) later. (D) ECG one week later with QS and deep negative T wave (Sagie *et al.* 1989. Reproduced with permission from the American College of Chest Physicians). Right: Patient with acute chest pain. (A) Three hours after the onset of chest pain. See ST depression plus very tall T wave. (B) Changes in QRS (QS and ST elevation) were not present until 18 hours after the onset of symptoms. (C and D) Progressive inversion of the previously high T waves (Reproduced with permission from Dressler and Roesler 1947) (see text).

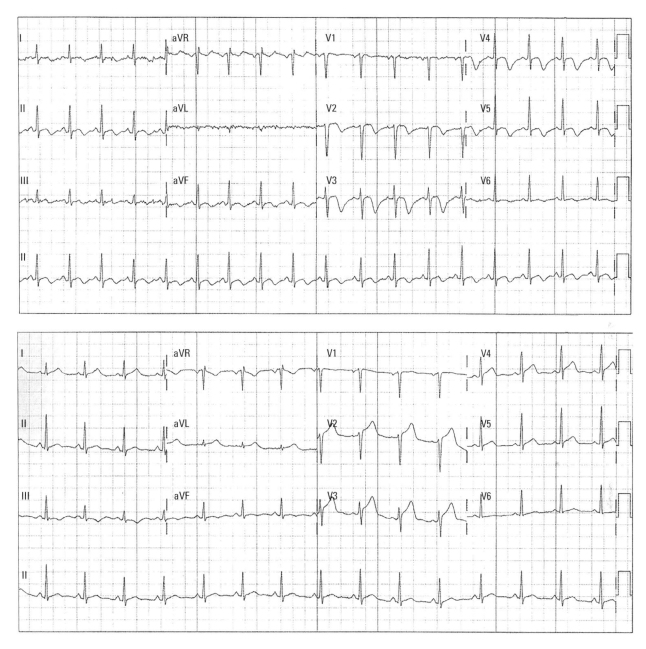

Figure 20.8 Top panel. ECG corresponding to a patient who reports prolonged anginal pain before hospital admission but who is currently asymptomatic. It is a typical post reperfusion pattern of the long anterior descending artery (the negative T wave also affects the inferior wall). Lower panel. ECG recorded during pain recurrence. An occlusion pattern of the anterior descending artery is observed.

(CMR) that in these cases of deep negative T waves in right precordial leads considered an atypical pattern of STEMI (Figure 20.4C), there is transmural evidence of myocardial edema in certain parts of the left ventricular wall (Migliore *et al.* 2011) (Figure 13.7E).

In the case that STEMI evolves to Q wave MI, obviously the pattern of deep negative T wave is observed, but with QS pattern and the negativity of T wave is due to recording of LV intraventricular pattern (see before) (Figure 13.6E).

Differential diagnosis

It is important to remember that without clinical information, even expert cardiologists will have problems in diagnosis of some cases of ST elevation (Jayroe *et al.* 2009). One of the most important problems is related to differential diagnosis of the asymptomatic cases with mild ST elevation and often with "r" in V1–V2. These cases may be seen in the Brugada syndrome, pectus excavatum, and in athletes (Figure 7.16).

Clinical and prognostic implications

The characteristics of the ST elevation and mirror patterns are relevant when localizing the occlusion and area at risk, quantifying of the ischemic burden, and detecting the grade of severity of ischemia.

Location of occlusion

Many authors (Birnbaum *et al.* 1993; Engelen *et al.* 1999; Tierala *et al.* 2009; Kanei *et al.* 2010), in addition to our group (Fiol *et al.* 2004, 2009, 2020) among others, have demonstrated the usefulness of **ECG-coronarography correlations to locate the place of culprit artery** and the site of occlusion. This has been discussed in detail in Chapter 13. Figure 13.38 shows the algorithm for predicting the LAD occlusion site in cases of an ACS with STE in the precordial leads and Figure 13.39 represents the algorithm to follow in cases of ACS with STE in the inferior leads to distinguish between RCA and LCX occlusion. Figures 13.40–13.52 show examples of different ECG patterns according to the coronary artery involved and the site of the occlusion. **In our experience, these ECG criteria have high statistical value** (see Figures 11.37 and 11.38), as has also been demonstrated by other investigators for the same or other algorithms (see Chapter 13).

Usually, the involvement of the LMT is expressed by suboclusion of the artery because acute complete occlusion in general rapidly triggers cardiogenic shock and ventricular fibrillation, and the patient dies before reaching the Emergency Department. However, some cases of complete occlusion of the LMT if arrive at Hospital very early may survive. Fiol *et al.* (2012) have documented 9 patients, 8 with ECG of STEMI, and 1 resembling the ECG of LMT suboclusion as a result of great collateral circulation. Four survived (Figure 20.3). The ECG pattern of STEMI is similar to proximal occlusion (before S1) of very long LAD, often with right bundle branch block (RBBB) and ST elevation in precordials and leads I and aVL, and ST depression in the inferior leads. Usually, in V1 and aVR, there is no ST elevation due to the involvement of LCX that depresses the ST in these leads and compensates the ST deviation (Figure 20.3), that usually is found in case of proximal LAD occlusion (see later), except in cases of large conal artery that also perfuses the high septum (Ben-Gal *et al.* 1997). In LMT occlusion, the hemodynamic state is poorest, especially in the absence of very dominant RCA.

All these criteria, that allows us to localize the culprit artery and even the place of occlusion in LAD, RCA, LCX, and LMT, have some limitations (Huang *et al.* 2011) that are a consequence of the varied anatomy of the coronary arteries, the cancellation of ST vectors, the quick change of location of occlusion during treatment, and also in cases of LAD occlusion the incorrect placement of precordial electrodes because the ECG pattern may change from one location to another (see Figure 13.79). Therefore, before trying to localize the culprit artery with the ECG, we have to take into account the following considerations:

• **In the case of proximal LAD occlusion before S1**, often there is no ST elevation in V1, in spite of proximal LAD occlusion to S1 (Figure 13.41). This occurs in cases with a large conal branch of the RCA (Ben-Gal *et al.* 1997) that perfuses the high septum together with the first septal branch (S1), and due to this double perfusion, the high septum does not become ischemic.

• If a very long LAD wrapping the apex and perfusing a large part of inferior wall is found, the ST vector of ischemia may points downward instead of upward, which usually happens in cases of LAD occlusion proximal to D1 (Figure 13.42), and consequently an ST depression in the inferior leads may not be present (Sasaki *et al.* 2001).

• Often in cases of proximal LAD occlusion (proximal to D1) (Figures 13.37 and 13.41), ST elevation takes place only in V1–V3, with ST depression in V5–V6. However, this does not always mean that the involved area is small (ST elevation only in V1–V3). The mirror pattern (ST depression) has to be considered as ST elevation equivalent. In some leads, even the lack of ST shifts may be the expression of a vector's cancellation (Zhong-Qun *et al.* 2009).

• **The ECG patterns usually change very quickly with treatment**. In a matter of minutes, ST elevation can change from being present in V1–V5 (extensive involvement), to ST elevation only in V1–V2 (Figure 20.9). In this figure, an extensive anterior involvement (A), probably proximal to S1 and D1, is shown to change into a limited anterior involvement probably distal to D1 (B). Therefore, the period of time between ECG recording and coronarography is crucial, because the site of occlusion can only be located using ECG if the tracing is recorded practically at the same time as the coronarography.

• Quantification of the ischemic burden based on ST deviation

Although the location of the occlusion may indicate the approximate area at risk, an understanding of how to quantify the ischemic burden and calculate the size of area at risk using different risk scores is important. ST deviations are an important parameter (TIMI score, PREDICT score, GUSTO score, GRACE score, etc.) (Fiol-Sala *et al.* 2020). A score based on the percentage of left ventricle area infarcted according to Selvester score has also been reported (Aldrich *et al.* 1988).

The TIMI risk score is the most commonly used system for prognosis and includes ST deviations as one of the parameters to be assessed (Antman *et al.* 2000; Morrow *et al.* 2000). The score derived from the GUSTO trial (Hathaway *et al.* 1998) for estimating 30-day mortality from initial clinical and ECG variables shows that despite the fact that some limitations exist, as seen in proximal RCA occlusion that may mask the spread of ischemia because of isodiphasic ST present in V1, the sum of the ST

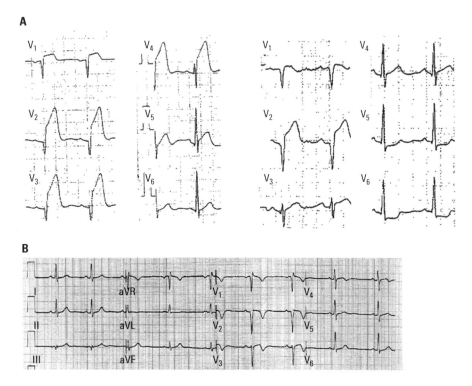

Figure 20.9 (A) Left: ECG of a patient in hyperacute phase of acute coronary syndrome (ACS) with great involvement of anteroseptal zone. Observe ST segment elevation from V1 to V5. Right: After an hour of fibrinolytic treatment, the area at risk decreases significantly, being limited exclusively to septum (ST segment elevation from V1 to V2 with ST segment depression in V5–V6). (B) In a chronic phase, the patient presented with an anteroapical infarction.

changes in all leads may estimate the degree myocardium at risk. More than 15 mm of ST deviation usually represents an important area at risk.

• Grade of severity of ischemia

The morphology of QRS-ST may indicate the degree of ischemia. According to the Birnbaum–Sclarovsky ischemic grading system (Birnbaum *et al.* 1993), grade I ischemia presents with a tall persistent T wave, generally without mild ST depression; grade 2 presents with an ST elevation without distortion of the QRS complex; and grade 3 presents with an ST elevation that sweeps the QRS complex upward and provokes a distortion of it and with ratio J point/R wave >0.5 (see Figure 20.36) (Figure 20.2).

The cases described by De Winter *et al.* (2008) that also present with a tall T wave as the most evident ECG change (predominant subendocardial involvement) are most likely more than grade I of ischemia. The presence of associated mild ST depression that often occurs before the tall T wave may be due to a higher grade of subendocardial ischemia than just tall T waves (Sagie *et al.* 1989).

Global prognostic value of ECG changes at admission (Fiol-Sala *et al.* 2020)

The in-hospital prognosis of both STEMI and NSTEMI has improved considerably with new thrombolytic and antiplatelet drugs and primary PCI. In both types of ACS, the GRACE score based on clinical ECG and blood tests (Eagle *et al.* 2004) has been recommended for risk stratification and the evaluation of best management.

We will now summarize **the most important ECG parameters that are useful for global prognosis**.

• The cases caused by a proximal occlusion of LAD, a very dominant RCA occlusion (especially when the obstruction is proximal to the right ventricle branches), or proximal very dominant LCX occlusion are the cases at higher risk.

• The sum in millimeters of the ST segment elevations and depressions is useful in assessing the size of the myocardial area at risk (Hathaway *et al.* 1998) (see above).

• ST segment morphology is also useful. Cases with the poorest prognosis are those presenting with a high ST segment elevation, with distortion of the final portion of the QRS complex (Figure 20.2C).

• ECG signs of poor prognosis in the STEMI evolution of a patient who has been admitted to the hospital with STEMI, the following ECG changes can depict prognosis both in the short and long term:

• Persistent sinus tachycardia or development of rapid supraventricular or ventricular arrhythmias has a poor prognosis.

• Persistent ST segment elevation without development of a negative T wave after one week is a marker of poor prognosis and of the potential for subsequent cardiac rupture (see Mechanical complications).

• Currently, the occurrence of primary ventricular fibrillation during the first week of evolution of an acute infarction with ST segment elevation does not influence the prognosis at follow-up. Therefore, the implantation of an ICD is not recommended (Bayés de Luna and Baranchuk 2017).

• The presence of wide QRS is a sign of poor prognosis. This especially includes the development of complete bundle branch block, especially RBBB in anterior infarctions or advanced atrioventricular (AV) block in inferolateral infarctions (Lie *et al.* 1975). The development of left bundle branch block (LBBB) is much rarer because the left bundle receives double perfusion. Currently, it is considered that LBBBs that do not present with the ST/T changes described by Sgarbossa *et al.* (1996) do not appear to represent a very bad prognosis, especially when LBBB is of transient nature.

• In general, the evidence of STEMI of the anteroapical zone is a strong determinant of lower ejection fraction (EF) and a poorer prognosis than STEMI of the inferolateral zone, even with similar amounts of myocardial necrosis detected by enzyme level assessment (Elsman *et al.* 2006). However, it has been reported that MI of the inferior wall presents with sudden death more often than MI of the lateral wall (Pascale *et al.* 2009).

• Evidence of an extensive Q wave infarction also implies a poor prognosis. Data may be derived from the ECG when a large number of involved leads are found. Furthermore, a high QRS score estimated in the first ECG after hospital admission is an independent predictor of incomplete ST recovery and 30-day complications in the STE-ACS treated with primary PCI (Uyarel *et al.* 2006).

• The presence of a Q wave does not always imply irreversible damage. Reperfusion therapy should not be ruled out simply because a Q wave is present (Wellens and Connover 2006).

• In patients with normal intraventricular conduction, a 30-day mortality is higher among those with an initial Q wave accompanying ST segment elevation in the infarct leads (Wong *et al.* 2006).

• Recently, Petrina *et al.* (2006) have identified the ECG changes in the admission ECG in patients with acute MI that better predict prognosis by means of a literature review. These include ST segment deviations, arrhythmias, and QRS duration (see Fiol-Sala *et al.* 2020).

• STEMI in patients with multivessel occlusion: Which is the culprit artery?

When an STEMI occurs in clinical practice, a critical occlusion has often developed in just one culprit artery although in many cases, multivessel disease is present. There is no general agreement how to proceed, but it seems the best approach is to open only the culprit artery in the first procedure (Widimsky and Holmes 2011). However, in the case of hemodynamic impairment or the presence of more than one critical occlusion, opening more than one artery may be indicated.

What is most important in the catheterization laboratory, when faced with STEMI and multivessel disease, is that the interventional cardiologist can, thanks to the correct and quick interpretation of the ECG, correctly select the coronary arteries in which the PCI must be performed. With the coronaroangiographic results at hand, the ECG provides important information for the identification of the culprit artery in these cases. Unfortunately, this information is often underused in clinical decision-making (Nikus *et al.* 2004). Figure 20.10 shows one example of the relevance of this approach.

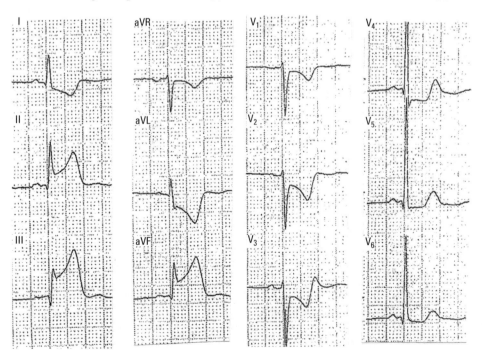

Figure 20.10 Case of right coronary artery (RCA) occlusion (ST depression, ST elevation III > II). However, there is ST depression from V1 to V6 that is unusual in isolated RCA occlusion. This suggests LAD involvement (95% proximal to D1). Therefore, in this case, it is advisable to perform double percutaneous coronary intervention (PCI) (RCA + LAD), although the culprit artery is the RCA because the LAD has a critical occlusion.

Close collaboration between clinicians, experts in ECG, and interventional cardiologists should be emphasized. Nowadays, with modern technology, it is possible to obtain an expert opinion on an ECG interpretation from a distance in seconds (Leibrandt *et al.* 2000). The transmission of ECGs directly to a consulting center with web-browsing capabilities may facilitate immediately starting a revascularization procedure in the appropriate culprit artery (Adams *et al.* 2006; Sejersten *et al.* 2008; Ting *et al.* 2008; Ducas *et al.* 2012; Al-Zaiti *et al.* 2013; Kerem *et al.* 2014).

ECG changes during fibrinolysis and percutaneous coronary intervention (Figure 20.11)

Fibrinolysis

During fibrinolysis, the most typical ECG changes are the following:

• Rapid resolution of ST segment elevation is a very sensitive sign of reperfusion, especially in anteroapical infarction. It has been recently published that the lack of resolution of concomitant ST depression in mirror leads is a prognostic marker of death at 90 days (Tjandrawidjaja *et al.* 2010).

• The early development (within the first 12 hours following fibrinolysis) of a negative and usually deep T wave in the leads in which an ST segment elevation was initially observed in patients with an anterior infarction is a specific marker of reperfusion and good prognosis (Doevendans *et al.* 1995).

• The presence of Q wave in the admittance ECG and lower ST segment resolution despite early infarct artery patency are markers of poor tissue reperfusion and epicardial recanalization (Wong *et al.* 1999).

• Efficient reperfusion of the RCA shows a highly specific association with sinus bradycardia and, sometimes, AV block (Zehender *et al.* 1991).

• The twofold increase in premature ventricular complexes (PVCs), the development of accelerated idioventricular rhythm, and runs of non-sustained ventricular tachycardia are indicative of successful reperfusion (reperfusion arrhythmias) (Wellens *et al.* 2003). In contrast, monomorphic sustained ventricular tachycardia is not a sign of reperfusion (Fiol *et al.* 2002).

• Vectorcardiographic dynamic monitoring of the QRS–T loop is a non-invasive technique that provides a higher positive predictive value for the detection of reperfusion (Dellborg *et al.* 1991).

Percutaneous coronary intervention (PCI)

The most typical ECG changes are the following:

• A few seconds after PCI, small changes in the ECG appear (lengthening of the QT interval immediately followed by the appearance of a symmetric T wave (Kenigsberg *et al.* 2007) (Figure 20.12). In some cases with a negative T wave, this may pseudonormalize (Figure 20.13), but only rarely does clear ST elevation appear. This indicates a transmural involvement (left ventricle not protected by collaterals).

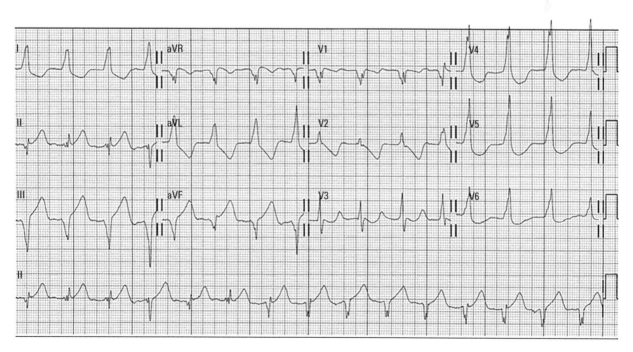

Figure 20.11 A 45-year-old man with occlusion of the posterior descending coronary artery. During the PCI procedure, intraluminal thrombus and the appearance on the 12-lead-ECG of accelerated idioventricular rhythm with frequent fusion beats. Note how in the narrower QRS complexes there is elevation of ST-T in II, III, aVF and a mirror image in V1–V3.

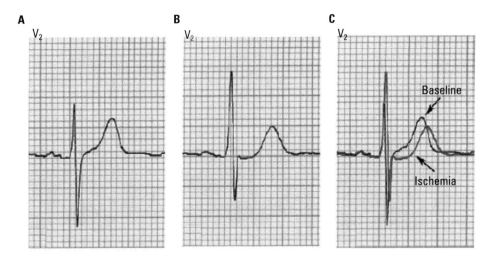

Figure 20.12 (A) Single ECG complex from lead V_2 obtained under baseline conditions, before the start of percutaneous coronary intervention (PCI) of the left anterior descending coronary artery (LAD). (B) Single ECG complex from the same lead shown in (A) is displayed 25 sec after balloon inflation in the proximal LAD. The QT interval is seen to prolong by 44 ms. (C) The two complexes seen in (A) and (B) are superimposed to better illustrate ischemia-induced changes showing prolongation of QT interval and symmetric T wave (Reproduced with permission from Kenigsberg *et al.* 2007).

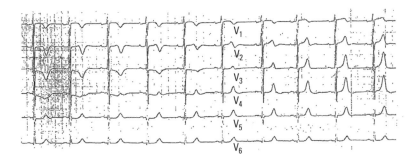

Figure 20.13 This patient presents with a negative T wave just during percutaneous coronary intervention (PCI) that pseudonormalizes the T wave during the inflation period (see text).

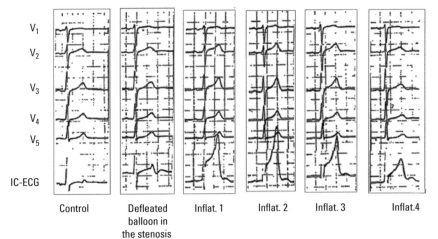

Figure 20.14 ECG recorded on precordial leads and intracoronary ECG that shows the small changes of T wave in precordial leads (see after inflation 1, peaked T wave that after successive inflations is less evident). However, the decrease of ST changes due to preconditioning after several inflations is much better seen in intracoronary ECG (IC-ECG) (Reproduced with permission from Koning *et al.* 1993).

• After successive and prolonged coronary occlusion during PCI, a progressive decrease in ST elevation (ischemia) due to collaterals or probably more to preconditioning can be seen with intracoronary ECG (equivalent to epicardial ECG) (Koning *et al.* 1993; Tomai *et al.* 1999) (Figure 20.14).

• When the presence of clear signs of localized wall motion abnormalities is noted during PCI, usually there is ST segment elevation, as seen in the ECG, and it has been shown that this is correlated with the extension of the asynergy (Cohen *et al.* 1987; Santoro *et al.* 1998).

• Occasionally, peri-procedural infarctions occur that are generally small but represent a marker of poor prognosis (see Peri-procedural myocardial infarction).

ECG in acute coronary syndrome with no ST elevation (NSTEMI) (Table 20.4)

Obviously, **all atypical cases of STEMI that present with non-STE changes have to be excluded** (see Figure 20.4). The depth of the negative T wave in atypical ECG patterns of STEMI, especially in case of LAD occlusion, is usually much more significant than in NSTEMI (compare Figures 13.11 with 13.12 and 20.15).

ECG patterns (see Chapter 13, ST segment in ACS and Figures 20.16–20.26)

According the new universal definition of MI (Thygesen *et al.* 2019), the **ECG manifestations of acute ischemia in patients with NSTEMI include** a new horizontal or downsloping ST depression ≥0.5 mm in two contiguous leads and/or new T wave inversion ≥1 mm in two contiguous leads with a prominent R wave, or R/S ratio > 1 and/or negative T wave in two or more contiguous leads (see Table 13.1). We would like to make some comments on this statement (see also Chapter 13, Changes of repolarization: T wave).

• The **presence of a persistent and negative/flat T wave in the evolution of NSTEMI** as an isolated finding without ST changes exists when anginal pain has already disappeared (Figures 13.12 and 20.25), and corresponds to a post-ischemic change not to acute crisis of ischemia. However, this does not signify the problem is over. Often, an important and even ulcerated subocclusion persists, even the artery is at least partially open, and not complete transmural involvement takes place. Therefore, a new crisis of acute ischemia may occur, indicating intensive treatment and hospitalization. Although coronarography is not needed as an emergency procedure, it should be performed as soon as possible (Figures 13.12 and 20.15).

• **During the appearance of dynamic ST depression,** changes may be seen in some leads from a positive T wave to flat/mildly negative T wave, but it is a dynamic and very transient change that is never found isolated, but rather is always accompanied in many leads by ST segment depression. This is clearly demonstrated using the MIDA method of recording (Figure 20.16).

ECG characteristics of NSTEMI with ST depression (see Chapter 13)

We consider two types according to the number of leads with ST depression: extensive involvement and regional involvement.

Table 20.4 ECG patterns in non-ST elevation myocardial infarction (50% of ACS). Non-STEMI: non-occluded artery and non-transmural involvement. Without pain, the ECG may change sometimes dramatically and even may be normal (Figure 20.17)

ST depression ≈ 70%	**Extensive involvement: ST↓ in ≥7 leads with ST↑ in 1–2 leads (aVR>V1):**
	• ST↑aVR: ST↑aVR >1 mm: severe LM or proximal 3VD subocclusion
	• ST↑aVR ≤1 mm: severe proximal LAD subocclusion or LCX subocclusion or less severe 3VD/LM
	• The ECG pattern of repolarization in precordial leads presents different grades of ST↓ morphology. The most possible correlation with the culprit artery, with limitations, to be confirmed in larger studies, are the following:
	Lead aVR · Mid-precordial leads
	A. ST↑ > 1 mm · A. LM (Figure 20.18) LM/3VD (Figure 20.19) 3VD (Figure 20.20)
	B. ST↑ ≤ 1 mm · B. Usually 3VD/may be non-severe LM Also ST↓ in I and aVL (Figure 13.30)
	C. ST↑ < 1 mm · C. Figure 20.21. Severe LAD proximal subocclusion
	D. ST↑ < 1 mm · D. LCX proximal subocclusion. Also, ST↓ in II and aVF
	Regional involvement: ST↓ in <7 leads
	• ST↓ in V1–V4. May be STEMI (LCX) or NSTEMI (usually proximal LAD subocclusion (see text))
	• ST↓ in inferior leads: RCA/LCX subocclusion (exceptionally occluded with collaterals/preconditioning) (Figure 20.22)
	• ST↓ in V4–V6: and often in some FP leads: The culprit artery is RCA or LCX. In some cases, distal LAD. Often there is 2/3VD (Figures 20.23–20.25)
Flat/negative T wave (≈15% of cases)	May be seen in different locations: V1–V3 proximal LAD (Figure 13.12); V4–V6 (distal LAD/LCX), etc.
Changes of U wave (<1%)	May be seen as a post-ischemic pattern in case of LAD involvement (Figure 20.15), and also in case of acute ischemia (negative U with pseudonormalization of T wave) (Figure 20.26)
ECG normal or unmodified (≈15%)	The ECG may be normal even during pain. Usually, ACS with normal ECG during pain has good prognosis. Many cases with 3VD or LM trunk without pain present with normal ECG (Figure 20.17)

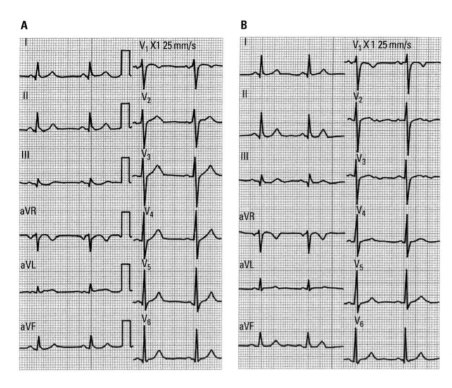

Figure 20.15 A 46-year-old patient with previous precordial pain. The ECG (B) without pain showed very discrete changes in V2–V3 leads (slightly negative U wave with somewhat positive T wave) (see V2–V3). These small changes are significant when compared with the previous ECG taken few months ago (A). The exercise stress test was positive and the coronary angiography showed proximal LAD stenosis resolved by percutaneous coronary intervention (PCI). The subsequent ECG was the same as the initial one (A).

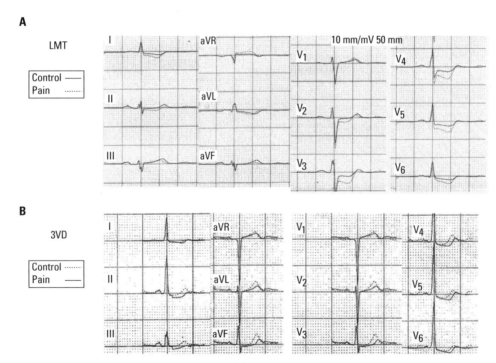

Figure 20.16 (A and B) Changes of ST/T during angina crisis in the case of left main trunk (LMT) subocclusion (A) and severe three-vessel disease (B). See the differences in (A) and (B) before and after pain. It is evident, especially in LMT subocclusion, that the increase of ST depression is accompanied by negative or nearly negative final T wave.

• **In the case of extensive involvement, in the presence of pain, there are ≥7 leads with ST depression and there is ST elevation in aVR and often V1 (aVR > V1)** (Kosuge *et al.* 2011; Yamaji *et al.* 2001). It is advised (Nikus *et al.* 2010, 2011) that the threshold for ST depression in precordial leads be adjusted for age and sex, and that the threshold for ST elevation in aVR be specified as 0.05 mV. In around 50% of cases, the ECG in the absence of pain will be normal or nearly normal (Figure 20.17).

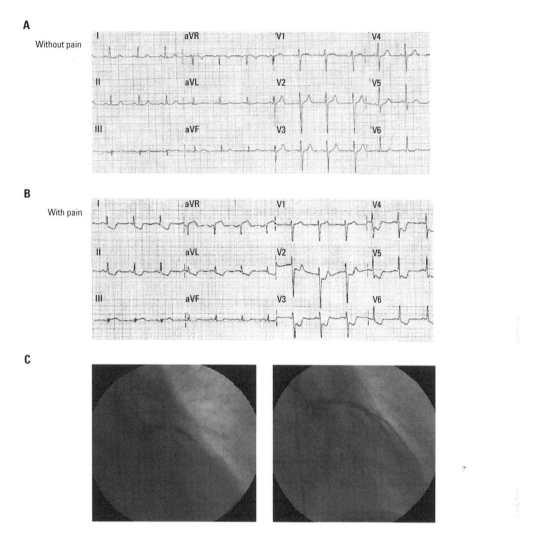

Figure 20.17 (A) ECG without pain is practically normal. (B) ECG during pain shows ST segment depression and inverted T waves in more than eight leads, maximally in leads V4–V5 where there is no positive T wave and ST segment elevation >1 mm in lead aVR (circumferential subendocardial involvement). (C) Coronary angiography shows tight stenosis in the left main coronary artery before and after primary percutaneous coronary intervention (PCI).

This ECG pattern may be seen in LMT subocclusion, three-vessel disease subocclusion, and isolated but tight and proximal LAD and rarely in proximal subocclusion of large LCX. The ST depression is seen especially in V3–V6 and I, II, and aVF and/or aVL; ST elevation in aVR exists in severe LMT/3VD, usually >1 mm (Figures 20.16–20.20). If there is an increased heart rate, the upsloping ST depression may be influenced by the tachycardia (Birnbaum *et al.* 2011). Although there is no definitive statement clarifying the culprit artery in the case of diffuse ST depression in >7 leads with ST elevation in aVR, we suggest, based on recent papers (Kosuge *et al.* 2011) and our experience, the following (Table 20.4).

• **Cases with severe LMT subocclusion** (>75%) and **LMT equivalent** (LAD+LCX proximal severe subocclusion) **or severe three-vessel disease subocclusion** (>90% stenosis LAD, LCX, and RCA) present during pain ST elevation in

aVR>1 mm (80% SE, 93% SP) (Kosuge *et al.* 2011) (Figures 20.17–20.19). It is important to remember that aVR is a mirror pattern of a lead located between I and II in which ST depression would always be present (see Figure 6.11) (Table 20.4). Usually, the final positive T wave in precordials if it exists is mild (Figure 20.17). In the case of LMT subocclusion, although sometimes the ST depression in precordials is ≤2 mm, the ST elevation in aVR is >1 mm (Figure 20.18).

• Cases with proximal three-vessel subocclusion/occlusion sometimes present with an important upsloping ST depression with a final tall positive T wave (Figure 20.10).

• Cases with less severe LMT or three-vessel disease may present ST depression in precordials with a small positive T wave and ST elevation in aVR<1 mm.

• Compared with severe LMT or three-vessel disease, **cases of severe proximal LAD subocclusion** (Figure 20.20) present with fewer changes in the frontal plane

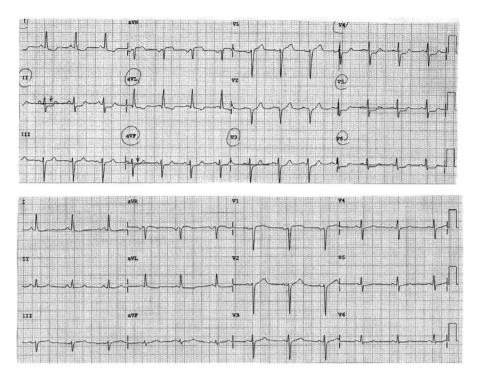

Figure 20.18 The ECG taken during pain shows ST segment depression not very prominent (<2 mm) in V2–V6 and I and aVL but with clear (>1 mm) ST elevation in aVR. The patient presented with severe left main trunk (LMT) subocclusion. The ECG after pain shows flat T wave in leads with previous ST depression.

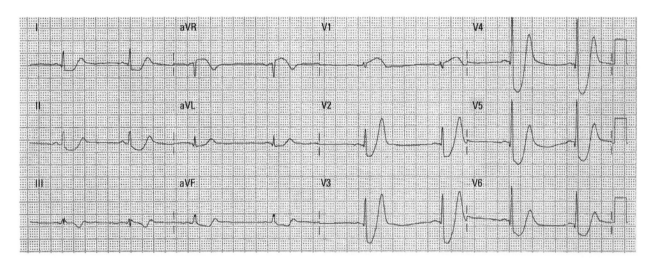

Figure 20.19 The ECG of a patient with an NSTE-ACS and three-vessel disease with proximal subocclusion of LAD and LCX that shows during angina a huge ST segment depression in many leads more prominent in precordial leads V3–V5 with tall positive T wave and with ST segment elevation in aVR and V1. This case is similar to that shown in Figure 20.21, but the presence of ST elevation in aVR > 1 mm in this case is in favor of proximal three-vessel disease.

(especially less ST elevation in aVR). In the horizontal plane, the ST depression in precordials is upsloping and in general not very important, followed by a final positive tall T wave. This pattern may be also seen in some cases of three-vessel disease, but in these cases, there is usually more ST elevation in aVR (compare Figures 20.20 and 20.27A) (Table 20.4). This type of ECG pattern indicates that despite severe occlusion, there is no transmural homogeneous involvement of the left ventricular wall by the ischemia. In fact, this pattern corresponds to the De Winter pattern (Figure 20.6B). Without treatment, or often despite treatment, it evolves to "q" wave and deep negative T wave and this means that NSTEMI has converted into a STEMI, and a Q wave of MI usually appears (Figures 20.8B), as happened with the cases reported by Dressler and Roesler (1947) in the pre-fibrinolytic era, which evolved to a Q wave extensive anteroseptal MI (Figure 20.7 right).

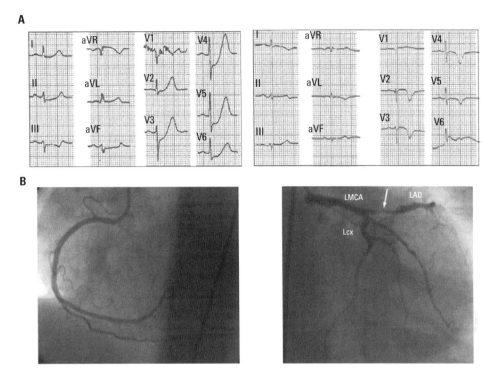

Figure 20.20 (A) ECG showing diffuse ST segment depressions with positive T waves in the inferior leads II, III, and aVF and in leads V2–V6 besides ST segment elevation in lead aVR. ST elevation in lead aVR not >1 mm. The ST segment in lead V1 cannot be reliably analyzed because of technical artifacts. (B) Right coronary artery with a large posterior descending (PD). No significant stenoses are present. (C) Left anterior oblique caudal angiographic view shows a very tight stenosis in the proximal LAD (arrow). (D) Discharge ECG of the patient showing Q wave in V1, V2, and inverted T waves in leads V2–V6 and in leads I and aVL. Probably the patient presented with STEMI with finally residual "q" in V1–V2 and a deep negative T wave in V2–V5 due to final transmural involvement (Adapted with permission from Gul and Nikus 2011).

• Cases of severe proximal predominant LCX subocclusion may also present with slight ST depression in mid-left precordials followed by a tall positive T wave. Compared with the De Winter pattern, a tiny "q" in V1–V3 never appears and ST depression always exist in the left precordials, usually with Rs pattern and especially with a smaller positive T wave (compare Figures 20.6B and 20.21).

Table 20.4 shows all these patterns. However, in spite of **all these considerations, their predictive accuracy still has to be confirmed in a larger trial**.

In cases of regional involvement, the culprit artery is in general a subocclusion of a proximal short LAD, distal LAD, or LCX/RCA. However, sometimes two- or three-vessel disease is responsible. Table 20.4 shows the three groups of pattern that may be found:

• Isolated ST depression in V1–V4 (Figure 20.22); ST depression in V1–V4 corresponds to LAD subocclusion (or total occlusion with collaterals/preconditioning). In general, ST depression in V1 is mild or non-existent (Figure 20.20). It is important to rule out STEMI equivalent (LCX occlusion) (ST depression evident in V1) without positive T wave in V2–V3 and sometimes the ST elevation in inferior or lateral leads is mild or non-existent (Figure 20.5).

• Isolated ST depression in inferior leads (Figure 20.22).
• ST depression in V4–V6 and often in some leads of the frontal plane (including ST elevation in aVR).
• A patient that presents with ST depression in left lateral leads and some frontal leads, without final evident positive T wave, will usually have two- or three-vessel disease and a poor prognosis (Barrabes *et al.* 2000; Nikus *et al.* 2004, Birnbaum and Atar 2006; Birnbaum *et al.* 2011).

In all the cases of regional involvement, it is practically impossible to identify the culprit artery with high predictive accuracy (Figures 20.23–20.25).

ECG characteristics of NSTEMI with flat or negative T wave and negative U wave.

The negative T wave is usually not deep (<2 mm) and is not diffuse. It is more frequently seen in leads with a dominant R wave (Figure 20.26A) but may be also seen in V1–V3 (rS pattern) (Figures 13.12 and 20.15). This type of T wave may become an ST depression with pain or exercise test (Figure 20.25B).

As previously mentioned, the prognosis is better than in cases of ST depression because it usually appears after the cessation of pain (post-ischemic change). If pain reappears, the prognosis depends on whether the ECG pattern remains unmodified (better prognosis) or an ST depression

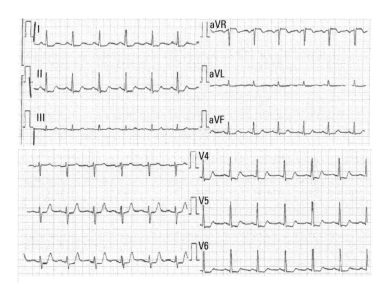

Figure 20.21 ECG of a patient with NSTE-ACS with ST depression in seven leads (V3–V6, I, II, aVF). This corresponds to the type D of Table 20.4 that is usually seen, as in this case, due to proximal subocclusion (95%) of the large left circumflex artery (LCX).

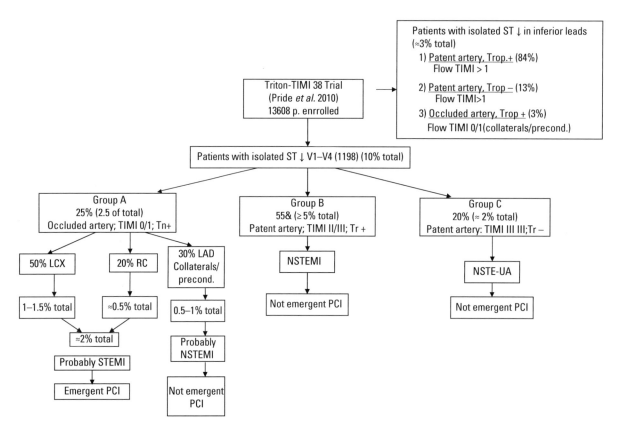

Figure 20.22 Patients of the Triton TIMI 38 trial presenting with isolated ST depression in V1–V4. Note the type of occluded artery, TIMI flow, and troponin levels (positive or negative) and presumably the ACS type, according to the results of the study (Adapted from Pride *et al.* 2010). The information about the presence or not of final positive T wave in the presence of ST depression and in which leads ST depression is more evident is lacking. Probably the cases of LCX or RC total occlusion are true STEMI and need emergent PCI. UA: unstable angina.

appears. However, non-emergency PCI is recommended in the presence of a T wave of these characteristics in the subacute phase of ACS because a coronary subocclusion often exists that sometimes may be tight (see above) (Figures 13.12

and 20.15). In general, biomarkers are negative or in resolution.

Sometimes in case of NSTEMI, the flat/mild negative T wave is accompanied by a negative U wave (Figure 20.15).

With pain

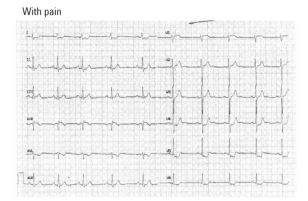

Figure 20.23 Patient with NSTE-ACS with ST depression in <7 leads. In this case, it is difficult to identify the culprit artery that is the right coronary artery (RCA) (95% occlusion).

If a patient who has presented with precordial pain arrives within a few hours at the Emergency Department with a very deep negative T wave without Q wave MI, and with normal or borderline biomarkers, but without pain at entrance, the most probable explanation is that it corresponds to atypical pattern of STEMI and not to an NSTEMI (Figure 20.26A). Sometimes, if pain reappears, the negative T wave pseudonormalizes and negative U wave may appear (Figure 20.26B–D).

Normal ECG

A patient with ACS and a normal ECG at entrance can later evolve to a clear ACS even with LMT subocclusion (Figure 20.17). The ECG may remain normal in 5–10% of cases during an ACS even during crisis of pain. Sometimes the changes of T wave are very subtle, and may be

advisable to compare, if possible, with previous ECG (Figure 20.15). The cases that maintain a normal ECG usually have a good prognosis.

Differential diagnosis

Abnormal ST depression may be seen in many other circumstances (see Table 13.5 and Figure 13.60).

Flat or usually mild negative T waves may also be seen under many other conditions (see Table 13.3 and Figure 13.16). It is important to emphasize that except in cases of perimyocarditis, in which the affected zone may be limited to the subepicardium, in cases such as ischemia or other causes, the ECG pattern of flat/negative T waves is a result of a transmural affected area of the left ventricle presenting with a delayed transmural repolarization (longer TAP) compared with the rest of the left ventricle (see Figures 13.6F and 13.7D).

The prognostic value of ECG changes at admission (Fiol-Sala et al. 2020)

General considerations

• We have already stated that the GRACE score is useful both in STEMI and NSTEMI patients (Eagle *et al.* 2004; Abu-Assi *et al.* 2010). In NSTEMI, to evaluate the risk of death at six months. If the risk is >3%, a coronariography before 96 hours is advised, and according with the results, we will proceed with medical treatment, PCI, or CABG.

• The differentiation between an unstable angina and a non-Q wave infarction is mainly based on the presence or not of increased biomarkers.

• The presence of confounding factors that are relatively frequently found in NSTEMI represents a poor prognosis.

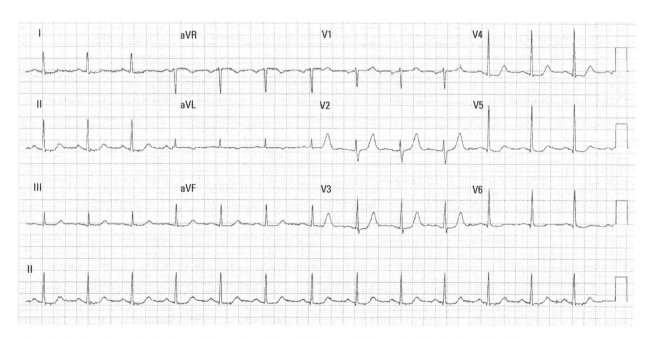

Figure 20.24 In this case that is similar to Figure 20.24, the culprit artery is 95% proximal occlusion of the left circumflex artery (LCX).

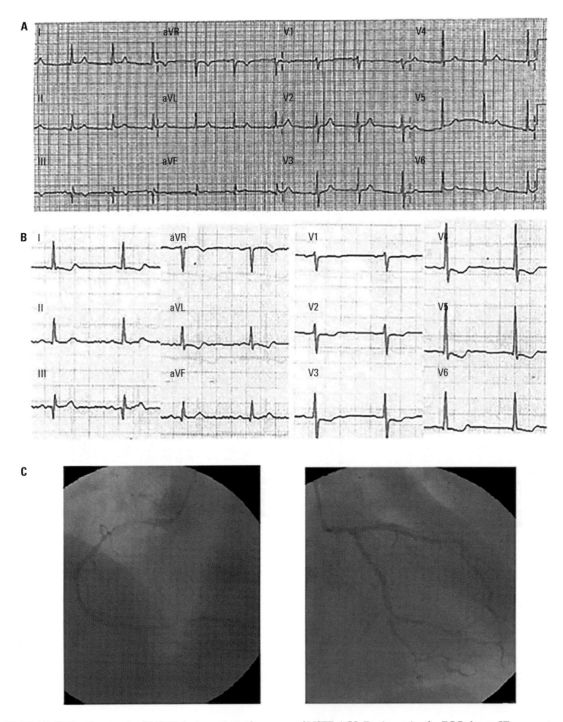

Figure 20.25 (A) ECG without pain. (B) ECG during pain in the course of NSTE-ACS. During pain, the ECG shows ST-segment depression (<3 mm) in V2–V6, I, and aVL. As there is no significant ST-segment depression in II, there is no ST elevation in aVR. (C) Coronary angiography shows three-vessel disease (left: RCA, right: left coronary artery).

- The recording of ST segment monitoring is important for observing changes at follow-up with and without pain.
- Patients may evolve to non-Q wave MI or unstable angina. The differential diagnosis is based on the clinical symptoms, the presence of more severe ECG signs and especially on the levels of biomarkers. In a few number of cases, patients evolve to Q wave MI (Figures 20.6B, 20.7B, and 20.20).

High-risk group
The most important ECG signs of risk are as follows:
- Overall, patients with NSTEMI and ST segment depression upon arrival to the hospital have a worse prognosis

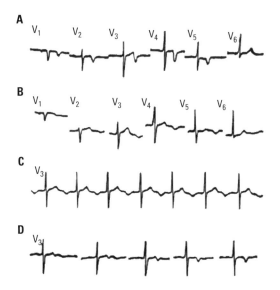

Figure 20.26 (A) Basal ECG (V1–V6) with ECG pattern of very deep negative T wave in a 65-year-old patient with daily crisis of variant angina that always appeared at the same hour. During a crisis (B, C), there is pseudonormalization of the ST segment with an evident negative U wave. A few seconds later, the ECG returns to the original situation (D). The five morphologies in the fourth strip are samples taken minute by minute, with a total duration of pain of 5 min that shows the changes in V3 from positive, T negative U wave during pain to negative T wave after the crises.

than patients with flat negative T wave. These patients often present with angina and more frequently have two- or three-vessel disease as well as many more complications than those presenting with a flat/slight negative T wave that usually are already asymptomatic.

• Patients with deeper ST segment depression in various ECG leads have the worst prognosis. In these patients, an early invasive strategy may reduce the risk of death or MI up to 50% (Holmvang *et al.* 1999).

• Cases that evolve to non-Q wave infarction generally refer more frequent crises of longer duration of angina, and their ECG recordings exhibit ST segment depression more frequently than negative T waves.

• Cases with a deep negative T wave in precordials (V1–V4–V5) present with proximal LAD occlusion already partially open and represent an atypical pattern of STEMI (reperfusion pattern) (Figure 20.4C) (see before).

• The presence of evident ST segment depression in seven or more leads with ST segment elevation in aVR > 1 mm and sometimes V1 (circumferential involvement) (Yamaji *et al.* 2001; Kosuge *et al.* 2011) suggests LMT severe subocclusion and indicates a pattern of bad prognosis (Figure 20.18) (Kosuge *et al.* 2011). The final part of the T wave in V4–V5 is often negative because it is involved in the important ST depression (see Table 20.4).

• There are high-risk patients with tight subocclusion of the proximal LAD and LCX (LMT equivalent), in whom

the ST segment depression is often also very large, but the final T wave is clearly positive in V3–V5 (Figure 20.29).

• The cases with ST segment depression in fewer than seven leads with the worst prognosis present with ST segment depression in V4–V6 and in some frontal leads without a positive T wave or only a mild positive T wave (Birnbaum and Atar 2006) (Figure 20.26).

Low-risk group

The ECG signs of low risk are as follows:

• The cases of NSTE-ACS with only mild flat or negative T waves have a better prognosis. However, non-emergency coronary angiography is recommended, especially when these small changes are present in V1–V3, because sometimes a tight proximal LAD occlusion is present and therefore the patient is at risk for acute ischemia.

• Patients with a normal ECG have the best prognosis (Fiol-Sala *et al.* 2020).

• Patients with unstable angina usually experience fewer pain episodes and their ECGs are less abnormal (flattened or slightly negative, T wave) with normal levels of troponins.

Changes from NSTEMI to STEMI ECG patterns and vice versa

We have explained that the ECG changes of **STEMI are due to transmural homogeneous involvement** usually with a completely occluded artery and that the ECG findings of **NSTEMI are due to incomplete transmural homogeneous involvement** with usually non-total, although it may be tight, occlusion. If, for any reason, a patient with predominant ST depression due to NSTEMI, often with positive terminal T wave, presents spontaneously (acute thrombosis, coronary spasm, or occlusion of a stent) with total occlusion and there is no collateral circulation/preconditioning, an absolute transmural involvement exists and the ECG pattern changes from NSTE to STE (see Figure 20.27). In fact, in the first minutes of STEMI, the only ECG change is a tall/wider T wave that evolves quickly to ST elevation (transmural homogeneous involvement). However, sometimes the subendocardial involvement that is important persists because the artery, usually the LAD, is not completely occluded, and the ECG not only presents with a tall T wave but also some ST segment depression. We have already mentioned that this pattern, which was described many decades ago by Dressler and Roesler (1947), usually evolves to STEMI (Figure 20.6B). We know that this change from NSTEMI to STEMI occurs when transmural and homogeneous ischemia exists (Figures 20.6B, 20.7, 20.20, and 20.27).

In contrast, sometimes a patient with ACS presents in the first phase with an ECG pattern of STEMI (Figure 20.28) (tall T wave in V1–V3 and ST elevation in I, aVL, and V2). In the first instance, only antithrombotic treatment was

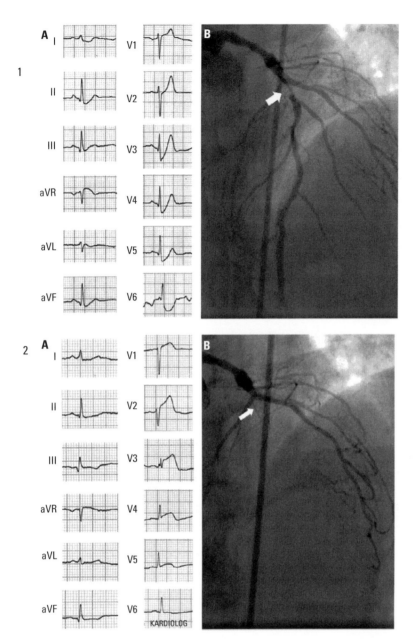

Figure 20.27 (1-A) ECG taken in a patient with NSTEMI and three-vessel disease. (1-B) Occlusion of RCA + LCX + LAD distal to big diagonal. Note ST depression from V3 to V6, I, II, aVF with a final positive T wave that is very tall in V3–V5 and ST elevation >1 mm in aVR (see Table 20.4). (2-A) ECG recorded during chest pain 18 hours after stent implantation in LAD. Note ST elevation in V1–V5 consistent with STEMI due to LAD occlusion (stent thrombosis), as demonstrated by coronarography (2-B) (see arrow) (Reproduced with permission from Stankovic *et al.* 2011).

given and the patient was sent to a reference center. On arrival, the treatment has partially opened the artery and the tall T wave in the precordials is now converted to clear ST depression (NSTEMI). Finally, the artery is opened with PCI and the ECG normalizes, showing only a mild negative T wave (Figure 20.28).

Acute coronary syndrome with confounding factors: left ventricular hypertrophy and wide QRS

These cases correspond to 20% of all ACS. **In cases of LVH** with a strain pattern and/or wide QRS complex, the diagnosis of ACS is more difficult, especially if concurrent with NSTE-ACS. Performing the recording of a sequential pattern may be useful (see Figure 13.58).

Bundle branch block and other situations with wide QRS

The presence of bundle branch block in patients with ACS is not frequent (≈2–3%), and usually indicates a bad prognosis, mostly LBBB. This is especially true: (i) when the bundle branch block has developed during the ACS; (ii) when the duration of QRS is very wide; (iii) if ST segment elevation resolution is delayed; and (iv) if the ST deviations are very striking.

The presence of new LBBB is less frequent than RBBB because the left bundle presents with double perfusion (LAD + LCX). In contrast, the right bundle receives perfusion only from the first septal branch. Therefore, an appearance of RBBB is a sign of a proximal LAD occlusion in the clinical setting of ACS.

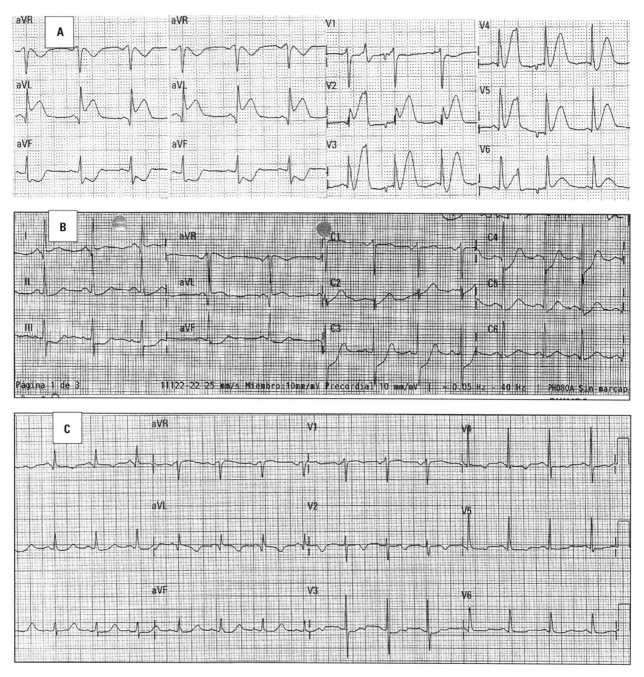

Figure 20.28 (A) A 59-year-old patient with acute coronary syndrome (ACS) and oppressive chest pain that lasts for more than 1 hour. The ECG corresponds to a first-stage STEMI (ST elevation in I and aVL and tall wide T wave from V2 to V5 of the hyperacute phase). The patient received antithrombotic treatment and was sent to reference hospital for percutaneous coronary intervention (PCI). On arrival (B), the patient still presented with precordial pain of lower intensity and the ECG has changed very much. Now the ST in I and aVL is only mildly elevated and in the precordial leads, there is a pattern of NSTE similar to the ECG pattern that may be seen in isolated tight subocclusion of LAD (ST depression V2–V5). In fact, the patient presents with tight subocclusion of the big first diagonal with LAD involvement that has been partially opened after treatment. The ST depression in the precordials means that at this moment there is no any part of the left ventricular walls with transmural involvement and that predominates subendocardial involvement (NSTEMI). Finally, after PCI, the ECG only presents negative T waves (C).

In the presence of RBBB, the diagnosis of STEMI is possible in a similar way to that in normal situations. RBBB does not interfere with the diagnosis of acute STEMI, and the ECG criteria for STEMI are the same as for patients with a narrow QRS. Diagnosing ST elevation in the anterior, inferior, and lateral leads can easily be done in patients with RBBB. However, the diagnosis of inferolateral STEMI equivalent in patients with RBBB and

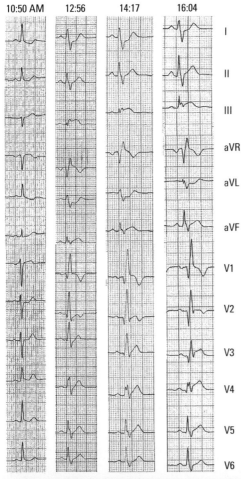

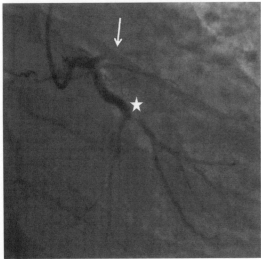

Figure 20.29 A 46-year-old man who presented to a health center for chest pain that started one hour before (at 9 AM). An ECG sequence is shown before reperfusion therapy. The indication of coronary angiography is in the second ECG that shows inferior ST-segment elevation (mainly in III) with reciprocal ST depression in I and aVL and appearance of RBBB with a wide symmetric T wave in the precordial leads. New RBBB is not commonly seen with RCA infarction, unless this is rate dependent. In some cases, the ECG sequence may end with the

baseline ST depression in V1–V3 is a challenge, and prospective studies are needed to define the threshold for ST deviations in this setting. Remember that in the presence of RBBB, the presence of symmetric negative T wave in precordial leads is always suspicious of abnormality (Figure 20.29).

New or "presumably new" LBBB

The left bundle branch (LBB) is a larger and less vulnerable structure than the RBB. The blood supply to the LBB is clearly of dual origin as the anterior fascicle is supplied mainly by anterior septal branches of the LAD and the posterior fascicle from the AV nodal artery, which originates from the RCA or the LCX depending on coronary artery dominance. Accordingly, severe two- or three-vessel disease should typically be present for a new LBBB to develop.

Sgarbossa *et al.* (1996) introduced three criteria to help in identifying acute MI in patients with LBBB (Sgarbossa *et al.* 1996). They were: (i) ST-segment elevation ≥1 mm and concordant with the QRS complex (5 points); (ii) ST-segment depression ≥1 mm in leads V1, V2, or V3 (3 points); and (iii) ST-segment elevation ≥5 mm and discordant with the QRS complex (2 points). A total score of three or more points was considered diagnostic of acute MI, whereas a score of 2 points suggests an acute MI. A meta-analysis reported the Sgarbossa criteria to be specific (98%) but with low sensitivity (20%) (Jain *et al.* 2011; Tabas *et al.* 2008). ST-segment elevation has proved to be the single-most specific criterion for the diagnosis of acute MI in the presence of LBBB, and improves the detection of this "STEMI equivalent" (Larson *et al.* 2007; Lopes *et al.* 2011). An adaptation of the Sgarbossa criteria, including ST elevation to S-wave ratio may be too complicated for use in the emergency setting (Smith *et al.* 2012).

In a study from the Minneapolis Heart Institute STEMI protocol (n = 3903), new or presumably new LBBB was present in 3.3% of the patients (Pera *et al.* 2018). The authors tested a hierarchical algorithm based on hemodynamic instability and Sgarbossa concordance criteria. The algorithm yielded high sensitivity (97%) and negative predictive value (94%) for identification of a culprit lesion, while specificity was 48%.

Another study from the United States reported new or presumably new LBBB in 69/802 (8.6%) in the hospital primary PCI laboratory activation database (Mehta

appearance of Q waves without a clear ST-segment elevation being observed. Coronary angiography shows a proximal total occlusion of the LAD (arrow) and diffuse disease in the LCX. In the LCX, there is also sub-total occlusion at the origin of the OM branch (star), which received collateral circulation from the LAD. Upon occlusion of the LAD, ischemia also appeared (elevated ST) in the territory irrigated by the LCX.

et al. 2012). Less than 30% of the patients with new or presumably new LBBB had troponin elevation, and 54% underwent emergent coronary angiography. Of these, 22% had a culprit vessel occlusion; the emergent revascularization rate was 11.6%.

The fourth Universal definition of myocardial infarction (Thygesen *et al.* 2019) states that in patients with LBBB, ST-segment elevation ≥1 mm concordant with the QRS complex in any lead may be an indicator of acute myocardial ischemia. The conclusion was that since the detection of ischemia by the ECG in LBBB is difficult, decisions concerning urgent reperfusion therapy should be based mainly on symptoms and hemodynamic parameters. The presence of concordant ST-segment elevation (i.e. in leads with positive QRS deflections) appears to be one of the best indicators of ongoing MI with an occluded infarct artery. Patients with a clinical suspicion of ongoing myocardial ischaemia and LBBB should be managed in a way similar to STEMI patients, regardless of whether the LBBB is previously known. It is important to remark that the presence of a (presumed) new LBBB does not predict an MI per se.

In contrast, the diagnosis of concurrent **NSTEMI in the presence of confounding factors may be even more difficult** because there are no visible changes in the ECG, or the changes may be confused with basal ECG changes (see Figure 13.58).

Mistakes performed in the ECG interpretation of ACS (Birnbaum *et al.* 2012; Fiol-Sala *et al.* 2020)

In our opinion, the most frequent mistakes made in the interpretation of ECG in the course of ACS are the following:

• **Considering cases of LCX occlusion that present with an ST depression in V1 to V3–V4 as the major change** (with often minimal ST elevation in some inferior/lateral leads) as **NSTEMI**. These are clear cases of STEMI that need to be treated with emergency PCI (Figures 20.5 and 13.51). In many papers (From *et al.* 2010), the number of cases of STEMI when the culprit artery is the LCX are much lower than those with other culprit arteries, although the cases diagnosed as NSTEMI due to LCX subocclusion present with higher levels of troponins and do not have good collateral flow. **It is clear that many cases of STEMI due to LCX occlusion are underdiagnosed**. There are no any logical explanation that the LCX artery may be less prone to plaque rupture leading to a fewer cases of STEMI (From *et al.* 2010). **We consider that the STEMI events due to LCX occlusion are underdiagnosed because the ECGs (ST depression in V1 to V3–V4) are often not well interpreted**. Posterior leads and body mapping (McClelland *et al.* 2003) may help to clarify the diagnosis (Figures 20.5B and 25.18). However, we believe that

the interpretation of subtle changes of ST in 12-lead surface ECGs may be of great help in performing a correct diagnosis and may avoid the use of other recording techniques (Figure 20.5A).

In the hiperacute phase of ACS, it is very important to perform the differential diagnosis between STEMI (LCX occlusion) and NSTEMI (LAD subocclusion) in the presence of ST depression in V1–V3–V4. In the first case (LCX occlusion), it is an emergency to activate the catheterization laboratory. The ECG usually solves the problem because in case of LCX occlusion presents ST depression already in V1, and there is not final positive T wave (or very small). On the contrary, in cases of LAD subocclusion, the ST depression in V1 is mild and in V2–V4, there is final evident positive T wave (see Figures 20.5 and 20.20). During the evolving process of LCX occlusion, a RS pattern with less ST depression and final positive T wave appears as a mirror pattern of lateral wall involvement.

• **Not knowing that the only change in the hyperacute phase of STEMI is often a change of T wave**, usually peaked, taller, and more symmetrical (Figure 20.4B).

• Interpreting **the presence of tall and peaked T wave when it is accompanied by some ST segment depression, as a typical NSTEMI** and therefore, not treating with emergency PCI. When this ECG pattern is present, it is true that there is no transmural homogeneous involvement, and in this moment, if the ST depression is evident that corresponds to NSTEMI (Figures 20.20 and 20.6). However, it is also clear that these patients probably need to be treated with emergency PCI, because the majority of them will evolve to a true STEMI (this needs to be considered in the guidelines) (Dressler and Roesler 1947; Sagie *et al.* 1989; De Winter *et al.* 2008; Zhong-qun *et al.* 2011) (Figures 20.6 and 20.7).

• **Considering that small negativity of T waves, especially in V1–V3**, in the course of ACS **do not represent danger of new events and that the presence of very deep T waves is always a sign of impending MI**. In this regard, we can state the following: (i) The presence either of flat/negative T wave ≤2 mm (Figure 13.12) or deep negative T wave (Figure 13.11) may be found in patients with critical LAD stenosis. (ii) The very negative T wave that appears in the course of an ACS is usually an atypical pattern of STEMI that at this moment represents a post-ischemic change (ischemia/reperfusions pattern) because usually the artery is open or many collaterals exist (no angina at this moment) (Figure 20.6B). However, it may suddenly evolve into pseudonormalization of negative T wave and an ST elevation. (iii) When the negative T wave is mildly deep (<2 mm) (Figure 13.12), it usually corresponds to NSTE-ACS and represents at this moment a post-ischemic change that may occur also in the presence of tight LAD occlusion. In this case an urgent, not emergency, PCI is recommended.

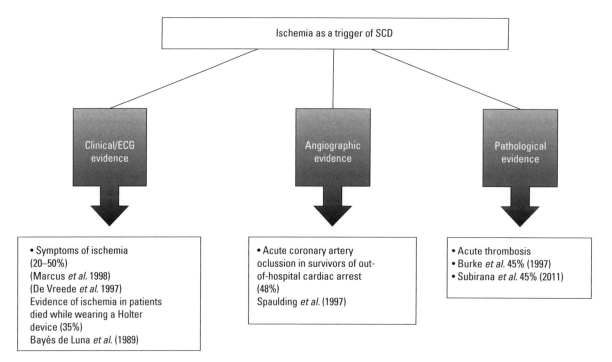

Figure 20.30 The importance of acute ischemia is a trigger of sudden death: clinical ECG, angiographic, and pathological evidence (see text) (Adapted from Marcus *et al.* 1988; de Vreede-Swagemakers *et al.* 1997; Bayés de Luna *et al.* 1989; Spaulding *et al.* 1997).

Arrhythmias in acute coronary syndromes

We do not discuss this topic in depth in this book (consult Fiol-Sala *et al.* 2020 and Bayés de Luna and Baranchuk 2017). However, it is necessary to point out that **acute ischemia frequently triggers ventricular arrhythmias which may lead to ventricular fibrillation and sudden death** (Figure 20.30 and Chapter 16, Ventricular fibrillation). In fact, in nearly 50% of cases of sudden death, acute ischemia is the trigger of the fatal event (Figure 20.30), and ischemic heart disease is the most frequently associated disease.

From an experimental point of view, ventricular arrhythmias have been shown to develop after ligature of a coronary artery in two phases. The first phase occurs after a few seconds, and is probably induced by a reentry mechanism; the second phase occurs after a few hours, and is most likely explained by post-potential (Janse 1982).

Severe ventricular arrhythmias, runs of ventricular tachycardia, and, occasionally, ventricular fibrillation appear in relation to most severe degrees of ischemia. This is especially true in case of long-lasting ischemia and hearts with poor ventricular function (Bayés de Luna and Baranchuk 2017). Cases with the most severe ischemia, such as a coronary spasm with total occlusion of a large epicardial vessel (Prinzmetal angina or ACS with grade III of ischemia), is accompanied by significant ST segment elevation or even a TAP morphology (Figure 20.45). In the most extreme cases, T wave or ST segment alternans is observed (Figure 20.48). In general, severe ventricular arrhythmias do not appear immediately after the acute occlusion, but rather after a few minutes. **Therefore, the**

danger of ventricular fibrillation is much more frequent in STE-ACS evolving to MI than in coronary spasm.

Ischemia and sudden death

Acute coronary syndromes, especially STEMI, often trigger sudden death. Nowadays, with current treatments available, the number of cases with long-term complications of MI, such as heart failure and low EF, is much lower than previously. However, acute and chronic ischemic heart disease is still often associated with sudden cardiac death, and this is probably the most important challenge in modern cardiology. In the United States, ischemic heart disease is present in 80–90% of cases of sudden death, but this association in the Mediterranean area is lower (Subirana *et al.* 2011). Globally (as is shown in Figure **20.30**), in fewer than 50% of cases of sudden death are there clinical (presence of angina) (Marcus *et al.* 1988; de Vreede-Swagemakers *et al.* 1997), electrocardiographic (ST changes in Holter recording) (Bayés de Luna *et al.* 1989), or coronarographic (acute thrombus) (Spaulding *et al.* 1997) findings that acute ischemia is the trigger of sudden death. Furthermore, in fewer than 50% of these cases is there pathologic evidence of acute infarction (fresh thrombus) (Burke *et al.* 1997; Subirana *et al.* 2011). These conclusions clearly clarify that around 50% of cases of sudden death are caused by acute ischemic attack. In the majority of other cases of sudden death in patients with IHD, the cause of death is sustained ventricular tachycardia/ventricular fibrillation (VT/VF) triggered by reentry around an old MI scar. It is interesting to point out that in the Mediterranean area, a higher

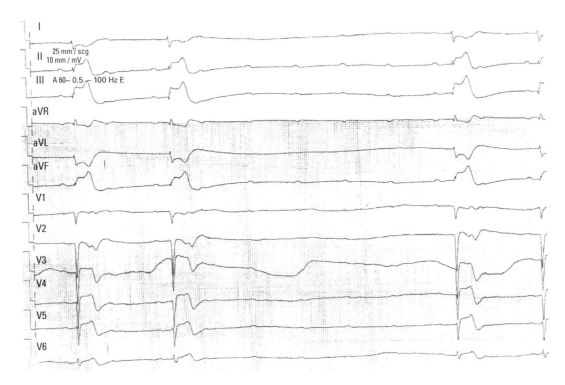

Figure 20.31 Patient with STE-ACS due to proximal occlusion of dominant RCA (ST depression in I, ST elevation III > II, ST isodiphasic in V1 and ST elevation in V6). The patient presented with 2 × 1 atrioventricular (AV) block and suddenly advanced AV block.

incidence of cases of sudden death associated with left ventricular hypertrophy has been found than in the United States (Subirana *et al.* 2011).

The most frequent supraventricular arrhythmia to occur during ACS is **atrial fibrillation**. **Atrial fibrillation** is a relatively frequent supraventricular arrhythmia (10–12% of cases of STE-ACS and arrhythmia), as other supraventricular arrhythmias are typically related to atrial involvement (Liu *et al.* 1961; Zimerman *et al.* 1968) and/or pericarditis. Atrial fibrillation usually occurs in the most extensive ACSs. However, in patients with ACS due to RCA occlusion, it may be explained by vagal overdrive and may be accompanied by AV block. Age, presence of abnormal P wave (Agrawal *et al.* 2014), chronic obstructive pulmonary disease (COPD), and heart failure are triggering factors. The incidence of atrial fibrillation has decreased in the post-thrombolytic era. Atrial fibrillation is usually self-limited; thus, electric cardioversion is advised only when the heart rate is rapid and causes hemodynamic impairment. P-wave analysis on signal-averaged ECG may aid in predicting atrial fibrillation in ACS (Rosiak *et al.* 2002).

Also all types of **passive arrhythmias** (sinus bradycardia, sinoatrial, and AV block–RCA occlusion) may be found. Figure 20.31 shows a third-degree AV block that has a different significance according to the location of the MI: inferior or anteroapical. When it occurs in association with inferior MI, it usually evolves from a first-degree block, the QRS complex is narrow, and the block is supra-

hisian. Thus, the prognosis is relatively good, though the mortality rate is higher than in cases with no advanced AV block with reperfusion therapy (Alnsasra *et al.* 2018).

Mechanical complications of an ACS evolving to myocardial infarction (Color Plate 5) (Fiol-Sala *et al.* 2020)

Fortunately, with the introduction of new treatments of acute phase, mechanical complications are much less frequent these days.

Free-wall rupture accompanied by cardiogenic shock may take place during the evolution of a Q wave acute MI. The persistence of ST segment elevation at the end of the first week without evolving to negative T wave as a sign of regional pericarditis is an indirect risk marker of cardiac rupture (Color Plate 5) (Reeder and Gersh 2000). This persistence of ST segment elevation, which is generally more persistent than significant, is seen more frequently in inferior and/or lateral wall MI than in anterior wall MI (Oliva *et al.* 1993). In general, the RCA and the LCX are more frequently involved than the LAD, and the lack of well-developed collateral circulation favors the occurrence of **transmural MI (Q wave or equivalent) with transmural homogeneous involvement of the entire wall**.

In patients with an evolving inferior acute MI, the presence of PR segment depression ≥1.2 mm in II, III, and aVF is associated with a higher risk of in-hospital mortality and free-wall cardiac rupture and/or atrial rupture when

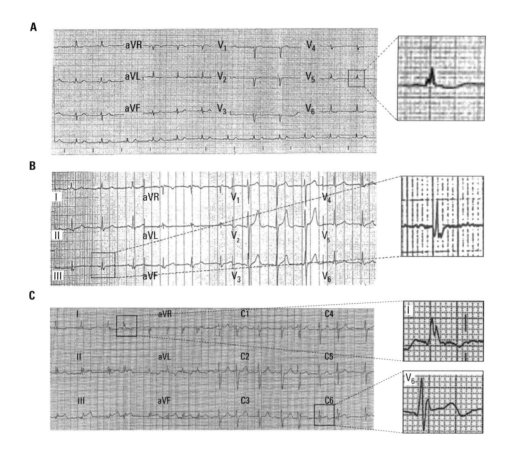

Figure 20.32 (A) A 55-year-old patient with previous myocardial infarction (MI) due to LCX occlusion who presents with a nearly normal ECG with low-voltage R wave in V5–V6 with evident "slurrings." (B) A 60-year-old patient with MI eight months previously. The coronary angiography demonstrates occlusion of the LCX. There are striking final "slurrings" in II, III, aVF, aVL, and the right precordial leads (V2–V3). The Q wave in the inferior leads and the "r" wave in V1 are narrow, and additionally the R/S ratio <0.5. This is a case of MI shown by striking final "slurrings" of QRS. (C) A 65-year old woman in atrial fibrillation with two previous MIs due to RCA and LCX occlusion who presented with a typical fragmented QRS pattern. The ST elevation in the chronic phase is very suggestive of left ventricular inferoapical aneurysm.

compared with patients without PR segment deviations (Jim *et al.* 2006).

Septal rupture usually occurs, in turn, in larger infarctions, especially due to a proximal LAD occlusion. A systolic murmur may be heard, suggestive of a ventricular septal defect. Frequently, the patient presents with cardiogenic shock if surgery is not carried out urgently.

The ECG may also show the persistence of ST segment elevation (Figure 22.11) with a higher incidence compared to Q wave infarction controls and the existence of RBBB with or without added superoanterior hemiblock (SAH), advanced AV block, and atrial fibrillation.

Finally, **papillary muscle infarction** is more frequent than previously thought (40% of STEMI), although its prognosis is better than expected in the absence of ruptures (Tanimoto *et al.* 2010). The rupture that occurs currently very rarely causes acute mitral regurgitation

frequently with acute pulmonary edema. Urgent surgery is often required. The posteromedial papillary muscle is more frequently involved, since its perfusion is derived only from the posterior descending artery (RCA or LCX), while the anterolateral papillary muscle has double perfusion (LAD and LCX). **In contrast to free-wall cardiac rupture, the infarct is frequently of the non-Q wave type (>50% of cases).**

With regard to **ventricular aneurysms**, their presence has been classically suggested by the persistence of ST segment elevation. In chronic patients, the sensitivity of this sign is poor. Just 10% of the patients in the postinfarction setting with ventricular aneurysm exhibit a higher than 0.1 mV ST segment elevation (East and Oran 1952). Also, it has been described that some changes of the mid-late part of QRS, including rsR' in left surface leads (Sherif 1970) and other morphologies (**fractioned QRS**), are very specific of ventricular aneurysm (Reddy *et al.* 2006) (Figure 20.32C).

Other ECG changes in acute coronary syndrome

P wave and PR segment

The deviations of the PR interval are especially seen in pericarditis (Figures 9.35) and atrial involvement in cases of MI (Figure 9.33).

The diagnosis of atrial infarction is based especially on the presence of PR segment deviations (elevation or depression in different leads) associated with reciprocal changes in other leads (especially ST segment elevation in aVR and ST segment depression in II) and any atrial arrhythmias (Liu *et al.* 1961).

Recently, it has been shown (Jim *et al.* 2006) (see above) that PR segment depressions ≥1.2 mm in patients with inferior STE-ACS (ST segment elevation in II, III, and aVF) are a marker for high risk of AV block, supraventricular arrhythmias, cardiac rupture, and in-hospital mortality.

Changes in the QRS complex

ACS with ST segment elevation and severe ischemia often present changes in the final portion of the QRS complex (**distortion of QRS**) (see Figure 20.2C). Severe ischemia may also induce QRS widening with or without classic patterns of intraventricular block. The importance of some of these changes from a prognostic point of view has already been discussed (see above).

QT interval

During the acute phase of ischemia, a lengthening of the QT interval (TAP) is the first manifestation of ischemia (Kenigsberg *et al.* 2007) (Figure 20.12) (see ECG changes during fibrinolysis and percutaneous coronary intervention). However, the change with respect to basal QT is difficult to identify.

The presence of an evident long QTc interval at admission in a patient with ACS has been shown to be a marker of poor prognosis. In addition, patients with non-Q wave infarction, in comparison with those with unstable angina, have longer QTc intervals overall (Rukshin *et al.* 2002). However, this is not useful when applied to an individual patient. Therefore, the troponin levels remain as the best way to distinguish whether an ACS with no ST segment elevation has evolved to a non-Q wave infarction or has remained as an unstable angina.

U wave changes (Table 20.4)

A normal U wave is always positive in the presence of a positive T wave and, under normal conditions, it is negative only in aVR. In patients with different clinical settings of IHD, U wave abnormalities may be recorded, generally as a negative U wave, while the T wave may be negative, positive, or flattened. The U wave may be positive when the T wave is negative (T–U discordance) (Reinig *et al.* 2005).

When the negative T wave is recorded in precordial leads in patients with IHD, it is highly probable that the LAD is involved.

A negative T wave may be present as acute ischemic events (STEMI or coronary spasm) (Figure 20.26) or during the post-ischemic phase usually in NSTEMI (Figure 20.15 and Table 20.4). It should be noted that: (i) a negative U wave may be the only ECG sign of ischemia; (ii) it sometimes precedes ST segment changes; and (iii) it may increase the sensitivity of the exercise stress test (Correale *et al.* 2004).

Changes in PVC morphology

Repolarization abnormalities may be more visible in the PVCs than in normal ones and sometimes even are seen in

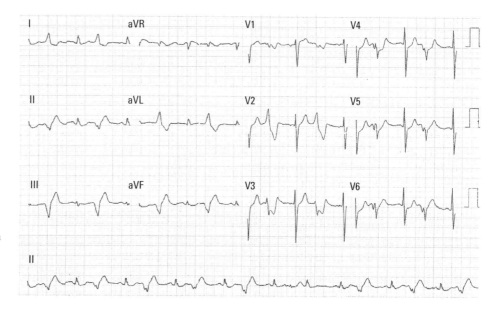

Figure 20.33 One example of exercise test in a patient with ischemic heart disease that demonstrates the presence of significant ST segment changes in premature ventricular complexes (see V3–V4) that were not so evident in normal sinus complexes.

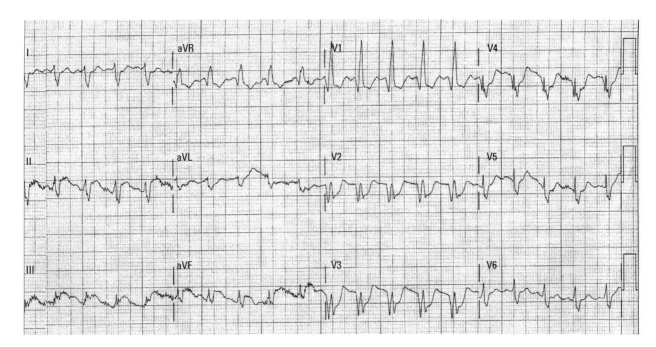

Figure 20.34 Recurrent acute coronary syndrome (ACS). A 75-year-old man with old anterior myocardial infarction complicated by right bundle branch block (RBBB), who presented with heart attack. Note the old Q wave from V1–V4, sinus tachycardia (pulmonary edema), and ST segment elevation in the inferior leads and ST segment depression in the right precordial leads due to occlusion of LCx.

PVC only (Figure 20.33). In addition, the ST segment depression in the PVCs in the exercise stress test has been shown to be more useful than the ST segment depression in normal complexes for predicting myocardial ischemia. The ST segment depression in the PVCs higher than 10% of the R wave amplitude in V4–V6 has a 95% sensitivity and a 67% specificity for predicting ischemia (Rasouli and Ellestad 2001). However, cases of repolarization abnormalities exist in the PVCs of healthy patients, and thus the test specificity is not very high.

Furthermore, a meticulous study of the QRS complex or the T wave morphology of the PVCs may suggest an old infarction (qR morphology, with a wide q wave or slurred QS complex and sometimes a symmetric T wave).

Recurrence of acute coronary syndrome

Recurrence refers to repeated episodes of ACS with or without ST segment elevation usually evolving into MI. It is not an infrequent event and usually appears after 2–3 years after the index MI, often in a different location and with the same type of ACS, suggesting that some patients present with factors that predispose to repeated episodes of STE or non-STE-ACS (Figure 20.34) (Fiol-Sala *et al.* 2020).

ECG in chronic myocardial infarction with narrow QRS

Evolutionary concepts

Before the era of reperfusion, it was relatively easy to predict the final Q wave infarction pattern according to the

acute phase of STE-ACS. With the current treatment strategies, if the treatment is started on time, the infarction may be faded (Figure 20.1).

In patients with chronic Q wave MI, it is currently impossible to determine, from the correlation with the Q wave pattern, the exact degree and location of the occlusion of the culprit artery at the moment of an acute attack, because the area at risk is initially larger and become smaller as reperfusion treatment is successfully applied (Figure 20.9). Therefore, in the chronic phase of Q wave MI, what may be presumed is the location of the occlusion that produced the Q wave, but not the place of the occlusion when the ACS starts.

In over 50% of cases of MI, the QRS complex does not show a Q wave of necrosis or equivalent (R in V1–V2). The MI without Q wave encompasses the classic non-Q wave MI and many other types, as shown in Table 20.5, including the masked MI (wide QRS with LBBB and others) that sometimes may present with a Q wave. Furthermore, in 25–30% of cases, more in inferior MI, the Q wave disappears at follow-up due to the presence of collaterals (Figure 20.35), the appearance of new necrosis (Color Plate 4), or new bundle branch block.

Until relatively recently, it was thought that MIs in an exclusive subendocardial location existed and were electrically mute. However, the concept that MI with Q wave is transmural and non-Q wave MI only involves subendocardial compromise is false. Now, it has been demonstrated from a pathologic point of view that infarctions

Table 20.5 Myocardial infarction without Q wave or equivalent

A. Non-Q wave MI: ST depression and/or negative T wave

B. Other types of MI without Q wave:

- Infarction located in an area that does not generate Q wave of necrosis:
  - Atria (never single infarction): usually extensive MI of inferolateral zone (associated Q wave)
  - Right ventricle. It is usually associated with an inferior wall MI. It is due to an occlusion of a proximal RCA before the RV branches and usually presents Q wave of inferior MI
  - MI of basal areas of LV (distal occlusion of the LCX or RCA). Usually without Q wave, but often with fractioned QRS pattern
  - Microinfarction (positive biomarkers). ECG usually normal
- Q wave MI, with Q that disappears during the follow-up (Figure 20.35)
- Aborted MI with Q wave: acute coronary syndrome with ST elevation (infarction in evolution) with early and efficient reperfusion (Figure 20.1). Rarely spontaneous thrombus resolution. Troponin level is decisive to separate unstable angina from MI without Q wave
- Masked Q wave:
  Left bundle branch block
  Wolff–Parkinson–White, Pacemaker} Often can present with an abnormal Q wave

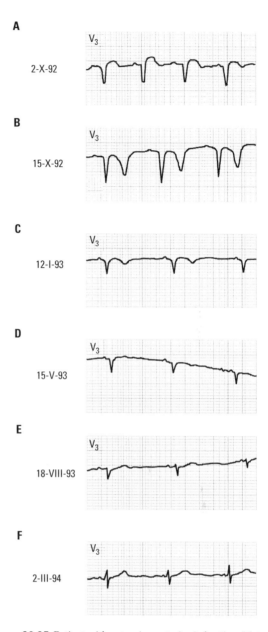

Figure 20.35 Patient with extensive anterior infarction. Note ECG normalization with Q wave disappearing and T wave becoming positive during 18-month follow-up. A to F.

usually do not have an exclusive subendocardial location and that infarctions with predominant subendocardial involvement may or may not develop a Q wave. Furthermore, some transmural MIs, such as those involving the basal areas of the left ventricle, may not exhibit a Q wave (Moon *et al.* 2004).

Contrast-enhanced cardiovascular magnetic resonance (CE-CMR) is the ideal technique for infarct identification, transmural characterization, and infarct localization and quantification. CE-CMR has demonstrated that the Q wave MIs are larger than non-Q wave ones, although they do not always have a deeper transmural extension. Therefore, **the terms Q wave and non-Q wave MIs are useful in the chronic phase from a prognostic point of view but not for determining whether a MI is or is not transmural** (see Chapter 13, Q wave of necrosis).

Q wave myocardial infarction with narrow QRS (see Chapter 13)

The evolution of the ECG pattern

Since the early days of the ECG, the pattern of established transmural infarction has been associated with the presence of pathologic Q wave or its equivalents. Figure 13.32 shows the evolutionary appearance of the Q wave and negative T wave in cases of Q wave MI without modern treatment. Today, the evolution of the ECG may be very different if quick current treatment is established (see Figures 20.1 and 20.36).

Diagnostic criteria of Q wave myocardial infarctions

The changes associated with prior MIs are described in Table 13.1. Table 13.6 shows the ECG criteria of pathologic (necrosis) Q wave that in the appropriate clinical context may be used to diagnose prior MI (Thygesen *et al.* 2019). The presence of fractioned QRS (Das *et al.* 2006) must be considered abnormal and in the adequate clinical setting suggestive of prior MI. Remember that there are many pathologic Q waves not secondary to MI (see Table 13.9).

To classify the ACS with narrow QRS and confounding factors in two groups—STEMI and non-STEMI—it is necessary to have a full understanding of the ECG patterns of each group (remember the atypical patterns of STEMI) and their various pathophysiological mechanisms.

The most important pathophysiological aspect that determines the appearance of ST elevation is the presence of **brusque and homogeneous transmural involvement in a territory without important subendocardial ischemia and collateral circulation**. The prototype of that is a coronary spasm. After resolution of important spasm, a reperfusion–post-ischemic–deep negative T wave often appears.

Currently, with modern treatment, a patient with ongoing STEMI (tall peaked T wave) may convert to NSTEMI (Figure 20.28) and conversely a patient with NSTEMI if not treated quickly or if some complications occur (thrombosis of stent) may convert to STEMI (Figures 20.6, 20.20, and 20.27).

All this information helps us to take the decision to treat as an STEMI (emergent PCI) some types of NSTEMI (ST depression + tall T wave) that much probably will evolve into STEMI without treatment (Figures 20.20 and 20.27).

Location of Q wave myocardial infarctions

A statement from the International Society for Holter and Noninvasive Electrocardiology (Bayés de Luna *et al.* 2006b) presented a new classification system for Q wave MI based on the correlation between the Q wave and the infarcted area as assessed by CE-CMR performed by our group and others (Bayés de Luna *et al.* 2006a; Cino *et al.* 2006; Rovai

et al. 2007; Van der Weg *et al.* 2009). We commented on this extensively in Chapter 13 (Figure 13.66).

The most important conclusions of these correlations are as follows:

• R/S≥1 in V1 is never caused by MI of the inferobasal (old posterior) wall, but rather is always due to infarction of the lateral wall (see Figures 13.66 and 13.76). Other new criteria for lateral MI (R/S>0.5 and S wave<3 mm in V1) that are more sensitive and maintain very high specificity have been published (Figure 13.75) (Bayés de Luna *et al.* 2008).

• Myocardial infarctions exclusive to the inferior wall always present small r in V1 (see Figures 13.72 and 13.75).

• A Q wave in aVL (and sometimes in I and a small q in V2–V3) is in our experience not due to high lateral infarction (LCX occlusion) rather to mid-anterior MI caused by occlusion of the first diagonal (see Figure 13.70) (extensive anterior of Figure 13.66).

• In the presence of MI of the anteroapical zone with a Q wave beyond V2, the presence of Q in I and/or aVL suggests that the infarction is more extensive than that of the apical zone (see Figure 13.69).

• It is difficult to differentiate some types of MI of the anteroapical zone, especially when the location depends on the presence or not of a Q wave in V3–V5. This is due to irregular methodology in the placement of electrodes (see Figure 13.78) as well as other problems such as body habitus, or type of coronary circulation, etc. Because of this, it is especially difficult to differentiate

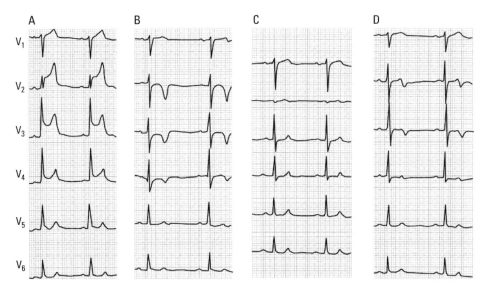

Figure 20.36 (A) A patient with acute coronary syndrome (ACS) with ST segment elevation with the ECG pattern found in cases of severe transmural ischemia (increase in R, disappearance of S wave, ratio J point/R wave >0.5). Troponin levels were normal. (B) The ECG after primary percutaneous coronary intervention (PCI) of proximal LAD shows a deep negative T wave from V2 to V4, suggestive of opened artery (reperfusion pattern). (C) Some hours after PCI, the patient presented with precordial pain with pseudonormalization of the ECG as a sign of re-occlusion (V2 lead shows artifacts). (D) A new PCI demonstrates intrastent thrombosis and a new stent was inserted, and again non-prominent negative T waves were recorded.

between septal and apical-anterior MI (types A-1 and A-2) (Figure 13.66) (Bayés de Luna *et al.* 2006b) (see Chapter 13).

Quantification of necrosis

Selvester *et al.* (1985) described a 31-point scoring system based on 50 criteria (e.g. the presence of Q wave in different leads or R wave in V1–V2 as a mirror pattern, etc.). The scores quantify the amount of infarcted tissue (3% of the left ventricular mass for each point). At the individual level, the standard error in myocardial damage quantification using this score is relatively large, resulting in limited clinical usefulness. The most important cause of errors with this scoring system comes from its inability to quantify basal infarcted areas, mainly the septal and lateral areas.

The prediction of final MI size based on the amount of ST deviation on the admission ECG was reported (Aldrich *et al.* 1988). However, recently it has been demonstrated that this score with current treatments has a low correlation with real infarction size, probably because this score is not stable in the acute phase over time (Bouwmeester *et al.* 2011).

Today, CE-CMR has been shown to be highly accurate in estimating the size of the infarcted mass, and has become the "gold standard" technique FOR damage quantification (Figure 20.37). However, it is still necessary to develop standards that may be consistently applied to CE-CMR measurements (Fiol-Sala *et al.* 2020).

Myocardial infarction without Q wave or equivalent

Concept

MI without Q wave or equivalent includes all of the MIs listed in Table 20.5, including: non-Q wave infarction, infarctions located in areas that do not generate a Q-wave, right ventricular infarction, and atrial infarction among others. It should also be noted that relatively often the Q wave disappears during follow-up especially in case of inferior MI (see Figure 20.35).

We should remember that **the presence of an R wave in V1 in patients post-MI may be equivalent to the Q wave** as a mirror image expression of the Q wave of the lateral infarction (Figures 13.75 and 13.76).

According to the new classification of MI developed by the European Society of Cardiology and the American College of Cardiology (Thygesen *et al.* 2019), the presence of increased enzymes allows differentiation of a non-Q wave MI from unstable angina. The masked Q wave MI in the case of wide QRS will be discussed in the following section.

Non-Q wave myocardial infarction

In these cases, the occlusion of the coronary artery is generally incomplete and the patient has usually had significant previous ischemia mainly in the subendocardial zone. Consequently, when the ischemia increases (ACS), a AP of poor quality is generated, predominantly in the subendocardium, accounting for the development of a subendocardial ischemia pattern (**ST segment depression**) that normalizes or at least decreased with time (Figure 13.25), or converts to flat/negative T wave (post-ischemic change).

However, it has already been noted that **there are transmural MIs without Q** if the transmural involvement is in the basal part of the left ventricle, **and that some predominant subendocardial MIs** with extension to the mid part of the wall present Q waves (Figure 13.6D). The importance of the presence of Q waves is **that the MI with a Q wave is larger** (Moon *et al.* 2004) (see before).

The abnormality of repolarization is sometimes an isolated negative or flattened T wave. These patterns much probably related to partial or total reperfusion and not to "acute" ischemia (see Chapter 13). This may explain the best prognosis of NSTEMI of "non-Q wave MI type" and negative T wave in the ECG.

Furthermore, troponin levels are decisive in assuring that an ACS has evolved to an MI when the ECG pattern may not give the correct answer. A non-Q wave infarction is an NSTEMI that produces increased enzyme levels.

The non-Q wave group of infarctions includes cases of large MI secondary to extensive involvement of the left ventricle but without homogeneous transmural involvement of the free LV wall, in cases of subocclusion of the LMT or three-vessel disease. However, most of them are small infarctions. Currently, they represent more than 50% of all MIs.

In the chronic phase, the ECGs of patients with non-Q wave infarction are usually normal or show mild abnormalities (flat mild negative T wave, slight ST segment depression, etc.) (Figure 13.25) (see above). The group of patients who present with important subocclusion of LMT may even present a normal or nearly normal ECG in approximately 50% of the cases in the acute phase in absence of pain (Figure 20.17). It has been demonstrated that in the chronic phase (Choi *et al.* 2011), lateral ST depression at discharge is a marker of risk, as also was shown in the ECG at admission (Barrabes *et al.* 2000). In the study of Choi *et al.* (2011), lateral ST depression was the only variable that independently predicted one-year major adverse complications (MACE).

Other types of MI without Q wave infarction located in areas that do not generate a Q wave

• **Infarction may involve the basal parts of the left ventricle (areas of late depolarization). We have to remember that these areas depolarize after 40 ms (Durrer *et al.* 1970) (see Figure 5.19), and therefore these** MIs do not generate a Q wave or its equivalent. In

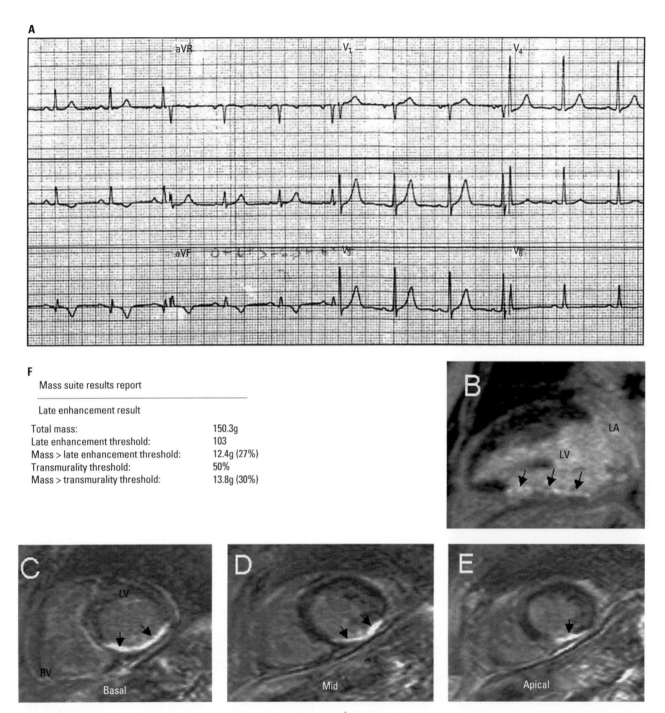

Figure 20.37 Inferior myocardial infarction (MI). (A) The ECG shows QR in leads DIII and R in aVF and rS in V1. (B) Contrast-enhanced cardiovascular magnetic resonance (CE-CMR) image in a vertical long-axis (sagittal-like) view confirming inferior MI as showed by delayed hyperenhancement (arrows). (C–E) Contrast-enhanced short-axis images show myocardial hyperenhancement (arrows) at basal (old posterior wall and the ECG in V1 is rS (see Figure 13.75)), mid, and apical levels of the inferior wall, indicating transmural myocardial infarction. (F) Quantification of myocardial necrotic mass.

contrast, various changes of the mid-late part of the QRS may appear (**fractioned QRS**) (see Figures 13.80 and **20.32**) (Das *et al.* 2006). The most frequent isolated infarctions involving the basal parts of the left ventricle are lateral MIs.

An apparently normal or near-normal ECG in the chronic phase may be considered probably abnormal if the following subtle changes are present in the ECG:
• evidence of amputation of the R wave in I aVL and/or V6 (low voltage) (Figure 20.39B);

- development of "slurrings" or "notches" in the final portions of the QRS complex in different leads (sometimes a "slurred" S wave in II, III, and aVF or an r' wave in V1 or rsr' in II and V4–V6 (Figure 20.32);
- a very striking low voltage of QRS in the frontal plane with dubious "q" wave (qrs, rsr'), in the inferior leads, in the absence of COPD, emphysema, heart failure, or other factors that may decrease the voltage of QRS;
- tall and peaked T waves or mild ST-segment depression (<0.5 mm) with normal QRS complex in V1–V2 (Figure 20.38); and
- the presence in V1–V2 of a peaked tall T wave and/or mild ST segment depression with normal QRS complex and lower R in V6 compared with previous ECG, suggest NSTEMI (Figure 20.39).

Right ventricular infarction (Figures 13.40 and 20.40)

In the acute phase of STEMI of the inferior wall (ST segment elevation in II, III, and aVF), right ventricular involvement may be suspected due to the presence of ST segment elevation in the extreme right precordial leads (V3R–V4R) with a positive T wave in V4R (Wellens and Connover 2006) (see Figure 13.39). In our experience, the isoelectric or elevated ST segment in V1 is also very useful for diagnosing extension of inferior MI to the right ventricular wall (Fiol *et al*. 2004) (Figure 13.47).

Atrial infarction

Atrial infarction never occurs in isolation. In the acute phase, the atrial ischemia (infarction) is expressed in different leads as PR depression and/or PR elevation (see Figure 9.33).

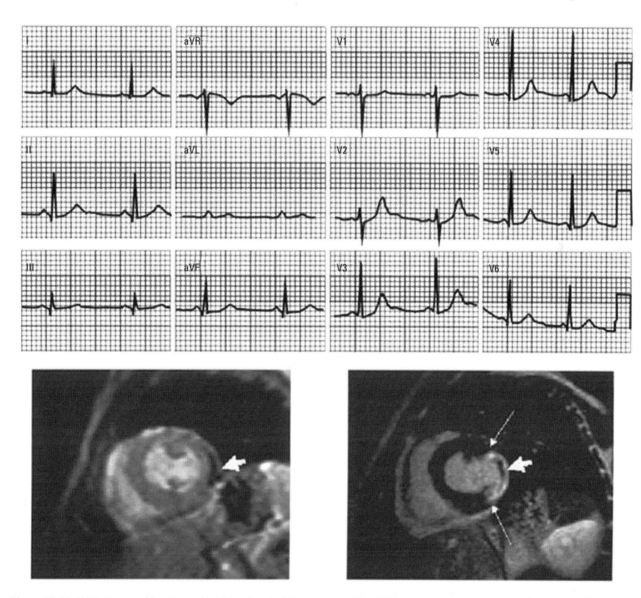

Figure 20.38 (A) A 46-year-old patient who had suffered a MI 2 years ago. The ECG does not show any abnormality in the QRS morphology and only mild ST-segment depression and positive and symmetric T wave in V2 with rS morphology can suggest lateral ischemia. (B) CMR revealed a lateral infarction.

A

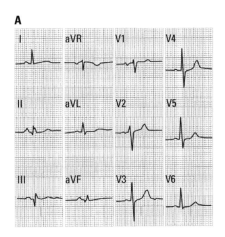

B

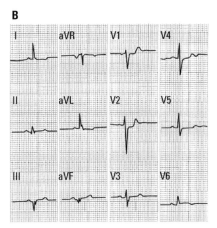

Figure 20.39 (A) ECG of 62-year-old patient with multivessel chronic coronary artery disease. (B) During an NSTEMI, an ST segment depression in V1–V2 and low-voltage R wave in V6 with flattened T wave, compared to pattern displayed in previous ECG (A), was observed. This patient presented with a non-Q wave MI due to obtuse marginal (OM) occlusion.

Other types of myocardial infarction without Q wave or its equivalent

Other types include the following:

• Myocardial infarction associated with PCI (type 4a myocardial Infarction), Stent/scaffold thrombosis associated with PCI (type 4b myocardial infarction), and Restenosis associated with PCI (type 4c myocardial infarction) (Thygesen *et al.* 2019);

• Myocardial infarction associated with coronary artery bypass grafting (type 5 myocardial infarction) (Thygesen *et al.* 2019);

• **aborted infarctions** (see Figures 20.1 and 20.36);

• **some MI with abnormal Q waves that disappear with time** (see Figure 20.35);

• **some MIs with confounding factors** (see Chapter 13 and below); and

• **masked Q wave by two MIs** (Color Plate 4 and Figure 20.41).

ECG in chronic myocardial infarctions in the presence of confounding factors (see Chapter 13)

We will briefly mention the diagnosis of MI in the chronic phase in the presence of ventricular blocks, pacemakers, and WPW pre-excitation. We have discussed extensively this topic in Chapter 13.

Right bundle branch block

Because cardiac activation begins normally, a Q wave MI may be generated in the chronic phase as it is in cases with a normal QRS complex (Figures 13.82 and 13.84).

Left bundle branch block

Due to changes of ventricular activation, even if important zones of the left ventricle are necrotic, the overall direction of the depolarization vector continues to point from the right to the left, and the Q wave of necrosis is usually not recorded. However, if the necrosis is extensive, sometimes an evident q wave in I, aVL, V5, or V6 and/or an r in V1 may be recorded (see Figures 13.85–13.88).

Hemiblocks (see Figures 13.89–13.99)

In general, in the presence of left anterior hemiblock, a Q wave of necrosis may be easily diagnosed. The loop–hemifield correlation (see Figure 13.97) explains how in the presence of a SAH in lead II, no terminal r wave is found while it is present in lead aVR, which is the opposite of the pattern that occurs in isolated inferior MI. This is an example of how the ECG may provide the same information as the VCG, something that was not considered possible in the past (Benchimol *et al.* 1972).

In Chapter 13, we discussed: (i) the diagnosis of association; (ii) how the hemiblock may mask Q waves; (iii) how Q waves of infarction may mask the hemiblocks, and (iv) false Q wave pattern due to hemiblocks.

Pre-excitation and pacemakers (Figures 13.100–13.103)

In both these cases, it may be difficult to diagnose the presence of a Q wave MI. In the case of pacemakers, the presence of a spike–qR pattern in V5–V6 confers high specificity but low sensitivity as a sign of necrosis.

ECG changes due to decreased blood flow not related to atherothrombosis (Table 20.1)

This section will discuss the ECG characteristics found in some cases of myocardial ischemia due to decreased flow usually acute, but not related to atherothrombosis although sometimes may occur associated to atherosclerotic plaque. Some of these are triggers of true ACS, and may lead to MI. We will comment on the most frequent. For more information, consult Fiol-Sala *et al.* (2020).

Hypercoagulability

Hypercoagulation state may be found especially in heaving smokers or as a consequence of drug-induced states (e.g. contraceptive drugs); and in pregnancy in women

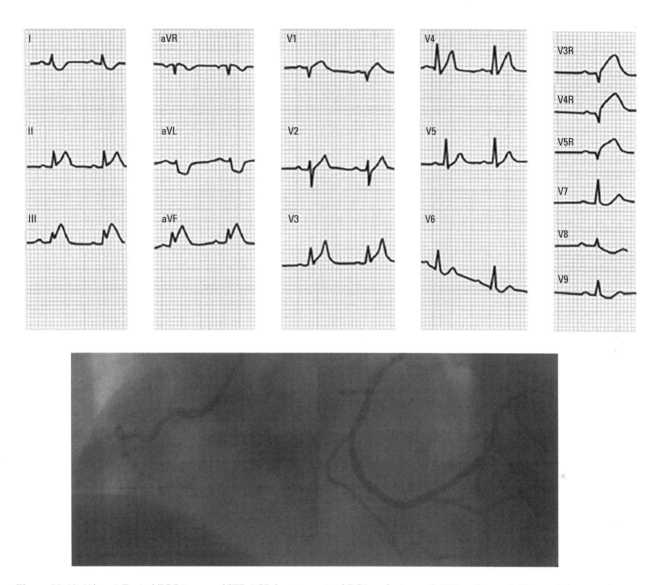

Figure 20.40 (Above) Typical ECG in case of STE-ACS due to proximal RCA occlusion with RV involvement. Observe ST-segment elevation in II, III, and aVF with III > II, ST-segment depression in I and aVL, and elevated ST in V1–V3 as well as in V3R–V4R leads with positive T wave. (Below) Coronary angiography before (left) and after (right) reperfusion showing right dominance.

with hereditary thrombophilia. In the latter case, even in the absence of atherothrombosis, ACS usually with ST elevation may occur, especially due to LAD thrombosis. There are no differential ECG signs.

Angina secondary to tachyarrhythmias

An episode of paroxysmal arrhythmia crisis, especially atrial fibrillation, may cause long-lasting chest pain, which may have anginal characteristics.

When an ECG is recorded during crisis of tachyarrhythmia, even supraventricular reciprocating tachycardia in young people, certain abnormalities, such as ST segment depression (Figure 19.7) or a negative T wave, at the end of an episode, may be found. These abnormalities usually do not represent true ischemic heart disease (Bayés de Luna and Baranchuk 2017). The ST segment

elevation evolving to Q wave MI is never found (see Chapter 15).

Coronary dissection (Figure 20.42)

STEMI may occur suddenly especially in young women, usually multiparous, during the postpartum period. This is caused by a collagen abnormality that favors dissection. The LAD is the most frequently involved artery (Roig *et al.* 2003).

Significant ST segment elevation, generally of the type found in LAD occlusion, may occur proximal to S1 and D1, with a mirror pattern in II, III, and aVF, or in the proximal RCA or LCX occlusion. If the coronary dissection affects LMT, ST segment elevation ACS usually appears because there is no previous subendocardial ischemia or collateral circulation. It is important to emphasize that

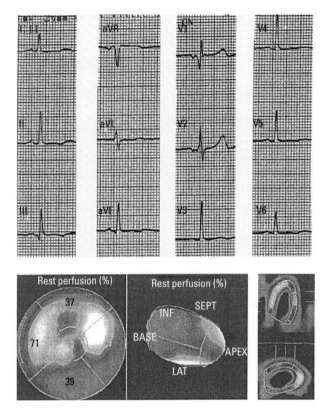

Figure 20.41 ECG of a patient with two myocardial infarction (MI), one apical and the other inferolateral. The presence of QR in V1, RS in V2, and qR with wide q in III is the abnormal QRS change. The QR pattern of V1 is explained by double infarction (apical + inferolateral). However, there are not many leads with Q wave in spite of clinical and isotopic evidence of double infarction, probably due to partial cancellation of infarction vectors. The final R in V1 and the R in V2–V3 are explained because the inferolateral infarction is more important than the apical infarction. The nuclear study clearly shows the presence of double infarction of inferolateral zone and smaller apical area.

although usually the ECG of LMT shows huge and diffuse ST segment depression (NSTEMI) because it is the expression of LMT subocclusion (Figure 20.17), total occlusion of LMT may also occur, showing ST segment elevation (STEMI) (Figure 20.3). Patients with STEMI due to coronary dissection (LMT or proximal LAD) often present with cardiogenic shock and may even need heart transplantation if ventricular fibrillation has not triggered sudden death.

Transient left ventricular apical ballooning (Tako–Tsubo syndrome) (Figure 20.43)

This pattern of apical dyskinesia is transient, involving coronary arteries that are normal or scarcely affected. The increase in coronary artery tone and/or catecholamine storm release rather than an authentic spasm, with little involvement of the vessel but probably with lysis of a thrombus accounts for the ACS (Ibáñez *et al.* 2004).

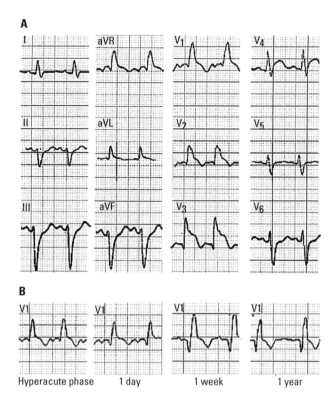

Figure 20.42 (A) ECG of a 35-year-old multiparous woman with a very serious acute coronary syndrome (ACS) due to dissection of LAD proximal to D1 and S1. Note the morphology of the advanced right bundle branch block (RBBB) + superoanterior hemiblock (SAH) together with evident ST segment changes (ST elevation in precordials due to occlusion in LAD), with ST segment depression in II, III, and aVF (occlusion proximal to D1), and ST segment elevation in aVR and V1 with ST segment depression in V6 (occlusion proximal to S1). (B) The evolution of the ECG patterns through time (V1).

Although the ECG alone should not be used to differentiate between TTS and ACS, there are distinct differences between these clinical entities with respect to the ECG findings at presentation. As in ACS, the ECG presentation in an individual patient with TTS is dependent on the time delay between symptom onset and the ECG recording. In the first 24 hours, ST elevation occurs, most frequently in leads V2–V6 and without mirror-image ST depression. ST elevation is followed by T-wave inversion and prolonged QTc interval. The QTc tends to peak on day 3, and it correlates with the risk of ventricular arrhythmias (Watson *et al.* 2019). ST depression occurs in less than 10% of TTS patients. Though, ST depression in lead aVR (=ST elevation in lead -aVR) is a typical finding in TTS, is also typical of ST-segment elevation myocardial infarction due to occlusion that is distal to D1 (Carrillo *et al.* 2010; Kosuge *et al.* 2011).

Congenital defects (Figure 20.44)

Coronary anomalies should be suspected when a very young person suffers from exertional anginal pain. The congenital defects causing more problems are located at

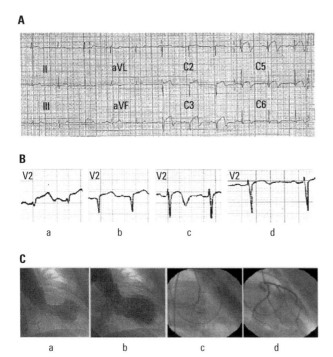

Figure 20.43 (A) Twelve-lead ECG in subacute phase in a patient with typical transitory apical ballooning (Tako–Tsubo syndrome). (B) ECG changes in V2 during the period of 3–4 days (a–d). Note the ECG pattern from ST elevation with Q wave to rS with deep negative T waves. (C) Typical angiographic image (a,b) and normal coronary tree (c,d).

the anomalous take-off of the left coronary artery, from the pulmonary artery.

Coronary spasm: Prinzmetal variant angina

Prinzmetal angina (vasospastic angina or variant angina), first described by Prinzmetal *et al.* (1959), is a clinical syndrome characterized by angina at rest induced by coronary artery vasospasm (Stern and Bayes de Luna 2009). A recent study conducted in the United States and included 97,280 admissions with an ICD-9 code 413.1 (Prinzmetal angina), reported that actually there was a significant increase in the number of hospitalization with Prinzmetal angina (3,678 in 2002 versus 8,633 in 2015; P trend <0.001) (Elbadawi *et al.* 2019). In-hospital mortality among patients with Prinzmetal angina has increased (0.24% in 2002 versus 0.85% in 2015; P trend = 0.02).

Prinzmetal angina can also be diagnosed by continuous Holter electrocardiographic monitoring (Bayes de Luna *et al.* 1985). Most of the patients (n = 19) were men and the mean age was 57 ± 7.5 years. A total of 121 episodes with ST elevation were recorded. These episodes were not associated with strenuous physical activity and were not clustered in a particular time of the day. Episodes started with an increase in the T wave amplitude, followed by ST elevation if ischemia persisted (Figure 20.46). In some episodes, only peaked positive T waves could be seen, with no ST elevation as an expression of first phase of coronary spasm

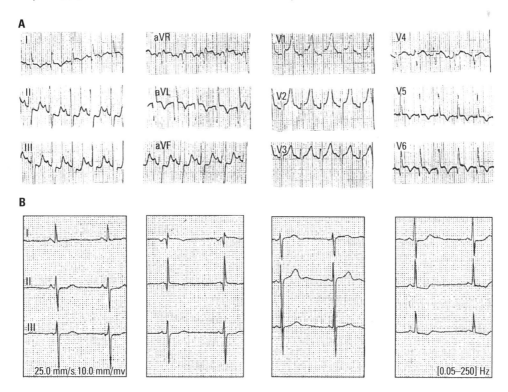

Figure 20.44 (A) A 3-year-old girl with abnormal origin of left coronary artery from pulmonary artery. ECG recording previous to a surgical intervention shows very abnormal Q wave, especially in aVL and V6. Ligature of left coronary artery was performed. (B) The same patient at 12 years of age. The abnormal q wave has practically disappeared. Currently, all the coronary perfusion depends on the huge RCA.

(peaked positive T wave of subendocardial ischemia). Episodes of ST elevation can last between 1 and 21 minutes. During episodes of ST elevation, changes in the terminal portion of the QRS, as later described by Sclarovsky and Birnbaum in the context of acute STEMI (Birnbaum *et al.* 2014), can be detected: increase of the R wave amplitude, and decrease of the S wave amplitude (Figure 20.45) (Bayes de Luna *et al.* 2014). Surface 12-lead ECG can depict reciprocal ST segment depression in leads facing away from the ischemic zone (Figure 20.45). The pattern of ST deviation enables to predict the location of the ischemic segment(s) and the site of the coronary artery spasm (Bayes de Luna *et al.* 2014). In some episodes, during the peak of ST elevation, the terminal part of the T wave becomes negative, giving an upsloping appearance to the T-Q segment (Bayes de Luna *et al.* 1985, 2014). This pattern has been suggested to reflect the most severe form of ischemia (grade IV) (Nikus and Birnbaum 2016). In a fifth of the episodes (n = 20), an alternans of the ST-TQ morphology was seen (Figure 20.48) (Bayes de Luna *et al.* 2014). This pattern was more prevalent in episodes with high-amplitude ST elevation.

When coronary spasm resolves, ST segment elevation rapidly disappears and the T waves can become negative, reflecting post-ischemic changes (Rey *et al.* 2016). The depth of the negative T waves after the ischemic episode depends on the severity and duration of the preceding ischemia and could last from minutes to hours (Bayes de Luna *et al.* 1985).

Yet, vasospastic angina can present with ST depression (Figueras *et al.* 2012), rather than ST elevation and there are episodes of pain without associated ST deviation (Bayes de Luna *et al.* 1985; Stern and Bayes de Luna 2009; Figueras *et al.* 2012). Interestingly; however, alternating episodes of ST depression and ST elevation have not been found, suggesting that the underlying pathophysiology could be different (Bayes de Luna *et al.* 1985, 2014).

Arrhythmias associated with Prinzmetal angina: Salermo *et al.* (1984) reported that among 56 patients with coronary spasm, ventricular arrhythmia (premature ventricular beats, ventricular tachycardia and ventricular fibrillation) was found during ischemia in 23 patients and during reperfusion in 10 patients. In a cohort of 20 patients, described by Bayes de Luna *et al.* (1985), ventricular arrhythmia were seen in most patients (n = 19); however, most episodes of ST elevation (64%) were not associated with arrhythmia. Reperfusion ventricular arrhythmias were seen in 37% of the episodes, whereas in 37% of the episodes, ventricular arrhythmias occurred between the beginning of ST elevation and the maximal ST elevation. Among 273 patients, admitted with rest angina and without significant coronary stenosis, ventricular fibrillation was detected in 14 (5.1%) and ventricular tachycardia in 14 (5.1%) (Figueras *et al.* 2012). Nishizaki *et al.* (2001) reported that Holter monitoring for an average of 42 hours revealed episodes of polymorphic ventricular tachycardia in eight out of 60 consecutive patients with vasospastic angina; in four of them, the ischemic episodes were silent. Second- or third-degree AV block has been described during vasospastic attacks, especially due to RCA spasm (Stern and Bayes de Luna 2009; Bayes de Luna *et al.* 2014).

A

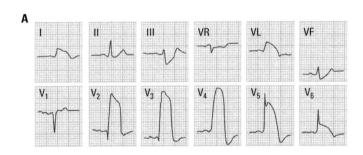

B

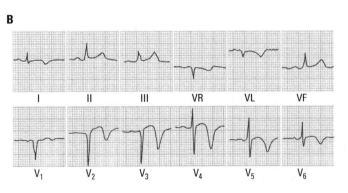

Figure 20.45 (A) Surface ECG of a 65-year-old patient with typical crisis of Prinzmetal angina that presents in the peak of pain an ST segment elevation like a transmembrane action potential (TAP). This case corresponds to a transitory complete proximal occlusion of the LAD above D1 (ST segment elevation from V1 to V6, I and aVL with ST segment depression in inferior leads, especially III and aVF). The lack of ST segment elevation in aVR, the small ST segment elevation in V1, and the clear ST segment elevation in V6—if the placement of V6 is well done—is against that the occlusion is also above S1 (see Figure 13.41). This is the first case of Prinzmetal angina seen by us in the early 1970s. Coronarography was not performed but enzymes were normal. (B) ECG after some hours of the crisis with a typical pattern of very negative T wave in all precordial leads (reperfusion pattern).

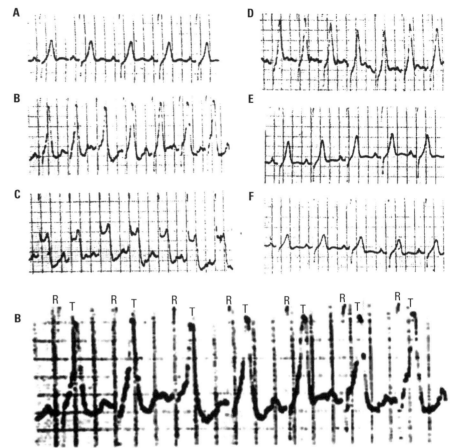

Figure 20.46 Crisis of coronary spasm (Prinzmetal angina) recorded by Holter ECG. (A) Control, (B) initial pattern of a very tall T wave (subendocardial ischemia), and (C) huge pattern of ST-segment elevation. (D–F) Resolution toward normal values. Total duration of the crisis was 2 minutes. (B) amplified to see well R and T.

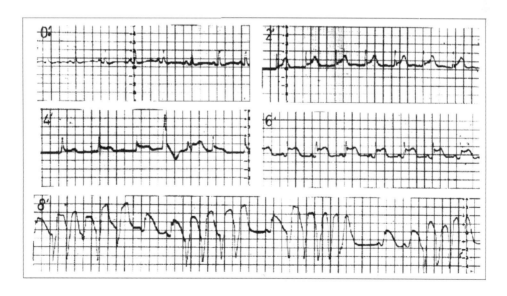

Figure 20.47 Sequence of a Prinzmetal angina crisis with the appearance of ventricular tachycardia runs at the moment of maximum ST segment elevation.

X Syndrome (Figure 20.49)

The more strict definition of CSX entails the following criteria (Kaski 2004; Lanza 2007; Agrawal *et al.* 2014): (i) Exercise-induced, angina-like chest discomfort, (ii) ST-segment depression during angina (Figure 20.49), rarely, ST segment elevation may occur, which is probably explained by multiple microcirculatory spasms, (iii) Normal or mild-to-moderate epicardial coronary artery stenoses (vascular

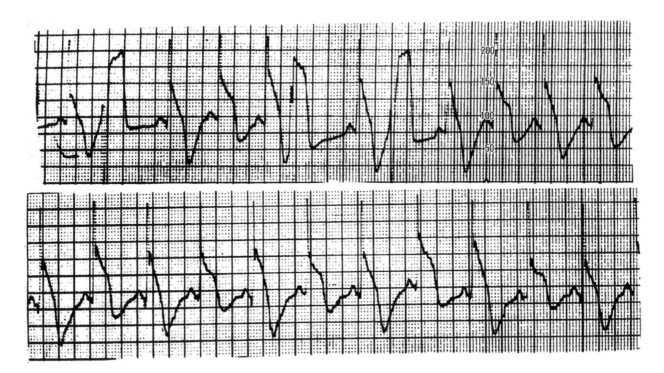

Figure 20.48 (A) Holter recording of a patient with a severe crisis of Prinzmetal angina. Observe the presence of clear ST segment and TQ alternans together with some premature ventricular complexes (PVCs).

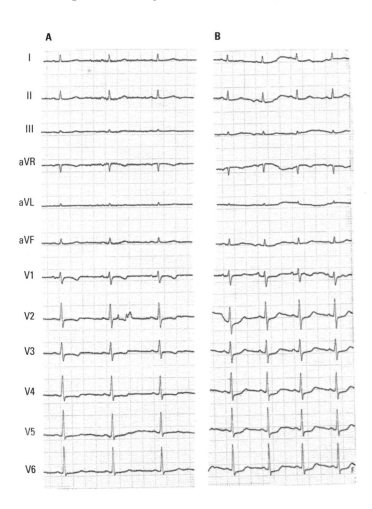

Figure 20.49 (A) A 60-year-old patient with typical X syndrome and normal coronary arteries. Observe the mild diffuse ST depression/flat T wave in the majority of the leads. (B) After exercise there is a clear ST depression, especially in horizontal leads.

irregularities or discrete very mild stenosis) (Lanza 2007) in angiography, (iv) No spontaneous or inducible epicardial coronary artery spasm upon ergonovine or acetylcholine provocation (Crea *et al.* 2014), (v) absence of cardiac or systemic diseases associated with microvascular dysfunction such as left ventricular hypertrophy, hypertrophic cardiomyopathy, aortic stenosis, and hypertensive heart disease, diabetes, or inflammation (such as myocarditis or vasculitis). The prognosis is generally good and, in general, does not evolve to MI.

Myocardial bridging

This is an anomaly of the course of the coronary arteries, especially the LAD, which partly penetrates the epicardial muscular mass. It is frequently, though not always, accompanied by atherosclerosis and/or coronary spasm.

The clinical picture often is stable exercise angina that may appear without ECG changes in a patient with usually normal basal ECG. On other occasions, the anginal pain appears at rest and is probably associated with coronary spasm related to myocardial bridging.

Rarely, cases of ACS with or without MI (with and without Q wave) have been described.

It has been exceptionally linked to sudden death, although in general the prognosis is good (Mohlenkamp *et al.* 2002).

Peri-procedural myocardial infarction
Cardiac surgery (Thygesen *et al.* 2019)

Criteria for CABG-related MI: 48 hours after the index procedure (type 5 MI) CABG-related MI is arbitrarily defined as elevation of cTn values >10 times the 99th percentile URL in patients with normal baseline cTn values. In patients with elevated pre-procedure cTn in whom cTn levels are stable (≤20% variation) or falling, the post-procedure cTn must rise by >20%. However, the absolute post-procedural value still must be >10 times the 99th percentile URL. In addition, one of the following elements is required:
- Development of new pathological Q waves[1]
- Angiographic documented new graft occlusion or new native coronary artery occlusion;
- Imaging evidence of new loss of viable myocardium or new regional wall motion abnormality in a pattern consistent with an ischemic etiology.

Percutaneous coronary intervention

According to Kenigsberg *et al.* (2007), the sudden occlusion of a coronary artery during PCI prolongs QTc in 100% of cases (Figure 20.13). This change is usually accompanied by rectified ST segment and symmetric T wave that is often taller than normal. Changes of T wave polarity (from negative to positive) and especially ST segment deviations are not frequent during short periods of ischemia (Figure 20.13). However, in intracoronary recordings, an evident ST elevation may be recorded in cases of only small changes of T waves in surface ECG recordings (Figure 20.14). The presence of ST segment deviations is a marker for very bad prognosis (Quyyumi *et al.* 1986; Björklund *et al.* 2005).

Criteria for PCI-related MI _ 48 hours after the index procedure (type 4a MI) (Thygesen *et al.* 2019)

Coronary intervention-related MI is arbitrarily defined by an elevation of cTn values more than five times the 99th percentile URL in patients with normal baseline values. In patients with elevated pre-procedure cTn in whom the cTn level are stable (≤20% variation) or falling, the post-procedure cTn must rise by >20%. However, the absolute post-procedural value must still be at least five times the 99th percentile URL. In addition, one of the following elements is required:
- New ischemic ECG changes;
- Development of new pathological Q waves[2];
- Imaging evidence of new loss of viable myocardium or new regional wall motion abnormality in a pattern consistent with an ischemic etiology;
- Angiographic findings consistent with a procedural flow-limiting complication such as coronary dissection, occlusion of a major epicardial artery or a side branch occlusion/thrombus, disruption of collateral flow, or distal embolization.[3]

Others

Other situations apart from atherothrombosis that may cause ACS and MI include (Fiol-Sala *et al.* 2020): (i) cocaine abuse (STEMI); (ii) carbon monoxide poisoning (may present with an ACS and sometimes a silent Q wave MI); (iii) anaphylactic crisis (ACS with Q or non-Q wave MI); (iv) acute anemia (clinical picture of NSTEMI); (v) pheochromocytoma; (vi) coronary arteritis (Takayasu's disease, Kawasaki's disease), etc.

---

1 Isolated development of new pathological Q waves meets the type 5 MI criteria if cTn values are elevated and rising but <10 times the 99th percentile URL.

2 Isolated development of new pathological Q waves meets the type 4a MI criteria if cTn values are elevated and rising but less than five times the 99th percentile URL.

3 Post-mortem demonstration of a procedure-related thrombus in the culprit artery, or a macroscopically large circumscribed area of necrosis with or without intra-myocardial hemorrhage meets the type 4a MI criteria.

ECG changes due to ischemia caused by increased demand (see Table 20.1)

Classic exercise angina in patients with ischemic heart disease

These patients present with angina during exercise. The most frequent cases of ischemia caused by increased demand are explained by a coronary atherosclerosis due to a fixed stable plaque that produces impairment of subendocardium perfusion at rest that is not usually so prominent as to change the basal ECG. However, frequently **ST segment depression** is present during exercise. This ECG change is typical of significant subendocardial ischemia without total occlusion and occurs because the vasodilatory capability of the subendocardium is low and therefore is more vulnerable to ischemia (see Chapter 13).

Exercise angina may appear with or without previous myocardial infarction (MI). Often in the presence of angina, the exercise tests presents ST depression but there are false-positive and false-negative results (see Chapter 25). The exercise test helps to establish the most adequate treatment (Fiol-Sala *et al.* 2020). In case of doubt, it is necessary to clarify the diagnosis with imaging techniques and/or coronariography.

These changes especially appear in leads with a predominant R wave. The ECG changes during exercise angina may also be detected by Holter monitoring (see Figure 13.27), and they may also be reproduced during exercise testing (see Figure 13.26). Rarely, a peaked T wave (Manankil *et al.* 2011) (first pattern of subendocardial ischemia) or even an ST elevation appears during exercise which is generally due to coronary spasm (Figure 20.50).

Other cases

There are various other situations (pulmonary hypertension, chronic anemia, tachyarrhythmias, left ventricular hypertrophy, coronary perfusion imbalance, carbon monoxide poisoning, etc.) in which angina may also appear due to increased demand and that may present with changes of repolarization. The most frequent changes are probably the appearance of ST depression and/or precordial discomfort during exercise, or if the heart rate increases too much in the case of atrial fibrillation.

ECG in chronic stable ischemic heart disease

Morphological changes and arrhythmias (see ECG in chronic MI with narrow QRS and in the presence of confounding factors).

A

B

C

D

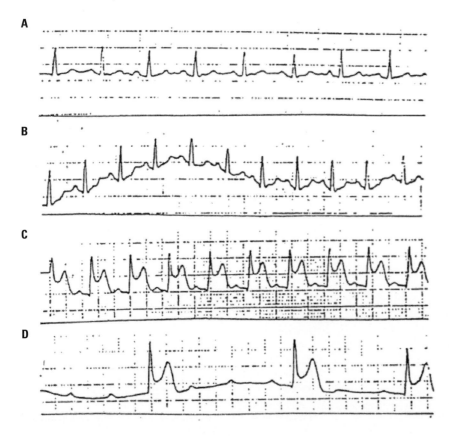

Figure 20.50 Exercise test in a patient with precordial pain. Before the exercise test (A) and during it (B), ST segment is normal. At the end, there is an important ST segment elevation, accompanied by precordial pain (C), which was followed by advanced AV block (D). This corresponds to a spasm of RCA before the branch that perfuses the AV node.

Patients with chronic stable ischemic heart disease (IHD) with or without previous MI may present normal basal ECG or different changes of QRS (Q wave or equivalent, or fragmented QRS), or ST/T changes (ST depression or elevation and/or flat/negative T wave).

The negative T wave that appears after Q wave MI (post-ischemic change) may disappear with time and it is a sign of good prognosis (Figure 20.35).

The persistence of flat/negative T wave or mild ST depression in leads without Q wave indicates the need to perform an exercise test to recognize if a clear ST depression appear. The presence of flat/mild negative T wave very often has a good prognosis and may persist for years (post-ischemic changes).

The persistence of ST elevation far from acute MI is suggestive of LV aneurysm (Figure 20.32C).

Finally, very often different types of intraventricular blocks appear as a consequence of IHD. These usually represent a marker of bad prognosis. In respect to arrhythmias (see Chapters 23 and 24), the presence of ventricular arrhythmias, especially frequent PVCs and runs of VT, represents a marker of risk, especially in the presence of LV dysfunction (consult Bayés de Luna and Baranchuk 2017; Fiol-Sala *et al.* 2020). We have already discussed (see Ischemia and sudden death) the importance of acute and chronic IHD in the occurrence of sudden death. The incidence of atrial arrhythmias, especially atrial fibrillation, is frequent and also is a marker of bad prognosis.

References

Abbas A, Boura J, Brewington S, *et al*. Acute angiographic analysis of NSTE-acute myocardial infarction. *Am J Cardiol* 2004; 24:907.

Abu-Assi E, García-Acuña JM, Peña-Gil C, *et al*. Validation of the GRACE risk score for predicting death within 6 months of follow-up in a contemporary cohort of patients with acute coronary syndrome. *Rev Esp Cardiol* 2010;63:640.

Adams GL, Campbell PT, Adams JM, *et al*. Effectiveness of prehospital wireless transmission of electrocardiograms to a cardiologist via hand-held device for patients with acute myocardial infarction (from the Timely Intervention in Myocardial Emergency, NorthEast Experience [TIME-NE]). *Am J Cardiol* 2006;98:1160

Agrawal S, Metha PK, Merz NB. Cardiac syndrome X-update 2014. *Cardiol Clin* 2014;32:463.

Aldrich HR, Wagner NB, Boswick J, *et al*. Use of initial ST-segment deviation for prediction of final electrocardiographic size of acute myocardial infarcts. *Am J Cardiol* 1988;61:749.

Alnsasra H, Ben-Avraham B, Gottlieb S, *et al*. High-grade atrioventricular block in patients with acute myocardial infarction. Insights from a contemporary multi-center survey. *J Electrocardiol* 2018;51:386.

Al-Zaiti SS, Shusterman V, Carey MG. Novel technical solutions for wireless ECG transmission & analysis in the age in the internet cloud. *J Electrocardiol* 2013;46:540.

Antman EM, Cohen M, Bernink PJ, *et al*. The TIMI risk score for unstable angina/non-ST elevation MI: a method for prognostication and therapeutic decision making. *JAMA* 2000;284:835.

Barrabes J, Figueras J, Moure C, Cortadellas J, Soler Soler J. Prognostic significance of ST depression in lateral leads on admission ECG in patients with first acute myocardial infarction. *J Am Coll Cardiol* 2000;35:1813.

Bayés de Luna A, Baranchuk A. *Clinical Arrhythmology*, 2nd edn. Wiley-Blackwell, 2017.

Bayés de Luna A, Carreras F, Cladellas M, *et al*. Holter ECG study of the electrocardiographic phenomena in Prinzmetal angina attacks with emphasis on the study of ventricular arrhythmias. *J Electrocardiol* 1985;18:267.

Bayés de Luna A, Coumel Ph, Leclercq JF. Ambulatory sudden cardiac death: mechanism of the basis of fatal arrhythmais from 157 cases. *Am Heart J* 1989;117:151.

Bayés de Luna A, Cino JM, Pujadas S, *et al*. Concordance of electrocardiograhpic patterns and healed myocardial infarction locaton detected by cardiovascular magnetic resonance. *Am J Cardiol* 2006a;97:443.

Bayés de Luna A, Wagner G, Birnbaum Y, *et al*. A new terminology for the left ventricular walls and for the location of myocardial infarcts that present Q wave based on the standard of cardiac magnetic resonance imaging. A statement for healthcare professionals from a committee appointed by the International Society for Holter and Non Invasive Electrocardiography. *Circulation* 2006b;114:1755.

Bayés de Luna A, Cino J, Goldwasser D, *et al*. New electrocardiographic diagnostic criteria for the pathologic R waves in leads V1 and V2 of anatomically lateral myocardial infarction. *J Electrocardiol* 2008;41:413.

Bayés de Luna A, Cygankiewicz I, Baranchuk A et al Prinzmetal angina: ECG changes and clinical considerations: A consensus paper. *Ann Noninvasive Electrocardiol* 2014; 19: 442-453.

Benchimol A, Desser KB, Schumacher J. Value of the vectorcardiogram for distinguishing left anterior hemiblock from inferior infarction with left axis deviation. *Chest* 1972;61:74.

Ben-Gal T, Sclarovsky S, Itzhak H, *et al*. Importance of the conal branch of the right coronary artery in patients with acute anterior wall myocardial infarction: electrocardiographic and angiographic correlation. *J Am Coll Cardiol* 1997;29:506.

Birnbaum Y, Atar S. Electrocardiogram risk stratification of non ST elevation acute coronary syndrome. *J Electrocardiol* 2006;39:558.

Birnbaum Y, Sclarovsky S, Blum, *et al*. Prognostic significance of the initial electrocardiographic pattern in a first acute anterior wall myocardial infarction. *Chest* 1993;103:1681.

Birnbaum Y, Zhou S, Wagner GS. New considerations of ST segment "elevation" and "depression" and accompanying T wave configuration in acute coronary syndromes. *J Electrocardiol* 2011;44:1.

Birnbaum Y, Bayes de Luba A, Fiol M *et al*. Common pitfalls in the interpretation of electrocardiograms from patients with acute coronary syndromes with narrow QRS: a consensus report. *J Electrocardiol* 2012;45:463.

Birnbaum GD, Birnbaum I, Birnbaum Y. Twenty years of ECG grading of the severity of ischemia. *J Electrocardiol* 2014;47:546.

Björklund E, Stenestrand U, Lindbäck J, *et al*. RIKS-HIA investigators. Prehospital diagnosis and start of treatment reduces time delay and mortality in real-life patients with STEMI. *J Electrocardiol* 2005;38:186.

Bouwmeester S, van Hellemond I, Maynard Ch, *et al.* The stability of the ST segment estimation of myocardial area at risk between the prehospital and hospital electrocardiograms in patients with ST elevation myocardial infarction. *J Electrocardiol* 2011;44:363.

Burke A, Farb A, Malcom GT, *et al.* Coronary risk factors and plaque morphology in men with coronary disease who die suddenly. *N Engl J Med* 1997;336:1276.

Carrillo A, Fiol M, García-Niebla J, *et al.* Electrocardiographic differential diagnosis between Takotsubo syndrome and distal occlusion of LAD is not easy. *J Am Coll Cardiol* 2010;56:1610.

Choi WS, Lee JH, Park SH, *et al.* Prognostic value of standard electrocardiographic parameters for predicting major adverse cardiac events after acute myocardial infarction. *Ann Noninvasive Electrocardiol* 2011;16:56.

Cino JM, Pujadas S, Carreras F, *et al.* Utility of contrast-enhanced cardiovascular magnetic resonance (CE-CMR) to assess how likely is an infarct to produce a typical ECG pattern. *J Cardiovasc Magn Reson* 2006;8:335.

Cohen M, Scharpf SJ, Rentrop KP. Prospective analysis of electrocardiographic variables as markers for extent and location of acute wall motion abnormalities observed during coronary angioplasty in human subjects. *J Am Coll Cardiol* 1987;10:17.

Correale E, Sattista R, Ricciardíello V, *et al.* The negative U wave: apathogenetic enigma but a useful, often overlooked bedside diagnostic and prognostic clue in ischemic heart disease. *Clin Cardiol* 2004;27:674.

Crea F, Camici PG, Bairey Merz CN. Coronary microvascular dysfunction: an update. *Eur Heart J* 2014;35:1101.

Das MK, Khan B, Jacob S, *et al.* Significance of a fragmented QRS complex versus a Q wave in patients with coronary artery disease. *Circulation* 2006;113:2495.

De Vreede-Swagemakers JJ, Gorgels AP, Dubois-Arbouw WI, *et al.* Out-of-hospital cardiac arrests in the 1990s: a population based study in the Maastricht area on incidence, characteristics and survival. *J Am Coll Cardiol* 1997;30:1500.

De Winter RJ, Verouden NJ, Wellens HJ, *et al.* Interventional Cardiology Group of the Academic Medical Center. A new ECG sign of proximal LAD occlusion. *N Engl J Med* 2008;359:2071.

De Zwan C, Bär H, Wellens HJ. Characteristic ECG pattern indicating a critical stenosis high in left anterior descending coronary artery in patients admitted because of an impending infarction. *Am Heart J* 1982;103:730.

Dellborg, M, Topol, EJ, Swedberg, K, *et al.* Dynamic QRS complex and ST segment vectorcardiographic monitoring can identify vessel patency in patients with acute myocardial infarction treated with reperfusion therapy. *Am Heart J* 1991;122:943.

Dixon W. Anatomic distribution of the culprit lesion in patients with NSTE-ACS undergoing PCI. *J Am Coll Cardiol* 2008; 62:1347.

Doevendans PA, Gorgels AP, van der Zee R, *et al.* Electrocardiographic diagnosis of reperfusion during thrombolytic therapy in acute myocardial infarction. *Am J Cardiol* 1995;75:1206.

Dressler W, Roesler H. High T waves in the earliest stage of myocardial infarction. *Am Heart J* 1947;34:627.

Ducas RA, Philipp RK, Jassal DS, *et al.* Cardiac outcomes trough-digital evaluation (CODE) STEMI project: prehospital digitally-assisted reperfusion strategies. *Can J Cardiol* 2012;28:423.

Durrer D, Van Dam R, Freud G, *et al.* Total excitation of the isolated human heart. *Circulation* 1970;41:899.

Eagle K, Lim M, Dabbous O, *et al.* for the GRACE Investigators. A validated prediction model for allf orms of acute coronary syndrome. Estimating the rist of 6-month postdischarge death in an international registry. *JAMA* 2004;291:2727.

East T, Oran S. The ECG in ventricular aneurysm following acute infarction. *Br Heart J* 1952;14:125.

Elbadawi A, Elgendy IY, Naqvi SY, *et al.* Temporal trends and outcomes of hospitalizations with Prinzmetal angina: perspectives from a national database. *Am J Med* 2019;132:1053.

Elsman P, Van't Hof AW, de Boer MJ, *et al.* Impact of infarct location on left ventricular ejection fraction after correction for enzymatic infarct size in acute myocardial infarction treated with primary coronary intervention. *Am Heart J* 2006;151:1239.

Engelen DJ, Gorgels AP, Cheriex EC, *et al.* Value of the electrocardiogram in localizing the occlusion site in the left anterior descending coronary artery in acute anterior myocardial infarction. *J Am Coll Cardiol* 1999;34:389.

Figueras J, Domingo E, Ferreira I, Lidon RM, Garcia-Dorado D. Persistent angina pectoris, cardiac mortality and myocardial infarction during a 12 year follow-up in 273 variant angina patients without significant fixed coronary stenosis. *Am J Cardiol* 2012;110:1249.

Fiol M, Barcena JP, Rota JI, *et al.* Sustained ventricular tachycardia as a marker of inadequate myocardial perfusion during the acute phase of myocardial infarction. *Clin Cardiol* 2002;25:328.

Fiol M, Cygankiewicz I, Bayés Genis A, *et al.* The value of ECG algorithm based on 'ups and downs' of ST in assessment of a culprit artery in evolving inferior myocardial infarction. *Am J Cardiol* 2004;94:709.

Fiol M, Carrillo A, Cygankiewicz I, *et al.* A new electrocardiographic algorithm to locate the occlusion in left anterior descending coronary artery. *Clin Cardiol* 2009;32:E1–6.

Fiol M, Carrillo A, Rodríguez A, *et al.* Electrocardiographic changes of ST-elevation myocardial infarction in patients with complete occlusion of the left main trunk without collateral circulation: differential diagnosis and clinical considerations. *J Electrocardiol* 2012;45:487.

Fiol-Sala M, Birbaum Y, Nikus K, Bayes de Luna A. *Electrocardiography in Ischemic Heart Disease: Clinical and Imaging Correlations and Prognostic Implications*, 2nd edn. Wiley Blackwell, 2020.

From A, Best P, Lennon R, *et al.* Acute myocardial infarction due to circumflex artery occlusion and significance for ST-segment elevation. *Am J Cardiol* 2010;106:1081.

Gorgels A. Explanation of the ECG in the subendocardial ischemia of the anterior wall of the left ventricle. *J Electrocardiol* 2009;42:248.

Gul E, Nikus K. An unusual presentation of left anterior descending artery occlusion: significance of lead aVR and T-wave direction. *J Electrocardiol* 2011;44:27.

Hathaway WR, Peterson ED, Wagner GS, *et al.* Prognostic significance of the initial electrocardiogram in patients with acute myocardial infarction. GUSTO-I Investigators. Global Utilization of Streptokinase and t-PA for Occluded Coronary Arteries. *JAMA* 1998;279:387.

Holmvang L, Clemmensen P, Wagner G, *et al.* Admission standard electrocardiogram for early risk stratification in patients with unstable coronary artery disease not eligible for acute revascularization therapy: A TRIM substudy. ThRombin Inhibition in Myocardial Infarction. *Am Heart J* 1999;137:24.

Huang HD, Tran V, Jneid H, Wilson JM, Birnbaum Y. Comparison of angiographic findings in patients with acute anteroseptal versus anterior wall ST-elevation myocardial infarction. *Am J Cardiol* 2011;107:827.

Ibáñez B, Navarro F, Farré J, *et al*. Tako-tsubo syndrome associated with a long course of the left anterior descending coronary artery along the apical diaphragmatic surface of the left ventricle. *Rev Esp Cardiol* 2004;57:209.

Jacobs A. Chair: ACC/AHA Task force members. Unstable angina/NSTEMI Guidelines revision. Circulation 2011:May 3.

Jain S, Ting H, Bell M, *et al*. Utility of left bundle branch block as a diagnostic criterion for acute myocardial infarction. *Am J Cardiol* 2011;107:1111.

Janse MJ. Electrophysiological changes in acute myocardial ischemia. In Julian DG, Lie KI, Wihelmsen L (eds). *What Is Angina?* Astra, 1982, p. 160.

Jayroe JB, Spodick DH, Nikus K, *et al*. Differentiating ST elevation myocardial infarction and nonishcemic causes of ST elevation by analyzing the presenting electrocardiogram. *Am J Cardiol* 2009;103:301.

Jim M-H, Siu C-W, Chan AO-O, *et al*. Prognostic implications of PR-segment depression in inferior leads in acute inferior myocardial infarction. *Clin Cardiol* 2006;29:36.

Kanei Y, Sharma J, Diwan R, *et al*. ST segment depression inVR as a predictor of culprit artery in inferior STE-MI. *J Electrocardiol* 2010;43:132.

Kaski JC. Pathophysiology and management of patients with chest pain and normal coronary arteriograms (cardiac syndrome X). *Circulation* 2004;109:568.

Kenigsberg DN, Khanal S, Kowalski M, *et al*. Prolongation of the QTc interval is seen uniformly during early transmural ischemia. *J Am Coll Cardiol* 2007;49:1299.

Kerem Y, Eastvold JS, Faragoi D, Strasburger D, Motzny SE, Kulstad EB. The role of prehospital electrocardiograms in the recognition of ST-segment elevation myocardial infarctions and reperfusion times. *J Emerg Med.* 2014:46:202.

Koning R, Cribier A, Korsatz L, *et al*. Progressive decrease in myocardial ischemia assessed by intracoronary electrocardiogram during successive and prolonged coronary occlusions in angioplasty. *Am Heart J* 1993;125:56.

Kosuge M, Ebina T, Hibi K, *et al*. An early and simple predictor of severe left main and/or three-vessel disease in patients with non-ST-segment elevation acute coronary syndrome. *Am J Cardiol* 2011;107:495.

Lanza GA. Cardiac X syndrome: a critical overview and future perspectives. *Heart* 2007;93:159

Larson D, Menssen K, Sharkey S, *et al*. False positive cardiac catheterization activation among patients with suspected STEMI. *JAMA* 2007;298:2754.

Leibrandt PN, Bell SJ, Savona MR, *et al*. Validation of cardiologist's decisions to inbitiate reperfusion therapy with ECG viewed on liquid crystal displays of cellular phones *Am Heart J* 2000;140:747.

Lie KI, Wellens HJ, Downar E, *et al*. Observations on patients with primary ventricular fibrillation complicating acute myocardial infarction. *Circulation* 1975;52:755.

Liu CK, Greenspan G, Piccirillo RT. Atrial infarction of the heart. *Circulation* 1961;23:331.

Lopes RD, Siha H, Fu Y, *et al*. Diagnosing acute myocardial infarction in patients with left bundle branch block. *Am J Cardiol* 2011;108:782.

Manankil MF, Wang T, Bhat PK. Transient peaked T waves during exercise stress testing: an unusual manifestation of reversible cardiac ischemia. *J Electrocardiol* 2011;44:23.

Marcus FI, Cobb LA, Edwards JE, *et al*. Mechanism of death and prevalence of myocardial ischemic symptoms in the terminal event after acute myocardial infarction. *Am J Cardiol* 1988;61:8.

McClelland A, Owens C, Menown I, *et al*. Comparison of 80 lead body surface map to 12 lead ECG in detection of acute myocardial infarction. *Am J Cardiol* 2003;92:252.

Mehta N, Huang HD, Bandeali S, *et al*. Prevalence of acute myocardial infarction in patients with presumably new left bundle-branch block. *J Electrocardiol* 2012;45:361.

Migliore F, Zorzi A, Perazzolo Marra M, *et al*. Myocardial edema underlies dynamic T-wave inversion (Wellens' ECG pattern) in patients with reversible left ventricular dysfunction. *Heart Rhythm* 2011;8:1629.

Mills JR, Yound E, Gorlin R, *et al*. The natural history of ST elevation after acute myocardial infarction. *Am J Cardiol* 1975;35:609.

Mohlenkamp S, Hort W, Ge J, *et al*. Update on myocardial bridging. *Circulation* 2002;106:2616.

Moon JC, De Arenaza DP, Elkington AG, *et al*. The pathologic basis of Q-wave and non-Q-wave myocardial infarction: a cardiovascular magnetic resonance study *J Am Coll Cardiol* 2004;44:554.

Morrow DA, Antman EM, Giugliano RP, *et al*. A simple risk index for rapid initial triage of patients with ST-elevation myocardial infarction: an InTIME II substudy. *Lancet* 2000;358:1571.

Nikus K, Birnbaum Y. About QRS prolongation, distortion and the acuteness score. *J Electrocardiol* 2016;49:265.

Nikus KC, Eskola MJ, Virtanen VK. ST-depression with negative T waves in leads V4–V5-A marker of severe coronary artery disease in non-ST elevation acute coronary syndrome. A prospective study of angina at rest, with troponin, clinical, electrocardiographic and angiographic correlation. *Ann Noninvasive Electrocardiol* 2004;9:207.

Nikus K, Pahlm O, Wagner G, *et al*. Electrocardiographic classification of acute coronary syndromes: a review by a committee of the International Society for Holter and Non-Invasive Electrocardiology. *J Electrocardiol* 2010;43:91.

Nikus K, Pahlm O, Wagner G, *et al*. Report of the third International Society for Holter and Noninvasive Electrocardiology working group on improved electrocardiographic criteria for acute and chronic ischemic heart disease—Lund, Sweden: June 2010. *J Electrocardiol* 2011;44:84.

Nishizaki M, Arita M, Sakurada H, *et al*. Polymorphic ventricular tachycardia in patients with vasospastic angina—clinical and electrocardiographic characteristics and long-term outcome. *Jpn Circ J* 2001;65:519.

Oliva Ps, Hammill SC, Edwards WD. Cardiac rupture, a clinically predictable complication of acute myocardial infarction: report of 70 cases with clinicopathologic correlations. *J Am Coll Cardiol* 1993;22:720.

Pascale P, Schlaepfer J, Oddo M, *et al*. Ventricular arrhythmia in coronary artery disease: limits of a risk stratification strategy based on the ejection fraction alone and impact of infarct localization. *Europace* 2009;11:1639.

Pera VK, Larson DM, Sharkey SW, *et al*. New or presumed new left bundle branch block in patients with suspected ST-elevation myocardial infarction. *Eur Heart J Acute Cardiovasc Care* 2018;7:208.

Petrina M, Goodman SG, Eagle KA. The 12-lead electrocardiogram as a predictive tool of mortality after acute myocardial infarction: current status in an era of revascularization and reperfusion. *Am Heart J* 2006;152(1):11.

Pride YB, Tung P, Mohanavelu S, *et al*. TIMI Study Group. Angiographic and clinical outcomes among patients with acute coronary syndromes presenting with isolated anterior ST-segment depression: a TRITON-TIMI 38 (Trial to Assess Improvement in Therapeutic Outcomes by Optimizing Platelet Inhibition With Prasugrel-Thrombolysis In Myocardial Infarction 38) substudy. *JACC Cardiovasc Interv* 2010;3:806.

Prinzmetal M, Kennamer R, Merliss R, *et al*. Angina pectoris. I. A variant form of angina pectoris; preliminary report. *Am J Med* 1959;27:375.

Quyyumi AA, Crake T, Rubens MB, *et al*. Importance of "reciprocal" electrocardiographic changes during occlusion of left anterior descending artery. Studies during percutaneous transluminal coronary angioplasty. *Lancet* 1986;1:347.

Rasouli ML, Ellestad MH. Usefulness of ST depression in ventricular premature complexes to predict myocardial ischemia. *Am J Cardiol* 2001;87:891.

Reddy CV, Cheriparambill K, Saul B, *et al*. Fragmented left sided QRS in absence of bundle branch block: sign of left ventricular aneurysm. *Ann Noninvasive Electrocardiol* 2006;11:132.

Reeder GS, Gersh BJ. Modern management of acute myocardial infarction. *Curr Probl Cardiol* 2000;25:677.

Reinig MG, Harizi R, Spodick OH. Electrocardiographic T- and U-wave discordance. *Ann Noninvasive Electrocardiol* 2005;10:41.

Rey F, Mock S, Frei A, Noble S. Vasospastic angina: a forgotten acute coronary syndrome and the usefulness of twelve-lead electrocardiogram monitoring in diagnosis. *Int J Cardiol* 2016;223:46.

Roig S, Gómez JA, Fiol M, *et al*. Spontaneous coronary artery dissection causing acute coronary syndrome: an early diagnosis implies a good prognosis. *Am J Emerg Med* 2003;21:549.

Rosiak M, Bolinska H, Ruta J. P wave dispersión and P wave duration on SAECG in predicting atrial fibrillation in patients with acute myocardial infarction. *Ann Noninvasive Electrocardiol* 2002;7:363.

Rovai D, Di Bella G, Rossi G, *et al*. Q-wave prediction of myocardial infarct location, size and transmural extent at magnetic resonance imaging. *Coron Artery Dis* 2007;18:381.

Rukshin V, Monakier D, Olshtain-Pops K, *et al*. QT interval in patients with unstable angina and non-Q wave myocardial infarction. *Noninvasive Electrocardiol* 2002;7:343.

Sagie A, Sclarovsky S, Strasberg B, *et al*. Acute anterior wall myocardial infarction presenting with positive T waves and without ST segment shift. Electrocardiographic features and angiographic correlation. *Chest* 1989;95:1211.

Salermo JA, Previtali M, Chimienti M, *et al*. Vasospasm and ventricular arrhythmias. *Ann N Y Acad Sci* 1984;427:222.

Santoro GM, Valenti R, Buonamici P, *et al*. Relation between ST-segment changes and myocardial perfusion evaluated by myocardial contrast echocardiography in patients with acute myocardial infarction treated with direct angioplasty. *Am J Cardiol* 1998;82:932.

Sasaki K, Yotsukura M, Sakata K, *et al*. Relation of ST-segment changes in inferior leads during anterior wall acute myocardial infarction to length and occlusion site of the left anterior descending coronary artery. *Am J Cardiol* 2001;87:1340.

Sejersten M, Sillesen M, Hansen PR, *et al*. Effect on treatment delay of prehospital teletransmission of 12-lead electrocardiogram to a cardiologist for immediate triage and direct referral of patients with ST-segment elevation acute myocardial infarction to primary percutaneous coronary intervention. *Am J Cardiol* 2008;101:941.

Selvester RH, Wagner GS, Hindman NB. The Selvester QRS scoring system for estimating myocardial infarct size. The development and application of the system. *Arch Intern Med* 1985;145:1877.

Sgarbossa EB, Pinski SL, Barbagelata A, *et al*. Electrocardiographic diagnosis of evolving acute myocardial infarction in the presence of left bundle branch block. GUSTO-1 (Global Utilization of Streptokinase and Tissue Plasminogen Activator for Occluded Coronary Arteries) Investigators. *N Engl J Med* 1996;334:481.

Sherif NE. The rsR' pattern in left surface leads in ventricular aneurism. *Br Heart J* 1970;32:440.

Smith SW, Dodd KW, Henry TD, *et al*. Diagnosis of ST-elevation myocardial infarction in the presence of left bundle branch block with the ST-elevation to S-wave ratio in a modified Sgarbossa rule. *Ann Emerg Med* 2012;60:766

Spaulding CM, Joly LM, Rosenberg A, *et al*. Immediate coronary angiography in survivors of out-of-hospital cardiac arrest. *N Engl J Med* 1997;336:1629.

Stankovic I, Ilic I, Panic M, *et al*. The absence of the ST-segment elevation in acute coronary artery thrombosis: what does not fit, the patient or the explanation?. *J Electrocardiol* 2011;44:7.

Stern S, Bayés de Luna A. Coronary spasm: a 2009 update. *Circulation* 2009;119:2531.

Subirana MT, Juan-Babot JO, Puig T, *et al*. Specific characteristics of sudden death in a mediterranean Spanish population. *Am J Cardiol* 2011;107:622.

Tabas JA, Rodriguez RM, Seligman HK, Goldschlager NF. Electrocardiographic criteria for detecting acute myocardial infarction in patients with left bundle branch block: a meta-analysis. *Ann Emerg Med* 2008;52:329.

Tamura A, Nagasi KM, Kriya Y, *et al*. Significance of spontaneous noramlization of negative T wave during healing of anterior myocardial infarction. *Am J Cardiol* 1999;84:1341.

Tanimoto T, Imanishi T, Kitabata H, *et al*. Prevalence and clinical significance of papillary muscle infarction detected by late gadolinium-enhanced magnetic resonance imaging in patients with ST-segment elevation myocardial infarction. *Circulation* 2010;122:2281.

Thygesen K, Alpert JS, Jaffe A et al; Joint ESC/ACCF/AHA/WHF Task Force for the Redefinition of Myocardial Infarction. Fourth Universal definition of myocardial infarction (2018). *Eur Heart J* 2019;40:237.

Tierala I, Nikus KC, Sclarovsky S, *et al*. Predicting the culprit artery in acute ST elevation MI: Correlation with coronary anatomy in the HAAMU trial. *J Electrocardiol* 2009;42:120.

Ting HH, Krumholz HM, Bradley EH, *et al*. Implementation and integration of prehospital ECGs into systems of care for acute coronary syndrome: a scientific statement from the American Heart Association Interdisciplinary Council on Quality of Care and Outcomes Research, Emergency Cardiovascular Care Committee, Council on Cardiovascular Nursing, and Council on Clinical Cardiology. *Circulation* 2008;118:1066.

Tjandrawidjaja MC, Fu Y, Westerhout CM, *et al*.; APEX-AMI Investigators. Resolution of ST-segment depression:a new prognostic marker in ST-segment elevation myocardial infarction. *Eur Heart J* 2010;31:573.

Tomai F, Crea F, Chiariello L, *et al*. Ischemic preconditioning in humans: models, mediators, and clinical relevance. *Circulation*. 1999;100:559.

Uyarel H, Cam N, Okmen E, *et al*. Level of Selvester QRS score is predictive of ST-segment resolution and 30-day outcomes in patients with acute myocardial infarction undergoing primary coronary intervention. *Am Heart J* 2006;151:1239.

Van der Weg K, Bekkers SCAM, Winkens B, *et al*., on behalf of MAST. The R in V1 in non-anterior wall infarction indicates lateral rather than posterior involvement. Results from ECG/MRI correlations. *Eur Heart J* 2009;30(suppl):P2981K.

Watson GM, Chan CW, Belluscio L, *et al*. Comparing the variants of takotsubo syndrome: an observational study of the ECG and structural changes from a New Zealand tertiary hospital. *BMJ Open*. 2019;5(9):e025253.

Wellens HJ, Connover HP. *The ECG in Emergency Decision-making*. WB Saunders Co, 2006.

Wellens HJ, Gorgels A, Doevendans PA. *The ECG in Acute Myocardial Infarction and Unstable Angina*. Kluwer Academic Publishers, 2003.

Widimsky P, Holmes DR Jr. How to treat patients with ST-elevation acute myocardial infarction and multi-vessel disease? *Eur Heart J* 2011;32:396.

Wong CK, French JK, Aylward PE, *et al*. Usefulness of the presenting electrocardiogram in predicting successful reperfusion with streptokinase in acute myocardial infarction. *Am J Cardiol* 1999;83:164.

Wong CK, Gao W, Raffel OC, *et al*. HERO-2 Investigators. Initial Q waves accompanying ST-segment elevation at presentation of acute myocardial infarction and 30-day mortality in patients given streptokinase therapy: an analysis from HERO-2. *Lancet* 2006;367:2061.

Yamaji H, Iwasaki K, Kusachi S, *et al*. Prediction of acute left main coronary artery obstruction by 12 lead electrocardiography. ST segment elevation in lead VR with les s ST segment elevation in lead VI. *J Am Coll Cardiol* 2001;48:1348.

Zehender M, Utzolino S, Furtwangler A, *et al*. Time course and interrelation of reperfusion-induced ST changes and ventricular arrhythmias in acute myocardial infarction. *Am J Cardiol* 1991;68:1138.

Zhong-qun Z, Wei W, Jun-feng W. Does left anterior descending coronary artery acute occlusion proximal to the first septal perforator counteract ST elevation in leads V5 and V6? *J Electrocardiol* 2009;42:52.

Zhong-qun Z, Nikus K, Sclarovsky S.Prominent precordial T waves as a sign of acute myocardial infarction: electrocardiographic and angiographic correlations. *J Electrocardiol* 2011;44:533.

Zimmerman HA, Bersano E, Dicosky C. *The Auricular Electrocardiogram*. Charles C Thomas Publisher. Sprinfield, Ilinois, USA, 1968.

Chapter 21
Inherited Heart Diseases

Introduction

The inherited heart diseases with risk of sudden death discussed in this chapter are listed in Table 21.1 (Bayés de Luna and Baranchuk 2017). In describing each of these processes, we will emphasize the importance of the ECG in reaching a diagnosis and in determining the clinical implications. Molecular, genetics, and many aspects related to sudden death are not considered in depth in this book (Ackerman *et al.* 2011). In this chapter, we include the heart diseases that are deemed to be due to inherited changes. Other heart diseases that are occasionally inherited, such as dilated cardiomyopathy (DC) or Wolff–Parkinson–White (WPW) syndrome, are discussed in other chapters. For more information, consult the general references (page XII).

Cardiomyopathies

Hypertrophic cardiomyopathy (Figures 21.1–21.4)
Concept and diagnosis

Hypertrophic cardiomyopathy (HCM) is usually a familial disease of genetic origin, characterized by alterations in proteins of the myocardial cells leading to myocardial fiber disarray, hypertrophy of the heart, and an increased incidence of sudden death. More than 500 mutations and 9 genes have been described. The more frequent mutations include troponin T (*TNNTZ*) and beta myosin heavy chain (*MYH7*).

The diagnosis is suggested by family history and ECG and is confirmed by echocardiography and other imaging techniques (Figure 21.3) (Maron *et al.* 2006).

The hypertrophy may cause a dynamic obstruction of the left ventricle outflow tract, and on some occasions it leads to DC and heart failure (HF). When the apex is preferentially involved in the cardiomyopathy, the ECG pattern shows typical features (Figure 21.2).

ECG findings (Figures 21.1–21.4 and Table 21.2)

Pathologic ECGs are observed in approximately 95% of cases, although there is no characteristic ECG alteration indicative of a specific mutation.

In contrast to what is observed in the inherited long QT syndrome, **in HCM, it is not possible to predict the different mutations based on the ECG changes**, and vice versa, except for some types of predominantly apical HCM (Arad *et al.* 2005).

However, there are **some electrocardiographic patterns clearly indicative of HCM**, in particular, a large negative and sharp T wave that is typical of apical HCM (Figure 21.2), as well as a narrow and deep Q wave associated with a positive T wave, suggestive of septal hypertrophy (Figure 21.1).

In patients with HCM, especially apical HCM, RS morphology may be observed in V1. This may be diagnosed mistakenly as right ventricular hypertrophy, but is in fact caused by septal hypertrophy. Thanks to the relationships between ECG and magnetic resonance imaging (MRI), it has become possible to locate the more hypertrophic areas with the ECG (Dumont *et al.* 2006).

Patients frequently show ECG signs of left ventricular enlargement, which are in some cases very characteristic (Figure 21.2). However, sometimes are impossible to distinguish from those found in other heart diseases. In these cases, imaging techniques play a major role in establishing the correct diagnosis (Figure 21.3).

The QRS voltage is usually increased with often clear criteria of LVH (Figure 21.2). However a low voltage associated with a higher incidence of DC during follow-up may be seen (Ikeda *et al.* 1999) (Figure 21.4). Fragmentation of the QRS (fQRS) has been proved to be a predictor of poor evolution and arrhythmias in patients with HCM (Femenia *et al.* 2013).

Clinical Electrocardiography: A Textbook, Fifth Edition. Antoni Bayés de Luna, Miquel Fiol-Sala, Antoni Bayés-Genís, and Adrián Baranchuk.
© 2022 John Wiley & Sons Ltd. Published 2022 by John Wiley & Sons Ltd.

Table 21.1 Inherited heart diseases with risk of sudden death

• Cardiomyopathies (alterations in myocardial protein)	• Hypertrophic cardiomyopathy
	• Arrhythmogenic right ventricular dysplasia/cardiomyopathy
	• Spongiform cardiomyopathy (non-compacted)
	• Dilated cardiomyopathy (sometimes)
• Specific conduction system involvement:	• Lenegre syndrome
• No structural involvement: channelopathies (isolated alterations in ionic channels)	• Long QT syndrome
	• Short QT syndrome
	• Brugada syndrome
	• Catecholaminergic ventricular tachycardia
	• Familial atrial fibrillation
	• Torsades de pointes ventricular tachycardia with short coupling interval (probably)
	• Idiopathic ventricular fibrillation (possible)
	• Others (possible)

(Bayés de Luna and Baranchuk 2017).

At times **the ECG alterations are observed before the echocardiogram shows any change**. Therefore, an abnormal ECG may be the only evidence suggesting the presence of HCM in a patient's relatives, or may oblige us to rule it out when it is a casual finding.

An increased interval T wave peak/T wave end may be a more significant risk marker of torsades de pointes ventricular tachycardia (VT) than the QT dispersion or even the corrected QT (QTc) (Yamaguchi *et al.* 2003).

Often patients with HCM present with **arrhythmias** in the ECG. The most frequent supraventricular arrhythmia is atrial fibrillation (≈10% of patients) (Britton *et al.* 2017). The resulting loss of the atrial contribution to the filling of a hypertrophied and stiff left ventricle results in clinical deterioration. The presence of premature ventricular complexes (PVCs) is also common; they are found in more than three-quarters of patients wearing a Holter device. Runs of non-sustained VT are found in one-quarter of patients and its presence has prognostic implications. However, the presence of sustained VT is infrequent.

Very often, **different types of blocks**, especially intra-ventricular blocks (left bundle branch block, LBBB), are present in advanced cases.

Clinical implications

Most patients with HCM will likely develop left ventricular outflow obstruction (Maron 2010), although a clear dynamic pressure gradient in the left ventricular outflow tract is only seen in ≈30%. Some patients with HCM present with predominant apical involvement, which is more frequently observed in Japan (Suzuki *et al.* 1993).

Often, patients with HCM present with progressive dyspnea, especially after 40–50 years, due to diastolic dysfunction. Sometimes it is related to the appearance of atrial fibrillation. However, only about 10–15% of HCM patients will develop DC. The underlying physiopathologic mechanism that explains this evolution is not known with certainty. However, it has been shown that at 10-year follow-up, the incidence of HF is higher in patients with low-voltage QRS complexes (SV1 + RV6 < 35 mm) (Figure 21.4). This is probably because the low voltage is a marker of increased fibrosis (Ikeda *et al.* 1999).

The few cases with normal ECG have a better prognosis (McLeod *et al.* 2009), even though some exceptions have been found in patients with troponin T alterations, family history, and evidence of fibrosis by MRI (see below).

The differential diagnosis with athlete's heart constitutes an interesting challenge. There are clinical, ECG, and echocardiographic data on which we could base our differential diagnosis (Maron *et al.* 1981). If necessary, other techniques may be used to diminish the doubtful cases (gray zone in Figure 21.5) (Bayés de Luna *et al.* 2000; Zhang 2014).

Sudden death is the most important risk in this patient population. The yearly mortality rate is around 1%. Sudden death usually occurs during exercise due to a sustained VT leading to ventricular fibrillation (VF). This is the most common cause of sudden death in athletes. However, based on the experience of Maron (2010), more than 30 years may elapse before another cardiac arrest occurs. The most useful main **risk factors of sudden death** (McKenna and Behr 2002; Maron 2003, 2010) are:

- familial history of sudden death;
- personal antecedents of unexplained syncope;
- multiple-repetitive non-sustained VT in Holter recordings;
- abnormal blood pressure response during exercise testing;
- massive right ventricle hypertrophy ≥20 mm, and especially ≥30 mm.

The presence of two, or even one for some authors (Maron 2010), of the abovementioned factors, especially when accompanied with genetic alterations (especially troponin T mutations), **is associated with an increased risk of sudden death** and requires implantable cardioverter defibrillator (ICD) implantation. Meanwhile, the absence of the abovementioned risk factors, especially family history of sudden death in patients older than 50–60 years, is indicative of a better prognosis.

In HCM, as happens in all other inherited heart diseases described in this chapter, **the advantages of ICD implant always have to be balanced with the risk of complications** (inappropriate shocks, infections, etc.) (Bayés de Luna and Baranchuk 2017).

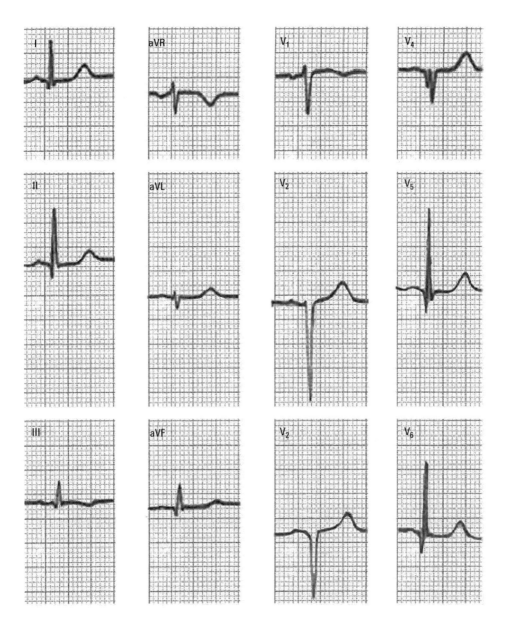

Figure 21.1 Hypertrophic cardiomyopathy (HCM). Deep "q" waves in anterolateral leads, which may be mistaken for those observed in ischemic heart disease. However, usually are narrow and fine.

Arrhythmogenic right ventricular dysplasia cardiomyopathy (Tables 21.3 and 21.4, Figures 21.6 and 21.7)

Concept and diagnosis

Arrhythmogenic right ventricular dysplasia cardiomyopathy (ARVC) is a familial disease of genetic origin, comprising both a recessive form and a dominant form. In 50% of cases, it is related to a mutation in the plakofilin gene. The disease is characterized by fatty infiltration and fibrosis localized especially in the right ventricle, leading to electrical instability and risk of sudden death. Frequently, left ventricle involvement exists as well.

The diagnosis must be made according to the criteria of the Task Force for Cardiomyopathy (McKenna *et al*. 1994).

Recently, revised Task Force Criteria (Marcus *et al*. 2010) have been published (Table 21.3).

ECG findings (see Table 21.3)

The following are the ECG signs most frequently observed in ARVC (Jain *et al*. 2009; de Alencar Neto *et al*. 2018):

- **Prolonged QRS complex width in lead V1 greater than V6** (Fontaine *et al*. 2004). This is due to late right ventricular depolarization and explains that late potentials are in fact frequently positive (see Chapter 25) (Figure 21.6). This is reported in 80% of the cases.

- **Atypical pattern of right bundle branch block (RBBB)**. This is generally manifest as a wide R wave of relatively low voltage in lead V1 (Figure 21.6). It is also due to late right ventricular depolarization. This is found in 35% of cases.

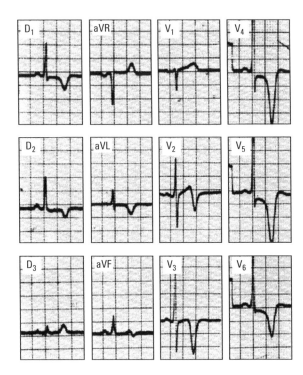

Figure 21.2 Apical hypertrophic cardiomyopathy (HCM). The large negative T waves lead us to make a differential diagnosis with ischemic heart disease (IHD).

• **Negative T wave in precordial V1 to V3–V5 leads and sometimes in inferior leads and usually symmetric** (Figures 21.6 and 21.7). Sometimes with mild ST segment elevation. This is observed in 50% of cases.

• Occasionally (≈10% of cases), the late depolarization of the upper right ventricular wall is recorded as separate from the end of the QRS complex, showing subtle notches/undulations (ε **wave**), especially in the right precordial leads and frontal plane leads (Figure 21.8).

• Abnormal P wave is seen in more than 10% of cases.

• It is important to remember that the ECG may be normal in 20% of cases.

• Frequently, ventricular arrhythmias are present. They originate in the right ventricle as isolated or repetitive PVCs (VT runs) with LBBB morphology, generally with left QRS axis deviation, although a right axis deviation is also possible (Figure 21.6 and Table 16.3). Sustained VT, sometimes at very high rate, is observed (Figure 21.7B), which may lead to aVF.

Clinical implications

ARVC may lead to a sustained and generally monomorphic VT with LBBB morphology, eventually leading to aVF and sudden death.

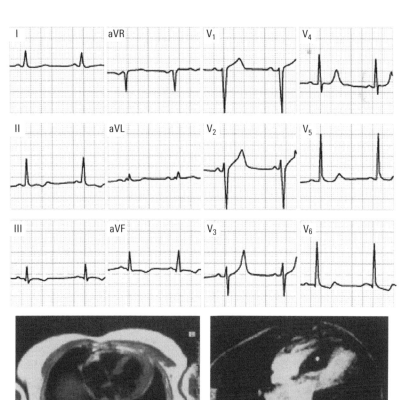

Figure 21.3 Top: ECG with left ventricular enlargement pattern not specific of any heart disease. Below: Cardiovascular magnetic resonance (CMR) (right) showing an asymmetric septal hypertrophy (asterisk), which confirms the diagnosis (HCM). Left: CMR with normal left ventricle image (for comparative purposes). It should be pointed out that echocardiography allows us to reach the same diagnosis.

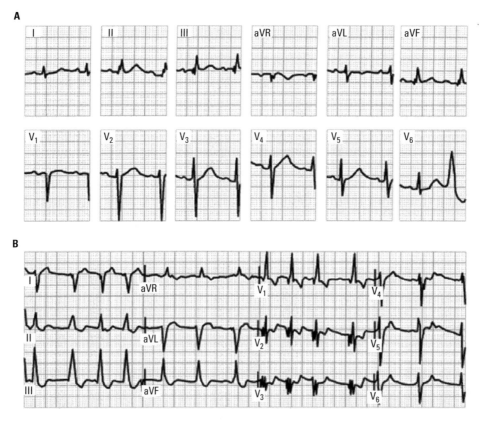

Figure 21.4 A 50-year-old patient with familial hypertrophic cardiomyopathy. (A) Note the low-voltage QRS and the diffuse repolarization alterations, as well as the presence of premature ventricular complexes (PVCs). Patients with hypertrophic cardiomyopathy usually exhibit a high voltage. It has been shown that the presence of relatively low voltages is associated with congestive heart failure (CHF) in the long-term follow-up. (B) In this case, after 15 years, the patient suffered from advanced CHF with atrial fibrillation, resulting in a very abnormal ECG: advanced right bundle branch block (RBBB) with pseudonecrosis q waves and a significant right QRS deviation due to right heart failure.

Table 21.2 ECG alterations in hypertrophic cardiomyopathy (Figures 21.1–21.4)

Abnormal ECG	Abnormal in 95% of the cases. Sometimes with normal or slightly changed echocardiogram
Signs of left ventricular enlargement	Frequent. Sometimes characteristic repolarization alterations are observed (Figure 21.2) (Large negative T wave, frequently very symmetrical and sharp). The ECG is frequently not distinguished from other processes which involve left ventricular enlargement (aortic stenosis, hypertension) (Figure 21.3) QRS voltage is usually increased. If it is relatively low (SV1 + RV6 < 35 mm), the patient is likely to suffer from heart failure in the future (Figure 21.4)
Pathological Q wave	Not very frequent It is observed in leads where it is usually not seen Narrow and sometimes very deep. Generally the T wave is positive (Figure 21.1)
Repolarization alterations	Very frequent (see above), sometimes with large negative but sharp T waves (Figure 21.2)

It is important to remember that small repolarization changes (Figure 21.7A) are enough to suspect the condition and that the ECG may be normal in about 20% of cases, and may initially mimic myocarditis (Pieroni *et al.* 2009).

When active arrhythmias of right ventricular origin are present (PVCs occurring frequently, above all during exercise, and runs of VT), and symptoms, such as syncope during exercise, are observed, a cardiac magnetic resonance (CMR) should be performed to confirm the ARVC. This technique is very useful in athletes to rule out or confirm this condition, and also HCM or an anomalous origin of the coronary arteries.

Frequently (>80% of cases), left ventricle involvement exists as well, often developing before the right ventricle is involved. Isolated left ventricular involvement is detected by the presence of a negative T wave in left lateral leads, PVCs of left ventricle origin, and imaging signs (CMR) of left ventricular dysfunction, without the evidence of right ventricular abnormalities (ECG, CMR) (Coats *et al.* 2009).

In the presence of sustained VT or frequent PVCs, ablation may be indicated, even though due to the presence of several foci frequent recurrences have been observed (Dalal *et al.* 2007) and for that its indication is controversial.

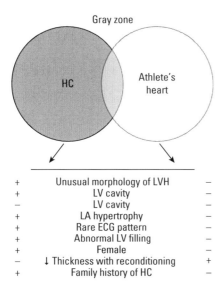

Gray zone

HC | Athlete's heart

+	Unusual morphology of LVH	−
+	LV cavity	−
−	LV cavity	−
+	LA hypertrophy	−
+	Rare ECG pattern	−
+	Abnormal LV filling	−
+	Female	−
−	↓ Thickness with reconditioning	+
+	Family history of HC	−

Figure 21.5 Criteria used to distinguish hypertrophic cardiomyopathy (HCM) from an athlete's heart when the left ventricular wall thickness is within the gray zone, consistent with both diagnoses (Adapted from Bayés de Luna *et al.* 2000).

Implantable cardioverter defibrillator (ICD) therapy is considered the best treatment option, particularly in patients with a history of sustained VT/VF, patients with extensive left ventricular involvement, and those with a history of syncope (consult p. XI).

Spongiform or non-compacted cardiomyopathy (Figure 21.9)

Concept and diagnosis

Spongiform or non-compacted cardiomyopathy is a rare familial cardiomyopathy of uncertain etiology, for which a genetic origin has been proposed (Murphy *et al.* 2005). From an anatomo-pathologic point of view, it is characterized by an increase in the trabecular mass of the left ventricle (non-compacted), contrasting with a thin and compacted epicardial layer that may be visualized with imaging techniques (echocardiography and, above all, CMR) that confirm the diagnosis.

ECG findings (Figure 21.9)

Initial diagnosis is based on the following surface ECG features (Steffel *et al.* 2009):
• intraventricular conduction disturbances (50%);
• repolarization disorders, manifest especially as negative T waves in precordial leads (70%);
• prolonged QT interval (50%);
• left ventricular hypertrophy (30%);
• normal ECG in 5% of cases.

Occasionally, the ECG is similar to that of some cases of ARVC (compare Figures 21.9 and. 21.7A). As the repolarization alteration disorder (negative T wave) is usually in the right precordial leads and not striking, it may be mistaken for normal ECG variations.

Table 21.3 ARVC: Summary of revised task force criteria (Marcus *et al.* 2010)

I Global or regional dysfunction and structural alterations	• By 2D echo, MRI or RV angiography: Regional RV akinesia, dyskinesia, or aneurysm • By MRI: ↓RV ejection fraction (<40%-major, 40–45% minor dysfunction)
II Repolarization abnormalities	• Major: Inverted T wave (V1–V3) or beyond in individuals >14 years. No RBBB (Figure 21.7A) • Minor: Inverted T wave only in V1–V2 in individuals >14 years. No RBBB • Inverted T waves in V1–V4 individuals >14 years in presence of RBBB (Figure 21.6)
III Depolarization abnormalities	• Epsilon wave in V1–V3 (Figure 21.8) • Localized prolongation of QRS in V1–V3 (>110 ms) compared with V6 (>20–30 ms) • Late potentials. In the absence, QRS ≥110 ms
IV Arrhythmias	• Non-sustained or sustained VT (LBBB morphology superior axis). Major criteria (Figure 21.7B) • Non-sustained or sustained VT (LBBB morphology inferior axis). Minor criteria. • >500 PVC per 24 hours. (Holter) Minor criteria
V Family history	• History of ARVC/D in a first-degree relative • Premature sudden death (<35 years of age) due to suspected ARVC/D in a first-degree relative • ARVC/D confirmed pathologically or by current Task Force Criteria in second-degree relative

ARVC: arrhythmogenic right ventricular dysplasia cardiomyopathy; MRI: magnetic resonance imaging; PVC: premature ventricular complex; RBBB: right bundle branch block; RV: right ventricle; VT: ventricular tachycardia.
(Adapted from Marcus *et al.* 2010).

Clinical implications

The patient may remain asymptomatic for many years, but this cardiomyopathy eventually evolves into DC and HF. Sometimes embolism and/or ventricular arrhythmias appear in the follow-up. Ventricular arrhythmias may trigger sustained VT/VF and sudden death.

Some cases need ablation, ICD, or even heart transplantation.

Specific conduction system involvement

Lenegre syndrome

Lenegre syndrome is a rare condition that consists of a **progressive intraventricular conduction block without**

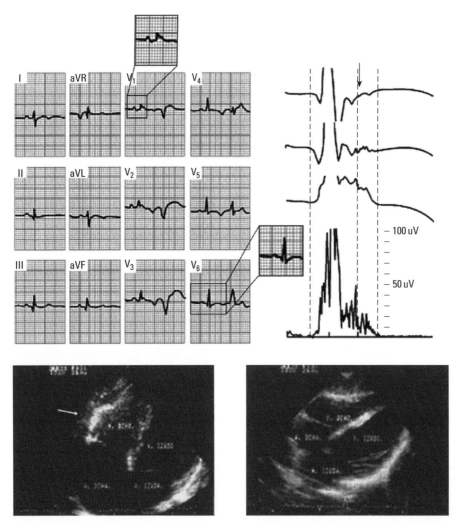

Figure 21.6 Typical ECG pattern of a patient with arrhythmogenic right ventricular cardiomyopathy (ARVC). Note the atypical right bundle branch block (RBBB), premature ventricular complexes (PVCs) from the right ventricle, and negative T wave in V1–V4. We also see how QRS duration is clearly longer in V1–V2 than in V6. The patient showed very positive late potentials (right). Below: typical echocardiographic pattern showing the distortion of the right ventricular contraction (arrow).

Table 21.4 QTc prolongation in different age groups, based on the Bazett formula: values within the normal interval, borderline values, and altered values

Value	1–15 years old	Adult (men)	Adult (women)
Normal	<440 ms	<430 ms	<450 ms
Borderline	440–460 ms	430–450 ms	450–470 ms
Altered (prolonged)	>460 ms	>450 ms	>470 ms

apparent heart disease. It appears in members of the same family at a relatively young age (Lenegre 1964).

From a genetic point of view, the Lenegre syndrome is caused by a Na channel dysfunction (decreased Na inflow into the cell). Histological studies show that a diffuse fibrotic degeneration of the whole intraventricular SCS exists, which may lead to an atrioventricular (AV) block without involvement of the sinus node and the fibrous skeleton of the heart. The presence of this evident pathologic involvement differentiates the Lenegre syndrome from channelopathies (see below).

Lenegre syndrome should be distinguished from Lev syndrome (Lev 1964), which is found in older patients and is caused by a non-inherited senile degeneration of the SCS and the fibrous skeleton of the heart.

Usually, pacemaker implantation becomes necessary during the course of both Lenegre and Lev syndromes.

Ionic channel disorders in the absence of apparent structural heart disease: channelopathies

Exclusive alterations of the ionic channels are observed in long and short QT syndrome, Brugada syndrome, and catecholamine-sensitive VT. They are also probably present in familial atrial fibrillation and other cases of sudden death due to other malignant ventricular arrhythmias, such as familial torsades de pointes VT and cases of VT

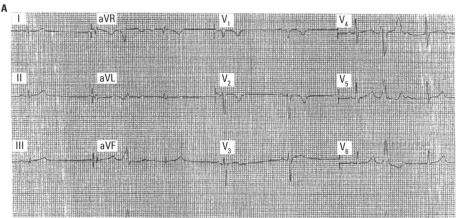

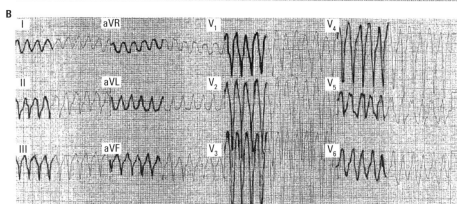

Figure 21.7 (A) Arrhythmogenic right ventricular cardiomyopathy (ARVC). Note that apart from the premature ventricular complexes (PVCs), the only ECG abnormality is the symmetric and negative T wave in V1–V2, with flat T wave in V3–V4. It is important to assess these subtle changes when suspecting the diagnosis. (B) Very fast and not well-tolerated ventricular tachycardia (VT) in the same patient. It is initiated in the apex (left VT ÂQRS), a different site from where PVCs are generated (see the different morphology in VF). Implantable cardioverter defibrillator implantation was performed.

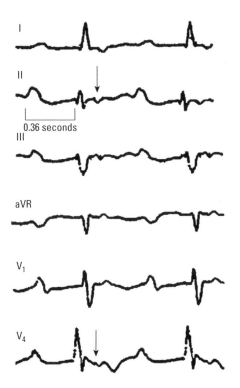

Figure 21.8 Example of delayed depolarization wave following the QRS complex with a small separation and, generally, low voltage (arrow). It is mainly observed in right precordial leads and in I, II, III, and aVR in some cases of arrhythmogenic right ventricular cardiomyopathy (ARVC). It is sometimes mistakenly taken for a very premature concealed atrial extrasystole. Note that in this case a high-voltage P wave is observed and that a first-degree atrioventricular (AV) block exists.

that until now were considered idiopathic VF (Marbán 2002).

Some of the best-known channelopathies show a typical phenotypic ECG pattern, which frequently allows for a correct diagnosis and even identification of the involved gene. There are some evidences showing that although initially isolated ionic alterations exist (true channelopathies), some ultrastructural changes may be present in the follow-up (see below) (Frustaci *et al.* 2009; Bayés de Luna and Baranchuk 2017).

All channelopathies may increase the risk of developing different types of VT/VF, eventually leading to sudden death.

Long QT syndrome (Figures 21.10–21.12)

Concept and diagnosis

We can only speak about long QT syndrome when a patient with apparent good health presents with a nonacquired long QT interval with syncopal attacks or recovered cardiac arrest due to torsades de pointes VT often leading to sudden death, or a family history of this syndrome.

The long QT syndrome is genetic channelopathy characterized by QTc prolongation in ECG and propensity to ventricular tachyarrhythmias (TdPVT, VF) leading to syncopal episodes and/or SCD. In about 10–15% of cases, QTc might remain within normal limit and in about 50% of cases, it will be categorized as borderline (between 440 and 470 ms). Table 21.5 lists ECG changes observed in the LQTS (Moss *et al.* 1985; Moss and Kan 2005).

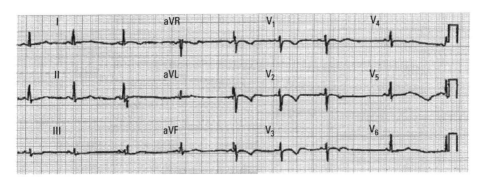

Figure 21.9 ECG of an 18 year-old patient with repetitive sustained ventricular tachycardia (VT). In sinus rhythm, a clear QT prolongation is observed (>500 ms), as well as a negative T wave up to lead V3 with a flat T wave in V4–V6. This ECG may be mistaken for a normal ECG variant in a healthy subject. However, the long QT interval, the negative T wave up to V3, and the flat T wave in V4–V6 raise the suspicion of abnormal pattern. The echocardiogram allows for the diagnosis of spongiform cardiomyopathy.

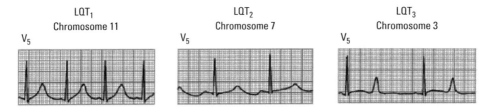

Figure 21.10 Three examples of ECG patterns in long QT syndrome clearly associated with different chromosomal alterations: LQT1, LQT2, and LQT3.

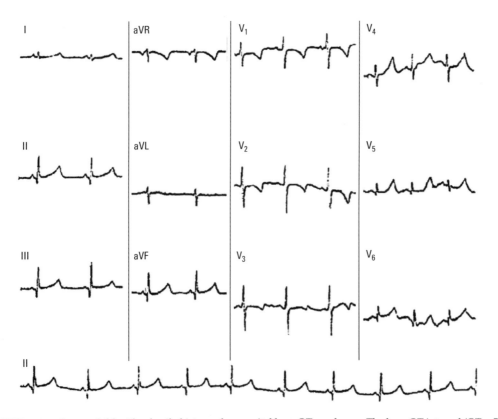

Figure 21.11 ECG pattern from a child with a family history of congenital long QT syndrome. The long QT interval (QT = 520) is clearly seen, and the ST-T abnormal morphology in this case allows us to reach a diagnosis of congenital long QT syndrome. This ECG pattern is not very consistent with any one of the three typical repolarization morphologies shown in Figure 21.10, although patterns like that may be seen in LQT3.

Long QT syndrome

Risk of VT/VF/SD*	Management
Very high risk 14%	Secondary prevention of SD • ICD + β Blockers
High risk 3%	QTc > 500 ms • β Blockers • ICD implant to be decided based on each particular case
Low risk 0.5%	QTc < 500 ms • β Blockers if no contraindications • Very effective in LQT1 • No ICD in absence of symptoms

Figure 21.12 Risk stratification in long QT syndrome (Based on Goldberger and Moss 2008).

* In some cases the prognosis may be different according the dysfunction that genetic mutations induce in ion channels (LQT1, LQT2).

Other therapeutic options may be necessary in some cases (left stelectomy, some drugs) (consult Bayés de Luna et al. *2012* and p. XII).

Table 21.5 ECG alterations in congenital long QT syndrome

QT prolongation (see Table 21.4)	3% of the genetic carriers may show a normal QT To record sequential ECGs in these cases is advisable
• QT dispersion (difference between the longest and the shortest QT in the 12 leads)	
• T peak/T end interval	Increased. Frequently >90 ms
• Morphological repolarization alterations (Zareba *et al.* 1998) (Figure 21.20)	
• Bradyarrhythmias	Generally sinus bradycardia. Sometimes due to a 2 × 1 block (bad prognosis)
• Tachyarrhythmias	Torsades de pointes VT (Figure 16.24). Sudden death may occur. The incidence is higher in LQT1 and LQT2 but they are more dangerous in LQT3

(Adapted from Zareba *et al.* 1998; Zareba *et al.* 2003; Zareba and Cygankiewicz 2008; Moss and Kan 2005 and Moss *et al.* 1985).

The ionic mechanism underlying the repolarization abnormalities in the LQTS varies depending on the type of underlying genetic mutation. There are over 12 genetic types of LQTS and related abnormalities of ion channels involve: slow and late activation of K channels (IKr, IKs), incomplete inactivation of Na⁺ channels, and Ca⁺⁺ channels with a late Ca⁺⁺ and Na⁺ inward current. The most common variants of LQTS in which there is a good genotype/ phenotype correlation (ECG expression) are LQT1, LQT2, and LQT3, which account for about 70–75% of LQTS cases (Figure 21.10 and Table 21.5) (Zareba *et al.* 1998, 2003; Zareba and Cygankiewicz 2008).

A "point score" diagnostic criteria for long QT syndrome has been proposed (Schwartz *et al.* 1993). These

Table 21.6 Long QT syndrome: diagnostic criteria

ECG findings[a]	Points
QTc[b]	
>480 ms	3
460–470 ms	2
450 ms (male)	1
Torsades de pointes[c]	2
T wave alternans	1
Notched T wave in 3 leads	1
Low heart rate for age[d]	0.5
Clinical history	
Syncope[3]	
With stress	2
Without stress	1
Congenital deafness	0.5
Family history[e]	
A. Family members with definite LQTS	1
B. Unexplained sudden cardiac death below age 30 among immediate family members	0.5

Score: <1 point = low probability of LQTS; 2–3 points = intermediate probability of LQTS; ≥3.5 points = high probability of LQTS.

[a] In the absence of medications or disorders known to affect these ECG features.

[b] QTc calculated by Bazett's formula where QTC = QT/√RR.

[c] Mutually exclusive.

[d] Resting heart rate below the 2nd percentile for age.

[e] The same family member cannot be counted in A and B.(Schwartz *et al.* 1993).

diagnostic criteria are listed in Table 21.6 with relative points assigned to various ECG, clinical, and familial findings. The score ranges from a minimum value of 0 to a maximum value of 9 points. The point score is divided into three probability categories: ≤1 point = low probability of long QT syndrome; >1–3.0 points = intermediate probability; and ≥3.5 points = high probability. As QTc overcorrects at fast heart rates, additional diagnostic caution is necessary when dealing with patients or infants with fast heart rates.

ECG findings (Figures 21.10 and 21.11 and Tables 21.5 and 21.6)

QTc values that are considered pathologic according to age and gender are listed in Table 21.4. QT interval measurement should be done in leads II and V5 or V6, taking the mean value of the QT interval measurements in five RR cycles, from the earliest QRS onset until the end of the T wave.

All the most important ECG alterations are found in Table 21.5.

It is very important to recognize a long QT when examining an ECG recording (Viskin *et al.* 2005).

The characteristic ECG alterations of LQT1, LQT2, and LQT3 syndromes are listed in Table 21.5 and shown in Figure 21.10 (Zareba *et al.* 1998; Moss 2002). Sometimes there are some poorly defined forms (Figure 21.11). All repolarization alterations (QT prolongation, QT dispersion T peak/T end interval, and other repolarization anomalies) are more striking than those observed in other pathologic conditions with a long QT.

The genotype/phenotype correlations (repolarization) in the long QT syndromes mentioned (LQT1, LQT2, and LQT3) are shown in Figure 21.10. Each shows a definitely long QTc (the longest QTc is observed in the LQT3 variant), and in many cases, the repolarization alterations allow for the recognition and identification of the genotype. LQT1 has wide, high-voltage T waves, while LQT2 features low voltage and frequently notched T waves, and LQT3 late T waves.

Fatal arrhythmia is the "torsades de pointes" VT leading to VF and sudden death (especially in LQT2 and LQT3).

Frequently, the VT begins in the presence of large negative (but not sharp) T–U waves after a premature ventricular complex, followed by a long pause before the onset of the torsades de pointes VT (Kirchhof *et al.* 2009).

Clinical implications

Figure 21.12 shows the global risk stratification in patients with long QT syndrome, including the three types of risk (yearly low, high, and very high risk of VT/VF). It is based on the studies carried out by the Moss group (Goldberger and Moss 2008).

The incidence of arrhythmias (especially torsades de pointes VT, see Chapter 16) that often induce syncopal attacks and unfortunately may trigger sudden death is higher in LQT1 and LQT2 types. However, arrhythmias observed in the LQT3 type are potentially more dangerous. Meanwhile, in LQT1, arrhythmias occur mainly as a result of physical exercise and stress (tachycardia-dependent arrhythmias), whereas in LQT2 and LQT3 types they are more related to rest, sleep, or acoustic stimuli (pause-dependent arrhythmias) (Schwartz *et al.* 2006). Competitive sports are contraindicated for patients with congenital long QT syndrome.

The best therapeutic approaches are the following: (i) beta blockers, which are especially effective in LQT1, and (ii) ICD implantation, which is indicated in patients at very high risk and in some high-risk patients (see text) (Figure 21.12).

Short QT syndrome (Figure 21.13)

Concept and diagnosis

A few years ago, two families showing a QT interval of ≤300 ms regardless of the heart rate with no apparent cause (i.e. electrolyte imbalance) were described (Gaita *et al.* 2003). As a result of the different degrees of shortening between the duration of subepicardial/midsubendocardial TAP, a voltage gradient is generated. This may trigger the occurrence of VT/VF through a reentrant mechanism in TAP phase 2 (see Figure 14.15).

This is a very infrequent, newly identified inherited disease in which mutations in various genes have been described, including: *HERG* (short QT syndrome 1), *KCNQ1* (short QT syndrome 2), and *KCNJ2* (short QT syndrome 3).

Recently, a score for diagnosis of short QT syndrome has been published (Gollob *et al.* 2011) (see Table 21.7).

ECG findings (Figure 21.13 and Table 21.7)

The short QT syndrome should be considered when the QT interval is between 320 and 350 ms without an apparent cause. The diagnosis is certain when a QT interval below 300 ms is confirmed.

A very tall and sharp T wave is recorded in virtually all cases of symptomatic short QT. The tall T wave presents especially in right precordial leads, almost equally in ascending and descending limbs (almost symmetrical T wave), with a J point–T peak distance <120 ms. This allows it to be differentiated from other asymptomatic short QT cases that show a J point–T peak interval >150 ms and healthy people (>200 ms) (Figure 21.13B) (Anttonen *et al.* 2009; Gollob *et al.* 2011).

Clinical implications

Sudden death triggered by VT/VF due to a reentry phase 2 mechanism is the most severe complication of short QT syndrome.

ICD implantation is the treatment of choice for high-risk cases (family history of sudden death and/or serious syncope).

Brugada syndrome (Figures 21.14–21.18)

Concept and diagnosis

The Brugada syndrome is a familial, genetically determined syndrome, characterized by an autosomal dominant inheritance and variable penetrance. More than 70 mutations usually related to Na⁺ channels have been

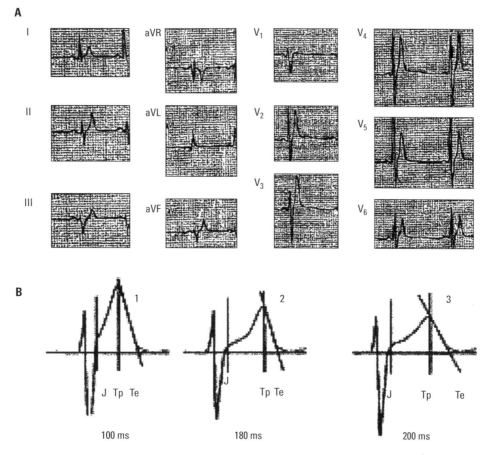

Figure 21.13 (A) Short QT syndrome. A typical ECG pattern with QT <300 ms and high, sharp T waves. (B) Symptomatic short QT pattern (1), asymptomatic (2), and normal QT (control) (3) (see text) (Adapted with permission from Anttonen *et al.* 2009).

described. In around 20% of cases, there are *SCN5A* mutations that explain the accelerated inactivation of Na channels.

The incidence rate is higher in young men without apparent structural heart disease (see below). Syncope or sudden death is usually triggered during rest or sleep, sometimes without any isolated, previous PVCs. Most often polymorphous VTs trigger VF because of a reentrant mechanism due to a voltage gradient between the different TAP length of layers of the right ventricle (see Figure 14.15) (Brugada and Brugada 1992).

There are currently two pathophysiologic hypotheses used to explain the ECG changes in the Brugada syndrome (Meregalli *et al.* 2009): (i) the repolarization hypothesis, involving the presence of voltage gradient due to transmural or transregional dispersion of TAP of different layers of right ventricle in the beginning of repolarization, consequent on loss of Na current and to dominant transient K current (I_{to}) (see Figure 14.14), and (ii) the depolarization hypothesis, involving a right ventricular conduction delay at the end of depolarization combined probably with subtle structural right ventricle anomalies. Recently has been

postulated the theory (Elizari *et al.* 2007) that both mechanisms may be explained by right ventricular outflow tract anomalies due to abnormal neural crest development.

The diagnosis is suggested by the clinical history in a patient with specific ECG patterns. Table 21.8 shows the diagnostic criteria of the Brugada syndrome. Brugada ECG pattern (BP) is a crucial part but not all for the diagnosis.

ECG findings (Table 21.9 and Figures 21.14–21.16)

Initially, the most used ECG criteria were the ones proposed by the consensus documents that, under the auspices of the ESC, were published within three years (Wilde *et al.* 2002; Antzelevitch *et al.* 2005). However, due to the small differences in morphology and the lack of prognostic implications between types 2 and 3, it was deemed not to be necessary to maintain this classification and type-3 was eliminated from the classification according to the third consensus (Bayes de Luna *et al.* 2012) (Figure 21.14B). The best criteria to diagnose types 1 and 2 BP are shown in Tables 21.9 and 21.10 (Bayes de Luna *et al.* 2012).

Table 21.7 Short QT syndrome: diagnostic criteria

ECG findings[a]	Points
QTc	
<370 ms	1
<350 ms	2
<330 ms	3
J point–T peak interval[b] <120 ms	1
Clinical history[c]	
History of sudden cardiac arrest	2
Documented polymorphic VT or VF	2
Unexplained syncope	1
Atrial fibrillation	1
Family history[d,e]	
First- or second-degree relative with high-probability STQS	2
First- or second-degree relative with autopsy-negative sudden cardiac death	1
Sudden infant death syndrome	1
Genotype[e]	
Genotype positive	2
Mutation of undetermined significance in a culprit gene	1

High-probability SQTS: ≥4 points, intermediate-probability SQTS: 3 points, low-probability SQTS: ≤2 points.

[a] Must be recorded in the absence of modifiers known to shorten the QT.

[b] Must be measured in the precordial lead with the greatest amplitude T wave.

[c] Events must occur in the absence of an identifiable etiology, including structural heart disease. Points can only be received for 1 of cardiac arrest, documented polymorphic VT, or unexplained syncope.

[d] Points can only be received once in this section.

[e] A minimum of 1 point must be obtained in the ECG section in order to obtain additional points.

VF: ventricular fibrillation; VT: ventricular tachycardia.(Gollob *et al.* 2011).

Table 21.8 Diagnostic criteria of the Brugada syndrome

1. Concave type I ST elevation in V1–V3 (Figure 21.14A) (usually in V1–V2) with no other cause accounting for the ST morphology. Remember that the ECG may be transient and more visible in high precordial leads. The ECG pattern is indicative of the syndrome if associated with one of the following ECG/clinical factors:
   - Survivors of cardiac arrest
   - Pliomorphic VF
   - Familial history of SD in patients <45 years old
   - Type I ST pattern in relatives
   - Inducible malignant ventricular arrhythmias
   - History of syncope
   - Non-concave type 2 ST elevation in V1–V2–V3 (Figure 21.14B), turning into type 1 after administering sodium channel blockers. The scenario is identical to the previous case

2. If there is an ST elevation ≥2 mm after drug administration but it is non-concave, the diagnosis is probable if any or more of the clinical criteria mentioned are present

3. If the morphology is unclear (either the baseline morphology or the morphology observed after drug administration), the diagnosis may be confirmed, apart from the ECG/clinical criteria put forward in the first paragraph, by the presence of the following parameters among others:
   - Other ECG criteria and findings (Table 21.9).
   - Other ECG methods (Exercise test, Holter, late potentials, VCG, EPS) (see Bayés de Luna and Baranchuk 2017 and recommended reading, p. XI)
   - Genetic test (Ackerman *et al.* 2011)

(Bayés de Luna *et al.* 2012).

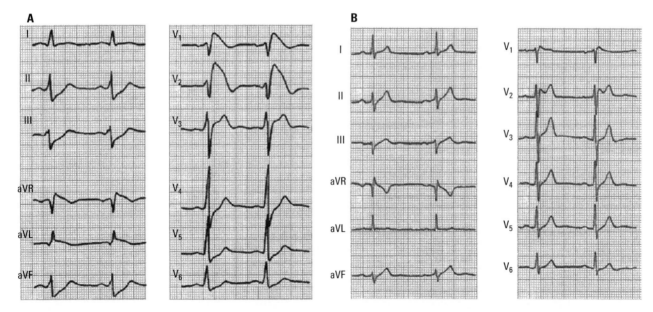

Figure 21.14 (A) Typical example of type 1 Brugada pattern. Note the morphology in V1–V2, with a concave ST downsloping elevation with respect to the isoelectric baseline, with no clear evidence of R′. (B) Typical example of type 2 Brugada pattern. See especially in V2 the wide r′, the ST elevated, and the positive T wave (see Tables 21.9 and 21.10) (Bayés de Luna *et al.* 2012).

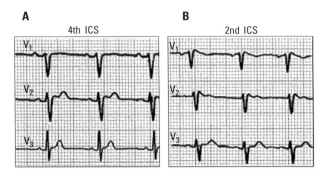

Figure 21.15 A patient with syncope episodes and an atypical ECG that present clearly more typical pattern of BP type 2 in second ICS than in the 4th ICS (see text and Table 21.2).

Tables 21.9 and 21.10 show the ECG criteria, especially the characteristics of ST-T in precordial leads in both types, as well as the mismatch in the duration of QRS in V1–V6 and the new ECG criteria recently reported (Corrado *et al.* 2010; Chevallier *et al.* 2011; Serra *et al.* 2012) that are explained in these tables. Also, other ECG findings are mentioned.

The ECG pattern is sometimes intermittent (Figure 21.16), although on other occasions it may be observed only in certain situations, such as fever, intoxication, vagal stimulation, and electrolyte imbalance (Antzelevitch and Brugada 2002; Samani *et al.* 2009). In contrast, there are some drugs that may produce a similar ECG morphology for no apparent reason (Yap *et al.* 2009).

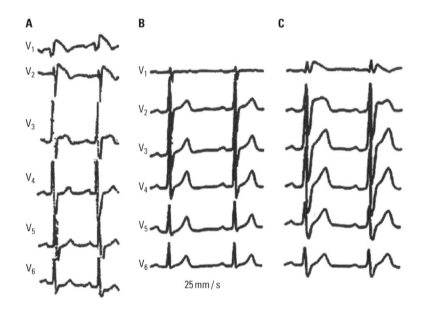

25 mm / s

Figure 21.16 (A) 12-lead ECG in a patient with the Brugada syndrome who lost consciousness some days before. A few days later, the ECG was normal (B), but it showed the characteristic features of Brugada syndrome after ajmaline administration (C).

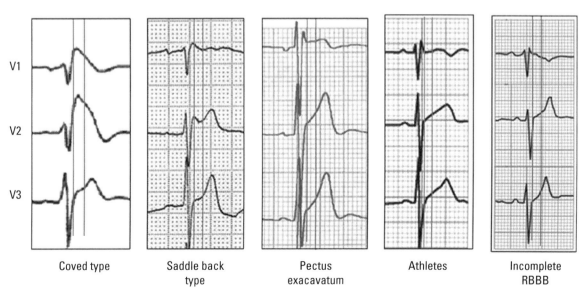

| Coved type | Saddle back type | Pectus exacavatum | Athletes | Incomplete RBBB |

Figure 21.17 The figure shows clearly the difference in the morphology of r′ in V1 between athletes and BP type 2 and the difference in duration of QRS in V1 and mild-left precordial leads that only is present in BP (see text). The second line, to measure the Corrado index in V1 or V2, is 80 ms later (see Table 21.9) than the end of QRS in V3.

Table 21.9 ECG alterations in the Brugada syndrome

A. ECG criteria

1. Changes in precordial leads

   1.- Morphology of QRS-T in V1–V3: ST elevation (sometimes only in V1 and exceptionally also in V3 (Brugada electrocardiographic pattern –BP-)

   – **Type 1 Coved pattern** (Figure 21.14A): initial ST elevation ≥2 mm, slowly descending and concave (sometimes rectilinear) respect to the isoelectric baseline, with negative symmetric T wave.

   – **Type 2 saddleback pattern** (Figure 21.14B): ST elevation, convex respect to the isoelectric baseline, with positive T wave in V2. The elevation, that usually is ≥1 mm, is preceded by an r′ wave, generally wide compared with the r′ wave in athletes or pectus excavatum (see Figure 21.17).

2. Duration of QRS:

   – Mismatch between the end of QRS pattern in V1–V2 (longer) and V6 (see text and Figure 21.17)

3. New ECG criteria (Figure 21.17)

   The ST is downsloping: The index: height of ST in V1–V2 at high take-off/at 80 ms. later >1 (in other cases is upsloping and the index is <1). The end of QRS (J point) usually is later (Bayés de Luna and Baranchuk 2017) than the high take-off of QRS-ST (according to Corrado coincides with J point – Corrado *et al.* 2010) but the index is still valid (Figure 21.17 and Table 21.10)

   – **The β angle formed by ascending S and descending r′ is >58° in type 2 BP** (in athletes is much lower) (Chevallier *et al.* 2011) (SE 79% SP 83%).

   – **The duration of base of triangle of r′** at 5 mm from the high take-off is much longer in BP type 2 than in athletes (usually >3.5 mm –SE:79.3% SP:84%) (Serra *et al.* 2012) (Table 21.10)

B. Other ECG findings:

1. QT generally normal. May be prolonged in right precordial leads (Pitzalis et a*l.* 2003).

2. Conduction disorders: Sometimes prolonged PR interval (long HV interval) or delayed RV conduction (VCG) (Pérez-Riera 2009).

3. Supraventricular arrhythmias. Especially atrial fibrillation (Schimpf *et al.* 2008; Pappone *et al.* 2009).

4. Some other ECG findings may be seen: Early repolarization pattern in inferior leads (Sarkozy *et al.* 2009), fractioned QRS (Morita *et al.* 2008), alternans of T wave after ajmaline injection (Tada *et al.* 2008), etc.

For more details, consult www.brugadadrugs.org (Postema *et al.* 2009).

Furthermore, in some cases, the ECG pattern is only evident or more evident in the upper precordial V1–V3 leads. The fact that an ECG pseudonormalization is observed when the electrodes are located in the correct position does not constitute any guarantee of diagnosis, especially if the ST elevation persists, albeit less markedly (Figure 21.15). For this reason, it is very important to put the electrodes in the same place when serial recordings are performed in order to allow comparative assessments (Coppola *et al.* 2019).

A Japanese population computerized diagnostic criteria for Brugada syndrome that has a reasonable accuracy has been published (type 1≈90%, type 2≈70–80%)

(Nishizaki *et al.* 2010). This study was based on the comparison with RBBB in apparently healthy people but not with athletes and people with pectus excavatum (see Figure 7.17).

One special aspect of the BP is that it can be unmasked by fever. Sodium channels are thermo-sensitive and fever has demonstrated to activate concealed ECG patterns, and anecdotally, to associate to higher risk of serious ventricular arrhythmias. During viral pandemics, the burden of people attending emergency rooms with fever dramatically increases, leading to more diagnosis of people with BP (Baranchuk and Simpson 2011; Wu *et al.* 2020).

Differential diagnosis

Table 21.11 shows some of more frequent conditions that present a BP like in right precordial leads. Sometimes the differential diagnosis of the cause of ST elevation for ECG alone may be difficult even for expert cardiologists. In asymptomatic patients, we have to perform the differential diagnosis especially with: Athletes (Figures 7.16 and 21.17), pectus excavatum (Figure 7.16), early repolarization (Chapter 24), and ARVD (see before).

In some doubtful cases, to determine the correct diagnosis, we may check if there are changes after the intravenous administration of Na channel blockers (ajmaline) (Figure 21.16). The assessment of the data shown in Table 21.8 is crucial in reaching a diagnosis of Brugada's syndrome.

Brugada phenocopies (BrP) are clinical entities that present with ECG patterns identical to those of BrS (Gottschalk *et al.* 2016), yet are caused by various clinical conditions (Baranchuk *et al.* 2012; Xu *et al.* 2019). Patients with BrP present with a Brugada ECG pattern in the context of an underlying clinical condition which normalizes upon treatment and resolution of that condition. The prognosis of BrP is benign and depends on the prognosis of the underlying condition.

Clinical implications

As with other inherited diseases, the most important factor is to evaluate the risk of sudden death and then to proceed to take a decision about ICD implantation. To do that, it is important to correlate the presence of family history, genetic studies, previous syncope, or cardiac arrest with the presence of spontaneous or provoked type I pattern. Also that prognosis is worst in men and in a window of age (15–60 years). With all that we must be aware of the approximate incidence of the yearly risk of sudden death and then we will be able to take the best decision for ICD implant.

The role of EPS to take this decision is under debate. Although in the series of Brugada's negative EPS support no implantation, there is not a general agreement about that (Benito *et al.* 2008; Anderson 2012; Priori *et al.* 2012).

Table 21.10 ECG patterns of Brugada syndrome in V1–V2

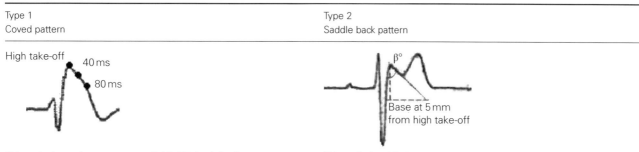

Type 1 Coved pattern	Type 2 Saddle back pattern

This typical coved pattern present in V1–V2 the following:
a. At the end of QRS an ascending and quick slope with a high take-off ≥0.2 mv followed by concave or rectilinear downsloping ST
b. There is no clear r' wave
c. The high take-off often does not correspond with the J point
d. At 40 ms of high take-off, the decrease in amplitude of ST is ≤0.4 mv (Nishizaki *et al.* 2010). In RBBB and athletes, the decrease is much higher
e. ST at high take-off > ST at 40 ms > ST at 80 ms
f. ST is followed by negative and symmetric T wave
g. The duration of QRS is longer than in RBBB and there is usually a mismatch between V1 and V6
h. The index of Corrado >1. In athletes is <1 (Figure 21.17 and Table 21.9)
i. There are few cases of coved pattern with a high take-off <2 mm >1 mm that needs, for clear identification of type 1 BP of complementary exams (Table 21.9)
	This typical saddle-back pattern present in V1–V2 the following:
	a. High take-off of r' (that not necessary coincides with J point) ≥2 mm
	b. Descending arm of r' coincides with beginning of ST (sometimes is not well seen)
	c. Minimum ST ascent ≥0.05 mv
	d. ST is followed by positive T wave in V2 (T peak > ST minimum > 0) and of variable morphology in V1
	e. The characteristics of triangle formed by r' allow to define different criteria useful for diagnosis
	  • β angle >58° (Chevallier *et al.* 2011)
	  • duration of the base of triangle of r' at 5 mm from the high take-off >3.5 mm (Serra *et al.* 2012)
	f. The duration of QRS is longer in BP2 than in other cases with r' in V1 and there is a mismatch between V1 and V6 (see text)
	g. The index of Corrado in V1–V2 > 1. In non-BP patients is <1 (Figure 21.17)

(Bayés de Luna *et al.* 2012).

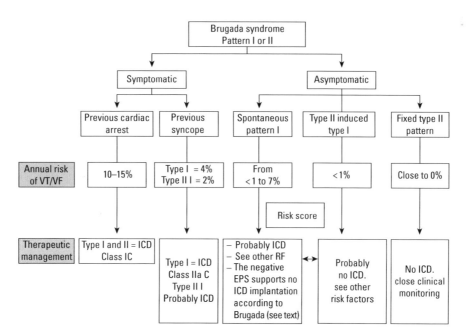

Figure 21.18 Decision tree algorithm for management of patients with the Brugada syndrome. Patients with type II induced type I pattern and with spontaneous asymptomatic pattern will benefit if score existed to determine candidacy for implantable cardioverter defibrillator implantation (Consult Bayés de Luna and Baranchuk 2017).

In any case a risk score would be useful in doubtful cases. New ECG markers of risk were advanced, and surface ECG still helps in determining which patients should be considered for further testing (Li *et al.* 2020). In the same manner, recent studies have confirmed the role of EPS to stratify risk (Hernandez-Ojeda *et al.* 2020).

Table 21.11 Most frequent conditions that can lead to Brugada-like pattern in right precordial leads (Bayés de Luna *et al.* 2012) (see Figures 7.16 and 21.17)

a. Right or left bundle branch block
b. Left ventricular hypertrophy
c. Acute ischemia
d. Pericarditis
e. Myocarditis
f. Pulmonary embolism
g. Hyperkalemia or hypercalcemia
h. Administration of certain drugs
i. ARVC (including the Naxos syndrome)
j. Early repolarization
k. Athletes
l. Pectus excavatum
m. Artifacts (incorrect H2 filter)
n. Miscellaneous: including a long number of different processes or situations (Consult 222.brugada.org).

(Based on Bayés de Luna *et al.* 2012).

Figure 21.18 summarizes the most important prognostic and therapeutic implications of the Brugada syndrome (Bayés de Luna and Baranchuk 2017).

Catecholaminergic polymorphic ventricular tachycardia
Concept and diagnosis (Priori *et al.* 2002)
Catecholaminergic polymorphic VT (CPVT) is a familial catecholaminergic autosomal dominant polymorphic VT. Genetic mutations in both the ryanodine cardiac receptor genes and the calsequestrin q2 gene have been described.

It has been shown that there are various mechanisms involved (triggered activity and rotors) in the genesis of sequential arrhythmias that appear with exercise and this confirms the diagnosis.

In general, an exercise or emotion-induced syncope constitutes the first clinical manifestation of the disease. Nevertheless, some cases of sudden death with no previous symptoms have been described.

ECG findings (Figure 21.19)
In general, after physical exercise or mental stress (Leenhardt *et al.* 1995), rapid supraventricular arrhythmias occur, followed by frequent PVCs, leading to runs of bidirectional VT that may be followed by polymorphic VT, VF, and sudden death, all despite a normal baseline ECG (Figure 21.19).

When CPVT is suspected, it is important to perform a Holter ECG to verify whether PVCs with bidirectional morphology are present. This information is enough to suspect the condition. It has recently been suggested that bradyarrhythmias may also be present.

Clinical implications
Because of the risk of sudden unexpected death, the prognosis is serious. Therefore, immediate treatment is required.

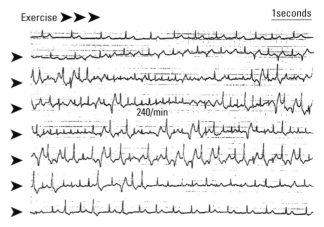

Figure 21.19 Continuous tracing during an exercise stress test of a patient with runs of catecholaminergic multiform ventricular tachycardia (VT). The sinus tachycardia is accompanied by bigeminal premature ventricular complexes (PVCs) along supraventricular tachyarrhythmia with runs of multiform PVCs, which lead to a run of bidirectional VT (sixth strip). Arrhythmias disappear shortly after discontinuing exercise in the last two strips (Adapted from Leenhardt *et al.* 1994) (see Figure 16.28).

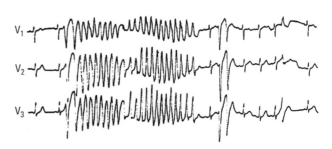

Figure 21.20 ECG (V1–V3) of a patient with runs of ventricular tachycardia (VT) with typical torsades de pointes morphology, although with a normal QT and a short coupling interval (270 ms). After one run of torsades de pointes VT, a second premature ventricular complex (PVC) is observed, but this time the coupling interval is not so short, not leading to another run of torsades de pointes VT (Reproduced with permission from Leenhardt *et al.* 1994).

Beta blockers should be administered. However, in about 40% of cases, beta blockers do not succeed in preventing recurrences during exercise testing. In these patients, as well as in patients with previous syncope and/or family history of syncope or sudden death, the implantation of an ICD is indicated.

Familial torsades de pointes ventricular tachycardia (Figure 21.20)
A rare form of familial torsades de pointes VT with a typical QRS complex morphology (see Chapter 16), without a long QT interval, and with a short coupling interval has been described (Figure 21.20) (Leenhardt *et al.* 1994). It has been reported in young people without heart disease and often leads to sudden death.

Because of the high incidence of fatal arrhythmias (torsades de pointes VT leading to VF), ICD implantation is indicated if the diagnosis is confirmed.

Atrial fibrillation

In the past few years, a genetic predisposition to atrial fibrillation has been proven. In fact, it is well known that familial atrial fibrillation is usually a monogenic disease. First, the locus was reported (Brugada *et al.* 1997) and later, various genes involved identified (Chen *et al.* 2003).

Familial atrial fibrillation appears in young people. Initially, it occurs as runs of tachycarrhythmia or frequent atrial extrasystoles with very short coupling interval. The presence of short QT syndrome should be ruled out in young patients with familial atrial fibrillation.

Other possible inherited heart diseases

It is possible that in the future, new genetic disorders with a characteristic phenotypic ECG pattern will be discovered. These patterns may include:

• some types of pre-excitation already genetically determined (Doevendans and Wellens 2001; Gollob *et al.* 2001) (see Chapter 12);
• some ECG patterns of early repolarization (see Chapter 24, Early repolarization pattern).

Finally, some other possible patterns include: (i) the presence of high and narrow QRS complexes (Wolpert *et al.* 2008) (see Chapter 24); (ii) cases of familial severe sinus bradycardia (Nof *et al.* 2007) (see Chapter 24), (iii) some cases of children presenting with intraventricular conduction blocks and VT (Iturralde-Torres *et al.* 2008), and (iv) cases of idiopathic VF in the presence of bradycardia-dependent intraventricular blocks (Aizawa *et al.* 1993).

References

Ackerman MJ, Priori SG, Willems S, *et al.* Heart Rhythm Society (HRS); European Heart Rhythm Association (EHRA). HRS/EHRA expert consensus statement on the state of genetic testing for the channelopathies and cardiomyopathies: this document was developed as a partnership between the Heart Rhythm Society (HRS) and the European Heart Rhythm Association (EHRA). Europace 2011;13(8):1077–109.

Aizawa Y, Tamura M, Chinushi M, *et al.* Idiopathic ventricular fibrillation and bradycardia-dependent intraventricular block. Am Heart J 1993;126:1473.

Anderson KP. Programmed electrical stimulation for risk assessment in brugada syndrome time to change the guidelines? J Am Coll Cardiol 2012;59:46–48.

Anttonen O, Junttila J, Maury F, *et al.* Differences in 12-lead ECG between symptomatic and asymptomatic subjects with short QT interval. Heart Rhythm 2009;6:267.

Antzelevitch C, Brugada R. Fever and Brugada syndrome. Pacing Clin Electrophysiol 2002;25:1537.

Antzelevitch C, Brugada P, Borggrefe M, *et al.* Brugada syndrome: report of the second consensus conference. Heart Rhythm 2005;2:429–440.

Arad M, Penas-Lado M, Monserrat L, *et al.* Gene mutations in apical hypertrophic cardiomyopathy. Circulation 2005;112:2805.

Baranchuk A, Simpson CS. Brugada syndrome coinciding with fever and H1N1 influenza virus. CMAJ 2011; 183(5):582.

Baranchuk A, Nguyen T, Ryu MH, Femenía F, Zareba W, Wilde AAM, Shimizu W, Brugada P, Pérez-Riera AR. Brugada Phenocopy: New terminology and proposed classification. Ann Noninvasive Electrocardiol 2012;17(4):299–314.

Bayés de Luna A, Furlanello F, Maron BJ, Zipes DP (eds). *Arrhythmias and Sudden Death in Athletes.* Kluwer Academic Publishers, 2000.

Bayés de Luna A, Brugada J, Brugada P, *et al.* Current ECG criteria for diagnosis of Brugada 1 and 2 patterns: a consensus document. J Electrocardiol 2012;45:454.

Benito B, Brugada R, Brugada J, Brugada P. Brugada syndrome. Prog Cardiovasc Dis 2008;51:1.

Britton S, Barbosa-Barros R, Alexander B, Baranchuk A. Progressive interatrial block associated with atrial fibrillation in a patient with hypertrophic cardiomyopathy. Ann Noninvasive Electrocardiol 2017;22(3):e12403.

Brugada P, Brugada J. Right bundle branch block, persistent ST segment elevation and sudden cardiac death: a distinct clinical and electrocardiographic syndrome. A multicenter report. J Am Coll Cardiol 1992;20:1391.

Brugada R, Tapscott T, Czernuszewicz GZ, *et al.* Identification of a genetic locus for familial atrial fibrillation. N Engl J Med 1997;336:905.

Chen Y, Xu SJ, Bendahhou S. KCNQ1 gen of function mutation in familiar atrial fibrillation. Science 2003;299:251.

Chevallier S, Forclaz A, Tenkorang J, *et al.* New electrocardiographic criteria for discriminating between Brugada types 2 and 3 patterns and incomplete right bundle branch block. J Am Coll Cardiol 2011;58:2290–2298.

Coats CJ, Quarta G, Flett AS, *et al.* Arrhythmogenic left ventricular cardiomyopathy. Circulation 2009;120:2613.

Coppola G, Corrado E, Curnis A, *et al.* Update on Brugada Syndrome **2019**.Curr Probl Cardiol 2019;23:100454.

Corrado D, Pelliccia A, Heidbuchel H *et al.* Recommendations for interpretation of 12-lead electrocardiogram in the athlete. Eur Heart J 2010;31:243.

Dalal D, Jain R, Tandri H, *et al.* Long-term efficacy of catheter ablation of ventricular tachycardia in patients with arrhythmogenic right ventricular dysplasia/cardiomyopathy. J Am Coll Cardiol 2007;50:432.

Nunes de Alencar Neto J, Baranchuk A, Bayés-Genís A, *et al.* Arrhythmogenic right ventricular dysplasia/cardiomyopathy: an electrocardiogram-based review. Europace 2018;20(FI1):f3–f12.

Doevendans PA, Wellens HJ. Wolff-Parkinson-White syndrome. A genetic disease? Circulation 2001;104:3014.

Dumont CA, Monserrat L, Soler R, *et al.* Interpretation of electrocardiographic abnormalities in hypertrophic cardiomyopathy with cardiac magnetic resonance. Eur Heart J 2006;27:1725.

Elizari MV, Levi R, Acunzo RS, *et al.* Abnormal expression of cardiac neural crest cells in heart development: a different hypothesis for the etiopathogenesis of Brugada syndrome. Heart Rhythm 2007;4:359–365.

Femenía F, Arce M, Van Grieken, J, *et al.* Fragmented QRS as a predictor of arrhythmic events in patients with hypertrophic obstructive cardiomyopathy. J Interv Card Electrophysiol 2013;38(3):159–165.

Fontaine G, Herbert JL, Probst-Squarcioni J, *et al.* Arrhythmogenic right ventricular dysplasia. ArchMal Cœur Vaiss 2004;97:1155.

Frustaci A, Russo MA, Chimenti C. Structural myocardial abnormalities in asymptomatic family members with Brugada syndrome and SCN5A gene mutation. Eur Heart J 2009;30:1763.

Gaita F, Giustetto C, Bianchi F, *et al.* Short QT syndrome. A familial cause of sudden death. Circulation 2003;108:965.

Goldberger I, Moss AJ. Long QT syndrome. J Am Coll Cardiol 2008;51:2291.

Gollob MH, Seger JJ, Gollob TN, *et al.* Novel PRKAG2 mutation responsible for the genetic syndrome of ventricular preexcitation and conduction system disease with childhood onset and absence of cardiac hypertrophy. Circulation 2001;104:3030.

Gollob MH, Redpath CJ, Roberts JD. The short QT syndrome: proposed diagnostic criteria. J Am Coll Cardiol 2011;57:802.

Gottschalk BH, Anselm DD, Brugada J, *et al.* Expert cardiologists cannot distinguish between Brugada Phenocopy and Brugada Syndrome ECG patterns. Europace 2016;18(7):1095–1100.

Hernandez-Ojeda J, Arbelo E, Jorda P *et al.* The role of clinical assessment and electrophysiology study in Brugada syndrome patients with syncope. Am Heart J 2020;220:213–223.

Ikeda H, Maki S, Yoshida N, *et al.* Predictors of death from congestive heart failure in hypertrophic cardiomyopathy. Am J Cardiol 1999;83:1280.

Iturralde-Torres P, Nava-Townsend S, Gómez-Flores J, *et al.* Association of congenital, diffuse electrical disease in children with normal heart: sick sinus syndrome, intraventricular conduction block, and monomorphic ventricular tachycardia. J Cardiovasc Electrophysiol 2008;19:550.

Jain R, Dalal D, Daly A, *et al.* Electrocardiographic features of arrhythmogenic right ventricular dysplasia. Circulation 2009;12(6): 477–487.

Kirchhof P, Franz MR, Bardai A, *et al.* Giant T-U waves precede torsades de pointes in long QT syndrome: a systematic electrocardiographic analysis in patients with acquired and congenital QT prolongation. J Am Coll Cardiol 2009;54:143.

Leenhardt A, Glaser E, Burguera M, *et al.* Short-coupled variant of torsades de pointes. A new electrocardiographic entity in the spectrum of idiopathic ventricular tachyarrhythmias. Circulation 1994;89:206.

Leenhardt A, Lucet V, Denjoy I, *et al.* Catecholaminergic polymorphic ventricular tachycardia in children. A 7-year follow-up of 21 patients. Circulation 1995;91:1512.

Lenegre J. Etiology and pathology of bilateral bundle branch block in relation to complete heart block. Prog Cardiovasc Dis 1964;6:445.

Lev M. Anatomic basis for atrioventricular block. Am J Med 1964;37:742.

Li KHC, Lee S, Yin C, *et al.* Brugada syndrome: a comprehensive review of pathophysiological mechanisms and risk stratification strategies. Int J Cardiol Heart Vasc 2020;26:100468.

Marcus FI, McKenna WJ, Sherrill D, *et al.* Diagnosis of arrhythmogenic right ventricular cardiomyopathy/dysplasia. Proposed modification of the task force criteria. Circulation 2010;121:1533.

Marbán E. Cardiac channelopathies. Nature 2002;415:213.

Maron BJ. Contemporary considerations for risk stratification, sudden death and prevention in hypertrophic cardiomyopathy. Heart 2003;89:977.

Maron BJ. Contemporary insights and strategies for risk stratification and prevention of sudden death in hypertrophic cardiomyopathy. Circulation 2010;121:445.

Maron BJ, Gottdiener JS, Epstein SE. Patterns and significance of distribution of left ventricular hypertrophy in hypertrophic cardiomyopathy. A wide angle, two dimensional echocardiographic study of 125 patients. Am J Cardiol 1981;48:418.

Maron B, Towbin JA, Thiene G, *et al.* Contemporary definitions and classification of the cardiomyopathies. An American Heart Association scientific statement from the council on clinical cardiology, heart failure and transplantation committee; Quality of care and outcomes research and functional genomics and translational biology interdisciplinary working groups; and Council on epidemiology and prevention. Circulation 2006;113:1807.

McKenna WJ, Behr ER. Hypertrophic cardiomyopathy: management, risk stratification, and prevention of sudden death. Heart 2002;87:169.

McKenna WJ, Thiene G, Nava A, *et al.* Diagnosis of arrhythmogenic right ventricular dysplasia/cardiomyopathy. Task Force of the Working Group Myocardial and Pericardial Disease of the European Society of Cardiology and of the Scientific Council on Cardiomyopathies of the International Society and Federation of Cardiology. Br Heart J 1994;71:215.

McLeod CJ, Ackerman MJ, Nishimura RA, *et al.* Outcomes of patients with hypertrophic CM and normal ECG. J Am Coll Cardiol 2009;54:229.

Meregalli PG, Tan HL, Probst V, *et al.* Type of SCN5A mutation determines clinical severity and degree of conduction slowing in loss-of-function sodium channelopathies. Heart Rhythm 2009;6:341.

Morita H, Kusano KF, Miura D, *et al.* Fragmented QRS as a marker of conduction abnormality and a predictor of prognosis of Brugada syndrome. Circulation 2008;118:1697.

Moss AJ. T wave patterns associated with the hereditary QT syndrome. Card Electrophysiol Rev 2002;6:311.

Moss AJ, Kan RS. Long QT syndromes: from channels to cardia arrhythmias. J Clin Investig 2005;15:2008.

Moss AJ, Schwartz PJ., Campton RS *et al.* The long QT syndrome: a prospective international study. Circulation 1985;71:17.

Murphy RT, Thaman R, Gimeno Blanes J, *et al.* Natural history and familial characteristics of isolated left ventricular noncompaction. Eur Heart J 2005;26:187.

Nishizaki M, Sugi K, Izumida N, *et al.* Classification and assessment of computerized diagnostic criteria for Brugada-type electrocardiograms. Heart Rhythm 2010;11:1660.

Nof E, Luria D, Brass D, *et al.* Point mutation in the HCN4 cardiac ion channel pore affecting synthesis, trafficking, and functional expression is associated with familial asymptomatic sinus bradycardia. Circulation 2007;11:463.

Pappone C, Radinovic A, Manguso F, *et al.* New-onset atrial fibrillation as first clinical manifestation of latent Brugada syndrome: prevalence and clinical significance. Eur Heart J 2009;30:2985.

Pérez-Riera, AR. *Learning Easily Frank Vectorcardiogram.* Editora e Gràfica Mosteiro. Sao Paulo, Brazil, 2009.

Pieroni M, Dello Russo A, Marzo F, *et al.* High prevalence of myocarditis mimicking arrhythmogenic right ventricular cardiomyopathy. J Am Coll Cardiol 2009;53:681.

Pitzalis MV, Anaclerio M, Iacoviello M. QT interval prolongation in right precordial leads in Brugada syndrome. J Am Coll Cardiol 2003;42:1632.

Postema PG, Wolpert C, Amin AS, *et al.* Drugs and Brugada syndrome patients: review of the literature, recommendations, and an up-to-date website (www.brugadadrugs.org). Heart Rhythm 2009;6:1335.

Priori SG, Napolitano C, Memmi M, *et al.* Clinical and molecular characterization of patients with catecholaminergic polymorphic ventricular tachycardia. Circulation 2002;106:69.

Priori SG, Gasparini M, Napolitano C, *et al.* Risk stratification in Brugada syndrome results of the PRELUDE (PROgrammed ELectrica stimUlation preDictive valuE) registry. J Am Coll Cardiol 2012;59:37–45.

Samani K, Wu G, Ai T, *et al.* A novel SCN5A mutation V1340I in Brugada syndrome augmenting arrhythmias during febrile illness. Heart Rhythm 2009;6:1318.

Sarkozy A, Cherchia G, Paparella G, *et al.* Inferior and lateral ECG repolarization abnormalities in Brugada syndrome. Circ Arrhythm Electrophysiol 2009;2:154.

Schimpf R, Giustetto C, Eckardt L, *et al.* Prevalence of supraventricular tachyarrhythmias in a cohort of patients with Brugada syndrome. Ann Noninvasive Electrocardiol 2008;13:266.

Schwartz PJ, Moss AJ, Vincent GM, Crampton RS. Diagnostic criteria for the long QT syndrome. An update. Circulation 1993;88:782.

Schwartz PJ, Spazzolini C, Crotti L, *et al.* The Jervell and Lange-Nielsen syndrome: natural history, molecular basis, and clinical outcome The Jervell and Lange-Nielsen syndrome: natural history, molecular basis, and clinical outcome Circulation 2006;113:783.

Serra G, Baranchuk A, Bayés-De-Luna A, *et al.* New electrocardiographic criteria to differentiate the Type-2 Brugada pattern from electrocardiogram of healthy athletes with r'-wave in leads V1/V2. Europace. 2014;16(11):1639–1645.

Steffel J, Kobza R, *et al.* ECG characteristics at initial diagnosis in patients with isolated left ventricle noncompaction. Am J Cardiol 2009;104:984.

Suzuki J, Watanabe F, Takenaka K, *et al.* New subtype of apical hypertrophic cardiomyopathy identified with nuclear magnetic resonance imaging as an underlying cause of markedly inverted T waves. J Am Coll Cardiol 1993;22:1175.

Tada T, Kusano KF, Nagase S. The relationship between the magnitude of T wave alternans and the amplitude of the T wave in Brugada syndrome. J Cardiovasc Electrophysiol 2008;19:56.

Viskin S, Rosovski U, Sands AJ, *et al.* Inaccurate electrocardiographic interpretation of long QT: the majority of physicians cannot recognize a long QT when they see one. Heart Rhythm 2005;2:569.

Wolpert C, Veltmann C, Schimpf R, *et al.* Is a narrow and tall QRS complex an ECG marker for sudden death? Heart Rhythm 2008;5:1339.

Wilde AA, Antzelevitch C, Borggrefe M, *et al.* Study Group on the molecular basis of arrhythmias of the European Society of Cardiology. Proposed diagnostic criteria for the Brugada syndrome: consensus report. Circulation 2002;106:2514.

Wu CI, Postema PG, Arbelo E *et al.* SARS-CoV-2, COVID-19, and inherited arrhythmia syndromes. Heart Rhythm 2020;17(9):1456–1462.

Xu G, Gottschalk BH, Pérez-Riera A, *et al.* Link between Brugada phenocopy and myocardial ischemia: results from the International Registry on Brugada Phenocopy. PACE 2019;42(6):658–662.

Yamaguchi M, Shimizu M, Ino H, *et al.* T wave peak-to-end interval and QT dispersion in acquired long QT syndrome: a new index for arrhythmogenicity. Clin Sci 2003;105:671.

Yap YG, Behr ER, Camm AJ. Drug-induced Brugada syndrome. Europace 2009;11:989.

Zareba W. Cygankiewicz I. Long QT syndrome and short QT syndrome. Prog Cardiovasc Dis 2008;51:264.

Zareba W, Moss AJ, Schwartz PJ, *et al.* Influence of genotype on the clinical course of the long-QT syndrome. International Long-QT Syndrome Registry Research Group. N Engl J Med 1998;339:960.

Zareba W, Moss AJ, Locati EH, *et al.* Modulating effects of age and sex on the clinical course of long QT syndrome by genotype. J Am Coll Cardiol 2003;42:103.

Zhang, L, Mmagu, O, Liu, L, *et al.* Hypertrophic cardiomyopathy: can the noninvasive diagnostic testing identify high risk patients? World J Cardiol 2014;6(8):764–770.

Chapter 22
The ECG in Other Heart Diseases

This chapter deals with the most important electrocardiographic abnormalities present in heart diseases other than ischemic heart disease (see Chapter 20) and inherited heart diseases (see Chapter 21).

Valvular heart diseases

Currently, the incidence of valvular heart diseases of rheumatic origin in developed countries is very rare and usually only found in immigrant populations. However, many cases of adults with rheumatic valvular heart disease acquired several decades ago still exist. The most frequent causes of valvular heart diseases are aortic stenosis and mitral regurgitation. Aortic stenosis is mainly due to degenerative calcification in the elderly but can be seen in younger patients with bicuspid aortic valve. Mitral regurgitation is mainly related with mitral valve prolapse and with dilated cardiomyopathy. The presence of left or right ventricular enlargement usually indicates that the disease is severe. The most frequent ECG findings and their clinical significance are explained below.

Mitral valve disease: ECG changes

Mitral stenosis typically presents with a P wave ± in V1 and a wide and biphasic P wave in other leads, especially I and II, as an expression of left atrial enlargement (P mitrale) (see Figure 9.35). We have to remember that for the evaluation of the P wave in V1, it is essential that the V1 electrode is correctly located. Throughout the natural evolution of mitral stenosis, atrial fibrillation is very common; the more abnormal the P wave, the more likely the appearance of this arrhythmia. In this sense, the presence of a P wave of ≥0.12 and ± in II, III, and aVF is a very specific marker of paroxysmal supraventricular arrhythmias in the future (Bayés de Luna *et al.* 1989). In

our experience, nearly every patient with valvular heart disease who presents this kind of interatrial block has presented paroxysmal arrhythmia, atrial fibrillation or flutter especially atypical flutter, within the first year (see Chapter 9). The presence of ECG signs of right ventricular enlargement (evident R wave ≥3mm in V1) suggests pulmonary hypertension (see Figure 10.4). A ratio QRS voltage in V2/QRS voltage in V1 >5 suggests right atrial and ventricular enlargement (see Figure 9.7). ECG signs of left ventricular enlargement suggest the possibility of other associated lesions (mitral regurgitation and/or associated aortic valve disease).

Non-severe mitral regurgitation, alone or associated with mitral stenosis, may alter the ECG slightly. When significant regurgitation is found, however, ECG signs of left ventricular enlargement associated with an abnormal P wave or atrial fibrillation are usually observed.

In **mitral valve prolapse,** repolarization abnormalities are frequently found in II, III, aVF, and left precordial leads. Atrial arrhythmias are common, especially frequent premature atrial complexes and atrial fibrillation, and ventricular arrhythmias might be seen (Figure 22.1), especially when mitral prolapse is severe, in which case the ECG is rarely normal.

Tricuspid regurgitation secondary to mitral stenosis with pulmonary hypertension usually shows in the ECG signs of right chamber enlargement (see Figures 10.34 and 10.35).

Aortic valve disease: ECG changes

Isolated aortic valve disease, except at advanced stages, is not typically accompanied by significant signs of left atrial enlargement or atrial fibrillation. Therefore, if these ECG signs are present in non-advanced cases, associated mitral valve disease must be suspected.

Clinical Electrocardiography: A Textbook, Fifth Edition. Antoni Bayés de Luna, Miquel Fiol-Sala, Antoni Bayés-Genís, and Adrián Baranchuk.
© 2022 John Wiley & Sons Ltd. Published 2022 by John Wiley & Sons Ltd.

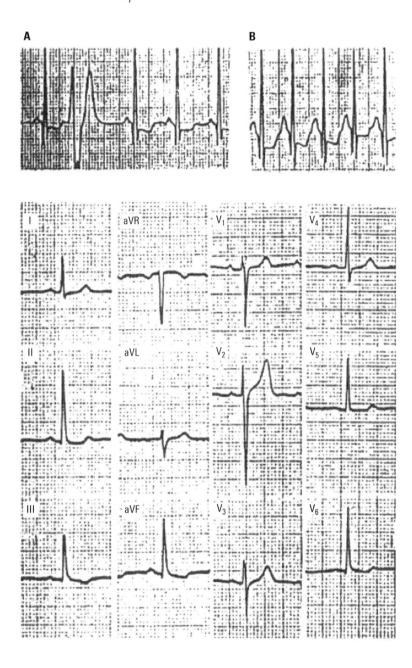

Figure 22.1 Bottom: A patient with mitral valve prolapse. Top: In the Holter recording, an ST-segment depression is seen at rest (A) and increases with exercise (B).

In the early stages of left ventricular enlargement, there is usually a pattern of qR morphology with positive T wave in left lateral leads, which is more evident with aortic regurgitation then with aortic stenosis (a deeper "q" wave and a taller T wave). This pattern has been considered (Cabrera and Mouroy 1952) a result of diastolic hemodynamic overload (see Chapter 10), but we now know that in advanced cases both aortic stenosis and aortic regurgitation generally show a similar morphology, known as "strain pattern" (see Figure 10.21) (somewhat depressed ST segment followed by a negative and asymmetric T wave). Although the ST segment/T wave pattern is similar in both cases, in aortic regurgitation, the R wave is often still preceded by a usually small Q wave, which usually decreases over time, whereas in aortic stenosis, QRS complex morphology tends to be a pure R wave (see Figure 10.21). Sometimes, a **mixed pattern is seen**, T wave more negative than usual and/or more symmetrical, or a more marked decrease of ST segment due to an added primary factor, such as associated ischemia or myocardial compromise or due to drug effects (see Figure 10.28).

The so-called pattern of diastolic overload is observed in the early stages of any type of ventricular enlargement due to aortic valve disease, but not in the ventricular enlargement of isolated aortic regurgitation. **The "strain pattern,"** named by Cabrera in 1956, is a pattern of systolic overload **observed in more advanced stages of aortic valve disease**, regardless of the predominance of stenosis or regurgitation. On the other hand, it has been proven that the presence or absence of a "q" wave in V5–V6 is more directly related to the degree of septal fibrosis (more fibrosis, less "q" wave) than the type of lesion (Bayés de Luna *et al.* 1983) (see Figures 10.22 and 10.23).

The presence of clear signs of left ventricular enlargement with a "strain" pattern indicates a severe and long-lasting aortic valve disease, is often correlated with the presence of symptoms, and is a marker of poor prognosis. Surgery is recommended in the presence of LV failure, syncope, or angina. However, it is not uncommon that patients with severe aortic stenosis with significant left ventricular enlargement have only discrete ECG abnormalities. This is not usually the case for patients with advanced aortic regurgitation.

Patients with advanced aortic valvular disease frequently present with ventricular arrhythmias and intraventricular blocks and atrioventricular (AV) block (calcification of the aortic valve), even more than those with advanced mitral valve disease, but the latter more frequently present atrial fibrillation.

The occurrence of new conduction abnormalities, including LBBB, has been reported to be the most frequent complication following transcatheter aortic valve implantation (TAVI) (Martinez-Selles *et al.* 2015). These conduction disturbances are mainly seen in the first 48 hours after TAVI (Kooistra *et al.* 2020) and their reasons and clinical significance are yet to be fully delineated. Specific procedure and patient-related factors may contribute to the development of LBBB and aberrant atrioventricular conduction following TAVI as well as its clinical consequences.

Myocarditis and cardiomyopathies

There are three major functional types of cardiomyopathies: dilated, hypertrophic, and restrictive. Hypertrophic cardiomyopathy (HCM) is usually inherited. Cardiomyopathies of inherited origin are explained in Chapter 21.

Myocarditis

Concept and evolution
Acute inflammatory myocarditis is caused by diverse infectious agents (most commonly viruses) or agents of unknown origin. This section is focused on ECG abnormalities seen in the acute stage of idiopathic or viral myocarditis.

Acute myocarditis may be severe, with signs of heart failure or even lethal evolution in a very short time, and may lead to dilated cardiomyopathy. However, the evolution is usually favorable and a *restitutio ad integrum* is often observed. It should be remembered that this state may appear isolated or as part of a generalized viral disease. In fact, many viral diseases, from the flu to hepatitis, show transient ECG abnormalities in 5–20% of cases.

ECG changes during the evolution and differential diagnosis
In the acute stage, sinus tachycardia, low-voltage, and various supraventricular arrhythmias, such as atrial fibrillation that may be transient, and ventricular arrhythmias, especially ventricular premature complexes, are common. Advanced AV block is generally transient. Cases with progression to dilated cardiomyopathy may present an intraventricular conduction block. Often, the evolution is favorable but a right or left bundle branch block can persist.

Also, repolarization abnormalities are frequently present, particularly flat or usually mild negative T waves, that may be deep or have a ± morphology, and/or an abnormal ST segment. These abnormalities are usually observed in many leads. The upsloping ST segment elevation is concave with respect to isoelectric line, at least in some leads (Figure 22.2). In some cases, differential diagnosis with ST-segment elevation acute coronary syndrome (ACS) may be difficult. During the evolution of acute myocarditis, Q wave ECG, or even QS pattern, may be present. Usually, it is not very deep, and is transient. The difficulty in making a diagnosis increases due to the presence of precordial discomfort, especially in cases of perimyocarditis and increase in biomarkers. Thus, it may be necessary to perform coronary angiography, multislice computerized tomography (MSCT), and/or magnetic resonance imaging.

The differential diagnosis is even more complicated with **Tako-Tsubo syndrome,** (see Figure 20.44) (Tsuchihashi *et al.* 2001). The diagnosis of Tako-Tsubo syndrome (see Chapter 20) is supported by: (i) marked upslope in the ST segment elevation; (ii) long QTc interval; (iii) "q" wave more frequently present, and less transient than in myocarditis; and (iv) deep negative T wave in the evolution (see Figures 13.11 and 20.4B). In clinical practice, the distinction is not easy to make and in some cases it is impossible without additional tests (see Chapter 20). However, persistent "q" wave is unusual in myocarditis, and the clinical presentation is frequently different.

When the acute phase is over, the evolution is usually good, and in these cases the ECG remains mildly changed (usually slight changes in the T wave) or becomes normal. Unfortunately, **some cases progress to dilated cardiomyopathy, even with a poor evolution in the short term**.

Restrictive cardiomyopathy
There are many etiologies for this infrequent type of cardiomyopathies (infiltrative including amyloid, sarcoid and Gaucher disease and non-infiltrative usually

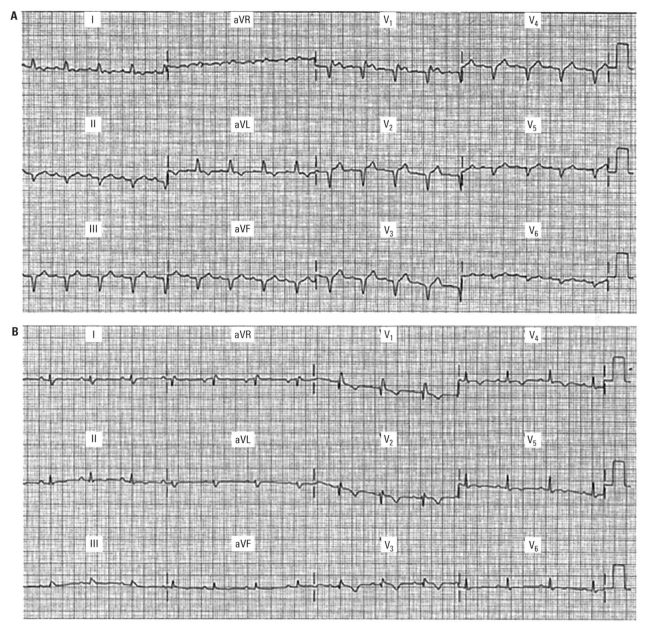

Figure 22.2 (A) Patient with acute myocarditis and ECG with signs of sinus tachycardia with RBBB plus LAHB and Q waves in many leads. After the acute phase (B), the Q waves and the LAHB disappear. In many leads, T wave inversion is still present. Observe the low voltage in both ECGs.

idiopathic processes, storage diseases, including hemochromatosis, Fabry disease due to deficiency of the lisozomal enzyme a-galactosidase A and all types of endomyocardial involvement). The hallmark is abnormal diastolic function usually with normal contractile function. Thus, restrictive cardiomyopathy bears some functional resemblance to constrictive pericarditis. The differential diagnosis is mandatory because of the potential surgical treatment of constrictive pericarditis.

Advanced restrictive cardiomyopathy **may display some striking ECG patterns** (Figure 22.3) including: (i) pseudo-necrosis "q" wave; (ii) obvious repolarization abnormalities; and (iii) a P wave with a significant brisk negative component in V1 due to the significant left atrial enlargement frequently found; (iv) intraventricular conduction disorders; (v) prominent R in V1; and (vi) LVH with "strain." All these parameters combined with echocardiography and clinical setting are useful for differential diagnosis (Hoigne *et al.* 2006) (Figure 22.3). Due to the presence of significant atrial dilation, atrial fibrillation is often present, even in young patients, and may be poorly tolerated. Heart transplant is often necessary but presents many problems due to frequent systemic involvement in infiltrative and storage diseases.

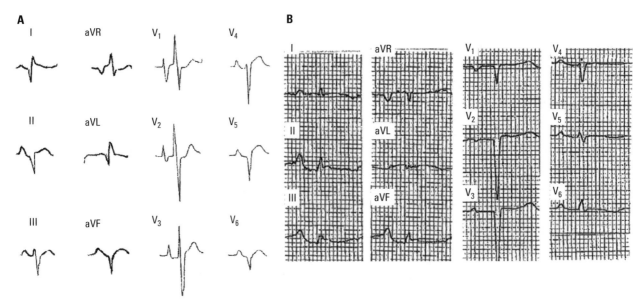

Figure 22.3 (A) A patient with advanced restrictive cardiomyopathy. Note the presence of clear QRS abnormalities simulating lateral necrosis. Evident P wave signs of very important bi-atrial enlargement are found in this type of a cardiomyopathy. (B) Patient of 56 years with cardiac amyloidosis that presents pathologic Q wave, low voltage, and abnormal repolarization (Hoigne *et al.* 2006).

Dilated cardiomyopathy and heart failure

Concept, etiology, and clinical syndromes

Dilated cardiomyopathy **is the most frequent type of cardiomyopathy. It is a syndrome characterized by cardiac enlargement and impaired systolic and/or diastolic function of the left or both ventricles. It is considered idiopathic when the cause is a primary disease of heart muscle. Over time, the symptoms of congestive heart failure usually appear.**

Its importance is great because it has a high incidence, especially if we include all cases of hypertensive, valvular, or ischemic origin evolving to a clinical picture of heart failure in a similar way to the idiopathic cases of dilated cardiomyopathy.

In a significant number of cases, the origin is unknown (idiopathic dilated cardiomyopathy). However, there is growing evidence that a relatively high number of idiopathic dilated cardiomyopathies are of genetic origin (around 30%).

The etiology of dilated cardiomyopathy is commonly infectious, (viral), **although in many cases there is no previous history of myocarditis. Furthermore, there are many causes of systemic, metabolic, or toxic origin, including alcohol and the administration of some chemotherapeutic drugs that can lead to a dilated cardiomyopathy. In South America, for example, Chagas cardiomyopathy continues to be a significant problem. It is caused by an acute myocarditis due to Trypanosoma cruzi, a flagellate protozoan present in jungle mammals and carried to humans via bites due to insects that typically dwell in the ceilings and walls of rural houses in Latin America (Mendoza and Acquatella** 2003). **In about 10–20% of cases, Chagas**

cardiomyopathy presents with different types of heart block and active arrhythmias and evolves to dilated cardiomyopathy with different degrees of heart failure. It is worth noting that in view of considerable existing immigration flows, there are certain to be many "silent" cases of Chagas cardiomyopathy, both in Europe and in the United States (Milei et al. 1992).

Patients with dilated cardiomyopathy present with signs of left ventricular impairment that often evolves to heart failure with depressed (systolic) or preserved (diastolic) left ventricular function. For this reason, we will examine the ECG changes of dilated cardiomyopathy together with those of heart failure.

Heart failure (HF) presents the most important challenge for cardiology in the twenty-first century, because it represents the final path of all heart diseases. It is of particular significance to recall that hypertension is the most frequent cause of heart failure, along with ischemic heart disease.

Heart failure occurs when the heart cannot efficiently pump blood to vital organs. The main symptom of heart failure is dyspnea, which is used to classify heart failure into different functional classes (NYHA).

Today, it is known that heart failure develops via two pathophysiological mechanisms: **heart failure with reduced ejection fraction,** and **heart failure with preserved ejection fraction**. Mid-range heart failure has also been introduced in Europe. B-type natriuretic peptide (BNP) plasmatic levels in patients with dyspnea are very useful for the diagnosis. Heart failure with preserved ejection fraction might also have by congestion, acute pulmonary edema, and sudden death (Varela-Román *et al.* 2002).

ECG changes and prognostic implications

It is quite rare that a patient with class III–IV heart failure does not present with ECG abnormalities. A normal ECG has a high negative predictive value (>90%) and almost rules out the presence of significant left ventricular dysfunction (Remme and Swedberg 2001). In advanced cases of high output heart failure (e.g. beriberi), the ECG does not exhibit many abnormalities (Figure 22.4). In patients with hypertrophic cardiomyopathy, on the other hand, it has been proven that a relatively low voltage could be a marker of heart failure in the medium term (see Figure 21.5) (Ikeda *et al.* 1999). In hypertrophic cardiomyopathy and arrhythmogenic right ventricular dysplasia, the ECG may be normal in some few cases (see Chapter 21). However, a normal ECG may not rule out diastolic dysfunction in patients with clinical suspicion of HF. In these cases, it has been demonstrated that a longer QT interval may predict LV dysfunction (Wilcox *et al.* 2011).

In patients with heart failure, the ECG may show signs of atrial and/or ventricular enlargement, intraventricular blocks (Escobar-Robledo *et al.* 2018) and/or Q wave even in the absence of ischemic heart disease.

The presence of low-voltage QRS complex in the frontal plane is a characteristic of dilated cardiomyopathy, although high voltage is found in the right precordial leads (Figures 11.27, 11.30, and 11.31). Cases with advanced heart failure, especially due to the presence of anasarca, may present with a low voltage of QRS, T and also P waves (Madias 2008) (see pericarditis) that can disappear with the improvement of the disease (Figure 22.5) (Madias *et al.* 2001).

QRS complexes are often notched and wide (with different degrees of left bundle branch block morphology). If advanced left bundle branch block (LBBB) is found, V3 voltage helps to differentiate idiopathic cardiomyopathy (with much higher QRS voltage) from ischemic cardiomyopathy (Figure 22.6) (Bayés-Genís *et al.* 2003). This sign is probably more useful than repolarization abnormalities or even pathologic Q waves in differentiating between ischemic and idiopathic cardiomyopathy.

The presence of advanced LBBB with very wide QRS complexes (≥170 ms) is an indicator of poor ventricular function (Das *et al.* 2001) and the presence of final R wave in aVR (QR) in advanced LBBB is a possible marker of RV dilation (Van Bommel *et al.* 2011) (see Chapter 11).

The heart rate is usually increased and atrial fibrillation and ventricular arrhythmias are common. The association of LBBB and atrial fibrillation present in at least 5% of patients with congestive heart failure is a marker of poor prognosis (Baldasseroni *et al.* 2002; Vazquez *et al.* 2009). Figures 10.30, 11.27, 11.30, and 11.31 show typical examples of patients with idiopathic dilated cardiomyopathy in advanced stages of heart failure.

It is estimated that approximately **40% of cardiovascular deaths reported in patients with heart failure are sudden**, whereas the remaining deaths may be attributed to heart failure progression. The three-year mortality rate in patients with heart failure (NYHA Classes II–III) is

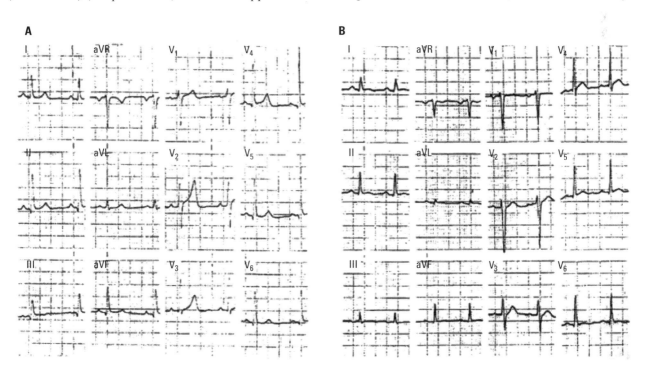

Figure 22.4 A 61-year-old patient with beriberi heart disease and heart failure who died in cardiogenic shock. (A) The ECG one month before death was normal. (B) The ECG two days prior to death. At that time, the QRS was still normal and only tachycardia and minor repolarization alterations could be seen.

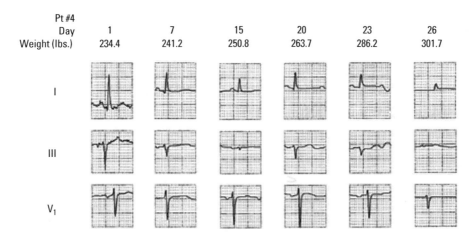

Figure 22.5 Serial weights and corresponding sum of the amplitudes of QRS complexes (SQRS) revealing the reciprocal relation of these two variables in this patient (Pt) (Reproduced from Madias *et al.* 2001, with permission from Elsevier).

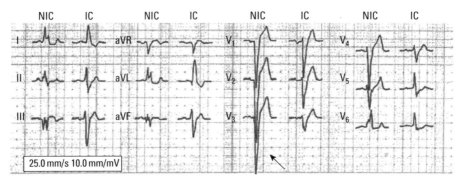

Figure 22.6 ECGs of two patients, one with non-ischemic cardiomyopathy (NIC) and the other with ischemic cardiomyopathy (IC). Both ECGs have a similar QRS width, left ventricular ejection fraction (LVEF) and left ventricular end diastolic diameter (LVEDD). Note the pronounced voltages of right precordial leads, particularly in V2 and V3 (arrow), observable in non-ischemic cardiomyopathy compared to ischemic cardiomyopathy.

20–30%. Half of these deaths can be attributed to sudden death ("a heart too good to die"). Cases of sudden death in patients with NYHA Classes II–III heart failure are mostly caused by ventricular arrhythmia (VT/ VF), whereas in NYHA Class IV patients, bradyarrhythmias play a more important role (Luu *et al.* 1989) (see Chapters 16 and 17). This may explain the inefficacy of antiarrhythmic drugs in preventing sudden death in Class IV patients.

Although some contradictory results exist, most studies (Vazquez *et al.* 2009) show that sudden death is more frequently observed in cases of heart failure with reduced ejection fraction, especially in patients with ischemic cardiomyopathy, than in cases of heart failure with preserved ejection fraction.

In contrast, there is considerable evidence indicating that several risk markers reflecting ANS alterations (heart rate variability [HRV], heart rate turbulence [HRT], sinus tachycardia) (Cygankiewicz *et al.* 2006, 2008) may play a role in the risk stratification of sudden death in heart failure patients, although the PPV is low. At the same time, it

has been demonstrated that one of the most extensively studied risk markers (T wave alternans) predicts sudden death (Bloomfield *et al.* 2004; Verrier *et al.* 2011). However, there is not enough evidence to use these risk markers to guide treatment.

The increase of sympathetic innervation, detected by Im-IBG images, correlates with an improvement in heart failure prognosis and a decrease in ventricular arrhythmias.

The MUSIC risk score for predicting death in heart failure (study) (Vazquez *et al.* 2009) includes 10 independent prognostic variables (Figure 22.7A). It should be emphasized that only atrial enlargement and NT-pro BNP levels were found to predict death, regardless of the mechanism involved (cardiac death, sudden death, or death due to heart failure progression). A combination of 10 of these variables allowed us to establish a risk score. Figure 22.7B shows the mortality curve according to the type of death studied. With this risk score, two different well-defined populations were found: one population group with a score < 20, considered a low-risk population,

A

	Total mortality	Cardiac mortality	Pump failure death	Sudden death
Prior AVE	3	3		8
Indexed LA size > 26 mm/m²	8	9	9	11
LV ejection fraction ≤ 35%	5	5	5	
Atrial fibrilation	3			
LBBB or IVCD				7
NSVT and frequent VPBs	3	4		7
eGFR < 60 ml/min/1.73 m²	4	4	5	
Hyponatremia ≤ 138 mEq/L	3	3	4	
NT-proBNP > 1000 ng/l	7	7	10	7
Troponin-positive	4	5	7	
Maximum possible risk score	40	40	40	40
High risk patient if score >	20	20	20	20

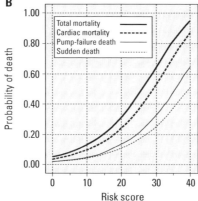

B

Figure 22.7 (A) Risk score for predicting different types of death. We see the parameters used to determine the score. (B) Mortality curves for the different types of death over a period of three years (Reproduced with permission from Vazquez *et al.* 2009).

and a second population group with a score > 20, considered a population with increasing high-risk. ST2 (Pascual-Figal *et al.* 2009)

It is reasonable to assume that the use of an implantable defibrillator (ICD) (Mirowski *et al.* 1980) is particularly advisable when in spite of best drug treatment the ejection fraction is below 30%, in patients assessed as Class II or III according to NYHA criteria, or in those with ischemic heart disease (sudden death is more frequent in coronary heart disease than in idiopathic heart disease). Cases with heart failure and a wide QRS complex (> 140 ms) and low ejection fraction (< 30–35%) may be good candidates for resynchronization therapy (biventricular pacemaker) plus ICD (ICD-CRT therapy) (Cazeau *et al.* 1994; Moss *et al.* 1996; Moss 2002; Moss *et al.* 2009). However, in some cases the only solution might be a heart transplant.

The transplanted heart ECG

Both recipient and donor P waves, the latter always being associated with the QRS complex, may be seen on the surface ECG. Sometimes, it is necessary to utilize a right atrial lead to view the recipient P wave (Figure 22.8). Usually, the donor P wave rate is higher than that of the recipient P wave, since the donor P wave is not under vagal control.

The ECG abnormalities most frequently observed in the transplanted heart ECG include: repolarization abnormalities, right bundle branch block (RBBB) morphology, atrial arrhythmias (flutter and fibrillation), and sinus bradycardia, which may be severe in some cases and even show evidence of sinus node disease (Martí *et al.* 1991). Ventricular hypertrophy, particularly apical ventricular hypertrophy, is also common (Vicent *et al.* 2020).

Pericardial disease
Concept and diagnosis

Pericardial disease encompasses: (i) acute inflammatory pericarditis, idiopathic or caused by different etiologies, presents frequently pericardial effusion, might be recurrent, and may progress to a chronic phase (constrictive pericarditis); (ii) pericarditis related to hypersensitivity or autoimmunity; (iii) other forms of pericardial disease (uremic, neoplasic, myxedema, post-myocardial infarction and post-pericardiotomy, etc.).

Clinical signs that are very much in favor of pericarditis are: (i) recent infection of upper respiratory tract; (ii) pain characteristics related to respiration and irradiated to the neck; (iii) pericardial rub; and (iv) ECG changes (see below).

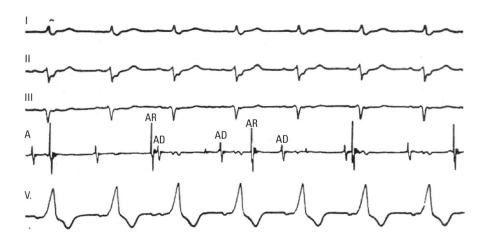

Figure 22.8 Leads I, II, III, V1, and right atrial leads (A) of a patient who underwent a heart transplant. Two atrial waves, that of the patient (AR) and of the donor (AD), are observed; the latter maintained cardiac rhythm.Pericardial disease

The differential diagnosis of acute pericarditis (perimyocarditis) must be performed with acute coronary syndrome (ACS), dissecting aneurysm, and early repolarization pattern, among other conditions. Table 19.3 shows the most important criteria, including the ECG, used to perform the differential diagnosis (see also myocarditis).

• Due to the presence of chest pain and ST segment elevation, it is mandatory to rule out ACS. This is not always easy, and myopericarditis may cause a moderate increase in troponin levels. Therefore, moderate increase in troponin levels is not effective for differentiating between pericardial disease and acute coronary syndromes because increased levels may be present in both.

• Quite frequently, a slight and convex notch at the end of QRS with some upward ST segment deviation with respect to the isoelectric line at the J point, known as early repolarization (Klatsky *et al.* 2003), once considered benign but recently shown to be a marker of bad prognosis in the presence of some specific characteristics (Chapter 23), has been confused with ST segment deviation of acute pericarditis, both by computerized ECG interpretation and by manual interpretation, especially when the ECG pattern pertains to a patient with atypical chest pain. The exercise stress test returns the ST segment elevation to normal in cases of early repolarization, but not in cases of pericarditis or coronary heart disease (Figure 19.6).

ECG changes

The ECG in idiopathic pericarditis

It has been documented that the **most characteristic ECG abnormalities** are from repolarization and **are presented in four stages** (Spodick 1982) (Figure 22.7): The first stage starts with a slight and extense ST segment elevation that is convex with respect to the isoelectric line, often accompanied by a PR segment elevation in aVR, with a mirror pattern of PR segment depression in the inferior and/or lateral wall (see Figure 9.20). Some days later (second stage), the ST segment returns to baseline, after which (third stage) the T wave becomes negative. Finally, a gradual return to normal in the ECG is observed (Figure 22.7). This four-step evolution is not commonly seen. Sometimes, the negative T wave is present from the beginning.

At other times, a fixed repolarization abnormality occurs, no negative T wave exists at all, or the repolarization abnormality is not diffuse or ST/T changes are more striking (perimyocarditis). In 15–20% of cases, different types of supraventricular arrhythmias, especially atrial fibrillation, may appear.

In acute pericarditis or during recurrences, as we have already commented, the presence of a PR segment shift (≥1 mm upward in aVR and downward in inferior leads) as an expression of atrial injury is frequently seen and sometimes it is the only indicator of the condition (see Figure 9.20).

As a summary from an electrocardiographic point of view, the diagnosis of idiopathic pericarditis is supported by the following data:

• **In the acute phase morphology and extension of ST segment elevation** (Figure 22.9A): In general terms, ST segment upward deviation in isolated pericarditis is mild (<2–3 mm), usually convex with respect to the isoelectric line, and quite diffuse. It must be remembered that in **myopericarditis**, the ST segment may have other morphologies (Figure 22.10).

• **Abnormalities of the PR segment**, typically upwardly deviated in aVR and downward in II, III, aVF, are quite common (see Figure 9.35). These abnormalities are also present in atrial infarctions, usually with evident Q waves and this is important for differential diagnosis (see Figure 9.33 and Chapter 20, Atrial infarction).

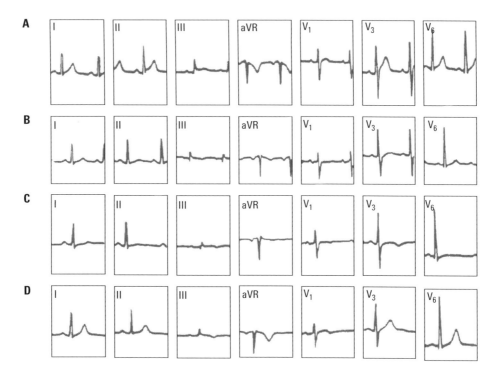

Figure 22.9 A 43-year-old male with acute pericarditis and the four ECG evolutive phases. The A, B, C, and D recordings were obtained at days 1, 8, 10, and 90. (A) The ST segment elevation convex respects the isoelectric line. (B) Flattening of the T wave. (C) Inversion of the T wave. (D) Normalization.

• **Evolution**: There is no Q wave and the image tends to disappear within a few days, with or without presence of a negative diffuse T wave (Figure 22.9), that may remain for a long time. This image demands a differential diagnosis with every other cause that may lead to a flat or negative T wave (see Table 13.4).

• **Associated myocarditis**: The changes in the ECG of patients with pericarditis partially depend on the presence of **associated myocarditis**, which could explain the more persistent and striking ST segment abnormalities: an ST segment that may be concave with respect to isoelectric line, a more negative T wave, and, in some cases, sinus tachycardia (Figure 22.10).

The ECG in other types of pericardial disease

In **constrictive pericarditis**, the ECG characteristically shows a diffuse and persistent repolarization disturbance that usually is not very striking and often shows abnormal P waves in the presence of atrial fibrillation (see Figure 13.17).

   In pericarditis with large pericardial effusion, diffuse repolarization abnormalities are often associated with low voltage in the QRS complex and T wave but not in the P wave. However, in cases of large peripheral edema of different etiologies, there is low voltage of QRS, T and also P wave (Madias 2008) (see heart failure).

   Sometimes, pericarditis may develop as a **post-operative complication of heart surgery.** ECG patterns of the QRS

complex may be confusing because of the associated disease, but the PR interval elevation in aVR (if present) and the morphology of the convex ST segment elevation with respect to the isoelectric line help determine the right diagnosis.

   The peri-MI pericarditis occurs in case of large MI. The ECG may present abnormalities of the PR segment. When the elevation of the ST segment persists after 48–76 hours in transmural Q wave infarctions without the T wave becoming negative, a **regional pericarditis**, which could be a prelude to **cardiac rupture,** must be suspected (Figure 22.11) (Reeder and Gersh 2000; lessons 13 and 20).

   The most specific sign of **pericardial tamponade** is the evidence of electric alternans of the QRS complex. In these cases, the study of pericardial effusion will assist in the diagnosis that unfortunately is not often due to idiopathic pericarditis (malignancy or rare infections) (Figure 22.12) (see Chapter 19).

Rheumatic fever

Rheumatic fever is a systemic inflammatory disease whose target organ is the heart. Therefore, it may develop in the acute stage, with significant joint involvement and, if untreated, carditis in 40% of cases that may cause tachycardia, heart failure, etc. Although rheumatic fever has

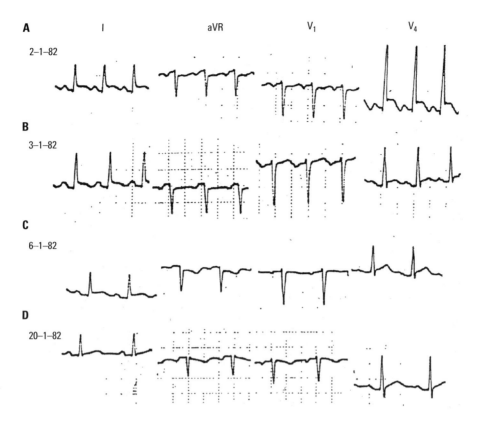

Figure 22.10 (A) A 54-year-old patient with precordial pain of pericardial characteristics. There is an ST elevation in some leads but without Q waves and with PR elevation in aVR and depression in II. The clinical history, the ECG, and the follow-up (B to D) with an ECG that shows a resolution of ST elevation without the appearance of a Q wave the diagnosis of pericarditis. The ST shift, however, is atypical (compare with Figures 19.4 and 22.9).

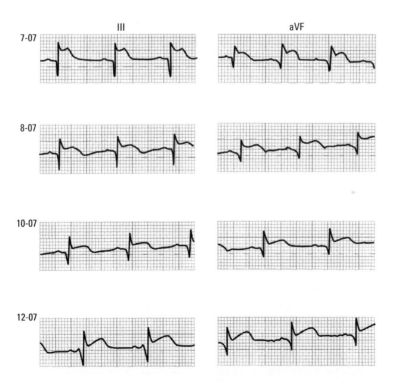

Figure 22.11 The ECG recordings (lead III and aVF) performed during one week of evolution of ST elevation myocardial infarction. ST segment elevation persists without the appearance of a negative T wave. This is a risk marker of cardiac rupture, which in fact occurred in this case.

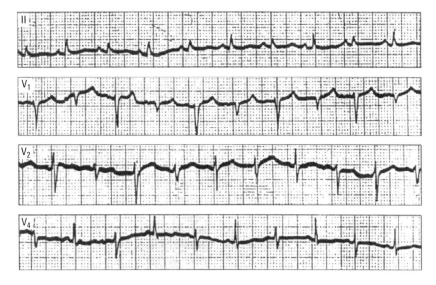

Figure 22.12 Typical morphology of electrical alternans in a patient with cardiac tamponade due to metastatic lung neoplasia.

been nearly eradicated in developed countries, its incidence still has an impact in developing countries as an etiological factor of valvular heart disease. Therefore, it is useful to recognize the ECG changes to diagnose this disease. The diagnosis of rheumatic fever requires the presence of two major, or one major and two minor, Jones criteria as well as evidence of previous streptococcal infection (Chávez Rivera 1986).

From an electrocardiographic standpoint, the most characteristic findings include: (i) **a prolonged PR interval**, which is a minor Jones criterion; (ii) **repolarization changes**, usually minor, which are observed in about 50% of cases; (iii) **more advanced degrees of AV block or bundle branch block and different types of arrhythmias**, which are not very common. These ECG abnormalities tend to disappear after the acute phase. If the disease has left valvular sequelae (**rheumatic heart disease**), they may cause different electrocardiographic changes over time (especially atrial and ventricular enlargement) (see valvular heart diseases).

Cor pulmonale

This section deals with: (i) **acute cor pulmonale** caused by pulmonary embolism or acute right-sided heart failure, usually with pre-existing cor pulmonale; (ii) **chronic cor pulmonale**, which tends to affect elderly people in particular and is often accompanied by emphysema; and (iii) cases of **primary pulmonary hypertension**, often in young and middle-aged people. Other types of pulmonary hypertension with right-chamber compromise seen in congenital and valvular diseases are described in different sections of this chapter and in Chapter 10.

Acute cor pulmonale (see Chapter 10)

Pulmonary embolism
Acute cor pulmonale caused by pulmonary embolism may present with a normal ECG in cases of mild embolism. However, this seldom occurs in the presence of a moderate/severe pulmonary embolism.

The most important diagnostic ECG signs, which tend to disappear if the condition improves and are not very sensitive but highly specific, are the following:
• McGinn–White sign (SI QIII generally with ST segment elevation with a negative TIII wave) (see Figure 10.15) (10% of cases);
• advanced RBBB, usually with upward ST segment deviation, which is seen in severe pulmonary embolism (see Figure 11.16) (15% of cases);
• significant ÂQRS rightward deviation (30% of cases);
• repolarization abnormalities (negative T wave) in the right precordial leads (40% of cases);
• commonly, sinus tachycardia (see Figure 10.16), except for certain patients, usually the elderly, with sinus node dysfunction; and
• a peaked P wave and clear signs of RVE.

Acute right-sided heart failure
This is triggered by respiratory infection or by a different process, usually in patients with pre-existing cor pulmonale. The ECG may show patterns similar to those observed in pulmonary embolism, particularly ÂQRS right deviation and a transient negative T wave in the right precordial leads (see Figure 10.14).

Chronic cor pulmonale
The term **chronic cor pulmonale** refers to the compromise of the right heart chambers caused by pulmonary hypertension secondary to diseases that primarily affect lung

function and/or structure, especially chronic obstructive pulmonary disease (COPD) caused by pulmonary emphysema or bronchitis. The diagnosis may be made when the pulmonary function test is abnormal (especially when a reduced forced expiratory volume in one second exists) and chest Rx findings of emphysematous hyperlucency are observed (Thomas *et al.* 2011).

The ECG may or may not show right ventricular enlargement, although the enlargement may exist but be undetectable by ECG (see Chapter 10). In fact, only 33% of patients with pulmonary hypertension secondary to chronic cor pulmonale present with an ECG that suggests right ventricular enlargement. Therefore, as previously mentioned in Chapter 10, the ECG is not very sensitive for detecting right ventricular enlargement.

ECG criteria that are more suggestive of chronic cor pulmonale include the following (see Chapter 10) (Spodick 1959; Zambrano *et al.* 1974):
• **Signs of right ventricular enlargement**, especially rightward-deviated ÂQRS and "rs," "qr," or a dominant R wave QRS complex morphology in V1, QRS V2/QRS V1 > 5 and/or with S ≥ R in V6 (see Figure 10.12).
• **ÂQRS to the right or with a SI, SII, SIII pattern** in the frontal plane (see Figure 10.13). It may be difficult to distinguish the morphologies from a normal variant using the ECG only (see Figure 10.13), although the abnormal changes of P and/or T wave may help.
• **The presence of the following signs suggesting right atrial enlargement**: AP deviated rightward, with a P wave that is flattened in lead I, peaked in II and III and quite often ± in V1, with a tall positive component > 1.5 mm.
• **Advanced RBBB** with special characteristics (a pure R wave with a slightly high voltage visible from V1 to V2–V3) (see Chapter 11).

• **ECG signs of pulmonary emphysema**: AP > 60° (SE = 62%; SP = 83%) (Thomas *et al.* 2011). Other ECG signs of emphysema are shortened QRS (< 75 mm) and low-voltage QRS.
• **Repolarization abnormalities**, especially in the inferior leads and/or right precordial leads (see Chapter 10).

Of all these ECG signs that suggest chronic cor pulmonale, those with **the worst prognosis are SI, SII, SIII** morphology and signs **of right atrial enlargement** (Chapter 9). The prognosis worsens if both signs are present, particularly if the alveoloarterial oxygen gradient (PAo$_2$–Pao$_2$) is above 48 mmHg with home oxygen therapy (Incalzi *et al.* 1999). The patients with chronic cor pulmonale whose ECG is normal or almost normal (> 50% of the total) have a better prognosis.

Primary pulmonary hypertension
Fortunately, this disease is rarely seen. It is a difficult disease to treat, although today there are new and promising agents available (prostaglandins and endothelin inhibitors).

The ECG typically shows a quite clear pattern of right ventricular enlargement, usually with R or R/S morphologies and negative T waves in the right precordial leads and sometimes till V5–V6. This pattern may be attenuated as the condition improves (Figure 22.13).

Congenital heart diseases

The imaging techniques are more effective than ECG for diagnosing congenital heart diseases. Nevertheless, certain ECG signs may be very suggestive of several congenital

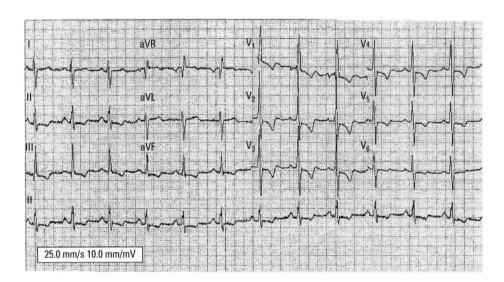

Figure 22.13 A 46-year-old man with primary pulmonary hypertension in a very advanced stage. The catheterization shows pulmonary hypertension of 100/60, with a mean of 75 mmHg. The ECG shows important signs of right ventricle enlargement similar to those found in Figure 22.15.

cardiac diseases. In front of diagnosis of abnormal ECG (morphological changes, arrhythmias), it is necessary to perform additional tests starting with the echocardiography.

Newborn ECG: suspected congenital heart disease

Some of the most interesting characteristics of the newborn ECG with respect to possible congenital heart disease are discussed in this section.

Many congenital heart diseases present with a normal ECG on the first day of life. Therefore, it is necessary to perform sequential ECGs to rule out congenital heart diseases.

The presence of negative P wave in lead I suggests **situs inversus** (right atrium to the left). However, a misplacement of electrodes and atrial ectopic arrhythmia has to be ruled out. **If there is a leftward-deviated ÂQRS (beyond +30°) in a newborn, congenital heart disease must be suspected.** Atrioventricular canal defects, tricuspid atresia, and single ventricle must be ruled out as possible causes of the deviation.

The association with an AV canal defect and/or corrected transposition of the great vessels should obviously be suspected in the presence of an AV block. **However, advanced congenital AV block usually appears as an isolated finding. Prognosis of the AV block and recommendations for the use of a definitive pacemaker will depend on the presence of an underlying cardiac disease and on heart rate characteristics (day and night mean, maximum and minimum, response to exercise, etc.) (see Figure** 17.15).

If a delta wave indicating Wolff–Parkinson–White-type pre-excitation is present, associated Ebstein's disease must be ruled out.

If the T wave is positive in V1 from the second day of life onward, right ventricular enlargement must be suspected.

The presence of a pure R wave in V1, usually < 15 mm, may be observed in newborns who are not affected by an underlying heart disease. A qR morphology in V1 is always suggestive of an underlying heart disease, except in post-term newborns (see Figure 7.39). In contrast, an rS morphology in V1 may be observed in premature newborns (see Figure 7.41).

The presence of a pathologic Q wave, especially in I and aVL, rules out right coronary artery of anomalous origin.

Atrial septal defect

The most characteristic ECG abnormalities of atrial septal defect are (see Figures 10.6 and 10.7):

• the presence of an rsR' morphology in V1, with a QRS complex < 0.12 sec;
• a lack of sinus arrhythmia in cases of large atrial septal defect;

• an extreme ÂQRS left deviation in the **ostium primum-type atrial septal defect** (see Figure 10.6);
• atrial fibrillation in adults.

Ventricular septal defect

The following are the most common ECG abnormalities in ventricular septal defect:

• a normal or almost normal ECG when **the ventricular septal defect is small**;
• signs of biventricular hypertrophy in **large ventricular septal defects with hyperkinetic pulmonary hypertension** with RSR' morphology in V1 and qRs in V6, and sometimes high voltages in intermediate leads (Katz and Watchell morphology) (Figure 22.14);
• a tall R wave in V1 if significant reactive pulmonary hypertension is found (**Eisenmenger syndrome**) (Figure 22.15).

Tricuspid atresia

The most common ECG abnormalities in tricuspid atresia include (Figure 22.16):

• extreme leftward ÂQRS deviation;
• P wave changes indicative of right atrial enlargement of the congenital type (slight leftward AP deviation);
• In rare cases, WPW-type pre-excitation.

Ebstein's disease

ECG abnormalities characteristic of Ebstein's disease include (Figures 22.17 and 11.10):

• P waves, usually high-voltage and sometimes markedly negative in V1. In Figure 22.17, the P wave in V1 (+/−) resembles a QRS complex with an rS morphology.
• Atypical RBBB morphology, often with an rsr', qR, or rsR's' morphology in V1–V3 and sometimes with a slight upward ST segment deviation in V1–V2;
• occasionally, a pathological Q wave;
• occasionally, WPW-type pre-excitation;
• commonly, a long PR interval;
• usually, paroxysmal supraventricular arrhythmias, especially after infancy.

Stenotic lesions

Right-sided stenotic lesions (isolated pulmonary valve stenosis and tetralogy of Fallot) and left-sided stenotic lesions (aortic stenosis and coarctation of the aorta) **may produce a morphology indicative of enlargement of the respective chambers; some of them are quite distinctive. Figures 10.8 and** 10.9 **show ECG differences between the pattern found in** pulmonary valve stenosis with intact ventricular septum **with strain pattern repolarization, named "barrier" systolic overload by the Mexican School (pure R wave from V1 to V2–V3 with "strain pattern"), and the image seen in** tetralogy of Fallot **(pure R wave in V1 with "strain pattern," rS morphology in V2 with positive ST/T known as "adaptative systolic overload"). In**

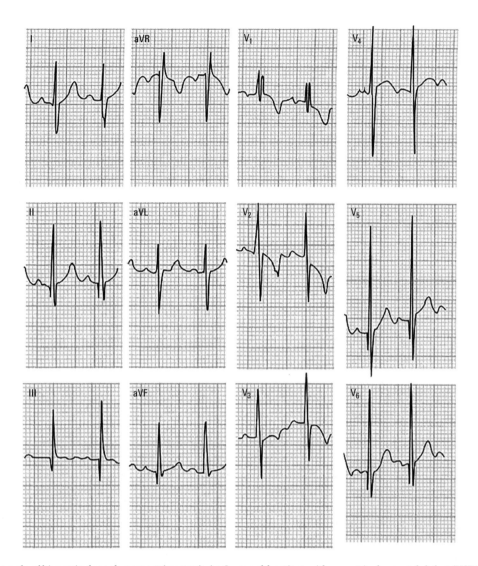

Figure 22.14 Example of biventricular enlargement (see text). An 8-year-old patient with a ventricular septal defect (VSD) and hyperkinetic pulmonary hypertension (Katz–Watchell pattern) (see text).

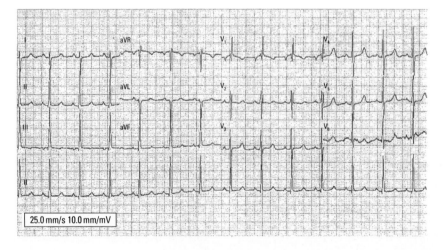

Figure 22.15 A 30-year-old woman with an ostium secundum-type atrial septal defect during the Eisenmenger phase. She was classified as NYHA class II–III and treated with bosentan and sildenafil. Right ventricle enlargement is very evident (QRS axis >90° and a unique R in V1 with RS morphology in V6). The P wave does not have very striking features.

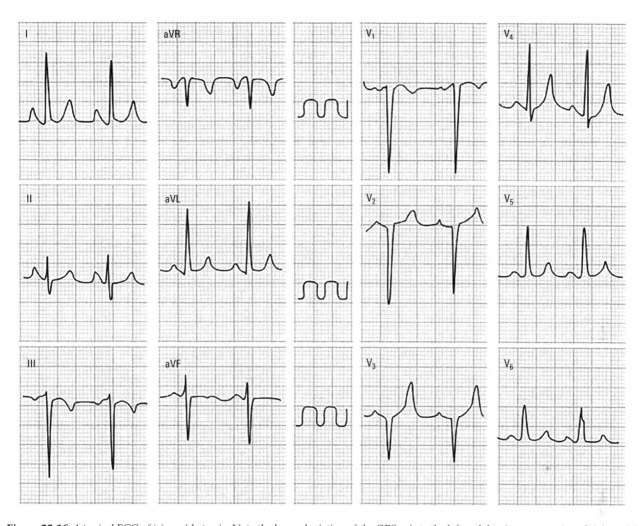

Figure 22.16 A typical ECG of tricuspid atresia. Note the hyperdeviation of the QRS axis to the left and the signs suggestive of right atrial and left ventricular enlargement.

children with moderate Fallot's tetralogy, an RS with a positive T wave may be seen (see Figure 10.10**). In newborns, right ventricular enlargement caused by severe pulmonary stenosis may be accompanied by a positive T wave.**

After reparative surgery is performed in cases **of tetralogy of Fallot** and other congenital heart diseases, advanced RBBB is often found and is usually due to a distal lesion of the specific conduction system caused by the surgery (see Figure 11.12). In such cases, the time from the beginning of ventricular depolarization to right ventricle apex (V-apex) activation is not prolonged (see Figure 11.9) (Sung *et al*. 1976). The opposite holds true in cases of proximal block, typically RBBBs occurring during acute infarction (Mayorga-Cortés *et al*. 1979) (see Chapters 10 and 11). After surgery for tetralogy of Fallot, ventricular arrhythmias may appear and rarely SD may occur (see later).

Aortic stenosis, even when severe, does not usually present with an image of left ventricular enlargement during the first years of disease, although it tends to progress to an image of left ventricular enlargement with strain pattern (see Figure 10.26A). The same can be said of **coarctation of the aorta.**

Mirror image dextrocardia

The arrangement of the cardiac chambers in mirror image dextrocardia is shown in Figure 22.18, as well as the changes produced in the frontal plane by the reorientation of the P wave, QRS complex, and T wave axes (A: normal; B: mirror image dextrocardia). Therefore, the ECG appearance resembles that seen when the arm leads are inverted and the precordial leads are located on the right side. This accounts for the negative P wave in lead I and the dwindling voltage of the precordial leads. In Chapter 6, all possible causes of negative P waves in lead I are discussed.

• Arrhythmias in congenital heart disease

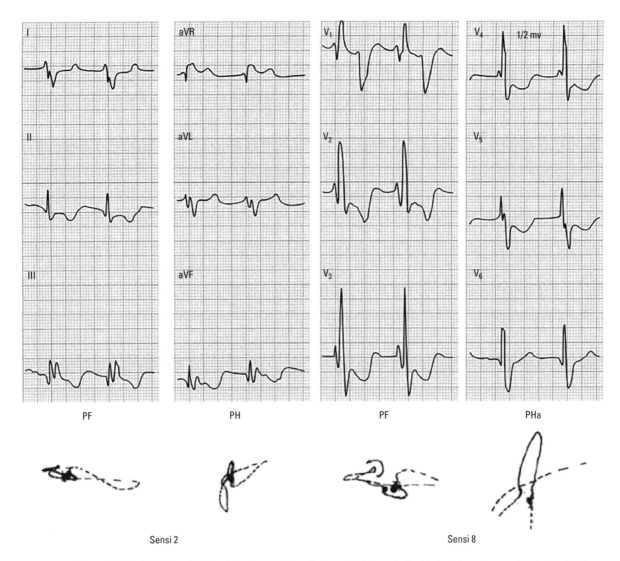

Figure 22.17 ECG and VCG of a child with Ebstein's disease. Note the long PR interval, the high-voltage P wave hidden in the T wave (+−, mimicking the rS in V1) and the atypical right bundle branch block morphology. FP: Frontal plane; HP: horizontal plane.

All the aspects related with this topic are discussed before (congenital heart diseases), in Chapter 23 (arrhythmias in children), and Chapter 24 (advanced congenital AV block).

Arterial hypertension

Effect of arterial hypertension on the heart

High blood pressure affects the heart via direct and indirect mechanisms (Bayés-Genís *et al.* 1995) (Figure 22.19). On the one hand, it causes left ventricular enlargement, which leads to hypertensive heart disease, and on the other hand, it is one of the most important risk factors in coronary artery atherosclerosis. Both mechanisms cause electrical instability (arrhythmias), ventricular dysfunction (heart failure), and myocardial ischemia (coronary heart disease).

The Framingham Study has clearly proven that high blood pressure is one of the most important risk factors in coronary heart disease, especially when it is associated with other risk factors (Figure 22.19) (Kannel 1976). Hypertensive patients are more frequently affected by ischemic heart disease than the general population, and there is also a greater occurrence of heart failure, atrial and ventricular arrhythmia, and sudden death (Levy *et al.* 1987, 1994). This is related to the fact that there are two mechanisms involved, as previously mentioned. Therefore, **the ECG in patients with high blood pressure** may reflect signs of both left ventricular enlargement and ischemic heart disease (Bayés-Genís *et al.* 1995).

ECG changes: clinical implications and prognosis

The ECG changes of LVH are secondary to changes in depolarization (reduced conduction delay) and repolarization

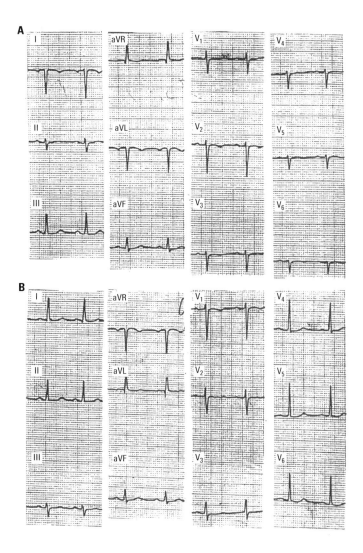

Figure 22.18 (A) Characteristic ECG of a patient presenting with mirror image dextrocardia as the sole heart abnormality. (B) When electrode positions are inverted, the ECG is recorded as normal.

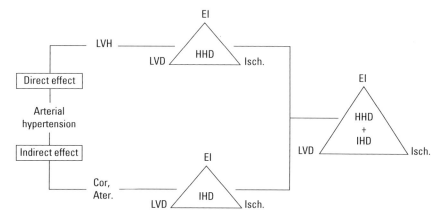

Figure 22.19 Direct and indirect effects of hypertension related to left ventricular hypertrophy (LVH) and coronary artery involvement. Cor ater: coronary atherosclerosis; EI: electrical instability; HHD: hypertensive heart disease; IHD: ischemic heart disease; Isch: ischemia; LVD: left ventricular dysfunction (Bayés-Genís *et al.* 1995).

(primary increase of AP duration). The contribution of both processes in the typical ECG pattern of LVH (strain pattern) has been recently studied in an experimental model (Bacharova *et al.* 2010). Often, influences in the ECG pattern other primary factors (ischemia, drugs) (see Chapter 10, repolarization changes).

ECG criteria for left ventricular enlargement in hypertensive patients shows also low sensitive as the general criteria for left ventricular enlargement discussed in Chapter 10 (see Table 10.4) (Levy *et al.* 1990).

The ECG criteria for left ventricular enlargement more commonly used in hypertension are shown in Table 22.1. Those with a higher sensitivity (≥80%) are: RV6/RV5 >0.65 and a QRS complex total voltage in 12 leads >120 mm (Rodriguez Padial 1991). However, these two criteria have low specificity, especially the first (21%). Most of the other criteria shown in this table, however, are highly specific (≥90%). The sensitivity of other ECG criteria may improve slightly when associated with other variables (sex, age, etc.) (Sheridan 1998) (see Chapter 10).

The sensitivity of ECG criteria for the diagnosis of left ventricular enlargement depends on whether the possibility of presenting with anatomical left ventricular hypertrophy in the group studied is high or not (Bayes' theorem) (Selzer 1981). Table 10.6 shows that in a group of 1000 patients with severe hypertension, of whom 90% have anatomical left ventricular enlargement, the patients with ECG signs of left ventricular enlargement have a high possibility of exhibiting hypertrophy from an anatomical point of view (720/740 = 97%). However, in a group of 1000 asymptomatic adults in whom only 1% present with anatomical left ventricular enlargement, the possibility of anatomical hypertrophy in patients with ECG signs of left ventricular enlargement is very low (8/206 = 4%).

Therefore, the utility of the ECG for diagnosing left ventricular enlargement is high for patients with severe hypertension and low for the general population.

ECG changes caused by left ventricular enlargement usually **correlate highly with the severity of hypertension** and its evolution. With treatment, these changes can be normalized or attenuated (Figure 22.20).

Quite often, an associated primary factor (medications, ischemia, etc.) that modifies repolarization and produces a mixed image similar to the one observed in ventricular enlargement of aortic valve disease is found (see Figure 10.26D). This repolarization abnormality may be transient. It is more likely to appear in coronary hypertensive patients with IHD, and its extent varies according to changes in heart rate and blood pressure. Different studies, both with experimental models and clinical trials, have shown a QTc interval prolongation in left ventricular hypertrophy (Baillard *et al.* 2000; Oikarinen *et al.* 2001).

There is no doubt that echocardiography and MR are the gold standard for diagnosing left ventricular enlargement **because of its high sensitivity and specificity, making it comparable to studies using anatomical correlation and also provides good information about LV function, and many others morphological aspects (valves, aorta, etc.).**

However, the ECG has a higher prognostic value than echocardiography; if a hypertensive patient exhibits clear signs of left ventricular enlargement, it indicates a high risk of developing cardiovascular complications (Levy *et al.* 1994). Physicians must always perform an ECG on hypertensive patients although may be also important to have an Echo image to study especially because is easy to perform and is not expensive.

Regarding the **association of arrhythmias and sudden death risk** in hypertensive patients, it is important to note the following:

• It has been demonstrated (Holter monitoring) that hypertensive patients, especially if exhibiting left ventricular enlargement, are more likely to present with arrhythmias, particularly atrial fibrillation and ventricular arrhythmias (generally, premature ventricular complexes and non-sustained ventricular tachycardia).

• Sudden death is more common in this group than in the general population. High blood pressure is a marker of sudden death, according to the Framingham Study (Figure 22.21).

• It has been proven that both the presence of left ventricular enlargement and asymptomatic ST segment depression

Table 22.1 Comparison of different ECG criteria for the diagnosis of left ventricular hypertrophy in systemic hypertension

ECG criteria	Sensitivity (%)	Specificity (%)
R wave in aVL >11 mm	11	93
Sokolow–Lyon voltage criteria (RV5 – 6 + SV1 > 35 mm)	22	100
Romhilt-Estes > 5 points	33	94
Cornell voltage criteria (RVL + SV3 >28 mm in males or 20 mm in females)	54	85
Cornell product. Cornell voltage criteria × QRS complex duration >2400 mm/m²	51	95
RV6/RV5 >0.65	89	21
Total QRS complex >120 mm	80	54

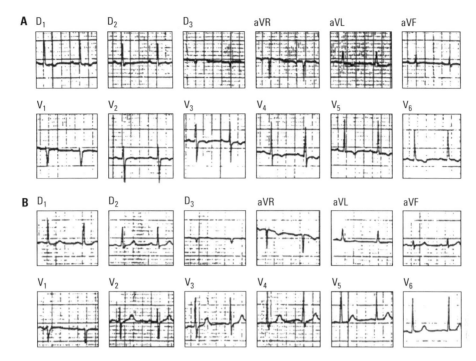

Figure 22.20 A 56-year-old male with hypertensive heart disease before treatment (A) and seven months later (B). Note the disappearance of the repolarization abnormalities of left ventricular enlargement.

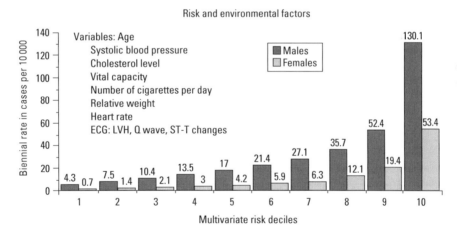

Figure 22.21 Risk of sudden death in the Framingham Study, according to multivariate risk (see inner note) in males and females (Kannel and McGee 1985).

(silent ischemia) detected using Holter monitoring are independent markers of poor prognosis in hypertensive patients. As previously mentioned, ECG has a low sensitivity for the diagnosis of left ventricular enlargement, especially when compared with echocardiography; however, the former is more effective from a prognostic point of view.

• The incidence of associated LVH by necropsic studies in cases of sudden death is higher in Mediterranean than in Anglosaxon countries (Subirana *et al*. 2011).

• In many cases, drugs that are being administered for hypertension therapy may decrease the left ventricular mass and improve the ECG (Figure 22.20). The drugs with a more favorable profile are angiotensin-converting enzyme (ACE) inhibitors, beta blockers, angiotensin II receptor blockers (AII), calcium channel blockers, and diuretics. Choosing one over the other as a first-line treatment depends on the associated heart disease. All of them may decrease the sequelae caused by high blood pressure, but none have been shown to decrease sudden death rates.

References

Bacharova L, Szathmany R, Mateasik A. Secondary and primary repolarization changes in LVH: a model study. *J Electrocardiol* 2010;43:628.

Baillard C, Mansier P, Ennezat PV, *et al.* Converting enzyme inhibition normalizes QT interval in spontaneously hypertensive rats. *Hypertension* 2000;36:350.

Baldasseroni S, De Biase L, Fresco C, *et al.* Cumulative effect of complete left bundle-branch block and chronic atrial fibrillation on 1-year mortality and hospitalization in patients with congestive heart failure. A report from the Italian network on congestive heart failure (in-CHF database). *Eur Heart J* 2002;23:1692.

Bayés de Luna A, Serra-Genís C, Guix M, *et al.* Septal fibrosis as determinant of Q waves in patients with aortic valve disease. *Eur Heart J* 1983;4(Suppl E):86.

Bayés de Luna A, Cladellas M, Oter R, et al. Interatrial conduction block with retrograde activation of the left atrium and paroxysmal supraventricular tachyarrhythmic treatment. *Int J Cardiol* 1989;22:147–150.

Bayés-Genís A, Guindo J, Viñolas X, *et al.* Cardiac arrhythmias and left ventricular hypertrophy in systemic hypertension and their influences on prognosis. *Am J Cardiol* 1995;76:54D.

Bayés-Genís A, López L, Viñolas X, *et al.* Distinct left bundle branch block pattern in ischemic and non-ischemic dilated cardiomyopathy. *Eur J Heart Fail* 2003;5:165.

Bloomfield DM, Steinman RC, Namerow PB, *et al.* Microvolt T-wave alternans distinguishes between patients likely and patients not likely to benefit from implanted cardiac defibrillator therapy: a solution to the Multicenter Automatic Defibrillator Implantation Trial (MADIT) II conundrum. *Circulation* 2004;110:1885.

Cabrera E, Mouroy J. Systolic and diastolic loading of the heart. *Am Hearet J* 1952;43:669.

Cazeau S, Ritter P, Bakdach S, *et al.* Four chamber pacing in dilated cardiomyopathy. *Pacing Clin Electrophysiol* 1994;17:1974.

Chávez Rivera I. Fiebre reumática. In Bayés de Luna A, Soler Soler J (eds). *Cardiología*. Ediciones Doyma S.A, 1986, pp. 507–512.

Cygankiewicz I, Zareba W, Vazquez R, *et al.* Relation of heart rate turbulence to severity of heart failure. *Am J Cardiol* 2006;98:1635.

Cygankiewicz I, Zareba W, Vazquez R, *et al.* Prognostic value of QT/RR slope in predicting mortality in patients with congestive heart failure. *J Cardiovasc Electrophysiol* 2008;19:1066.

Das MK, Cheriparambil K, Bedi A, *et al.* Prolonged QRS duration (QRS >/=170 ms) and left axis deviation in the presence of left bundle branch block: a marker of poor left ventricular systolic function? *Am Heart J* 2001;142:756.

Escobar-Robledo LA, Bayés-de-Luna A, Lupón J, *et al.* Advanced interatrial block predicts new-onset atrial fibrillation and ischemic stroke in patients with heart failure: the "Bayes' Syndrome-HF" study. *Int J Cardiol* 2018;271:174.

Hoigne P, Attenhofer Jost C, Duru F, *et al.* Simple criteria for differentiation of Fabry disease from amyloid disease and other causes of left ventricular hypertropy. *Int J Cardiol* 2006;111:413.

Ikeda H, Maki S, Yoshida N. *et al.* Predictors of death from congestive heart failure in hypertrophic cardiomyopathy. *Am J Cardiol* 1999;83:1280.

Incalzi RA, Fuso L, De Rosa M, *et al.* Electrocardiographic signs of chronic cor pulmonale: a negative prognostic finding in chronic obstructive pulmonary disease. *Circulation* 1999;99:1600.

Kannel WB. Some lessons in cardiovascular epidemiology from Framingham. *Am J Cardiol* 1976;37:269.

Kannel WB, McGee DL. Epidemiology of sudden death: insights from the Framingham study. *Cardiovasc Clin* 1985;15:93.

Klatsky AL, Oehm R, Cooper RA, Udaltsova N, Armstrong MA. The early repolarization normal variant electrocardiogram: correlates and consequences. *Am J Med* 2003;115:171.

Kooistra NHM, van Mourik MS, Rodríguez-Olivares R, *et al.* Late onset of new conduction disturbances requiring permanent pacemaker implantation following TAVI. *Heart* 2020; 106:1244.

Levy D, Anderson KM, Savage DD, *et al.* Risk of ventricular arrhythmias in left ventricular hypertrophy: the Framingham heart study. *Am J Cardiol* 1987;60:560.

Levy D, Labib SB, Anderson KM., *et al.* Determinants of sensitivity and specificity of electrocardiographic criteria for left ventricular hypertrophy. *Circulation* 1990;81:815.

Levy D, Salomon M, D'Agostino RB, Belanger AJ, Kannel WB. Prognostic implications of baseline electrocardiographic features and their serial changes in subjects with left ventricular hypertrophy. *Circulation* 1994;90:1786.

Luu M, Stevenson WG, Stevenson LW, Baron K, Walden J. Diverse mechanisms of unexpected cardiac arrest in advanced heart failure. *Circulation* 1989;80(6):1675–1680.

Madias J. The importance of P waves in the differentiation of alternation of the QRS voltage due to pericardial effusion versus to peripheral edema. *J Cardiac Failure* 2008;14:55.

Madias JE, Bazaz R, Agarwal H, *et al.* Anasarca-mediated attenuation of the amlitude of electrocardiogram complexes: a description of a heretofore unrecognized phenomenon. *J Am Coll Cardiol* 2001;38:756.

Martí V, Ballester M, Oter R, Obrador D, Bayés de Luna A. Recovery of sinus node function after pacemaker implant for sinus node disease following cardiac transplantation. *Pacing Clin Electrophysiol* 1991;14:1205.

Martinez-Selles M, Bramlage P, Thoenes M, *et al.* Clinical significance of conduction disturbances after aortic valve intervention: current evidence. *Clin Res Cardiol* 2015;104:1–12.

Mayorga-Cortés A, Rozanski JJ, Sung RJ, Castellanos A, Myerburg RJ. Right ventricular apical activation times in patients with conduction disturbances occurring during acute transmural myocardial infarction. *Am J Cardiol* 1979;43:913.

Mendoza I, Acquatella H. Miocarditis y miocardiopatías. In Bayés de Luna A, López-Sendón JL, Attie F, Alegría Ezquerra E (eds). *Cardiología clínica*. Masson S.A, 2003, pp. 561–580.

Milei J, Mautner B, Storino R, *et al.* Does Chagas' disease exist as an undiagnosed form of cardiomyopathy in the United States?. *Am Heart J* 1992;123:1732.

Mirowski M, Reid PR, Mower MM *et al.* Termination of malignant ventricular arrhythmias with an implantable automatic defibrillator in human beings. *N Engl J Med* 1980;303:322.

Moss AJ. MADIT-II and implications for noninvasive electrophysiologic testing. *Ann Noninvasive Electrocardiol* 2002;8:179.

Moss AJ, Hall WJ, Cannom DS *et al.* Multicenter automatic defibrillator implantation trial investigators. Improved survival with an implanted defibrillator in patients with coronary disease at high risk for ventricular arrhythmia. *N Engl J Med* 1996;335:1933.

Moss AJ, Hall WJ, Cannom DS *et al.* Cardiac resynchronization therapy for the prevention of heart failure events. *N Engl J Med* 2009;361:1329.

Oikarinen L, Nieminen MS, Viitasalo M, *et al*. Relation of QT interval and QT dispersion to echocardiographic left ventricular hypertrophy and geometric pattern in hypertensive patients. The LIFE study. The Losartan Intervention for Endpoint Reduction. *J Hypertens* 2001;19:1883.

Pascual-Figal DA, Ordoñez-Llanos J, Tornel PL, *et al*. Soluble ST2 for predicting sudden cardiac death in patients with chronic heart failure and left ventricular systolic dysfunction. *J Am Coll Cardiol* 2009;54:2174.

Reeder GS, Gersh BJ. Modern management of acute myocardial infarction. *Curr Probl Cardiol* 2000;25:677.

Remme WJ, Swedberg K. Guidelines for the diagnosis and treatment of chronic heart failure. *Eur Heart J* 2001;22:1527.

Rodriguez Padial L. Usefulness of total 12-lead QRS voltage for determining the presence of left ventricular hypertrophy in systemic hypertension. *Am J Cardiol* 1991;68:261.

Selzer A. The Bayes theorem and clinical electrocardiography. *Am Heart J* 1981;101:360.

Sheridan DJ. *Left Ventricular Hypertrophy*. Churchill Livingstone, 1998.

Spodick DH. Electrocardiographic studies in pulmonary disease. II. Establishment of criteria for the electrocardiographic inference of diffuse lung diseases. *Circulation* 1959;20:1073.

Spodick DH. Acute pericarditis: ECG changes. *Primary Cardiol* 1982;8:78.

Subirana MT, Juan-Babot J, Puig T, *et al*. Specific characteristics of sudden death in a mediterranean Spanish populaiton. *Am J Cardiol* 2011;107:622.

Sung RJ, Tamer DM, García OL, *et al*. Analysis of surgically-induced right bundle branch block pattern using intracardiac recording techniques. *Circulation* 1976;54:442.

Thomas AJ, Apiyasawat S, Spodick DH. Electrocardiographic detection of emphysema. *Am J Cardiol* 2011;107:1090.

Tsuchihashi K, Ueshima K, Uchida T, *et al*. Transient left ventricular apical ballooning without coronary artery stenosis: a novel heart syndrome mimicking acute myocardial infarction. Angina Pectoris-Myocardial Infarction Investigations in Japan. *J Am Coll Cardiol* 2001;38:11.

Van Bommel R, Marsan N, Delgado V, *et al*. Value of the surface ECG in detecting right ventricular dilatation in the presence of left bundle branch block. *Am J Cardiol* 2011;107:736.

Varela-Román A, González-Juanatey JR, Basante P, *et al*. Clinical characteristics and prognosis of hospitalised inpatients with heart failure and preserved or reduced left ventricular ejection fraction. *Heart* 2002;88:249.

Vazquez R, Bayes-Genis A, Cygankiewicz I, *et al*. The MUSIC risk score: a simple method for predicting moratlity in 100 ambulatory patients with chronic heart failure. *Eur Heart J* 2009;30:1088.

Verrier RL, Klingenhebern T, Malik M, *et al*. Microvolt T-wave alternans physiological basis, methods of measurement, and clinical utility–concensus guideline by International Society for Holter and Noninvasive Electroscardiology. *J Am Coll Cardiol* 2011;58:1309.

Vicent L, Fernandez-Yañez, Mateos R, *et al*. Apical ventricular hypertrophy in the transplanted heart: a 20-year single-center experience. *Rev Esp Cardiol (Engl Ed)* 2020. Doi: https://doi.org/10.1016/j.rec2020.06.029. Online ahead of print.

Wilcox J, Rosenberg J, Vallakati A, *et al*. Usefulness of ECG-QT interval to predict left ventricular diastolic dysfunction. *Am J Cardiol* 2011;108:1760.

Zambrano SS, Moussavi MS, Spodick DH. QRS duration in chronic obstructive lung disease. *J Electrocardiol* 1974;7:35.

Chapter 23
The ECG in Other Diseases and Different Situations

This chapter will review the different ECG characteristics in non-cardiac processes and other situations, which are sometimes striking.

Cerebrovascular accidents

Cerebrovascular accidents, and particularly **subarachnoid hemorrhage,** frequently show general repolarization abnormalities of the T wave, which can be highly negative or highly positive but are generally wide, and with long QT and mirror patterns in frontal plane leads (Figure 23.1). Even transient evident ST segment elevation with or without a negative T wave, very similar to an acute coronary syndrome, can be observed (Figure 23.2).

Endocrine diseases

Due to the presence of myocardial and infiltration in **myxedema,** the following ECG signs can be found: low QRS complex voltage, bradycardia, and flattening or even inversion of the T wave (Figure 23.3). In **hyperthyroidism,** in addition to sinus tachycardia, the presence of supraventricular arrhythmias, particularly atrial fibrillation, is frequent.

In the case of decompensated **diabetes** (ketoacidosis), repolarization abnormalities can often be observed, including even an ST segment elevation in the absence of a known clinical heart disease (Figure 23.4) (Chiariello *et al.* 1985). Furthermore, the ECG, if there is associated ischemic heart disease, shows more alterations in cases of type II diabetes than in non-diabetic patients. It has been proven that diabetic patients have the same risk of cardiovascular complications as patients who have suffered a myocardial infarction. Consequently, risk factors (hypertension, high cholesterol levels, smoking, etc.) should be more intensively treated in these cases. (Hypertension in Diabetes Study (HDS): II 1993).

Respiratory diseases

Numerous lung diseases may cause involvement of the right chambers both: (i) in the acute setting, acute cor pulmonale due to pulmonary embolism (see Figures 10.15 and 10.16) or acute decompensation of chronic obstructive pulmonary disease (COPD) (see Figure 10.14); and (ii) in the chronic phase, emphysema and chronic cor pulmonale (see Figure 10.12). The usefulness of the ECG in the diagnosis and prognosis of acute and chronic cor pulmonale, and **primary pulmonary hypertension** (see Figure 22.13), has been discussed in Chapter 22.

With regard to lung diseases that do not directly involve the right chambers, the ECG can be altered in the presence of a **pneumothorax,** particularly if it occurs on the left side. The alterations observed are probably a result of the interpositioning of air and displacement of the heart, together with a sudden increase in intrathoracic pressure. In the case of a left pneumothorax, an ÂQRS deviated to the right is usually observed, as well as a reduction in the QRS complex voltage which, in some cases, causes morphologies with a decreasing reduction in the R wave voltage in the precordial leads, which may mimic an anterior infarction. Confusion with ischemic heart disease may also be caused by the occasional presence of symmetric negative T waves in the precordial leads. A PR interval elevation has also been described and, rarely, a sometimes striking ST segment elevation in leads II, III, and aVF, with a reciprocal descent in leads I, aVL, and aVR, which may mimic an acute coronary syndrome (Figure 23.5).

ST segment upward deviation is probably caused by hypoperfusion and/or coronary spasm, and is shown in leads II, III, and aVF because the cardiac inferior wall of the LV is in contact with the collapsed lung. PR segment elevation might be seen due to atrial injury (Strizik and Forman 1999; Monterrubio Villar *et al.* 2000). In general, all these alterations are temporary and disappear when the condition is resolved.

Clinical Electrocardiography: A Textbook, Fifth Edition. Antoni Bayés de Luna, Miquel Fiol-Sala, Antoni Bayés-Genís, and Adrián Baranchuk.
© 2022 John Wiley & Sons Ltd. Published 2022 by John Wiley & Sons Ltd.

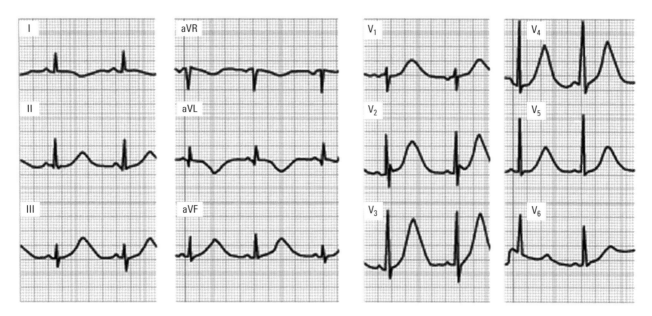

Figure 23.1 A 30-year-old patient with subarachnoid hemorrhage. The ECG shows quite significant repolarization changes, with a very long QT interval mainly at the expense of a very wide T wave, positive in some leads (precordial and inferior leads) and negative in others (I, aVL).

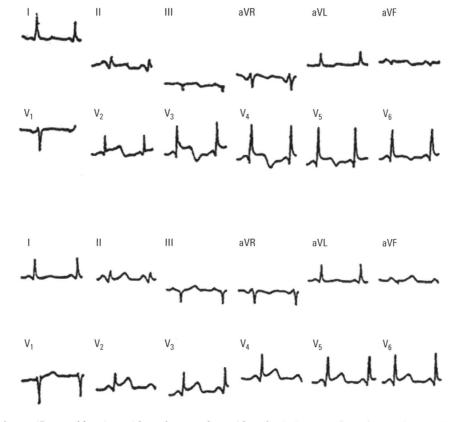

Figure 23.2 ECG from a 65-year-old patient with cerebrovascular accident that in its acute phase shows subepicardial injury morphology of the type observed in the acute phase of an acute coronary syndrome with ST segment elevation, or in some cases of perimyocarditis. Enzymes were negative, the patient never complained of chest pain, and the ECG returned to normal (B) on the following day, coinciding with the improvement of the clinical picture.

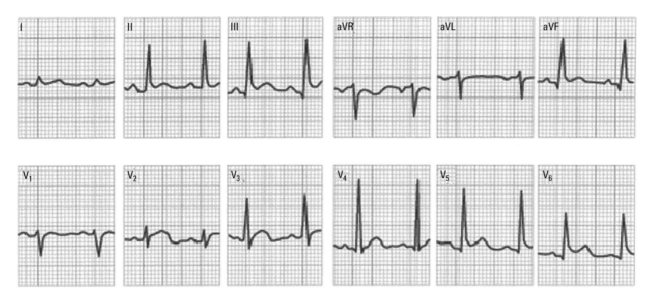

Figure 23.3 ECG from a 60-year-old patient with myxedema presenting with the typical abnormalities found in this process: slow baseline rhythm, generalized low voltage, and diffuse repolarization changes.

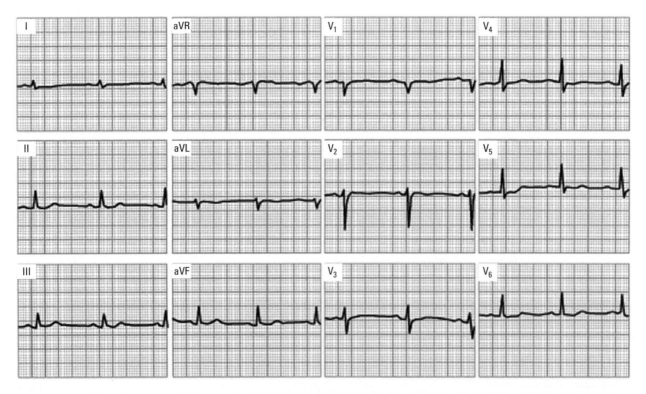

Figure 23.4 A 24-year-old patient with decompensated diabetes and asymptomatic ketoacidosis with an ECG tracing showing an ST segment elevation, particularly visible in precordial leads and II, III, aVF. This pattern disappeared when the decompensation was resolved a few days later.

Other diseases (see Chapter 22)

There are many other pathological processes in which the ECG shows alterations that may go from slight repolarization changes to patterns of evident chamber enlargement, bundle branch block, or even patterns suggesting myocardial ischemia or necrosis, as well as different active or passive arrhythmias. A description of the most characteristic findings occasionally observed during some of these conditions is discussed in the following paragraphs (see references p. XI).

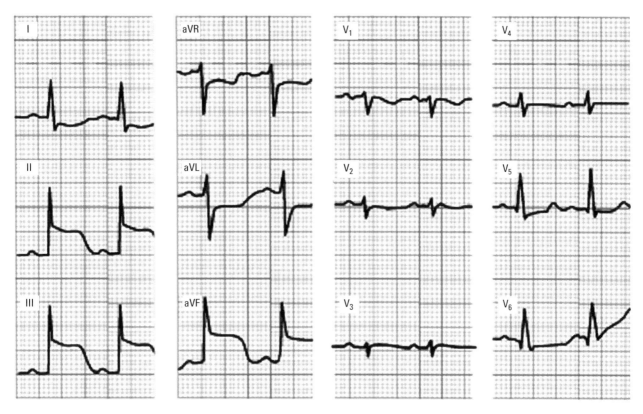

Figure 23.5 Striking elevation of the ST segment in leads II, III, and aVF with a mirror image in I, aVL, and aVR, and low voltage in the precordial leads in a patient with a left pneumothorax. Following evacuation of the pneumothorax, the ECG was almost normalized.

Infectious diseases

It has already been mentioned, when discussing myocarditis (Chapter 22), that infectious diseases of viral origin or having other etiologies may occasionally cause alterations in the ECG, in particular in repolarization, which are generally not very evident, and transient, and of no clinical significance. In the presence of septic shock, the alterations can be much more striking and may even cause malignant ventricular arrhythmias.

Hepatic cirrhosis

Often, a generalized low voltage with sometimes flat or slightly negative T waves is found in association with hepatic cirrhosis.

Anemia

In anemia, there is often sinus tachycardia and occasional repolarization changes, usually slight and in the form of a flat or somewhat negative T wave, as well as a usually slight ST segment depression (see Chapter 20).

Pheochromocytoma

Hypertensive crises, may be frequent, but not occur in more than 50% of cases of pheochromocytoma. Patients frequently exhibit symptoms such as headaches, palpitations, sweating, etc., but at least 10% of the crises are completely asymptomatic. The ECG is abnormal in almost 75% of the cases. Different active arrhythmias may appear as a result of the increase in the concentration of catecholamines, ranging from sinus tachycardia to supraventricular and ventricular tachyarrhythmias, and sometimes also a shortening of the PR interval. Also, left ventricular enlargement can be observed, as well as left bundle branch block, repolarization abnormalities, and Q waves compatible with necrosis, particularly in cases with myocarditis or dilated cardiomyopathy. Some of these findings are reversible, at least partially, once the process is resolved.

Systemic diseases (especially amyloidosis, sarcoidosis, and hemochromatosis)

All of these systemic diseases may cause a more or less significant ventricular myocardial involvement, which can result in a cardiomyopathy and/or involvement of the specific conduction system. As a result, the ECG may show pattern of: (i) atrial and/or ventricular enlargement; (ii) different types of atrioventricular (AV) or bundle branch block, (iii) alterations of repolarization and (iv) necrosis Q waves. These patients may also sometimes exhibit serious ventricular arrhythmias (sustained ventricular tachycardia) (see Chapter 22, restrictive CM).

Neuromuscular diseases

The ECG in neuromuscular diseases is often pathological and presents with P wave, QRS complex, and/or ST/T changes, as well as a series of different arrhythmias. **In Duchenne's progressive** muscular dystrophy, the ECG is almost always abnormal. The occurrence of patterns suggesting ventricular enlargement, particularly right ventricular enlargement, and/or a usually partial right bundle branch block (RBBB), is frequent (Figure 23.6). In **Steinert's disease** (myotonic muscular dystrophy), the most frequently found changes are signs of chamber enlargement, repolarization abnormalities, conduction disorders, pathologic Q waves, and arrhythmias, especially atrial fibrillation (Figure 23.7). In **Friedreich's ataxia,** there are usually necrosis Q waves and diffuse negative T waves.

Rheumatic diseases

Most rheumatic diseases with systemic involvement, particularly rheumatoid arthritis, sclerodermia and lupus erythematosus, present ECG pattern related to coronary heart disease, pericardial and/or myocardial involvement, as well as different types of arrhythmias, more frequently than in a healthy population.

Kidney diseases

The most striking ECG alterations in kidney disease are a consequence of the **hypertension** that usually affects these

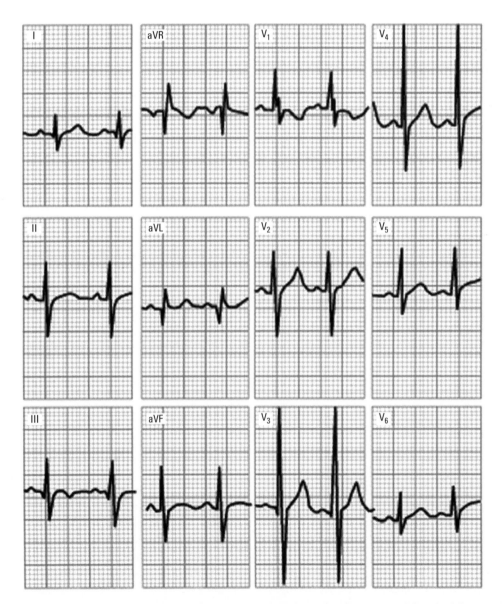

Figure 23.6 A 15-year-old patient with Duchenne disease. Note the SI, SII, SIII morphology, Rs in V1 with negative T wave, and RS morphology in V6 with positive T wave. All of this is the result of myocardial involvement with an ECG morphology showing mainly right ventricular enlargement.

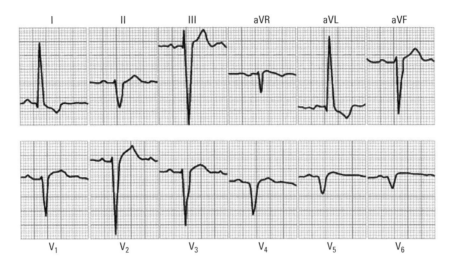

Figure 23.7 A 27-year-old patient with Steinert disease. This ECG displays pathological characteristics and evident signs of significant left ventricular enlargement (R in aVL ≥ 25 mm), diffuse left intraventricular conduction disorder (QRS ≥ 0.12 sec), but with an evident involvement of the superoanterior division area (ÂQRS −50°) and QS morphology in left precordial leads.

patients. In addition, due to chronic renal failure, other ECG anomalies can be observed, usually as a result of associated ionic abnormalities (**hyperkalemia**) (see below).

Psychiatric diseases

Various psychiatric diseases, including anorexia nervosa (Vázquez *et al.*, 2003), are accompanied by **ECG alterations either related or not to ionic alterations**. These include sinus bradycardia, a long QT interval, arrhythmias, and even sudden death.

Athletes (Figures 23.8–23.11) (Corrado *et al.* 2010); Uberoi *et al.* 2011)

We have already remarked (Chapters 7 and 9) the QRS–ST–T changes that may be found in athletes, and especially how to perform the differential diagnosis of ECG pattern with rSr' and/or ST elevation in V1–V2 found relatively often in athletes, with variants of normality such as thoracic malformation, especially pectus excavatum, and with Brugada pattern, especially type II (see Figure 7.16).

Now, we will comment on the global ECG changes that may be found in athletes in surface ECG, divided into:
i. frequent ECG findings that may be training related and
ii. uncommon ECG findings that are not training related.

Surface ECG morphology changes

Training-related ECG findings
The morphology of ECG in athletes very frequently shows **findings that may be training related** and require no additional evaluation, such as:
• sinus bradycardia;

• first-degree AV block, or even Wenckebach-type second-degree AV block during rest (see below);
• partial RBBB pattern (see Figures 7.14 and 23.9);
• high voltage of R wave in precordial leads in the absence of other criteria for left ventricular hypertrophy;
• isolated premature ventricular complexes (PVCs) (see below);
• early repolarization (ER) pattern. In this case, we have to remember that this pattern has been recently associated with sudden death (Haïssaguerre *et al.* 2008) although this is exceptional in the benign type of ER usually found in athletes (see Chapter 24, Early repolarization pattern). A crista supraventricularis pattern is also common (Martinez-Sellés *et al.* 2020).

Non-training related ECG findings (Figures 23.9 and 23.10)
In contrast, uncommon and non-training related ECG findings that may indicate further evaluation are:
• negative T waves ≥ two adjacent leads;
• ST segment depression;
• pathologic Q waves;
• important atrial abnormalities;
• short or long QT interval;
• advanced bundle branch block or hemiblocks;
• evident criteria of right or left ventricular hypertrophy;
• abnormalities of QRS–ST in V1 suggestive of Brugada pattern (see Figure 7.16 and Chapter 21);
• the presence of some arrhythmias (runs or sustained ventricular tachycardia, vagal atrial fibrillation, advanced second- or third-degree AV block) (see below).

Figure 23.8 shows the most frequent repolarization abnormalities found in well-trained athletes (Plas 1976), which make it necessary to rule out hypertrophic cardiomyopathy and other possible causes.

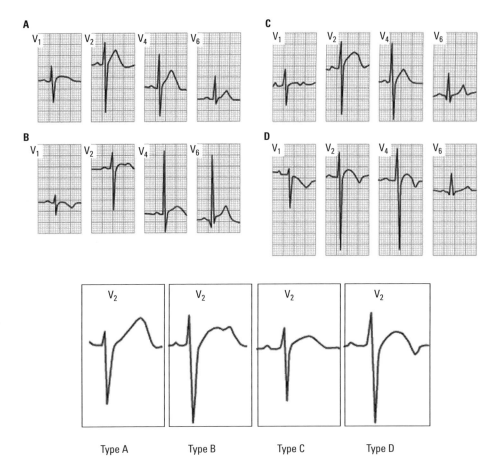

Figure 23.8 Different types of repolarization abnormalities found in athletes (A to D). These are usually benign, but it is compulsory to perform an echocardiogram to rule out hypertrophic cardiomyopathy (Based on Serra-Grima *et al.* 2000).

Arrhythmias

The most frequent arrhythmias found in athletes are the following:

- **PVCs**: These are not infrequent in healthy athletes, although they usually disappear with exercise. More than one PVC in a surface ECG must be referred for a further evaluation. Runs of ventricular tachycardia (VT) and especially sustained VT have to be considered definitively pathologic and need to be carefully studied.
- **Atrial fibrillation** (AF): Whereas paroxysmal AF is rarely seen in young athletes, the incidence of AF paroxysmal or chronic in adult athletes or ex-athletes is more frequent than in the normal population (Mont *et al.* 2009).
- **Some benign bradyarrhythmias**, such as sinus bradycardia often with junctional escapes and/or first- and even second-degree Wenckebach-type AV block may be found, occurring especially at night (Figures 23.10 and 23.11).
- **Advanced AV block**: This should not be assumed to be training-related and requires further evaluation.
- **Sudden death**: Although the incidence of sudden death among athletes is low, it constitutes a serious social problem, and extremely intense sports might increase the risk of sudden death (Martínez-Sellés and Lucia 2019). In young competitive athletes, the incidence of sudden death is approximately 1/100 000 people/year (Maron *et al.* 1980, 1995). In athletes over 35 years of age, the most frequent cause is ischemic heart disease (Vicent *et al.* 2018), whereas in younger athletes, the conditions most frequently associated with sudden death are hypertrophic cardiomyopathy, coronary anomalies, arrhythmogenic right ventricular dysplasia (ARVD), Brugada syndrome, myocarditis, coronary artery anomalies, and many others (Maron *et al.* 1980) (Figure 23.12). It has been recently demonstrated that the use of doping agents (androgenic anabolic steroids) may cause a significant shortening of the QT interval ($\approx 350\,\text{ms}$), albeit without reaching the values of short QT syndrome. This is related to the increase in I_{to} and I_k currents, resulting in a shortened repolarization (Bigi *et al.* 2009).

Table 23.1 shows cardiac abnormalities found in 161 elite athletes with arrhythmias considered pathologic after arrhythmologic study (Bayés de Luna *et al.* 2000). More than 40% had underlying heart abnormalities, four (2.5%) had documented recovered cardiac arrest, and three presented with sudden death.

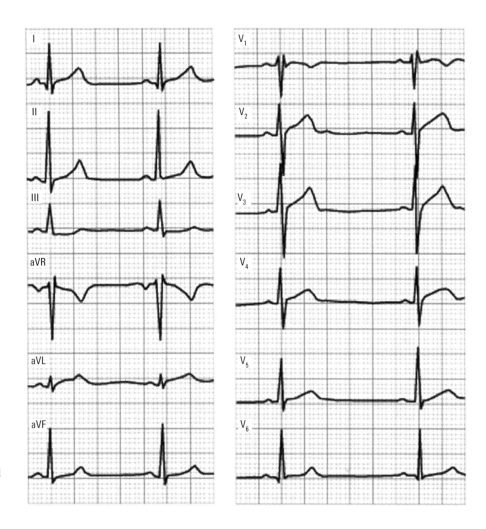

Figure 23.9 Athlete with normal ECG with sinus tachycardia and rSr′ pattern of benign characteristics in V1.

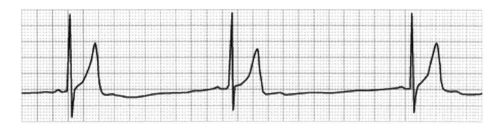

Figure 23.10 Very important sinus bradycardia during the night (28 bpm).

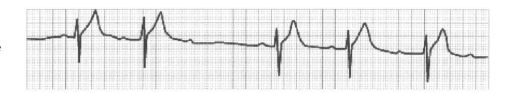

Figure 23.11 Another athlete with sinus bradycardia and Wenckebach AV block 3 × 2 during the night.

Athletes should undergo a cardiology check-up that includes a complete personal and family history and physical examination, a good interpretation of the ECG, and is very much recommended an echocardiogram, a key diagnostic tool in determining the presence of valvular heart disease and hypertrophic cardiomyopathy. The differential diagnosis with hypertrophic cardiomyopathy is especially important. Figure 21.5 shows the most important differential diagnostic clues. In the presence of syncope or other symptoms, especially during exercise, if

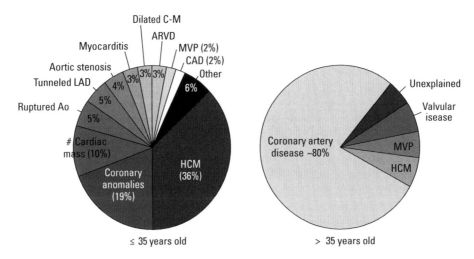

Figure 23.12 Estimated prevalence of cardiovascular diseases responsible for sudden death comparing young (≤35 years old) (left) and older (>35 years old) (right) trained athletes. ARVD: arrhythmogenic right ventricular dysplasia; MVP: mitral valve prolapse; CAD: coronary artery disease; HCM: hypertrophic cardiomyopathy (Based on Maron *et al.* 1980).

Table 23.1 Cardiac abnormalities in 161 elite athletes with arrhythmias

Disease	Total athletes with abnormalities	% of total elite athletes	Sudden death	Cardiac arrest
Arrhythmogenic ventricular dysplasia	12	7.5		1
Mitral valve prolapse	27	16.7		1
Wolff–Parkinson–White syndrome	15	9.3		1
Dilated cardiomyopathy	3	1.9	1	1
Hypertrophic cardiomyopathy	1	0.6		1
Mitral regurgitation (severe)	1	0.6		
Aortic valvular disease	3	1.9		
Myocarditis	4	2.5		
Coronary artery disease	1	0.6	1	
Unknown cardiomyopathy	1	0.6	1	
Total	68	42.2	3	4

Reproduced with permission from Bayés de Luna *et al.* 2000.

the diagnosis is not clear, imaging techniques, such as a multislice scanner and especially cardiovascular magnetic resonance imaging (CMRI) should be used. If necessary, electrophysiologic study (EPS) or even genetic testing and right ventricular biopsy should be performed, especially in the presence of exercise syncope or an "atypical" ECG. Using each of these techniques, hypertrophic cardiomyopathy, ARVD, other cardiomyopathies, coronary and aorta anomalies and even channelopathies may be diagnosed. In the presence of bicuspid aortic valve, the practice of isometric exercise, such as weight-lifting, is not recommended because of the danger of problems due to frequent association with aneurysm of the ascending aorta.

Drug administration

Drugs and ECG morphology

Many drugs alter the ECG morphology. Some examples have been discussed throughout this book. **In general, abnormalities occur in repolarization** (amiodarone—Figure 23.13, digitalis—Figures 23.14 and 23.15), etc. Also, **intraventricular and AV conduction** may be found (most antiarrhythmic agents, digitalis), **and sinus node dysfunction** as well (beta blockers) (Bayés de Luna and Cosin 1980).

Proarrhythmic effects of drugs

In addition, many drugs, whether used to treat heart diseases or not, such as erythromycin, some antidepressant and antihistaminic agents, and even some antiarrhythmic drugs among others, have the capability of causing arrhythmias (**arrhythmogenic effect**) (Horowitz and Zipes, 1987; Bayés de Luna *et al.* 1990; Bayés de Luna and Baranchuk 2017). This depends on the previous cardiovascular state and the dosage and interactions of any drug, but it is especially related to the **non-homogeneous lengthening of the QT interval induced by the drug** (see Tables 19.1 and 19.2). The most dangerous effect is the induction of ventricular tachycardia in the form of torsades de pointes, which can cause sudden death. The recent experience with QT prolongation, torsades de pointes and sudden death with short courses of chloroquine or hydroxychloroquine as used in the COVID-19

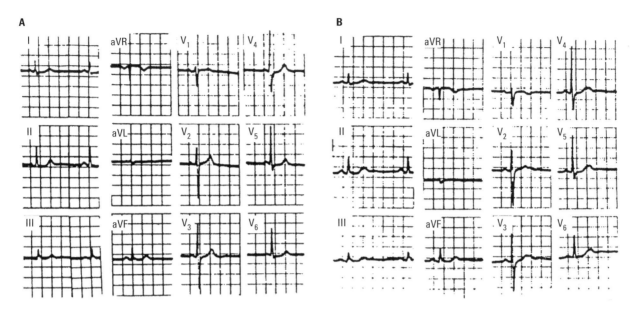

Figure 23.13 (A) A 57-year-old man with systemic hypertension and paroxysmal supraventricular tachycarrhythmias. (B) After three months of treatment with amiodarone, a change in the T wave morphology is visible, especially in right and mid-precordial leads in which split and flat T wave appear (see in V2 and V4).

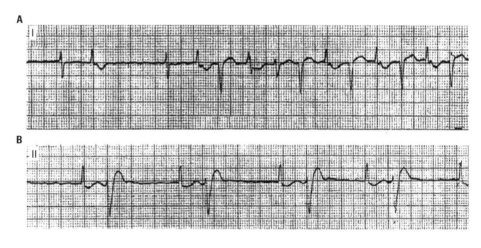

Figure 23.14 Patient with digitalis intoxication and atrial fibrillation (AF). (A) After two bigeminal premature ventricular complexes (PVCs), an episode of bidirectional ventricular fibrillation (VF) starts. (B) The same patient presented with bigeminal rhythm due to PVCs. Note the typical ST segment morphology.

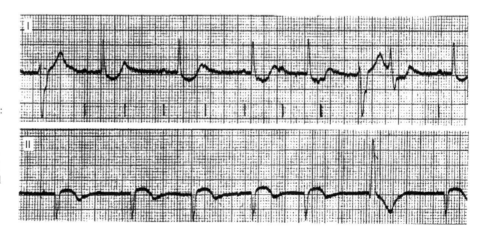

Figure 23.15 Digitalis intoxication: note the typical morphology of ST depression due to the digitalis effect with a shortened QT interval. This is a case of irregular junctional escape rhythm with some sinus and ectopic P waves, premature ventricular complexes (PVCs), and ventricular escape complexes.

pandemic is a good example of this menacing effect (Jankelson *et al.* 2020). This is especially related to the increase of the QT interval duration and the dispersion of refractory periods. Drugs that uniformly prolong repolarization, such as amiodarone, do not have this proarrhythmic effect; on the contrary, they are antiarrhythmic. The CAST (Cardiac Arrhythmia Suppression Trial) Investigators (1989) demonstrated in post-infarction patients with ventricular dysfunction that the administration of type I antiarrhythmics (quinidine, flecainide, and participate in the trial, and propafenone does not) increases mortality due to a proarrhythmic effect. The administration of type I antiarrhythmics is therefore contraindicated in patients with ventricular dysfunction. Propaphenon has the benefit of doubt.

Drugs that prolong repolarization therefore have to be carefully prescribed, in particular in heart disease patients and when have they to be used over long periods of time. Also, the presence of ionic disbalance, which may be induced by some drugs, may be dangerous. Very strict guidelines elaborated by American (FDA) and European (EMEA) medication agencies are currently available in order to control the use of new drugs under study to ensure that they do not cause an increase in the QT interval and do not have proarrhythmic effects. This danger is probably related to concealed and still little-known genetic mutations. Currently, drug agencies (FDA/EMEA) strictly monitor new drugs, especially in relation to QTc lengthening and the appearance of torsades de pointes VT/VF. To better understand the effects of different drugs on the QT interval, consult www.drugsqtlong.org.

Drugs that also shorten repolarization, such as digitalis, may induce practically all types of arrhythmias and even sudden death. Even before digitalis arrives to toxic dosage, its effect modifies the ECG, inducing QT shortening and changes on the ST segment (concave depression) that are very easily detected in the surface ECG (Figure 23.15). We recommend performing frequently blood levels control of digitalis, to detect early cases of toxicity.

Digitalis toxicity is often expressed by ectopic atrial, junctional tachycardia, and ventricular arrhythmias (Kelly and Smith 1992). PVCs are often the first sign of digitalis toxicity. This may be initially manifest by isolated PVCs or ventricular bigeminy. Ventricular tachycardia, sometimes bidirectional (Figure 23.14), and ventricular fibrillation may occur if digitalis toxicity is not recognized and treated. Digitalis intoxication also triggers atrial and junctional ectopic tachycardia relatively often. In both cases, the presence of AV dissociation is relatively frequent (see Figure 23.15). The most frequent passive arrhythmias found in digitalis intoxications are slow AV junctional rhythms, sinus bradycardia, sinoatrial block, and any degree of AV block. In the past, digitalis intoxication was more common. The most frequent arrhythmias

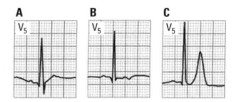

Figure 23.16 Typical examples of a notched (bimodal) T wave (A), a depressed T wave (B), and a peaked T wave (C), which can be observed in a chronic alcoholic patient.

found were PVCs: 80%; VT: 20%; atrial and junctional arrhythmias: 90%; and different degrees of AV block: 40% (Bayés de Luna and Cosin 1980).

Alcoholism (Figures 23.16–23.18)

It should be noted that small doses of alcohol (<30 g/day) can be considered a protecting mechanism against ischemic heart disease. However, higher doses, or even low ones, particularly in women as well as in cardiac patients and genetically predisposed individuals, may be deleterious and may account for the appearance not only of arrhythmias but also of some cases of dilated cardiomyopathy and sudden death.

From an electrocardiographic viewpoint, in **chronic alcoholics** with no heart failure, higher and symmetric (peaked) T waves can be found or, more characteristically, low-voltage T waves, sometimes bimodal (notched) or even negative, but not very deep (negative), that are generally persistent (Figure 23.16) (Evans 1959). Alcoholics with heart failure exhibit typical alterations frequently found in dilated cardiomyopathies of other etiologies (see above). Furthermore, drinking wine in a sporadic fashion, and even in **healthy non-alcoholics**, can occasionally cause **transient repolarization abnormalities. Also, on occasion, the repolarization abnormalities detected in chronic alcoholics may disappear with abstinence** (Figure 23.18).

It has already been mentioned that **alcohol can trigger, especially in some individuals, a series of arrhythmias**, particularly premature ventricular and atrial complexes, and often atrial fibrillation crises, especially at nighttime. All these arrhythmias can disappear with abstinence, although this is not always the case (Figure 23.17) (Ettinger *et al.* 1978). Abstinence also normally improves deteriorated ventricular function (Bayés de Luna 1977), and decreases the number of recurrences in cases of atrial fibrillation.

Ionic disorders

Changes in serum potassium concentrations, such as hyperkalemia or hypokalemia, cause very distinct repolarization abnormalities (Surawicz 1967). Figures 23.19

		ISO ABN			SUC ABN							ISO ABN			SUC ABN			
	Time	TOT QRS	TOT / HR	MAX RT	TOT / HR	CPL / HR	>2 /HR	% ABN			Time	TOT QRS	TOT / HR	MAX RT	TOT / HR	CPL / HR	>2 /HR	% ABN
1	13:30	5.043	396	47	37	14	3	0.50		1	* 13:30	6.190	0	0	0	0	0	0.00
2	14:30	5.106	823	46	47	10	3	17.03		2	* 14:30	5.703	0	0	0	0	0	0.00
3	* 15:30	4.955	1915	44	10	5	0	38.04		3	* 15:30	5.951	0	0	0	0	0	0.00
4	* 16:30	4.478	1182	38	0	0	0	26.39		4	* 16:30	4.984	0	0	0	0	0	0.00
5	17:30	4.265	482	27	8	4	0	11.40		5	* 17:30	4.818	0	0	0	0	0	0.00
6	* 18:30	4.773	1189	29	0	0	0	24.91		6	* 18:30	5.316	0	0	0	0	0	0.00
7	* 19:30	4.705	1555	43	6	3	0	33.17		7	* 19:30	5.054	0	0	0	0	0	0.00
8	20:30	4.805	1703	46	198	97	1	39.56		8	* 20:30	4.360	0	0	0	0	0	0.00
9	* 21:30	4.588	1673	42	140	70	0	39.51		9	* 21:30	4.565	0	0	0	0	0	0.00
10	* 22:30	4.522	1321	41	244	82	18	34.60		10	* 22:30	4.556	0	0	0	0	0	0.00
11	23:30	4.919	1320	47	150	65	6	29.88		11	* 23:30	4.405	0	0	0	0	0	0.00
12	00:30	4.086	198	40	6	3	0	4.99		12	* 00:30	3.655	0	0	0	0	0	0.00
13	01:30	3.992	696	41	43	18	2	10.51		13	* 01:30	3.427	0	0	0	0	0	0.00
14	02:30	3.877	812	43	16	0	0	21.35		14	* 02:30	3.423	0	0	0	0	0	0.00
15	* 03:30	4.047	1270	39	12	6	0	31.67		15	* 03:30	3.342	0	0	0	0	0	0.00
16	04:30	4.297	1891	38	125	57	3	46.91		16	* 04:30	3.432	0	0	0	0	0	0.00
17	05:30	4.246	1946	38	157	66	7	49.52		17	* 05:30	3.430	0	0	0	0	0	0.00
18	06:30	5.102	2312	54	257	96	19	50.35		18	* 06:30	3.491	0	0	0	0	0	0.00
19	07:30	6.196	1596	53	44	22	0	26.46		19	* 07:30	2.313	0	0	0	0	0	0.00

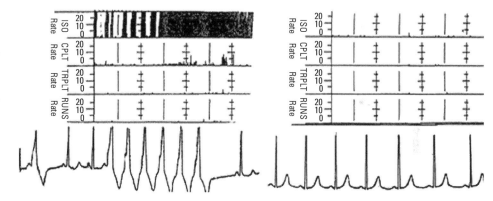

Figure 23.17 Left: Alcoholic patient with no heart failure complaining of palpitations. The Holter recording demonstrated the existence of different premature ventricular complexes—even in runs—which are very frequent, sometimes up to 2000 per hour. Right: The Holter study performed after one month of abstinence proved that there were no premature ventricular complexes in the 24-hour recording (Based on Ettinger *et al.* 1978).

and 23.20 illustrate the electrophysiological basis for the ECG changes found with hyperkalemia and hypokalemia.

In hyperkalemia, the T wave in some leads becomes too tall and peaked, sometimes with a striking elevation of the segment (Figure 23.19). Subsequently, the QRS complex becomes wider and the P wave may disappear. The evolutionary ECG changes in patients with extreme hyperkalemia due to severe renal failure are shown in Figure 23.20, from the moment (A) in which an extremely slow rhythm with a very wide QRS caused by ventricular escape or concealed sinus rhythm with **sinoventricular conduction occurs** (see Figure 7.2), until the moment (F) in which normality is almost regained.

With hypokalemia, on the other hand, there is a depression of the ST segment, and the QT seems long due to appearance of a U wave while the T wave flattens (see Figure 23.21).

Likewise, ECG changes related to serum **calcium** concentrations can also occur. **Hypocalcemia** causes the QT

to be prolonged at the expense of the ST segment, with the T wave being of low voltage, whereas **hypercalcemia** causes a short QRS and QT segment and a tall T wave. It has been described (Nierenberg and Rausee 1999) that the QT interval is an marker of hypercalcemia.

ECG changes associated with **magnesium** concentrations can also occur. It is difficult to find isolated alteration of magnesium concentrations. Electrolytic abnormalities, such as hypokalemia and hypomagnesemia, may be triggered by the administration of certain drugs (digitalis, diuretic agents, etc.), especially when renal function is not quite normal or in the setting of septic shock or severe metabolic abnormalities. All these circumstances may result in malignant arrhythmias, especially torsades de pointes, which, if not rapidly addressed, may lead to **sudden death** (Figure 24.7). Also, the ECG changes of combined hypercalcemia and hypermagnesemia have been described (Mosseri *et al.* 1990).

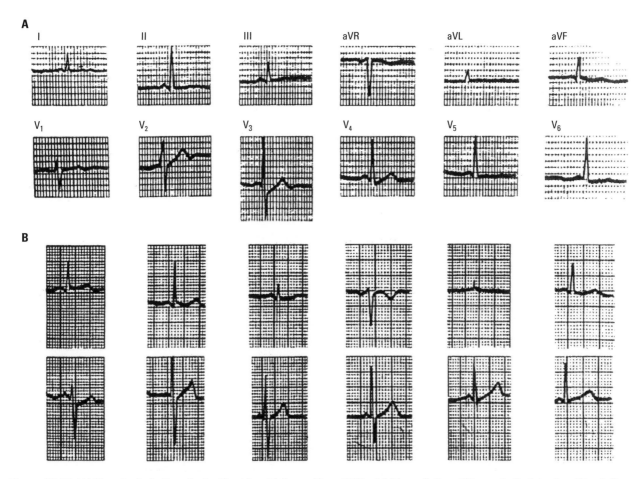

A

B

Figure 23.18 (A) Chronic alcoholic patient without heart failure with an ECG exhibiting a flattened T wave in the lateral wall leads (I, aVL, V5, V6), which disappeared with abstinence (B).

Hypothermia

Moderate and severe hypothermia produce **typical changes in the ECG tracing** (Figure 23.22) (Clements and Hurst 1972; Kanna and Wani 2003). The most common changes are:

- baseline with irregularities;
- slow heart rate;
- lengthening of the PR and QT intervals;
- reduction in the P wave and the T wave voltage in the diaphragmatic leads;
- appearance, as the most characteristic manifestation, of a J wave (Osborne wave, slurring of the final portion of the QRS complex).

Also a variety of supraventricular and ventricular arrhythmias can occur, particularly with severe hypothermia. The ECG changes disappear on improvement of the patient's clinical condition (Figure 23.22B).

Recently, the cases of acquired and inherited J waves that include cases with danger of sudden death have

been included in the named **J wave syndromes** (Antzelevitch and Yan 2010) (see Chapter 24).

Pregnancy and puerperium

During a **normal pregnancy**, the ÂQRS gradually deviates to the left and the heart rate increases. The heart often has a characteristic rotation (dextrorotation and horizontalization with the apex deviated forward), with an ECG recording similar to that seen in obesity (see Figure 18.6). On occasion, repolarization changes can be found, which are usually meaningless from a clinical standpoint, but which should be followed to check that they are indeed transient. Sometimes, ventricular and supraventricular arrhythmias can also be seen which are, in general, of a benign nature.

Peripartum cardiomyopathy is a potential complication during pregnancy with an uncertain prognosis, although it is rare. A good clinical setting and ventricular

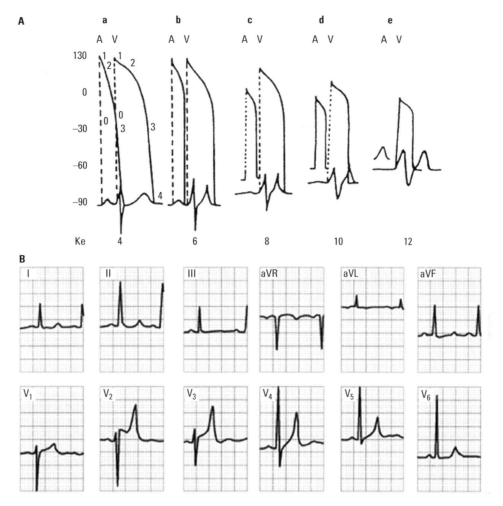

Figure 23.19 (A) Schematic representation of the ECG changes observed in successive stages of hyperkalemia. Atrial and ventricular transmembrane action potentials (TAP) are overlapped. Extracellular potassium levels increase (see below), causing a decrease in the diastolic transmembrane potential (DTP) (see image on the left), a decrease in height of the TAP 0 phase and of its upstroke velocity (the dots of the dotted line are closer together). The increased QRS complex duration is shown in the surface ECG; also, the abolishment of the P wave is shown (adapted from Surawicz 1967). (B) A 20-year-old male with chronic renal failure subjected to periodic hemodialysis during the last two years. Hypertension is significant (210/130 mmHg). Serum potassium levels are high: 6.4 mEq/l. Note the high and peaked T wave, as well as the ST segment elevation in V2 and V3. The QT interval duration is relatively long in leads I, II, and III at the expense of the ST segment due to the associated hypocalcemia.

function, the presence of mild symptoms, and a normal or near-normal ECG recording, are all factors that point toward a good evolution.

Rarely, during puerperium, due to connective tissue disruption associated with lack of fibrin, cases of **coronary dissection** usually in LAD coronary artery, may occur. These appear as severe STEMI that may induce cardiogenic shock and/or need for heart transplant (see Chapter 20 coronary dissection).

Anesthesia and surgery

Pre-operative ECG

A pre-operative ECG recording is performed in most hospitals in order to rule out any possible surgical contraindication. However, the ECG recording will only serve as a guide, and in all cases a correlation of the ECG with the clinical history and the other pre-operative tests (blood tests, X-ray) should be made in order to produce a final report.

Often, decisive importance is attributed to a normal ECG, which leads to a false sense of reassurance. It should always be borne in mind that, on occasion, the ECG may be normal or may show just minimal changes in the presence of a pulmonary embolism or an acute coronary syndrome. Also, it is quite common for an ECG to return to normal just a few months after a myocardial infarction.

The ECG does not always provide information about the need for treatment with cardioactive drugs, nor as regards the possibilities of toxic effects with some drugs. However, its usefulness in the detection of arrhythmias and conduction disorders, and in the overall assessment of the patient, is unquestioned.

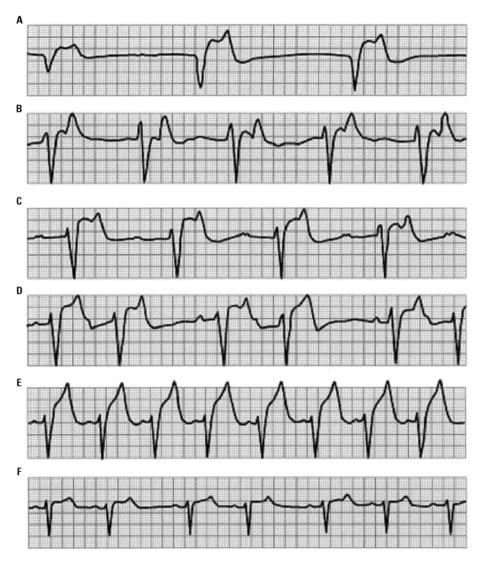

Figure 23.20 An 82-year-old patient with chronic renal failure and significant hyperkalemia (9.2 mEq/l) upon arrival (A) with a diagnosis of a severe renal failure and presyncope. The QRS is very wide and no P waves are seen. This is probably a ventricular escape rhythm, but the possibility of a slow sinus node rhythm with sinoventricular conduction cannot be ruled out, since this kind of conduction disorder may be observed with hyperkalemia (Bellet and Jedlicka 1969). From (B) to (F), a progressive normalization of the ECG tracing after the improvement of the clinical picture with dialysis. Serum potassium level was normal in (F).

Furthermore, a reference tracing is extremely important in order to assess potential abnormalities that might appear during a surgical procedure, especially considering that a post-operative myocardial infarction usually occurs without pain or its symptoms might be masked by analgesics or post-operative discomfort.

In **patients with ischemic heart disease,** the clinical and ECG situation should be assessed very carefully since the risks associated with anesthesia and surgery are increased and vary from one patient to another. Thus, a history of myocardial infarction during the three months prior to surgery is regarded as a risk factor, and therefore any kind of surgical intervention is not recommended, particularly during the first month, except for those cases of an urgent nature. The risk is mild in patients with stable angina, but it increases significantly in patients during or in a recent phase after acute coronary syndrome. In addition, patients with heart failure should always be treated to a maximum level before surgery.

Actually, there are **very few absolute surgical contraindications based on an ECG.** However, it may happen that, thanks to the practice of an overall pre-operative evaluation, specific problems such as, for example, a rapid atrial fibrillation, runs of non-sustained ventricular tachycardia, and a sick sinus syndrome, may be discovered and can be solved.

When the implantation of a pacemaker is indicated for surgery, it is generally preferable to implant a permanent pacemaker, since the selection is usually based on a clinical situation that is not going to revert after surgery.

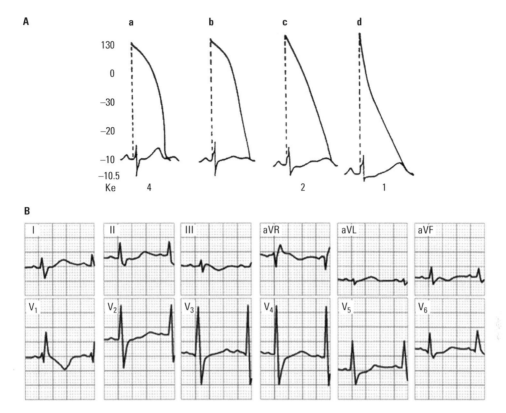

Figure 23.21 (A) Schematic representation of the ECG changes observed in the evolving stages of hypokalemia. The ventricular transmembrane action potential (TAP) has been drawn superimposed on the surface ECG. The diastolic transmembrane potential (DTP) value is to the left and the extracellular K$^+$ level is shown below. Note that as extracellular K$^+$ level progressively decreases, the ventricular TAP duration increases at the expense of the phase 3 velocity decrease. The U wave in the ECG tracing is gradually seen more clearly while the T wave tends to decrease, together with an apparent ST segment depression (adapted from Surawicz 1967). (B) This belongs to a 45-year-old patient with advanced mitroaortic heart valve disease treated with excessive doses of digitalis and diuretics. Extracellular K$^+$ level is 2.3 mEq/l. The ECG change corresponding to phase C of the scheme shown in Figure 23.21 can be clearly seen, particularly in V2–V4.

ECG during anesthesia and surgery

During anesthesia and surgery, the patient should be monitored correctly and continuously. The ECG recorded in the operating room is different from the conventional one in two aspects: on the one hand, because of the frequent presence of artifacts, and on the other, because of the sudden changes that may arise and that are a consequence of the effect of different drugs, as well as of the surgery and anesthesia themselves (intubation, change of position, etc.).

In healthy individuals and in the absence of hypoxia and electrolyte imbalance, ECG alterations during surgery are scarce. However, several arrhythmias, even severe, have been described. Continuous ECG monitoring is particularly useful in detecting the risk of cardiac arrest, and, if the event occurs, in knowing whether it is secondary to a ventricular fibrillation or to an asystole. The average incidence of cardiac arrest during anesthesia is one case in every 3000, and is higher (1/1000) in elderly or high-risk patients. **In the past, it was considered that in** 20% of cases, the anesthesia is totally or partially responsible for the cardiac arrest, although with the latest

advances in the field this figure is much lower nowadays. In general, prior to cardiac arrest, several warning signs can be identified, which may go from ventricular tachycardia to sinus bradycardia and are usually related to the presence of hypoxia, hypotension, hypercapnia, etc.

The occurrence of arrhythmias during anesthesia usually indicates that a disorder that should be corrected is present. In this case, the following measures should be taken: (i) control in the administration of anesthetic agent; (ii) improvement of oxygenation, which is extremely important; (iii) achievement of a suitable removal of carbon dioxide; and (iv) suppression of reflexogenic maneuvers. In cases of potentially dangerous arrhythmias, antiarrhythmic agents should only be administered once the corresponding measures for the correction of the hypoxia and hypotension have been taken, and after all possible reflexogenic stimuli, such as traction of the mesentery or pleura, have been removed. In urgent cases, electric cardioversion should be resorted to.

Arrhythmias are more frequent at two specific moments—during intubation and during tracheal aspiration. Bradyarrhythmias are triggered by drugs that cause

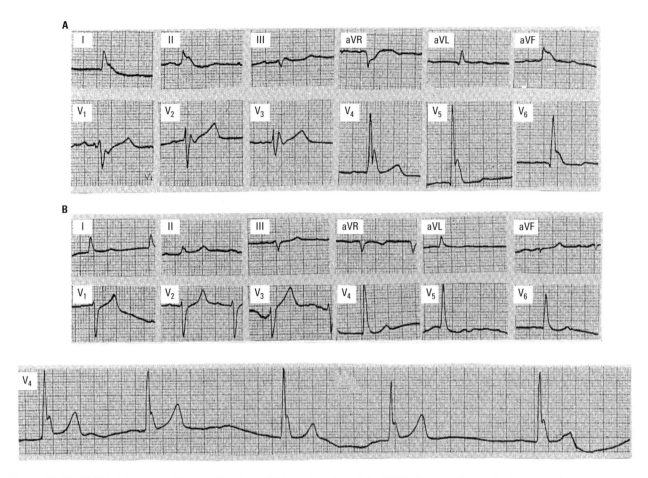

Figure 23.22 (A) This belongs to a 76-year-old patient with hypothermia and the ECG is the recording typically seen in this condition. Note the J, or Osborne, wave, typical of hypothermia, at the end of the QRS complex, sinus bradycardia, long QT interval, and an irregular baseline (lower strip). (B) When the problem was resolved after warming the J wave disappeared completely.

vagal stimulation, but this can be counteracted with atropine.

Environmental arrhythmias, especially all premature atrial or ventricular complexes, usually decrease when the patient is correctly anesthetized and oxygenated, and are less frequent with general anesthesia than with epidural anesthesia.

The appearance of the following ECG signs during anesthesia and surgery require careful surveillance, the suppression of the unleashing factors and urgent action, if necessary:

• tachycardia above 160/min;
• bradycardia below 45/min;
• bigeminy or multifocal ventricular complexes;
• marked repolarization changes (ST segment depression or elevation, inversion of the T wave, presence of high and peaked T waves with a long QT interval;
• appearance of an AV block or an advanced bundle branch block.

Post-surgical electrocardiography

In patients with heart disease it is convenient to perform at least one ECG control during the first days after the intervention. Patients with ischemic heart disease occasionally

(1–2%) develop a post-operative myocardial infarction, often in the absence of chest pain. In higher risk cases, monitoring should be performed after surgery.

During the post-operative period, an ECG should be immediately practiced under the following circumstances:

• in the event of unexplained hypotension;
• in the event of symptoms of heart failure (rales, gallop);
• in the event of arrhythmias (for example, rapid or slow rhythms);
• in case of chest pain, or pain in the arms or back;
• in the case of dyspnea or syncope.

In all of these cases, serial ECGs should be performed in order to rule out the possibility of a myocardial infarction, even if the first tracing is normal.

Arrhythmias in children

The incidence of arrhythmias increases very much with age, and the two biggest problems in arrhythmology—atrial fibrillation and sudden death—are very infrequent in children and even in young people. However, there are some types of arrhythmias that have already been described throughout this book that may be present sometimes at an early age, and even in newborns and fetus, and some of these arrhythmias are very characteristic of this age. We will make just a brief summary of the most frequent arrhythmias and some clinical considerations. For more information consult Bayés de Luna and Baranchuk 2017 and general references (Recommended Reading).

Premature ventricular complexes

PVCs are very infrequent in children. They may express just a sympathetic overdrive or expression of some type or myocardial problem (hidden myocarditis). It is necessary to rule out some type of inherited heart disease (see Chapter 21).

Incessant idiopathic ventricular tachycardia

Incessant idiopathic ventricular tachycardia is a rare arrhythmia which usually presents between three months and 3 years of age. It may arise in the left ventricle and also in the right ventricle. Sometimes, is very rapid and is present in > 10% of the time. It has been related to myocardial microscopic focus and may be often controlled with amiodarone. It usually resolves with time. Adenosine may help in diagnosis because it unmasks the AV dissociation.

Junctional ectopic tachycardia

Sometimes, junctional ectopic tachycardia may be seen in infants, and may be very rapid and badly tolerated. It may be necessary to perform a catheter ablation, which represents some risk of AV block (see Chapter 15).

Incessant junctional reciprocating tachycardia

Incessant junctional reciprocating tachycardia (IJRT) is a rare type of orthodromic junctional reentrant tachycardia (see Chapter 15) with retrograde arm in an anomalous pathway (see Figure 15.15) that in the majority of cases presents in childhood. Sometimes, it induces dilated cardiomyopathy. The differential diagnosis includes especially incessant type of ectopic atrial tachycardia (Chapter 15). Spontaneous resolution is uncommon and frequently catheter ablation is recommended.

Paroxysmal reentrant junctional tachycardia

As already discussed (see Chapter 14), there are two typical cases of paroxysmal reentrant junctional tachycardia: (i) involving only AV junction in the circuit (AVNRT) and (ii) with participation of an accessory pathway (AVRT). The latter is part of the **Wolff–Parkinson–White (WPW) syndrome** and is probably the most frequent paroxysmal

tachycardia found in children and even newborns. The AVNRT appears later in life and is probably caused by some inflammatory process that appears after childhood (Chapter 15).

Atrial fibrillation and flutter

Atrial fibrillation is a rare arrhythmia in children. Usually is due to inherited origin and it is necessary to rule out the short QT syndrome (Chapter 21) are also all types of pre-excitation (Chapter 12). Atrial flutter is frequently observed after repair of congenital heart diseases, especially atrial septal defect (ASD) and also in Ebstein's disease (see Figure 15.40).

Bradyarrhythmias

The most frequent cause of slow heart rate in newborns and children is advanced congenital AV block. This topic is discussed in Chapter 24.

Sudden death

The cases of sudden death in children, apart from congenital AV block, are related to ventricular tachyarrhythmias, in the majority of cases in the presence of some inherited heart diseases, especially long QT syndrome and polymorphic catecholaminergic VT. The Brugada syndrome window of danger of sudden death usually appears after 15 years, although some cases in childhood have been reported, and the same may occur in case of other inherited cardiomyopathies.

Also, in some cases, a fulminant myocarditis or ventricular arrhythmias related to surgical procedures in congenital heart diseases such as tetralogy of Fallot and great vessel transposition may occur sometimes after many years post-surgery.

References

Antzelevitch C, Yan GX. J wave syndromes. Heart Rhythm 2010;7:549.

Bayés de Luna A. *Alcohol y corazón*. Editorial Científico-Médica, 1977.

Bayés de Luna A, Cosin J. *Diagnosis and Treatment of Cardiac Arrhythmias*. Pergamon Press, 1980.

Bayés de Luna A. Baranchuk A *Clinical Arrhythmology*. 2nd edn. Wiley-Blackwell, 2017.

Bayés de Luna A, Guindo J, Viñolas X. The possible role of bradyarrhythmia explaining late proarrhythmia in CAST study. Cardiovasc Drugs Ther 1990;4:651.

Bayés de Luna A, Furlanello F, Maron B, Zipes D. *Arrhythmias and Sudden Death in Athletes*. Kluwer Academic, 2000.

Bellet S, Jedlicka J. Sinoventricular conduction and its relation to sinoatrial conduction. Am J Cardiol 1969;24:831.

Bigi MA, Aslani A, Aslani A. Short QT interval: a novel predictor of androgen abuse in strength trained athletes. Ann Noninvasive Electrocardiol 2009;14:311.

CAST (Cardiac Arrhythmia Suppression Trial) Investigators. Preliminary report: effect of encainide and flecainide on mortality in a randomized trial of arrhythmia suppression after myocardial infarction. N Engl J Med 1989;321:406–412. doi: https://doi.org/10.1056/NEJM198908103210629.

Chiariello M, Indolfi C, Cotecchia MR, *et al*. Asymptomatic transient ST changes during ambulatory ECG monitoring in diabetic patients. Am Heart J 1985;110:529.

Clements SD, Hurst JW. Diagnostic value of electrocardiographic abnormalities observed in subjects accidentally exposed to cold. Am J Cardiol 1972;29:729.

Corrado D, Pelliccia A, Heidbuchel H, *et al*. Section of Sports Cardiology, European Association of Cardiovascular Prevention and Rehabilitation; Working Group of Myocardial and Pericardial Disease, European Society of Cardiology. Recommendations for interpretation of 12-lead electrocardiogram in the athlete. Eur Heart J 2010;31:243.

Ettinger PO, Wu CF, de la Cruz C, *et al*. Arrhythmias and the "Holiday heart": alcohol-associated cardiac rhythm disorders. Am Heart J 1978;95:555.

Evans W. The electrocardiogram of alcoholic cardiomyopathy. Br Heart J 1959;21:445.

Haïssaguerre M, Derval N, Sacher F, *et al*. Sudden cardiac arrest associated with early repolarization. N Engl J Med 2008;358:2016

Horowitz LN, Zipes DP. A symposium: perspectives on proarrhythmia. Am J Cardiol 1987;59:1E.

Hypertension in Diabetes Study (HDS): II. Increased risk of CV complications in hypertensive type 2 diabetic patients. J Hypertens 1993;11:319–325. doi:https://doi.org/10.1097/00004872-199303000-00013.

Jankelson L, Karam G, Becker ML, Chinitz LA, Tsai MC. QT prolongation, torsades de pointes, and sudden death with short courses of chloroquine or hydroxychloroquine as used in COVID-19: a systematic review. Heart Rhythm 2020;17(9):1472–1479. doi: https://doi.org/10.1016/j.hrthm.2020.05.008.

Kanna B, Wani S. Giant J wave on 12-lead electrocardiogram in hypothermia. Ann Noninvasive Electrocardiol 2003;8:262.

Kelly RA, Smith TW. Recognition and management of digitalis toxicity. Am J Cardiol 1992;69:108G.

Maron B, Roberts W, Epstein S. Sudden death in young athletes. Circulation 1980;62:218.

Maron B, Pelliccia A, Spirito P. Cardiac disease in young trained athletes. Insights into methods for distinguishing athlete's heart from structural heart disease, with particular emphasis on hypertrophic cardiomyopathy. Circulation 1995;91:1596.

Martínez-Sellés M, Lucia A. Exercise and heart. In medium virtus est? Int J Cardiol 2019;286:143–144.

Martinez-Sellés M, Diaz-Gonzalez L, Lucia A. Right ventricular remodeling in athletes and crista supraventricularis pattern. Clin Cardiol 2020;43:657.

Mont L, Elosua R, Brugada J. Endurance sport practice as a risk factor for atrial fibrillation and atrial flutter. Europace 2009;11:11.

Monterrubio Villar J, Fernández Bergés D, Alzugaray Fraga RJ, *et al*. Elevación del ST y neumotórax a tensión. Rev Esp Cardiol 2000;53:467.

Mosseri M, Porath A, Ovsyshcher I *et al*. ECG manfisetations of combined hypercalcemia and hypermagnesemia. J Electrocardiol 1990;23:235.

Nierenberg B, Rausee B. QT interval as a clincial indicator of hypercalcemia. Am J Card 1999;44:243.

Plas F. *Guide du cardiologie du sport*. Bailliere, 1976.

Serra-Grima R, Estorch M, Carrio I, *et al*. Marked ventricular repolarization abnormalities in highly trained athletes' electrocardiograms: clinical and prognostic implications. J Am Coll Cardiol 2000;36:1310.

Strizik B, Forman R. New ECG changes associated with a tension pneumothorax: a case report. Chest 1999;115:1742.

Surawicz B. Relationship between electrocardiogram and electrolytes. Am Heart J 1967;73:814.

Uberoi A, Stein R, Perez MV, *et al*. Interpretation of the electrocardiogram of young athletes. Circulation 2011;124:746.

Vázquez M, Olivares JL, Fleta J, Lacambra I, González M. Alteraciones cardiológicas en adolescentes con anorexia nerviosa. Rev Esp Cardiol 2003;56:669.

Vicent L, Ariza-Solé A, González-Juanatey JR, *et al*. Exercise-related severe cardiac events. Scand J Med Sci Sports 2018;28:1404.

Chapter 24
Other ECG Patterns of Risk

Introduction

In this chapter, we summarize the ECG patterns of risk of important arrhythmias and sudden death that have not been fully discussed in previous Chapters 14 to 17 (arrhythmias), 20 (ischemic heart disease), and 21 (inherited heart diseases).

Severe sinus bradycardia

When pacemaker activity of the sinus node, or stimulus conduction from the sinus node to the atria, is diminished, passive arrhythmias occur, such as sinus bradycardia due to a decrease of automaticity and/or a sinoatrial block (see Chapter 17). In many situations—such as myxedema, drugs (beta blockers, some other antiarrhythmic agents), and ionic and metabolic disturbances—severe but often asymptomatic; sinus bradycardia may be present. Some asymptomatic cases of inherited severe bradycardia (related to HCN4 ion channel mutation) have been reported (Nof *et al.* 2007). These cases are usually associated with a good prognosis, and do not require pacemaker implantation in the long term.

If there is a significant sinus bradycardia and symptoms are present (dizziness, syncope), a diagnosis of **sick sinus syndrome** is suspected (Figure 24.1). The most important cause of symptomatic sick sinus syndrome (SSS) is idiopathic fibrosis of the sinus node, which appears more frequently in elderly individuals. SSS is also related to many heart diseases, especially ischemic heart disease. The effects of some drugs must be ruled out at all times (see above, consider beta blockers, calcium blockers, digoxin, timolol eye-drops, etc.). Bradyarrhythmias due to sinus node disease (significant sinus automaticity depression and/or sinoatrial block) are not associated with severe symptoms if a normal junctional escape rhythm exists. Most of the symptoms are caused by co-existent associated

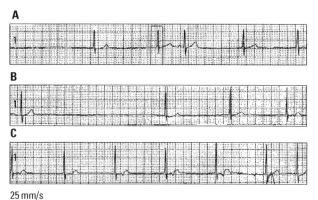

25 mm/s
10 mm/mV

Figure 24.1 Holter recording from a patient with sick sinus syndrome (SSS). (A) Note that the escape rhythm is quite slow with some sinus captures. In the first and fourth T-waves, a sinus P is probably concealed (see Figure 6.8). The last QRS escape complex is retrogradely conducted to the atria. (B) A pause > 3.5 seconds between the first and second QRS escape complexes. The last QRS complex is also conducted to the atria. (C) Junctional slow escape rhythm, with slow atrial retrograde conduction.

alterations: junctional automaticity depression (resulting in a slower escape rhythm) and/or atrioventricular (AV) block. If a normal escape rhythm exists, the patient could be virtually asymptomatic or have only mild symptoms (tiredness, mild dizziness).

Sick sinus syndrome is frequently associated with supraventricular arrhythmias, which alternate with significant bradyarrhythmias (**bradycardia–tachycardia syndrome**) (Figures 24.2 and 24.3). Indeed, patients with SSS often experience intermittent supraventricular arrhythmias, especially atrial fibrillation (AF), and marked or very marked pauses are frequently found at the end of these crises (Figure 24.2). If this occurs, concerning symptoms may be present (presyncope or syncope, low cardiac output, paroxysmal dyspnea, etc.). In these cases, the immediate implantation of a pacemaker is recommended.

Clinical Electrocardiography: A Textbook, Fifth Edition. Antoni Bayés de Luna, Miquel Fiol-Sala, Antoni Bayés-Genís, and Adrián Baranchuk.
© 2022 John Wiley & Sons Ltd. Published 2022 by John Wiley & Sons Ltd.

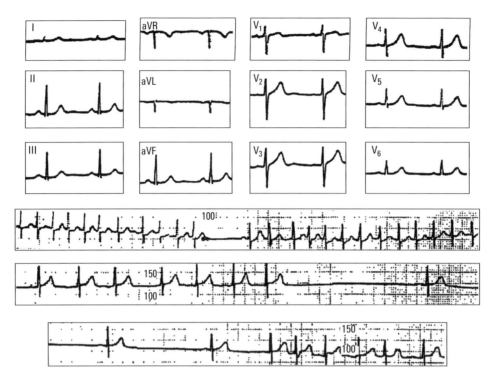

Figure 24.2 A 65-year-old man with a normal baseline ECG (above) and a history of fainting falls. The ECG Holter recording showed a typical bradycardia–tachycardia syndrome (three bottom strips).

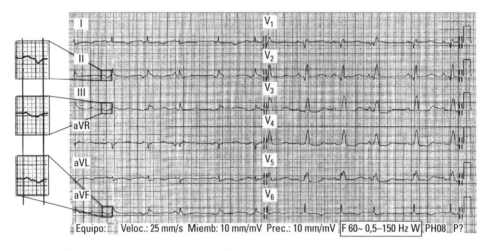

Figure 24.3 A characteristic ECG pattern of advanced interatrial block in a 60-year-old patient with Ebstein's disease. Note that the P ± is very wide in II, and in III and aVF. The patient also suffers from frequent episodes of supraventricular tachyarrhythmia (Bayés syndrome).

The pacemaker has a dual effect: first, it prevents bradyarrhythmia, and second, if tachyarrhythmia episodes persist, an appropriate antiarrhythmic treatment may be safely administered to prevent future episodes by having appropriate back-up provided by the pacemaker.

The implanted pacemaker should provide: (i) normal ventricular activation whenever possible (avoid unnecessary ventricular pacing), (ii) physiologic AV synchrony, and (iii) physiologic chronotropic competence (heart rate increase). This may be achieved with an atrial single-chamber pacemaker (AAI) when no AV block is present. However, as mentioned in Chapter 17, often a DDDR (universal dual chamber rate responsive) pacemaker should be implanted. This occurs especially when there is uncertainty about the appearance of an AV block in the future. About 2% of patients with SSS will develop AV block at 1–2 years (Andersen *et al.* 1998) (see Chapter 17, Choosing the best pacemaker).

Advanced interatrial block with left atrial retrograde conduction (Figures 24.3–24.5)

This type of advanced interatrial block produces a ± P-wave in leads II, III, and aVF, with a duration ≥ 0.12 sec (Bayés de Luna *et al.* 1985) (see Figure 9.18). This infrequent morphology (≈1/1000 ECG taken in the University Hospital Sant Pau, Barcelona) is explained because right atrial activation has a craniocaudal sense, but the left atrium is activated retrogradely from the mid-lower part of the septum. This retrograde activation of the left atrium occurs because the Bachman region, which is normally the way to cross the stimulus from the right to the left atrium, is blocked (see Figure 9.21). If the first part of the P-wave has a very low voltage, due to atrial fibrosis the atrial wave seems negative in II, III, aVF, mimicking a junctional rhythm (Bayés de Luna *et al.* 2019).

In the presence of this type of atrial block, the incidence of supraventricular tachyarrhythmias, especially AF, is very common (see Figures 24.4, and 24.5)(Bayés de Luna and Baranchuk 2017). Therefore, it has been considered that **the combination of advanced interatrial block** with left atrial retrograde conduction (P wave ± in II, III, and aVF) and **supraventricular arrhythmias constitutes a new arrhythmogenic syndrome** (Daubert 1996; Bayés de Luna *et al.* 1999) now called **Bayes' syndrome** (Conde and Baranchuk 2014).

Interatrial conduction block is generally present in patients with advanced heart disease who usually do not tolerate well fast atrial arrhythmias. Recently, has been demonstrated the association with stroke and dementia (Martínez-Sellés *et al.* 2020a, 2020b; Herrera *et al.* 2020) of elderly patients with A-IAB and structural heart disease. Therefore, in patients with this type of P-wave (P-wave ± in II, III, and aVF), may be advisable strict cardiac monitoring and antiarrhythmic or invasive approaches to control for rapid AF (Bayés de Luna *et al.* 1989; Baranchuk *et al.* 2014). Finally, a randomized trial (NOA vs placebo) is necessary to prove the potential benefit of anticoagulation in these patients.

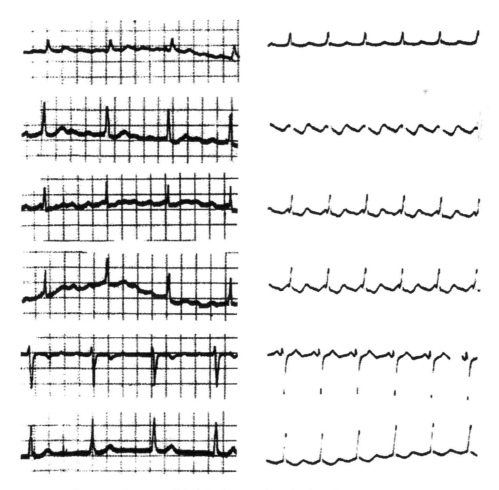

Figure 24.4 In this patient with advanced interatrial block, both types of atrial tachyarrhythmias (atrial fibrillation) and atrial flutter are observed.

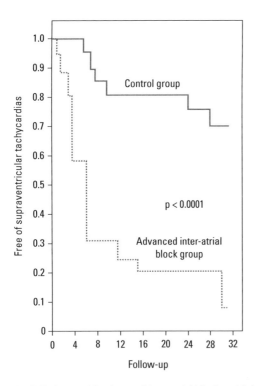

Figure 24.5 Patients with advanced interatrial block and left atrial retrograde activation show many more supraventricular paroxysmal arrhythmias during follow-up when compared with patients from the control group with the same ECG and clinical characteristics (Bayés de Luna *et al.* 1988).

Intraventricular conduction disturbances

High-risk bundle branch block

A bundle branch block is a marker of bad prognosis in patients with heart disease, especially left bundle branch block (LBBB). The presence of LBBB, or even right bundle branch block (RBBB), in post-infarction patients with ventricular dysfunction/heart failure (HF) is a marker of higher risk of sudden death, and, in the case of LBBB, it is also a marker for all-cause mortality (Bogale *et al.* 2007). Patients with HF and LBBB who present with AF have the worst prognosis (Baldasseroni *et al.* 2002; Vázquez *et al.* 2009) (see Chapter 15, Atrial fibrillation).

The "de novo" appearance of an advanced RBBB in the course of a serious acute episode with precordial pain and/or dyspnea **constitutes a marker of bad prognosis.** This situation obliges us to consider a diagnosis of acute coronary syndrome or pulmonary embolism. Naturally, in the course of an acute coronary syndrome with ST-segment elevation in precordial leads (STEMI), a RBBB pattern is observed when the left anterior descending coronary artery proximal to the first septal branch is occluded. This is the artery branch perfusing the right bundle (see Figure 13.53) (Wellens *et al.* 2003; Fiol-Sala *et al.* 2020). Additionally, the diagnosis of pulmonary

embolism when a new RBBB pattern occurs in patients with an acute episode of dyspnea should be entertained (Digby *et al.* 2015). In this case, the ECG may also show an ST-segment elevation in different leads, as well as sinus tachycardia, apart from the advanced RBBB pattern. The presence of a new RBBB is indicative of a massive pulmonary embolism, and thus is associated with a very poor prognosis. The cause of death is not usually a primary arrhythmia, but rather a hemodynamic failure with progressive impairment of automaticity leading to cardiac arrest (Qaddoura *et al.* 2017) (see Figure 10.16).

Special attention to rule out RBBB aberrancy in relation to sinus tachycardia (tachycardia-dependent block) should be given. In this case, the prognosis would not depend on the appearance of RBBB. Therefore, to determine the prognosis, it is important to know whether the patient had previously had an intermittent RBBB related to an increased heart rate (sometimes very difficult to prove).

High-risk combined intraventricular blocks

The possibility of progression to advanced AV block in the case of bifascicular block (i.e. RBBB plus superoanterior or inferoposterior hemiblock (SAH or IPH)) remains controversial (see Figures 11.50 and 11.54). Pacemaker implantation seems to reduce recurrence of syncope in comparison to monitoring with implantable loop recorders (Krahn *et al.* 2012). However, in asymptomatic individuals, pacemakers may not be indicated in cases of bifascicular block. However, close follow-up is recommended.

Classic masquerading bifascicular block (see Chapter 11)

It is a special type of bifascicular block with a particular bad prognosis. The diagnosis of masquerading bifascicular block is confirmed when in the presence of a tall and wide R-wave in lead V1 (**the ECG is suggestive of advanced RBBB**), no S-wave is recorded in leads I and aVL. The presence of extreme left axial deviation is explained by an associated superoanterior hemiblock (see Figure 11.51) (Bayés de Luna *et al.* 1989). At first glance, in an ECG of this type, it seems that LBBB is present in the frontal plane (FP), whereas in the horizontal plane (HP), RBBB is observed. The fact that an R-wave is recorded in lead V1 but no S-wave is seen in leads I and aVL is due to a significant left ventricular enlargement and/or associated conduction block in the left ventricular free wall. The final activation forces (see Figure 11.53) are not directed forward and rightward, as in the classic bifascicular block (Vector 1), but forward and leftward (Vector 2).

The masquerading bifascicular block rarely occurs intermittently (García-Moll *et al.* 1994) (see Figure 11.52).

In these cases, **prognosis** is poor regardless of whether a pacemaker is implanted or not (Bayés de Luna *et al.* 1989) because this type of block is usually detected in patients with advanced heart disease. Hence, the diagnosis in itself is a marker for poor prognosis (Elizari *et al.* 2013).

Masquerading RBBB pattern in the presence of advanced LBBB pattern

Masked RBBB in a patient with an LBBB ECG pattern may be diagnosed if there is a QR pattern in lead aVR and high R-wave in lead V1. In the presence of HF, this morphology may be explained by delayed activation of the basal part of the right ventricle (RV) (Van Bommel *et al.* 2011). In the absence of HF, this is probably explained by associated truncal partial RBBB pattern (Kukla *et al.* 2014).

RBBB with alternating block in the two sub-divisions of the left bundle

In 1968, Rosenbaum et al. described a type of intraventricular block that could lead to sudden death and that required urgent pacemaker implantation. Several consecutive ECGs showed RBBB and anterosuperior block, alternating with RBBB with posteroinferior hemiblock (Rosenbaum *et al.* 1968) (see Figure 11.56). This diagnosis, which usually has evident clinical characteristics (dizziness, near-syncope, etc.), is named **Rosenbaum–Elizari syndrome** (Bayés de Luna and Baranchuk 2017). **Pacemaker implantation is indicated** and improves patient's outcome. In the absence of advanced underlying heart disease, the prognosis can be excellent.

Alternating bundle branch block

In this case, the ECG alternatively shows LBBB and RBBB pattern, with or without associated hemiblocks, in the same patient (see Figure 11.49).

In most cases, the patient presents with symptoms (dizziness, syncope), and it is necessary to implant a pacemaker as soon as possible because of the potential risk of complete AV block and sudden death. After pacemaker implantation, patients may have a good prognosis in the long-term follow-up when the block is due mainly to the involvement of the specific conduction system and there is no structural heart disease.

Advanced atrioventricular block

Obviously, the **presence of an acquired AV block requires pacemaker implantation in most cases**. There may be exceptions, such as cases of AV block due to a reversible cause (ischemia, toxic substances, drugs, sarcoidosis, Lyme carditis, etc.) (Yeung and Baranchuk 2019).

The implantation of a pacemaker for congenital AV blocks is a questionable procedure. This condition is already present at birth, often related to a systemic disease of the mother during pregnancy (presence of Ro/SS-A and La/SS-B antinuclear antibodies in the mother's blood), which results in fetal myocarditis involving the specific conduction system. Using fetal kinetocardiography, it has been demonstrated (Rein *et al.* 2009) that 10% of fetuses whose mothers carried these antibodies experienced first-degree AV block at 20–30 weeks' gestation. When dexamethasone was prescribed, AV conduction was normalized and the infant showed no AV block or evidence of heart disease at birth. This type of AV block has sometimes been found in different members of the same family, although its genetic origin has not been demonstrated to date.

Immune-mediated cardiomyopathy has been recognized in infants born of mothers with antinuclear antibodies. The natural history of patients with isolated congenital AV block that requires pacing depends on their antibody status. If it is positive, it has been demonstrated that it is a predictor of HF and death. The cases with negative antibody status in a long follow-up have a survival free of new HF after pacemaker implant (Sagar *et al.* 2010).

Patients with advanced congenital AV block have a certain risk of sudden death. Although it is difficult to decide the best moment to implant a pacemaker, the tendency is to recommend pacemaker implantation even in the absence of symptoms if the escape rhythm is very slow (Friedman 1995).

Pacemaker implantation is usually not indicated during childhood: (i) if the baseline rate is ≥50 bpm with a narrow escape rhythm, (ii) if the nighttime rate (Holter recording) is never < 30–35 bpm with a mean 24-hour ventricular rate > 45–50 bpm, (iii) if the heart rate during an exercise test is > 100 bpm, (iv) if there is no lengthening of the QT interval, and (v) if there are no important ventricular arrhythmias (see Figure 17.15). If the previously mentioned parameters worsen during follow-up, or if the patient becomes symptomatic, pacemaker implantation is recommended (Figure 24.6).

The presence of ventricular arrhythmias in chronic heart disease patients

The presence of premature ventricular complexes (PVCs) in the surface ECG in patients with chronic heart disease, especially ischemic heart disease, indicates that probably they are occurring frequently. In this case, Holter recordings (or event monitors) and exercise testing to establish their characteristics is recommended. In fact, the presence of any PVC in a routine 10 sec ECG in patients with

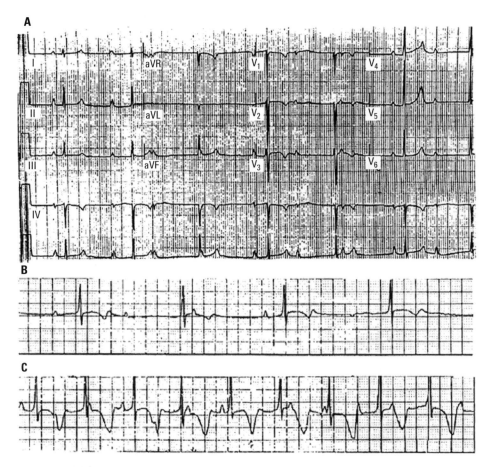

Figure 24.6 A 12-year-old child with congenital complete atrioventricular (AV) block and no heart disease in whom the following findings were observed. (A) At rest, the heart rate, which was always greater than 60 bpm, now decreased to 45 bpm; (C) during the exercise stress testing, it did not exceed 80 bpm; and (B) at night (Holter), it frequently decreased to <35 bpm. These findings, along with the occurrence of exercise dyspnea, suggest pacemaker implantation.

moderate HF is a powerful predictor of cardiovascular mortality (Van Lee *et al*. 2010).

PVC morphology may sometimes suggest the presence of necrosis (QR pattern, for example) (see Chapter 15, Premature ventricular complexes). It may even be more sensitive than sinus QRS complexes (ST depression) in detecting ischemia (Rasouli and Ellestad 2001) (see Figure 20.33). More recently, a comprehensive algorithm to detect the origin of idiopathic PVCs was published (Enriquez *et al*. 2019). The sensitivity and specificity of this algorithm needs to be tested.

PVCs associated with poor prognosis include:
• PVCs occurring in patients with acute ischemia, specifically those depicting R/T phenomenon, as they may trigger ventricular fibrillation (VF) (see Figure 16.31);
• PVCs occurring frequently or repetitively, especially in the presence of advanced heart disease and poor ventricular function mainly in post-infarction patients, as they may lead to sustained ventricular tachycardia (VT) and sudden death (see Figure 16.34A);

• PVCs with a "q" (QR especially with symmetrical T-wave), which are more often found in patients with associated necrosis and/or a low ejection fraction (dilated cardiomyopathy) and, therefore, have a poor prognosis (see Figure 16.6);
• very wide and notched PVCs >40 ms (see Figure 16.6);
• PVCs that may show more marked repolarization alterations (ST depression) indicative of ischemia during an exercise testing when compared with QRS complexes of the sinus rhythm (see Figure 20.33) (Rasouli and Ellestad 2001) (see above).

Sustained VT in patients with heart disease is associated with bad outcomes. In cases showing a low ejection fraction and in patients with inherited heart diseases (see Chapters 21 and 22), ICD therapy is usually advisable (Bayés de Luna and Baranchuk 2017). The cases of sustained VT in patients without apparent heart disease, if repetitive, must also be considered serious cases. New episodes should be first prevented either with pharmacologic treatment or ablation (Bayés de Luna and Baranchuk 2017).

Acquired long QT (see Chapters 7 and 19)

Acquired long QT interval is more frequent than congenital long QT syndrome. Frequently, there is an evident cause, but a genetic predisposition may also exist. Acquired long QT syndrome usually shows a heterogeneous repolarization dispersion, as does congenital long QT syndrome (see Figure 14.19), which is the triggering factor of torsades de pointes VT/VF. However, on certain occasions, such as with amiodarone administration, the prolongation of repolarization is homogeneous and the long QT is not associated with a potential risk of arrhythmias.

Table 24.1 shows the most important predisposing factors for long QT syndrome, including other ECG alterations, which may foster VT/VF. The ECG premonitory signs of TP/VF have already been described. They occur in patients with bradyarrhythmia, usually with an ionic imbalance and/or the administration of some drugs (Drew *et al.* 2010; Digby *et al.* 2011) (Chapter 16, Polymorphic ventricular tachycardia: Torsades de pointes).

The TP/VF may be seen in different inherited (hypertrophic cardiomyopathy, channelopathies, etc.), and acquired (dilated cardiomyopathy, ischemic heart disease, and others) heart diseases, and also as a consequence of septic, toxic, or metabolic shock or associated significant ionic imbalance, and after the administration of certain drugs that may induce abnormal lengthening of QT (see Table 24.2). The risk of developing TP/VF is evident when drugs lengthen the QT interval >60 ms and/or QTc is >500 ms. A QT lengthening >30 ms is already considered pathologic.

In most of these cases, long QT syndrome is due to the inhibition of the K currents (I_{kr}', I_{ks}) by drugs, leading to repolarization delay. This may explain some cases of sudden death. Torsades de pointes in a drug-induced long QT syndrome usually takes place after the occurrence of a premature complex, followed by a long pause, which is similar to what happens in the LQT2 syndrome (Kirchhof *et al.* 2009; Drew *et al.* 2010) (see Chapter 21, Long QT syndrome).

Table 24.1 Predisposing factors for QT interval prolongation

- Heart disease: Ischemic heart disease, heart failure, etc.
- ECG alterations: baseline prolonged QT, abnormal U wave, T-wave alternans, deep and negative T-wave, significant bradycardia
- Acute neurological accidents
- Ionic and metabolic alterations: diabetes, anorexia, hypoglycemia, hypothyroidism, obesity
- Septic shock
- Female sex
- Advanced age
- Hypothermia
- Intoxications

Table 24.2 Drugs associated with QT prolongation and potential arrhythmogenic risk (for more details, please consult www.qtdrugs.org)

Antiarrhythmic drugs:	Generally, types I and III. Also recently studied drugs (azimilide, ibutilide). Propafenone is probably less risky, in the absence of heart failure. A drug with less antiarrhythmic effect, despite the fact it significantly prolongs the QT interval, is amiodarone and dronadorone (see text) Type II and IV drugs are safe
Macrolide antibiotics:	Azithromycin, clarithromycin, erythromycin
Fluoroquinolones:	Ciprofloxacin, levofloxacin, etc.
Antidepressants:	Amitriptyline, disopyramide, fluoxetine, imipramine, paroxetine, etc.
Antipsychotics:	Haloperidol, risperidone
Antihistaminics:	Terfenadine (withdrawn)
Digestive tract:	Cisapride (withdrawn)

Due to the potential risk that certain drugs may lengthen the QT interval and initiate arrhythmias such as torsades de pointes, drug agencies (FDA, EMEA) now carefully examine each new drug's potential to increase dispersion of repolarization, especially when it concerns the effect on HERG channels (i.e. QT interval). Cases of sudden death that occurred with two apparently harmless drugs (cisapride and terfenadine) are especially relevant. As already mentioned, Table 24.2 shows some of the drugs that most frequently prolong the QT interval and which have been shown to cause torsades de pointes VT. Monitoring of the QT interval, and particularly when drugs that prolong cardiac repolarization are been used, was of utmost importance during the COVID-19 pandemic (Zaidel *et al.* 2020).

The CAST trial (Echt *et al.* 1991), which assessed the efficacy of different antiarrhythmic drugs (including flecainide and quinidine) for the prevention of post-infarction sudden death, had to be stopped because more cases of sudden death were observed in the active treatment group than in the control group. Meanwhile, the majority of the new antiarrhythmic agents studied (azimilide, dofetilide, and ibutilide and recently dronedarone) are not widely used due to the associated side effects, especially the risk of VT/VF and/ or depression of LV function, hepathotoxicity (dronadorone), etc. In this sense, amiodarone is the safest pharmacologic treatment to prevent VT/VF recurrences. More information on this subject may be obtained at www.qtdrugs.org.

The use of a long QT interval as a marker of poor prognosis in post-infarction patients is controversial, although more results supporting this hypothesis have been published (Schwartz and Wolf 1978). It has been reported (Chugh *et al.* 2009) that an abnormally long QT increases the risk of sudden death fivefold in chronic ischemic heart disease patients.

We have also reported that post-infarction patients showing QT peaks > 500 ms in a Holter recording have a poor prognosis (Homs *et al.* 1997).

In all these cases, the QT interval, although long, does not reach the values observed in congenital long QT interval syndrome, nor those related with certain significant ionic or metabolic alterations, such as septic shock (Figure 24.7). Furthermore, other repolarization alterations (i.e. abnormal or alternating T-wave morphology) that may exist in congenital long QT are usually not found in cases of acquired long QT (Kirchhof *et al.* 2009) (see Figure 21.10 and Tables 21.4–21.6).

Electrical alternans (see Table 18.1 and Figure 18.9)

Concept

This is characterized by a beat-to-beat alternans of the QRS complex morphology on an every-other-beat basis. Electrical alternans occurs when the changes of QRS–T are due to myocardial intrinsic changes, or at least are not explained by periodic changes in ventricular activation, or they are not due to a coincidence with the periodic presence of some arrhythmia. The latter may refer to pseudo-alternans (see Table 18.1).

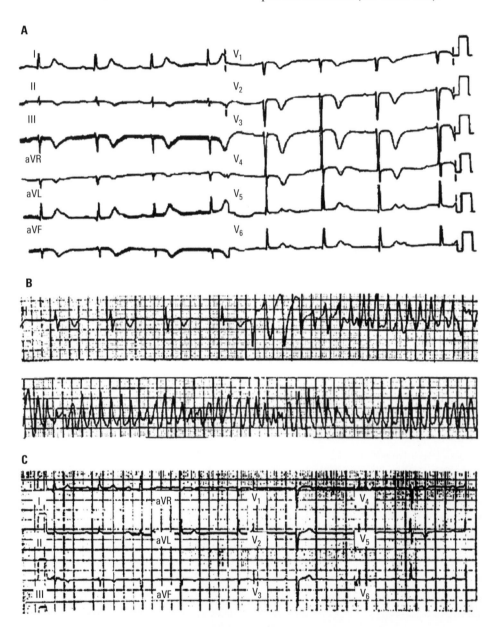

Figure 24.7 A 58-year-old patient hospitalized in an intensive care unit due to sepsis with a very pathologic ECG (A) with a long QT interval and deep negative T wave in anterior and inferior leads. The coronarography showed a normal pattern, whereas the ionogram showed hypokalemia and hypomagnesemia. The patient also showed runs of torsades de pointes ventricular tachycardia (VT), which led to ventricular fibrillation (VF) (B). Once the clinical and ionic alterations were solved, the QT interval was normalized and the ECG showed only a flat and somewhat negative T wave in inferior leads and in V4–V6 (C).

QRS alternans

We have already discussed (see Chapter 18, QRS-T complexes of variable morphology) that **QRS electrical alternans** may be seen in sinus rhythm in cases of cardiac tamponade and during a narrow AV junctional reentrant tachycardia with an accessory pathway. Cases that may be considered pseudo-alternans are: (i) bigeminal PVC in the PR interval, (ii) alternans pre-excitation, and (iii) alternans bundle branch block.

Repolarization alternans

Cases of **repolarization electrical alternans** are associated with a higher risk of developing VT/VF. It has been suggested that microscopic T wave alternans is a risk marker of sudden death in post-infarction patients (Rosenbaum *et al.* 1994; Nieminen and Verrier 2010), and in other situations. Here, we will refer to the cases in which these electrical alternans are visible in the surface ECG. In our experience, there are three well-defined clinical situations that show evident ST/T alternans in the surface ECG accompanied by VT/VF:

- T-wave alternans sometimes precede a torsades de pointes VT episode in patients with long QT syndrome (see Figure 18.7C);
- T-wave alternans associated with an acquired long QT, as observed in cases of shock and/or significant ionic disorders (see Figure 18.7D);
- ST/T alternans indicative of severe and hyperacute ischemia, as observed in cases of acute coronary syndrome involving a large ischemic area and also in cases of severe coronary spasm of a proximal artery (see Figure 18.7B).

New ECG patterns of risk for sudden death

Early repolarization pattern

The early repolarization (ER) pattern was defined as a positive and sharp notch (J wave) or slur at the end of QRS/beginning of the ST segment, with some elevation of ST (Miyazaki *et al.* 2010). Tikkanen *et al.* (2009) also include all cases of J point elevation (>1–2 mm) that were either a notched (clear positive J deflection inscribed on the S wave–typical early repolarization pattern) or a "slurred" pattern in at least two consecutive leads, in the concept of early repolarization pattern.

The typical early repolarization pattern occurs in 2% of population without acute disease and is usually seen at the end of the positive QRS complex, especially in mid-left precordial leads, but may also be seen in inferior (II, III, aVF) and lateral (V5, V6, I, aVL) leads. Sometimes the J-wave and slurs may be seen without ST-segment elevation and have been considered part of QRS complex (late depolarization not early repolarization). Therefore, recently Surawicz and Macfarlane (2011) considered that

the early repolarization term is not the most appropriate to describe this notch or deflection at the end of QRS.

It has been postulated that the mechanism of the early repolarization pattern occurs at the beginning of repolarization process, and is the consequence of a transient dominant I_{to} current. When compared with the Brugada syndrome, however, this I_{to} current is not accompanied by a decrease in an inward Na current, and occurs in all myocardium, not only in the RV. The J wave of hypothermia has similar origin but is of a higher intensity. It has been reported that some transient early I_{to} currents may participate in the genesis of ST-segment elevation in cases of STEMI, and in the triggering of VF in acute myocardial ischemia (Yan *et al.* 2004).

The first case study demonstrating that early repolarization pattern (J point elevation or J wave >1 mm, especially in inferior leads) has a higher prevalence among patients with a history of idiopathic VF was published by Haïssaguerre and colleagues in 2008 (Haïssaguerre *et al.* 2008). The subjects were mostly men with a mean age of 35 years. Characteristically, PVC origin was concordant with the location of the J-wave (usually J-waves in inferior leads and PVCs with negative QRS in the same leads), and usually a clear accentuation of early repolarization pattern (J-wave) appeared before the final event (Figure 24.8). Similar results were obtained by Rosso *et al.* (2008) and Merchant *et al.* (2009).

More recently (Tikkanen *et al.* 2009), the prognostic significance of the early repolarization pattern (J point elevation) in the general population has been studied. It has been shown that an early repolarization pattern in inferior leads, especially if ≥2 mm, is associated with risk of death from cardiac causes ($P < 0.001$) and from arrhythmias ($P < 0.01$) in middle-aged subjects (mean age 45 years). However, the absolute risk of death is very small in cases with a J point < 2 mm. Death from cardiac causes occurs late after the baseline ECG. The survival curves started to diverge 15 years after the first ECG, whereas in primary VF studies, this is most commonly observed in younger patients. It is possible that the early repolarization pattern increases vulnerability to fatal arrhythmia in the presence of acute ischemic attack, which is the first cause of death at this age in the Finnish population (Tikkanen *et al.* 2009). It has recently been suggested (see above) that in early acute STEMI, phase 2 reentry caused by loss of dome of epicardial transmembrane action potential is related to the transient outward potassium current (I_{to}) that occurs during ischemia and can produce an R-on-T PVC, triggering VF (Yan *et al.* 2004).

Antzelevitch and Yan (2010) **include early repolarization patterns in the term "J-wave syndromes."** This term encompasses all syndromes related to an abnormal J-wave: inherited (Brugada syndrome and three types of early repolarization syndromes) and acquired (ischemia-mediated VT/VF and hypothermia-mediated VT/VF).

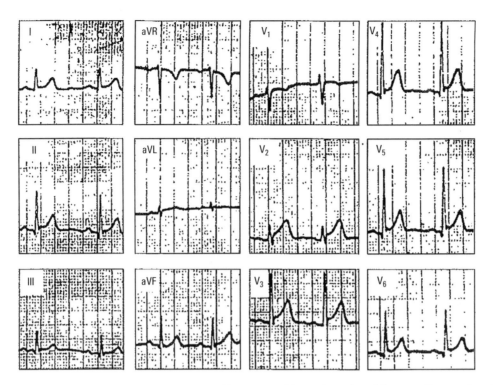

Figure 24.8 Example of an early repolarization pattern in a healthy 40-year-old man. Note the mild pattern (J wave < 1 mm), seen particularly in the intermediate left precordial leads. This corresponds to a benign pattern. Early repolarization pattern seen especially in inferior leads with a J point of ≥ 2 mm corresponds to a dangerous pattern (see Figure 7.15).

Table 24.3 J wave syndromes: similarities and differences

	Inherited ER pattern I	ER pattern II	ER pattern III[a]	Brugada syndrome	Acquired Ischemia-mediated VT/VF	Hypothermia-mediated VT/VF
Leads displaying J point/J wave abnormalities	I, V4–V6		Inferior and sometimes inferolateral leads Global	V1–V3	Any of the 12 leads	N/A
Anatomic location of ECG alterations	Anterolateral left ventricle	Inferior LV	Left and right ventricles	Right ventricle	L and R ventricles	L and R ventricles
Possibility of VF	In marginal Cases Commonly seen in healthy men and athletes	Higher risk especially in some cases (see text)	Yes Probably Brugada variant	Yes	Yes	Yes

[a]According to some data reported in Antzelevitch paper, these cases may correspond to a variant of Brugada syndrome.

ER: early repolarization; VF: ventricular fibrillation; VT: ventricular tachycardia.

Adapted from Antzelevitch and Yan (2010).

The early repolarization pattern and the Brugada syndrome may be related to the dominant and transient outward potassium current I_{to}. Table 24.3 summarizes the most important clinical differences between all these syndromes according to the Antzelevitch hypothesis. At first glance, it would seem that the early type III repolarization patterns of this table represent a variant of Brugada syndrome, and that type II patterns may be also considered dangerous, especially if appearing in inferior leads and J point > 2 mm and/or the amplitude changes abruptly. More information is needed to draw specific conclusions about risk when looking at an ECG with an early repolarization pattern. What we need to do is: (i) to check the voltage and location of the pattern and also if the pattern is fixed or changes abruptly, (ii) to know the family history, including personal antecedents of syncope or severe arrhythmia, and (iii) to be sure about the technical aspects of the ECG recording. It is surprising, for example, that

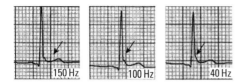

Figure 24.9 A 40-year-old man with a typical early repolarization pattern with small J wave. It should be noted that the low-pass filter at 40 Hz may cause it to disappear.

the early repolarization pattern virtually disappears when a 40 Hz low-pass filter is used (García-Niebla *et al.* 2009) (Figure 24.9).

At present, epidemiologic evidence suggests that the presence of an early repolarization pattern in young adults without family history of sudden death increases the risk of VF from 4.5/100 000 to 11/100 000 (Rosso *et al.* 2008). This is a negligible difference. Therefore, the incidental finding of an ER pattern (J-wave) during screening without the specific signs already shown (see before) should not be interpreted as a marker of increased risk. This is reassuring information, both for physicians and patients. This benign prognosis of concave upward ST elevation with J wave or slurring in asymptomatic ambulatory population has been recently strongly reasserted (Uberoi *et al.* 2011). A position paper (Macfarlane *et al.* 2015) summarizes all aspects of the early repolarization pattern, and we strongly recommend its lecture for a comprehensive understanding of this fascinating ECG manifestation.

Other ECG patterns

It has also been suggested that a tall and narrow QRS complex with a certain degree of repolarization alteration that is generally non-significant could be a marker of sudden death (Wolpert *et al.* 2008) (Figure 24.10). This possible association requires further investigation.

Finally, Aizawa *et al.* (1993) described the occurrence of idiopathic VF in patients with bradycardia-dependent intraventricular block, and Iturralde *et al.* (2008) also show the association between intraventricular blocks and VT in children (see Chapter 21, Other possible channelopathies).

Risk of serious arrhythmias and sudden death in patients with normal or nearly normal ECG

It is important to emphasize that a normal ECG does not exclude the presence of advanced heart disease or the risk of sudden death. On the one hand, we see the possible existence of an undiagnosed channelopathy or an idiopathic VF, as already discussed. On the other hand, it is not possible to know when a heart disease patient with a normal ECG will show a significant electrical instability

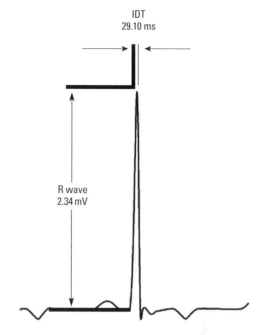

Figure 24.10 High-voltage QRS complex with abrupt peak of R wave. IDT: intrinsicoid deflection time (Wolpert *et al.* 2008).

leading to a high risk of sudden death. This is due to a combination of factors. The ECG does not allow us to determine when a patient has a vulnerable plaque likely to break and trigger an acute coronary syndrome, or when a subtle repolarization abnormality may represent a real danger in an asymptomatic patient. These cases show the limitations of ECG. We should, however, remember that we can get a great deal of information from the ECG if we are able to identify subtle alterations, such as flat or a not-very-deep negative T wave in leads V1 to V3–V4, which, although not posing a risk by itself, may be significant, especially if compared with previous ECGs.

We would also like to emphasize that in the presence of precordial chest pain, normal or nearly normal ECGs, or an unchanged ECG (compared with previous ECGs), should not lead us to rule out the presence of an acute coronary syndrome. The changes may be minor and go unnoticed (see Figure 20.15). For this reason, successive ECG recordings are necessary to carefully evaluate how the apparently normal morphologies evolve, especially the tall T-waves in leads V1–V2, as they may be the manifestation of a hyperacute phase of an acute coronary syndrome, eventually evolving into an infarction with ST elevation and a pathologic Q wave (STEMI), triggering VF.

Patients with a normal ECG may also suffer from other conditions (aortic rupture, pulmonary embolism, etc.), which may lead to sudden death (Bayés de Luna and Baranchuk 2017).

To summarize, (i) **apparently normal ECGs may,** in fact, demonstrate the presence of potentially dangerous pathologies (long or short QT syndrome, spongiform myocardiopathy, Brugada syndrome, early repolarization, etc.), and (ii) **the correlation of the clinical data with previous ECGs, as well as a detailed analysis of family history, will help to determine the significance of apparently normal ECG morphologies**. The presence of a **wide and high T-wave in leads V1–V2**, especially if the ST-segment is rectilinear or slightly depressed, could be a manifestation of the hyperacute phase of an acute coronary syndrome. Thus, the interpretation of the ECG, taking into account the clinical setting, is very important (see above).

References

Aizawa Y, Tamura M, Chinushi M, *et al*. Idiopathic ventricular fibrillation and bradycardia-dependent intraventricular block. Am Heart J 1993;126:1473.

Andersen HR, Nielsen JC, Thomsen PE, *et al*. Atrioventricular conduction during long-term follow-up of patients with sick sinus syndrome. Circulation 1998;98(13):1315–1321.

Antzelevitch C, Yan GX. J wave syndromes. Heart Rhythm 2010;7:549.

Baldasseroni S, De Biase L, Fresco C, *et al*. Cumulative effect of complete left bundle-branch block and chronic atrial fibrillation on 1-year mortality and hospitalization in patients with congestive heart failure. A report from the Italian network on congestive heart failure. A report from the Italian network on congestive heart failure (in-CHF database). Eur Heart J 2002;23:1692.

Baranchuk A, Conde D, Enriquez A, Bayés de Luna A. P-wave duration or P-wave morphology? Interatrial Block: seeking for the Holy Grail to predict AF recurrence. Ann Noninv Electrocardiol 2014;19(4):406–408.

Bayés de Luna A, Baranchuk A. *Clinical Arrhythmology*. 2nd edn, Wiley-Blackwell, UK, 2017.

Bayés de Luna A, Fort de Ribot R, Trilla E. Electrocardiographic and vectorcardiographic study of interatrial conduction disturbances with left atrial retrograde activation. J Electrocardiol 1985;18:1.

Bayés de Luna A, Cladellas M, Oter R, *et al*. Interatrial conduction block and retrograde activation of the left atrium and paroxysmal supraventricular tachyarrhythmia. Eur Heart J 1988;9:1112.

Bayés de Luna A, Cladellas M, Oter R, *et al*. Interatrial conduction block with retrograde activation of the left atrium and paroxysmal supraventricular tachyarrhythmias: influence of preventive antiarrhythmic treatment. Int J Cardiol 1989;22:147.

Bayés de Luna A, Guindo J, Viñolas X, *et al*. Third-degree interatrial block and supraventricular tachyarrhythmias. Europace 1999;1:43.

Bayés de Luna A, Platonov PG, García-Niebla J, Baranchuk A. Atypical advanced interatrial block or junctional rhythm? J Electrocardiol 2019;5:85–86.

Bogale N, Orn S, James M, *et al*. Usefulness of either or both left and right bundle branch block at baseline or during follow-up for predicting death in patients following acute myocardial infarction. Am J Cardiol 2007;99:647.

Chugh SS, Reinier K, Singh T, *et al*. Determinants of prolonged QT interval and their contribution to sudden death risk in coronary artery disease: the Oregon Sudden Unexpected Death Study. Circulation 2009;119:663.

Conde D, Baranchuk A. Interatrial block as anatomical-electrical substrate for supraventricular arrhythmias: Bayes´ Syndrome. Arch Mex Cardiol 2014;84(1):32–40.

Daubert J. IJC Atrial flutter and interatrial conduction block. In Waldo A, Touboul P (eds). *Atrial Flutter: Advances in Mechanisms and Management*. Futura Publishing Co 1996, p. 331.

Digby G, Pérez Riera AR, Barbosa Barros R, *et al*. Acquired long QT interval: a case series of multifactorial QT prolongation. Clin Cardiol 2011;9(34):577–582.

Digby GC, Kukla P, Zhan Q, *et al*. The value of Electrocardiographic Abnormalities in the Prognosis of Pulmonary Embolism: a consensus paper. Ann Noninv Electrocardiol 2015;20(3):207–223.

Drew BJ, Ackerman MJ, Funk M, *et al*. on behalf of the American Heart Association Acute Cardiac Care Committee of the Council on Clinical Cardiology, the Council on Cardiovascular Nursing, and the American College of Cardiology Foundation. Prevention of Torsade de Pointes in Hospital Settings: A Scientific Statement. Circulation 2010;121:1047.

Echt DS, Liebson PR, Mitchell LB, *et al*. Mortality and morbidity in patients receiving encainide, flecainide, or placebo. The Cardiac Arrhythmia Suppression Trial. N Engl J Med 1991;324:781.

Elizari MV, Baranchuk A, Chiale PA. Masquerading Bundle Branch Block: a Variety of Right Bundle Branch Block with Left Anterior Fascicular Block. Expert Rev Cardiovasc Ther 2013;11(1):69–75.

Enriquez A, Baranchuk A, Briceno D, Saenz L, Garcia F. How to use the 12-lead ECG to predict the site of origin of idiopathic ventricular arrhythmias. Heart Rhythm 2019;16(10):1538–1544.

Fiol-Sala M, Birnbaum Y, Nikus K, Bayés de Luna A. *Electrocardiography in Ischemic Heart Disease. Clinical and Imaging Correlations and Prognostic Implications*. 2nd edn. Willey-Blackwell, 2020.

Friedman RA. Congenital AV block. Pace me now or pace me later? Circulation 1995;92:283.

García-Moll X, Guindo J, Vinolas X, *et al*. Intermittent masked bifascicular block. Am Heart J 1994;127:214.

García-Niebla J, Llontop-García P, Valle-Racero JI, *et al*. Technical mistakes during the acquisition of the electrocardiogram. Ann Noninvasive Electrocardiol 2009;14:389.

Haïssaguerre M, Derval N, Sacher F, *et al*. Sudden cardiac arrest associated with early repolarization. N Engl J Med 2008;358:2016.

Herrera C, Bruña V, Abizanda P, *et al*. Relation of interatrial block to cognitive impairment in patients ≥70 years of age (from the CAMBIAD case-control study). Am J Cardiol 2020;136:94–99.

Homs E, Marti V, Guindo J, *et al*. Automatic measurement of corrected QT interval in Holter recordings: comparison of its dynamic behavior in patients after myocardial infarction with and without life-threatening arrhythmias. Am Heart J 1997;134:181.

Iturralde P, Nava S, Gómez J, *et al*. Association of congenital, diffuse electrical disease in children with normal heart sick sinus syndrome intraventricular conduction block and monomorphic ventricular tachycardia. J Cardiovasc Electrophysiol 2008;5:550.

Kirchhof P, Franz MR, Bardai A, *et al*. Giant T-U waves precede torsades de pointes in long QT syndrome: a systematic electrocardiographic analysis in patients with acquired and congenital QT prolongation. J Am Coll Cardiol 2009;54:143.

Krahn AD, Morillo CA, Kus T, *et al.* Empiric pacemaker compared with a monitoring strategy in patients with syncope and bifascicular conduction block--rationale and design of the Syncope: Pacing or Recording in the Later Years (SPRITELY) study. Europace 2012;14(7):1044–1048.

Kukla P, Baranchuk A, Jastrzębski M, Bryniarski L. Masquerading bundle branch block. Kardiol Pol 2014;72(1):67–69.

Macfarlane PW, Antzelevitch C, Haissaguerre M, *et al.* The Early Repolarization Pattern: a Consensus Paper. J Am Coll Cardiol 2015;66(4):470–477.

Martínez-Sellés M, Elosua R, Ibarrola M, *et al.* for the BAYES Registry Investigators. Advanced interatrial block and P-wave duration are associated with atrial fibrillation and stroke in older adults with heart disease: the BAYES registry. Europace 2020a;22:1001–1008.

Martínez-Sellés M, Martínez-Larrú E, Ibarrola M, *et al.* Interatrial block and cognitive impairment in the BAYES prospective registry. Int J Cardiol 2020b;321:95–98.

Merchant F. Reddy V, *et al.* Ability of terminal QRS notching to distinguish benign for malignant ECG forms of early repolarization. Am J Cardiol 2009:104;1402.

Miyazaki S, Shah AJ, Haïssaguerre M. Early repolarization syndrome - a new electrical disorder associated with sudden cardiac death. Circ J 2010;74(10):2039–2044.

Nieminen T, Verrier RL. Usefulness of T-wave alternans in sudden death risk stratification and guiding medical therapy. Ann Noninvasive Electrocardiol 2010;15:276.

Nof E, Luria D, Brass D, *et al.* Point mutation in the HCN4 cardiac ion channel pore affecting synthesis, trafficking, and functional expression is associated with familial asymptomatic sinus bradycardia. Circulation 2007;116:463.

Qaddoura A, Digby G, Kabali C, Kukla P, Zhan ZQ, Baranchuk A. The Value of Electrocardiography in Prognosticating Clinical Deterioration and Mortality in Acute Pulmonary Embolism: a Systematic Review and Meta-analysis. Clin Cardiol 2017;40(10):814–824.

Rasouli ML, Ellestad MH. Usefulness of ST depression in ventricular premature complexes to predict myocardial ischemia. Am J Cardiol 2001;87:891.

Rein AJ, Mevorach D, Perles Z, *et al.* Early diagnosis and treatment of atrioventricular block in the fetus exposed to maternal anti-SSA/Ro-SSB/La antibodies: a prospective, observational, fetal kinetocardiogram-based study. Circulation 2009;119:1867.

Rosenbaum M, Eelizari M, Lazzari J. *The Hemiblocks.* Editorial Paidos, 1968.

Rosenbaum DS, Jackson LE, Smith JM, *et al.* Electrical alternans and vulnerability to ventricular arrhythmias. N Engl J Med 1994;330:235.

Rosso R, Kogan E, Belhassen B, *et al.* J-point elevation in survivors of primary ventricular fibrillation and matched control subjects: incidence and clinical significance. J Am Coll Cardiol 2008;52:1231.

Sagar S, Shen WK, Asirvatham SJ, *et al.* Effect of long-term right ventricular pacing in young adults with structurally normal heart. Circulation 2010;121:1698.

Schwartz PJ, Wolf S. QT interval prolongation as predictor of sudden death in patients with myocardial infarction. Circulation 1978;57:1074.

Surawicz B, Macfarlane P. Inappropriate and confusing electrocardiographic terms. J-wve syndromes and early repolarization. J Am Coll Cardiol 2011;57:1584.

Tikkanen JT, Anttonen O, Juntila MJ, *et al.* Long-term outcome associated with early repolarization on electrocardiography. N Engl J Med 2009;361:2529.

Uberoi A, Jain N, Perez M, *et al.* Early repolarization in an ambulatory clinical population. Circulation 2011;124:2208.

Van Bommel RJ, Marsan NA, Delgado V, *et al.* Value of the surface electrocardiogram in detecting right ventricular dilatation in the presence of left bundle branch block. Am J Cardiol 2011;107(5):736–740.

Van Lee V, Mitiku T, Hadley D, *et al.* Rest premature ventricular contractions on routine ECG and prognosis in heart failure patients. Ann Noninvasive Electrocardiol 2010;15:56.

Vázquez R, Bayés-Genis A, Cygankiewicz I, *et al.* The MUSIC risk score: a simple method for predicting mortality in ambulatory patients with chronic heart failure. Eur Heart J 2009;30:1088.

Wellens HJJ, Gorgels A, Doevedans P. *The ECG in Acute Myocardial Infarction and Unstable Angina.* Kluwer Academic Press, 2003.

Wolpert C, Veltmann C, Schimpf R, *et al.* Is a narrow and tall QRS complex and ECG marker for sudden death? Heart Rhythm 2008;5:1339.

Yan GX, Joshi A, Guo D, *et al.* Phase 2 reentry as a trigger to initiate ventricular fibrillation during early acute myocardial ischemia. Circulation 2004;110:1036.

Yeung C, Baranchuk A. Diagnosis and Treatment of Lyme Carditis. J Am Coll Cardiol 2019;73(6):717–726.

Zaidel EJ, Wyss Quintana FS, Sosa Liprandi A, *et al.* Hidroxicloroquina. Mensajes desde la Cardiología en tiempos de pandemia por Coronavirus. Rev Medicina 2020;80(3):271–274.

Chapter 25
Limitations of the Conventional ECG: Utility of Other Techniques

Introduction

Throughout this book, we have discussed the value of the conventional surface ECG for the diagnosis of heart diseases in different situations. We have emphasized the need for a comprehensive approach to diagnosis, to always perform the interpretation of the surface ECG in light of the patient's clinical setting. This approach is essential and sufficient in many cases, but in other circumstances, as demonstrated, it may not provide the necessary information for the correct diagnosis with the highest sensitivity, specificity, and overall predictive value. Furthermore, it is often not sufficient for risk stratification and for arriving at therapeutic decisions. For that, the use of other diagnostic techniques may be necessary. We will now make some comments about the importance of the clinical context for ECG interpretation, and later we will briefly describe the utility of other electrocardiologic techniques.

Interpretation of the surface ECG in light of the patient's clinical setting

As discussed throughout the text, the following examples illustrate the need to use information related to the patient's clinical setting for the interpretation of the ECG:
• The importance of premature ventricular impulses is strongly related to the patient's clinical characteristics (see Chapter 16).
• The correlation of the voltage of ECG complexes with left ventricular enlargement (LVE) is related to the presence of anatomic LVE according to Bayés' theorem and other characteristics (see Chapter 10).
• The various patterns of bundle branch block have various prognostic and diagnostic implications according the clinical setting (Chapters 11 and 20).
• For the differential diagnosis of a tachycardia with a wide QRS, the presence of underlying structural heart disease suggests the ventricular origin (see Chapter 16).

• The prognosis for a ventricular tachycardia is related more to the patient's clinical setting than the ECG morphology (see Chapter 16).
• With precordial chest pain, a normal ECG (or an ECG with minimal repolarization changes) does not exclude an ischemic origin (see Chapters 13 and 20).
• The importance of most repolarization changes (e.g. ST shifts/T wave inversion) should be evaluated in relation to the clinical setting. In the absence of underlying heart disease, they may be non-specific or unimportant. However, it is necessary to first rule out their relation to ischemic heart disease or other diseases (see Chapter 13).

The abnormal ECG in the absence of heart disease and patients with normal ECG and advance heart disease (Bayés de Luna et al. 2020a)

Patient with advanced heart disease and normal ECG

The ECG can be normal even just before the patient experiences sudden death. This can occur in the following circumstances:

1. Inherited heart disease. This can occur in some cases of hypertrophic cardiomyopathy, arrhythmogenic right ventricular dysplasia, and non-compaction cardiomyopathy. It is important to bear in mind that the morphology with r' in V1 can be normal, and also the presence of negative T in V1–V2 is frequently normal if it is asymmetric, but is usually abnormal if it is symmetric (Nunes de Alencar Neto *et al.* 2018).

2. The Brugada Syndrome. In some occasions, the r' in V1 may be considered normal. It is convenient is some cases to perform a flecainide test.

3. A accurate measurement of the QT interval must be made, especially in the case of a family history of short-long QT syndrome.

Clinical Electrocardiography: A Textbook, Fifth Edition. Antoni Bayés de Luna, Miquel Fiol-Sala, Antoni Bayés-Genís, and Adrián Baranchuk.
© 2022 John Wiley & Sons Ltd. Published 2022 by John Wiley & Sons Ltd.

4. Ischemic heart disease. An ECG may be normal just before sudden death from ventricular fibrillation or AV block appears in a patient with acute ischemic heart disease. Sometimes, the only ECG finding in a patient with ST-elevation ACS is the appearance of a tall and symmetric pointed T wave, especially in the right precordial leads (V1–V2).

5. Other clinical changes that may accompany severe arrhythmias and sudden death that present a normal ECG are: a) pulmonary embolism; b) rupture of an aortic aneurysm; and c) many patients with heart disease may have a normal ECG or with small changes. This is less frequent in patients with valvular or congenital heart disease.

Patients without heart disease and with abnormal ECG

a. Due to incorrect ECG recording, consequence of bad placement of electrodes or inappropriate filters.

b. Presence of Q waves that could be pathological, but are not, such as the abnormal Q wave in lead III that disappears with deep inspiration.

c. Athletes can present altered repolarization without evident pathology.

d. The alteration of repolarization that can be seen in electrolytes.

e. The presence of the high voltage of R can be seen without LV enlargement in athletes and other normal patients, especially with vertical heart.

f. The presence of r' can be seen in patients with heart disease, but also in normal people, especially if the electrode of V1 is located high.

g. Presence of atrial or ventricular arrhythmias that appear sporadically.

Additional value of other techniques

We will briefly discuss different techniques that may help us when the information derived from the clinical setting and conventional ECG are not sufficient to arrive at correct diagnosis, projecting the prognosis and/or developing a therapeutic approach in each case.

We will assume that the reader is familiar with the most important features of each technique. However, we will give now a brief discussion on the most widely used.

Unified interpretation of the ECG: computerized interpretation and the use of ECG classification systems

We made some comments about computerized ECG interpretation systems in Chapters 3 and 10. More information on that is beyond the scope of this book.

With regard to the ECG classification systems, the most widely known are the Minnesota Code (MC) (Figure 25.1) and the Nova code (Nova). Both are valuable and useful for clinical trials and epidemiological studies. For more information about computers and classification systems, please consult Macfarlane (2010).

Vectorcardiography (Figures 25.2 and 25.3)

Vectorcardiography (VCG) is a technique that records the cardiac electrical activity as closed loops: the atrial depolarization (P loop), ventricular depolarization (QRS loop), and ventricular repolarization (T loop) loops. VCG curves originate from X, Y, and Z leads (Figure 25.2A), which are three orthogonal leads that are perpendicular to each other. The X lead is right–left (similar to lead 1), Y is supero-inferior (similar to aVF), and Z is postero-anterior (similar to V2). These leads are generally recorded with the Frank system by means of different electrodes located on various points of the body. Inscription of the curves is done with a preamplifier system that magnifies the voltage of the currents coming from the heart through the lead systems, and a cathodic X-ray tube by which the vectorcardiographic curve is seen.

VCG machines interrupt the current every 5 ms, 2.5 ms, or 1 ms using an oscillator; the VCG continuous curves are thus divided into tears or comma-shaped fragments, the head of which represents the direction of the electri-

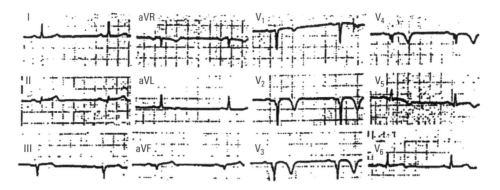

Figure 25.1 An ECG interpretation using the Minnesota Code: 1.1. 7 (sign of necrosis); 2.1, frontal plane axis −30°, 5.1, repolarization disorder; negative T wave; 8.8, sinus bradycardia. In this case, our interpretation would be: sinus bradycardia, old anteroseptal myocardial infarction with inferior extension, anterolateral subepicardial ischemia, and mild inferolateral subepicardial injury.

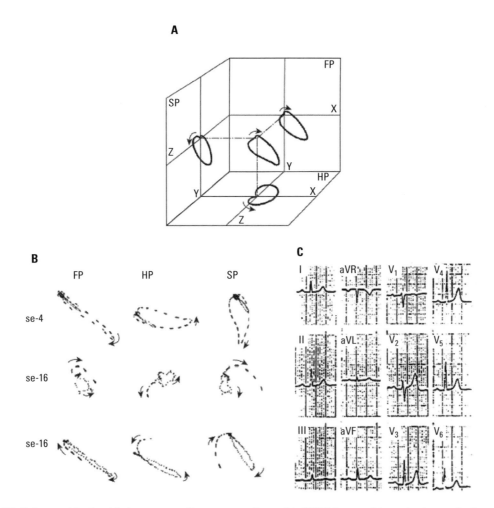

Figure 25.2 (A) Orthogonal leads with the corresponding vectorcardiographic (VCG) loop and its projection on the frontal, horizontal, and right sagittal planes. (B) Normal VCG corresponding to ECG of (C). At a sensitivity of 4, the P and T loops are poorly seen and the entire QRS loop is clearly visible (upper part of B). In the middle and lower panels of (B), the P and T loops with the respective onset and end of the QRS loop with amplified sensitivity may be seen.

cal current (Figure 25.2B). Figure 25.2C shows the ECG morphology that corresponds to the VCG of Figure 25.2B. We draw the loops as continuous lines when we use the VCG curves to aid in the comprehension of the ECG.

Characteristics of different loops
- **P loop**: The normal morphology, rotation, and orientation of the P loop are shown in Figure 25.3. This loop starts at point E and finishes at point O of the figure.
- **QRS loop**: This loop begins at point O and terminates at point J, where the T loop begins. The normal morphology, orientation and rotation of this loop are shown in Figure 25.3. The intermediate part is inscribed more rapidly. Three zones can be distinguished: the Q loop (initial vectors), R loop (intermediate vectors), and S loop (terminal vectors). The QRS loop has a centrifugal or efferent part, and a centripetal or afferent part.
- **T loop**: This loop extends from point J to point E. The centrifugal branch is inscribed more slowly. The loop is usually twice as long as it is wide. Figure 25.3 shows

the normal morphology, orientation, and rotation of the T loop on three planes.

Usefulness of vectorcardiography
Vectorcardiography is useful both as a clinical and teaching tool, especially for training in electrocardiography. Electrocardiography should be integrated with VCG, as described in this text; one should be able to deduce ECG morphology from the VCG curve, and vice versa.

Table 25.1 shows the classical usefulness of VCG (Benchimol *et al.* 1972). However, currently the clinical utility of vectorcardiography has progressively decreased, and as we have explained in Chapter 3 with the correlation of the morphology of the loops with the hemifields and ECG curves, most of the advantages of VCG loops may be found in the surface ECG. In recent years, the possible usefulness of spatial QRS–T angle for risk stratification and some other utilities of VCG have been described. However, the most important contribution of VCG nowadays is its use, as we have done in this book, for teaching purposes (see Chapter 3).

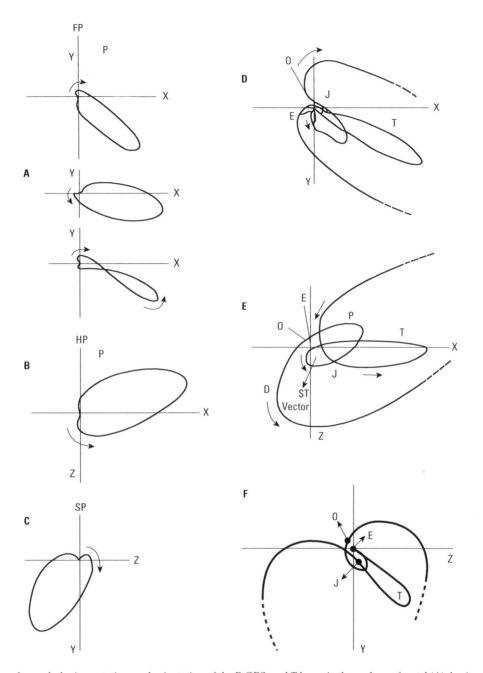

Figure 25.3 Normal morphologies, rotation, and orientation of the P, QRS, and T loops in three planes: frontal (A), horizontal (B), and sagittal (C). The QRS loop in the frontal plane may have clockwise rotation with an upward initiation (sometimes it forms a figure-of-eight) or, less often, counterclockwise rotation with an inferior onset. The latter is seen especially in obese subjects. EO = P loop; OJ = QRS loop; JE = T loop. The onset of the ST vector begins at point E, and the termination, at point J.

Table 25.1 Classical clinical usefulness of vectorcardiography (see text)

- To better study atrial activity, as the P loop may be amplified
- To confirm the presence of pre-excitation when it is not clear on the surface ECG
- For better evaluation of intraventricular conduction disorders and repolarization alterations
- For improved diagnosis of certain types of necrosis and the association of necrosis and left bundle branch block
- As a useful non-invasive tool (continuous VCG recording) for detecting effective reperfusion after thrombolytic treatment

Exercise testing (Figures 25.4 and 25.5)

Exercise is considered isotonic or dynamic when several muscle groups alternately contract and relax, as in running, and isometric or static, when few muscle groups contract for more prolonged periods against a fixed force, as in weightlifting. Isotonic exercise such as that on a bicycle or treadmill is the most appropriate form of exercise to assess cardiac functional capacity.

Exercise testing represents more than the establishment of ECG changes during exercise. Hemodynamic or metabolic (O_2 consumption, quantity of exercise, changes

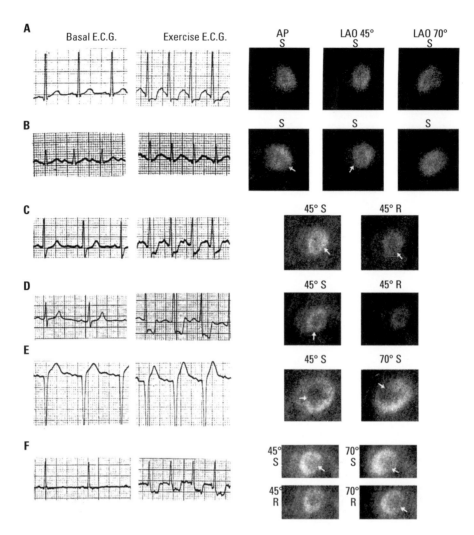

Figure 25.4 Six examples of exercise ECG–thallium scintigraphy correlation (S = exercise image, R = redistribution image). (A) Positive exercise testing in an asymptomatic patient with negative thallium and normal coronary angiography. (B) Patient with exercise angina, with a negative exercise test and stress images showing a mild defect in the lower septum, with complete redistribution. (C) A patient with an inferolateral infarction with a positive exercise test and exercise thallium image showing an inferolateral defect without redistribution. (D) Patient with angina, with a positive exercise test from V2 to V6 and 1, 11, VL, and thallium images showing an inferolateral defect with complete redistribution. (E) Patient with anterior myocardial infarction, without significant change in exercise testing. The thallium images show the existence of an anteroseptal defect without redistribution and marked dilatation of the left ventricle. (F) Patient with inferolateral myocardial infarction, with a positive exercise test in the lateral leads. Thallium images show an inferoposterolateral defect with only lateral redistribution (positive for inferoposterior necrosis and lateral ischemia).

in blood pressure, and heart rate, etc.) and clinica1 changes (presence of anginal pain, dyspnea, etc.) should also be evaluated.

Methodology

The bicycle and treadmill are equally useful for exercise testing. There is no ideal protocol, but the Bruce protocol is the most widely used (Table 25.2). The following general principles should be taken into account: (i) The intensity of exercise should be increased gradually, not suddenly. Increments are generally made at a minimal interval of 3 minutes. (ii) Patients should be monitored for symptoms (precordial pain, etc.), ECG changes, and hemodynamic changes (blood pressure and heart rate) during the exercise and for at least 6–8 minutes after the test. (iii) Exercise should not be stopped abruptly. Exercise capacity is described using the product of heart rate and blood pressure, which is the so-called double product.

A submaximal exercise test (85–90% of theoretical maximum heart rate for the patient's age and sex) is adequate for clinical purposes and is much easier to perform for patients with ischemic heart disease. Metabolic equivalents (METS) (multiples of basal metabolic requirements) are used to express the work performed at different stages of the exercise test. In patients with ischemic heart disease, a workload of 8 METS is usually sufficient to evaluate angina. Healthy sedentary individuals do not usually

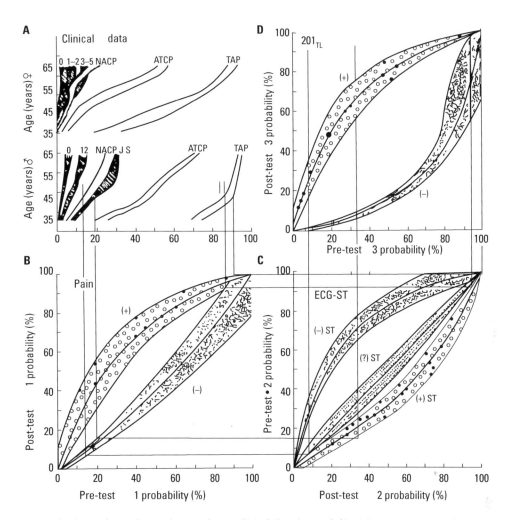

Figure 25.5 Diagnosis of ischemic heart disease by correlating clinical data (upper left) with exercise test results. Counterclockwise from the upper left, presence or absence of chest pain on the treadmill (lower left) (B); positive exercise ECG test with ST depression (ECG-ST) (lower right) (C); or positive thallium imaging (upper right) (D). Shaded curves indicate the mean (± standard deviation) for 96 patients. Different shaded curves represent positive (+) or negative (−) results; non-diagnostic ECG–ST results are shown by a question mark. For clinical data (upper left), the age and sex are shown on the vertical axis versus the probability of ischemic heart disease on the horizontal axis. Separate curves are shown according to the number of risk factors (0, 1–2, or 3–5) for asymptomatic patients (men and women). Symptomatic patients are classified as having no angina (NACP), atypical chest pain (ATCP), or typical angina pectoris (TAP). The post-test probability of ischemic heart disease according to each test becomes the pretest probability of the next test in sequence, moving counterclockwise. The lines represent the range of probabilities of ischemic heart disease (IHD) for two patients. Patient 1 is a 45-year-old man with no typical symptoms but three risk factors, and patient 2 is 45-year-old man with chest pain typical of angina pectoris. (Reproduced with permission Patterson *et al.* 1984).

Table 25.2 Bruce protocol for exercise (treadmill) ECG test

Stage	Speed (mph)	Grade (%)	Duration (min)	METS (units)	Total time (min)
1	1.7	10	3	4	3
2	2.5	12	3	6–7	6
3	3.4	14	3	8–9	9
4	4.2	16	3	15–16	12
5	5.0	18	3	21	15
6	5.5	20	3	—	—
7	6.0	22	3	—	—

METS: metabolic equivalents.
(Based on Benchimol *et al.* 1972).

exceed 10–11 METS, while athletes usually achieve more than 16 METS.

The exercise testing should be interrupted when: (i) significant symptoms or arrhythmias appear, (ii) significantly abnormal ST segment changes are detected, or (iii) the target heart rate is reached.

Usefulness

Exercise testing is very useful in patients with ischemic heart disease to arrive at the diagnosis, to evaluate functional capacity, and to monitor the response to treatment. It can also be useful in other heart diseases and in the evaluation and assessment of cardiac arrhythmias. The most important indications and contraindications of exercise testing are listed in Tables 25.3 and 25.4.

The most important indication is to determine the presence of ischemia (positive test) in patients with dubious precordial pain and in post-infarction patients to stratify prognosis. The combination of the appearance of anginal pain or other clinical or hemodynamic signs (Table 25.5)

and electrocardiographic ST depression confirms the diagnosis. If it is only electrocardiographically positive, the diagnosis can only be suggested, although other tests (another exercise test with isotopic methods and on occasions, coronary angiography) are needed to clarify the problem and to exclude false positive results. The degree of abnormality of the exercise test is very important. If it is clearly positive (early and/or important ST depression, and/or precordial pain or hypotension, etc.), coronary angiography is recommended. If it is equivocal for ischemia (minor ST depression at the final stage of the Bruce protocol) without severe clinical findings (angina, hypotension), we recommended other techniques (isotopic or CV), magnetic resonance studies of perfusion, to assure the diagnosis of ischemia. If these tests are positive for ischemia, coronary angiography or multislice scanner is recommended.

Pathological responses to exercise

Changes may be observed with exercise testing in patients with ischemic heart disease. Ischemia can be detected by: (i) ECG alterations, (ii) hemodynamic changes, and/or (iii) clinical signs and symptoms (Table 25.5). Table 25.6 lists the ECG criteria of positivity and Table 25.7 shows the potential causes for false positive and false negative responses.

Isotopic studies with thallium-201 or isonitriles can increase the sensitivity of exercise testing. Figure 25.4 shows

Table 25.3 Main indications for exercise testing

Diagnostic indications	Doubtful precordial pain. Early detection of ischemic heart disease
Functional	Arrhythmias and exercise
	Prognosis in patients with ischemic heart disease (post-myocardial infarction patients)
	Severity of ischemic heart disease
	Functional capacity of patients with heart disease
	Therapeutic effectiveness
	Behavior, with exercise, of known arrhythmias
	Level of physical training in asymptomatic patients and athletes
Other indications	Rehabilitation
	Research

Table 25.4 Contraindications for exercise testing

Absolute	Acute myocardial infarction
	Acute coronary insufficiency
	Severe aortic stenosis
	Acute endo- and myocardial diseases
	Acute pulmonary embolism
	Acute and severe non-cardiac disease and chronic handicapping diseases
Relative	Marked hypertension (systemic and pulmonary) (individual decision)
	Severe heart failure
	Significant physical and psychic handicaps
	Important electrolyte disorders
	Digitalis intoxication
	Drugs that can impede evaluation of the results
	Markedly altered basal ECG

Table 25.5 Exercise ECG: pathological responses

ECG changes	Diagnostic ST segment alterations
	Other repolarization alterations
	Appearance of AV or ventricular block
	Appearance of evident increase in the number of arrhythmias
Hemodynamic changes	Hypotension
	Poor heart rate response
	Marked hypertension
Symptoms and signs	Symptoms: severe chest pain (anginal) and/or dyspnea
	Signs: appearance of abnormal changes in palpation and/or auscultation

Table 25.6 Classic ECG criteria for positive stress test

- Horizontal or downsloping ST depression > 1 mm
- ST segment elevation > 1 mm
Also very suggestive are:
- Horizontal or downsloping ST segment depression > 1 mm
- Upsloping ST segment depression ≥ 1 mm
- Inverted U wave
- Appearance of important ventricular arrhythmias with light exercise (< 70% of maximal heart rate)
- Rarely may appear peaked T wave.

Table 25.7 False positive and False negative ECG tests

False-positive
- Drugs: digitalis, diuretics, antidepressant drugs, sedatives, estrogen
- Heart diseases: cardiomyopathy, valvular heart disease, pericarditis, hypertensive heart disease, ECG alterations (ventricular block, ventricular enlargement, WPW, repolarization alterations)
- Miscellaneous: thoracic abnormalities (pectus), female sex, hyperventilation (may explain false positive exercise test. Repeat ECG with hyperventilation at rest), glucose ingestion, hypokalemia
False negative
- Drugs: beta-blocking agents, antianginal drugs
- Inadequate exercise: premature termination of the test, poor physical training
- Technical problems.

six examples of the correlation of changes in the ECG and isotopic studies during exercise testing. Figure 25.5 shows how the correlation during exercise testing of clinical data and ECG and isotopic changes can influence the diagnosis of ischemic heart disease. If a patient has anginal pain, sequential ECG changes and the results of the isotope study must be considered. A positive response is of lesser value in a young woman than in an adult male with many risk factors (for further explanation, see Figure 25.5).

Holter ECG monitoring and related techniques

Holter ECG monitoring

Holter ECG monitoring is a continuous ECG recording with accelerated interpretation of data invented by the physicist N. Holter more than 50 years ago. This technique is to the conventional ECG what cinema is to photography. Thanks to this technique, we can determine cardiac electrical activity during daily activities (Bayés de Luna *et al.* 1983).

Holter ECG monitoring is very useful for the diagnosis and evaluation of arrhythmias (Table 25.8 and Figures 25.6–25.9). It may be used to quantify the number as well as the characteristics of arrhythmias, the point in time at which they occur, their relationship to exercise, emotions, and sleep, and 24 hour (or longer) heart rate behavior, in addition to being used to stratify the risk of sudden death (Bigger *et al.* 1984) and to identify the arrhythmia that triggers it (Bayés de Luna *et al.* 1989). Today, with digital recording systems, data interpretation may be done through the Internet, subsequently saving

Table 25.8 Usefulness of Holter monitoring

• Determination of the prevalence of the different arrhythmias in healthy subjects and in the different diseases
• Determination of a possible correlation between the symptoms the patient shows (dizziness, palpitations, syncope, etc.) and the presence of arrhythmias
• Assessment of the antiarrhythmic pharmacologic treatment and post-ablation treatment
• Assessment of the electrophysiologic mechanism of arrhythmias
• Determination of the arrhythmia responsible for the sudden death (Bayés de Luna and Baranchuk 2017)
• Sudden death stratification risk
• Control of the pacemaker function
Repolarization alterations:
• Repolarization alterations not due to IHD
• Repolarization alterations due to IHD: secondary angina vs. primary angina
• Silent ischemia
• Control of treatment for angina
• Post-infarction risk stratification

IHD, ischemic heart disease.

money and time (Figure 25.6). Currently, prolonged recordings of up to seven days are available, and they are especially useful to detect the incidence of paroxysmal atrial fibrillation (AF) and to assess whether they have disappeared after ablation. On certain occasions, Holter ECG monitoring may also be useful in studying repolarization alterations (Table 25.8).

Holter technology allows us to assess various disturbances of the autonomic nervous system (ANS) based on the study of different parameters, such as RR interval variability (HRV), dynamic QT behavior, and heart rate turbulence (HRT), among others. Many published studies show the potential utility of these parameters for risk stratification in patients post infarction and in patients with heart failure, in addition to other clinical situations (Cygankiewicz *et al.* 2006, 2008).

Related techniques

Conventional systems for the telephone transmission of ECG data are available, well known, and obviously useful, especially if no physician is available or if a pacemaker is to be controlled. Systems related to Holter ECG monitoring, which allow for ECG recording at the time when certain symptoms occur, are particularly interesting (**event analyzer**). These data are subsequently transmitted by telephone or through the Internet for interpretation. This is of great interest in the study of sporadic symptomatic arrhythmias (Figure 25.6).

It was published in 2004 that **implantable loop recorders** (Krahn *et al.* 2004) allow us to more frequently determine the cause of unexplained syncope occurring sporadically in patients who usually have good ventricular function but whose life may be at risk (Reveal Medtronic). In the RAST trial (Krahn *et al.* 2001), it was demonstrated that the implantable loop recorder is more effective, in terms of diagnosing the cause of unexplained syncope, than the conventional method (conventional event analyzer + tilt table test + intracavitary electrophysiological study (IES)).

Telemetry home monitoring of the implanted device (Ricci *et al.* 2008) has been shown to be very useful for patient follow-up after pacemaker and implantable cardioverter defibrillator (ICD) implantation, as well as for the detection of paroxysmal arrhythmias (Alexander and Baranchuk 2020).

The ambulatory cardiac telemetry (ACT) device consists of a small sensor and electrodes worn on the chest, which record the heart rhythm and transmit automatically, without requiring patient action, and wirelessly to a cellular phone monitor in which the transmission is analyzed by an algorithm, and the information is transmitted to a central station for review and appropriate interpretation. It has been demonstrated (Kadish *et al.* 2010) that 1% of patients wearing ACT for routine clinical indications experienced severe life-threatening arrhythmias over a three-week monitoring period.

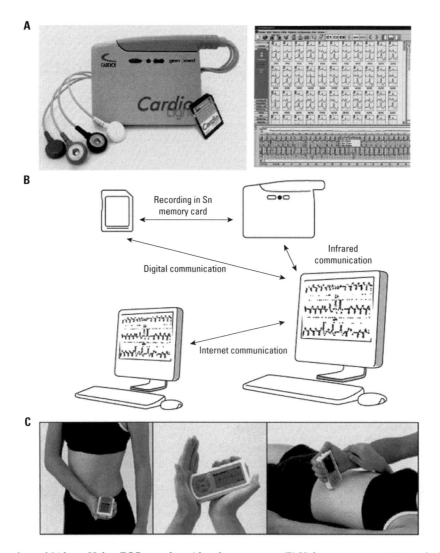

Figure 25.6 (A) Three-channel 24 hour Holter ECG recorder with software screen. (B) Holter remote acquisition platform. (C) Event analyzer.

Current state of techniques for long-term time ECG recording

Nowadays, small devices like watches for example, allow to constant follow up of cardiac rhythm and for the presence of arrhythmias and other ECG changes like bundle branch block or ST-segment changes facilitating rapid recognition ECG alterations. Also currently, thanks to recent advances in digital technology, we dispose of subcutaneous implantable loop recorder that can monitor arrhythmias for up to three years. Some of them may even be capable of also monitoring respiratory rate, and other parameters. Obviously, these new implantable recorders are very useful for the detection of both paroxysmal active and passive arrhythmias, helping in the decision to implant a pacemaker in case of paroxysmal AV block or start anticoagulation in the presence of paroxysmal AF. In fact, these subcutaneous devices with long recording capability have demonstrated that AF is not the direct cause of stroke but rather another risk factor, as it happens with the recognition of A-IAB (Chapters 7

and 9), because in patients with paroxysmal AF and stroke, there is no time-related coincidence between the onset of AF paroxysm and the stroke manifestation (Bayés de Luna *et al.* 2020a, 2020b). For more information, consult Victor Bazan 2020.

Intracavitary ECG and electrophysiologic studies

Intracavitary ECG and electrophysiologic studies (EPSs) allow for a better assessment of cardiac electrical activity. To perform this study, it is necessary to insert various catheters into the heart, which stimulate and record intracavitary electrograms (Figure 25.10) (Josephson 2008; Zipes and Jalife 2004). This includes: (i) electrical activity recording in different areas of the atria and ventricles, including the bundle of His and branches, which has allowed us to better understand

A

Time Period	Total PAC	Isolated PAC	Runs of PAC	Beats in Runs of PAC	Total pauses	Max ST mm	Min ST mm	Max ST slope degrees
1–13:15	426	255	44	171	2	0.8	−1.5	42
1–14:15	36	33	1	3	2	0.8	−1.1	22
1–15:15	2	2	0	0	2	1.1	−1.3	22
1–16:15	6	6	0	0	2	1.1	−1.1	27
1–17:15	7	3	1	4	5	1.3	−1.3	17
1–18:15	1	1	0	0	5	1.1	−0.8	17
1–19:15	6.093	2	8	6.091	0	1.5	−0.8	35
1–20:15	10.052	0	14	10.052	0	1.5	−0.8	45
1–21:15	1.048	0	13	1.048	0	1.7	−1.7	40
1–22:15	3	3	0	0	0	1.3	−2.1	27
1–23:15	0	0	0	0	0	1.3	−1.7	27
2–00:15	1	1	0	0	0	0.8	−0.6	17
2–01:15	3	3	0	0	0	0.8	−0.6	17
2–02:15	3	3	0	0	0	1.1	−0.2	11
2–03:15	13	10	1	3	1	1.3	−0.4	11
2–04:15	0	0	0	0	1	1.1	−0.2	14
2–05:15	5	5	0	0	0	0.8	−0.2	11
2–06:15	4	0	1	4	0	1.3	−0.6	17
2–07:15	4	4	0	0	1	1.1	−0.4	22
2–08:15	1	1	0	0	1	1.1	−0.4	17
2–09:15	1	1	0	0	0	0.8	−0.8	22
2–10:15	2	2	0	0	0	0.8	−0.8	27
2–11:15	2	2	0	0	0	0.8	−1.1	22
2–12:15	0	0	0	0	0	0.6	−0.8	17
	17.713	337	83	17.376	22	1.7	2.1	45

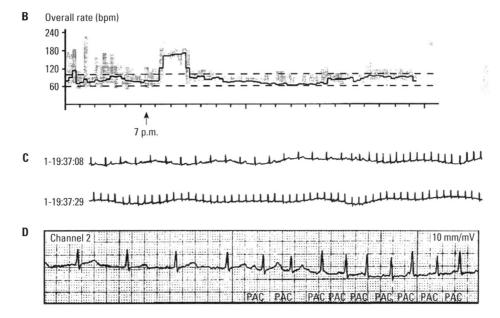

Figure 25.7 (A) Time schedule of premature atrial complexes (PACs), isolated or in runs (it is observed that at 7–9 p.m., a paroxysmal tachycardia episode occurs). The number of pauses and ST elevations are also recorded. There are no premature ventricular complexes (PVCs). (B) Heart rate trend in which it is observed how during the paroxysmal tachycardia episode, the heart rate increases abruptly and stays unchanged for two hours. (C and D) Onset of the paroxysmal tachycardia episode.

the activation sequence of the heart, both in normal and pathologic situations; and (ii) programmed electrical stimulation, including pacing techniques at increasing heart rates, and the application of extra stimulus at progressively shorter intervals with respect to the baseline rhythm, to study the refractory periods of the stimulated area (Figure 25.11).

These techniques are very useful in clinical arrhythmology (Table 25.9 and Figures 25.12–25.15) (Bayés de Luna and Baranchuk 2017). In many situations,

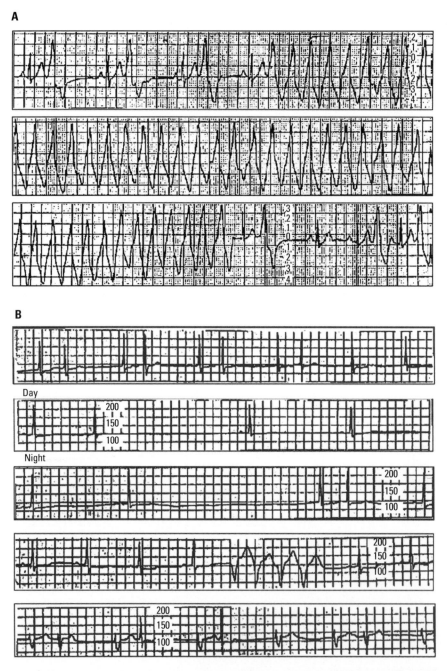

Figure 25.8 (A) A 50-year-old patient with palpitations and frequent premature ventricular complexes (PVC, often bigeminal PVC) and runs of ventricular tachycardia (VT), some of which are particularly long (>15 minutes), with a heart rate >150 bpm. (B) A 75-year-old patient with palpitations. The ECG Holter recording showed a sick sinus node (asymptomatic pauses >4 min) and frequent premature atrial complexes (PACs), sometimes bigeminal, which are part of a bradycardia-tachycardia syndrome, requiring a pacemaker implantation. Also a run of VT is recorded.

despite the large amount of information obtained by the surface ECG, performing an intracavitary ECG and carrying out EPS is essential, not only to confirm the diagnosis, but also to determine the best treatment for each type of arrhythmia. Some paradigmatic cases, for example, are:

(i)   determining the exact location of an AV block (Figure 25.12);

(ii) the study of sinus function (Figure 25.13);

(iii) the mechanisms of a wide QRS tachycardia (Figures 25.14 and 25.15);

(iv.) the best area for catheter ablation of VT, AF, or atrial flutter, or precisely identifying the circuit involved in a reentrant AV junctional tachycardia, including WPW syndrome; VT circuit, definition of scar by voltage maps, etc.

Thanks to these techniques, surface ECG diagnosis has advanced considerably so that we are able to apply the data obtained by intracavitary studies to the conventional ECG (and vice versa).

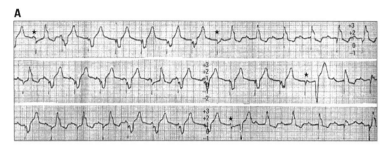

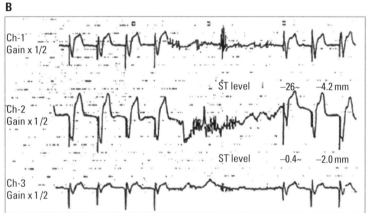

Figure 25.9 (A) Stimulation failure (spikes not followed by QRS) (stars) detected by the ECG Holter. (B) Long pause detected by the ECG Holter due to myopotentials, as a result of interferences caused by muscular contractions (the most frequent cause of oversensing).

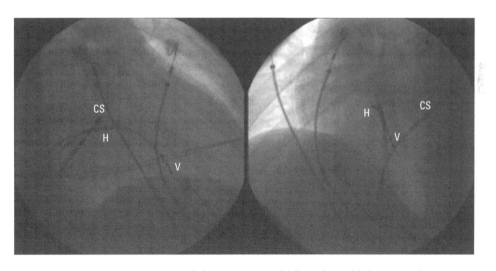

Figure 25.10 Catheter location for ablation. Right arterial oblique position (RAO) (right) and left anterior oblique position (LAO) (left). The coronary sinus catheter gives us information on electrical activity of the left side without arterial access. CS: coronary sinus; H: His; V: apex of the right ventricle.

Wave amplification and filtering techniques

Wave amplification techniques, sometimes along with ECG recording at a faster speed, may be useful to better determine atrial activity or make it more visible when not apparent and to diagnose the presence of AV dissociation, which, in turn, is crucial for the differential diagnosis between VT and aberrant supraventricular tachycardia (see Figures 15.37 and 16.13). These valuable techniques are not universally used due to lack of knowledge.

T wave filtering techniques allow us to visualize the P wave when it is concealed in the preceding T wave (Goldwasser *et al.* 2011). At present, T wave filtering techniques help to diagnose the location of atrial

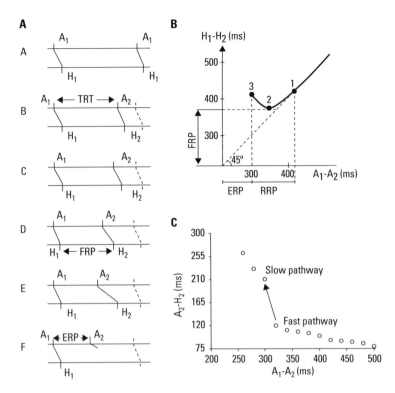

Figure 25.11 Diagram showing the different tissue refractory periods, in particular the atrioventricular (AV) node refractory period. (A) Response sequence to increasingly premature stimuli (A2). (B) Curve obtained from A1–A2 and H1–H2 values under normal conduction conditions. TRT (total recovery time) = shortest distance between the basal impulse (A) and the extra stimulus, with the latter being normally conducted (A2 H2 = A1 H1) (see B in A). FRP (functional refractory period): the shortest H1–H2, regardless of the A1–A2 distance (see D in A and 2 in B). Effective refractory period (ERP): the longest A1–A2 distance that is not followed by a hisian deflection (see F in A and 3 in B). Relative refractory period (RRP) starts when A2–H2 > A1–H1, that is to say, at the end of the TRT, and lasts until the beginning of the ERP (3 in B). (C) Confirmation of AV conduction through both α and β pathways. Note the A2–H2 response (AV conduction), to increasingly shorter A1–A2 (see A). With A1–A2 = 300 ms, the pathway ERP is reached, resulting in an abrupt and significant A2–H2 increase, as conduction is then only through the α pathway, up to 250 cm, where the ERP of the α pathway is reached.

Table 25.9 Utility of intracavitary electrophysiologic studies

- Study of the refractory periods of the different zones of the heart
- Topographic location of the AV block
- Study of the AV and VA conduction characteristics
- Study of the sinus function
- Study of the accessory pathways characteristics
- Study of the mechanisms of a wide QRS tachycardia and their differential diagnosis
- Pharmacoelectrophysiology
- Mapping of complex VT, PVCs integration of non-contact mapping, etc.
- Improvement of diagnostic precision of conventional ECG and determination of best possible invasive approach

AV: atrioventricular.
(Bayés de Luna and Baranchuk 2017).

waves, which may be very useful to better diagnose different types of supraventricular tachyarrhythmias (Figure 25.16). There are also promising results offering the possibility of detecting AV dissociation in patients with broad QRS tachycardia.

Other ECG leads

On occasion, the recording of a **bipolar precordial lead** (Lewis lead) may also be useful. This is obtained by placing the right arm electrode in the second right intercostal space and the left arm electrode in the fourth right intercostal space (Bakker *et al.* 2009).

The esophageal leads: The recording of ECG through a lead located in the esophagus was attempted in the early days of electrocardiography by Cremer in 1906 (Pehrson 2004). In fact, in spite of its importance from a research point of view, its use in clinical practice has not been very much expanded since due to the relative time investment necessary to record it properly.

Transesophageal recording may be useful from a diagnostic point of view in the following circumstances: (i) to study the atrium in normal and different types of atrial blocks (Bayés de Luna *et al.* 1985) (see Figure 9.19); (ii) to distinguish between AVNRT and AVRT in the case of paroxysmal narrow QRS tachycardia (Figure 25.17) (Gallagher *et al.* 1982); and (iii) to perform differential diagnosis in the case of wide QRS tachycardia between supraventricular or ventricular origin with aberrancy, demonstrating the relationship between atria and ventricles or the presence of AV dissociation, unmasking the atrial activity hidden in the QRS–T. With the improvement of filters on current ECG machines, these techniques are rarely used.

Transesophageal stimulation may be used from a clinical point of view in circumstances such as: induction and termination of supraventricular tachycardias, assessment of sinus node function, and emergency pacing. Again, due to the invasive nature of the procedure and the pain associated with the voltage needed for capture, this technique is rarely used.

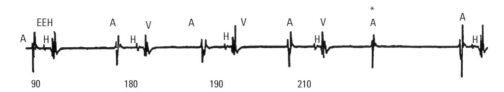

Figure 25.12 Electrophysiologic studies (EPS) in a patient with Wenckebach-type 5×4 AV block with pre-hisian block. Note the progressive prolongation of the AH interval, until the fifth A˙ is not conducted. The more significant conduction delay occurs between the first and second AH intervals (Bayés de Luna and Baranchuk 2017).

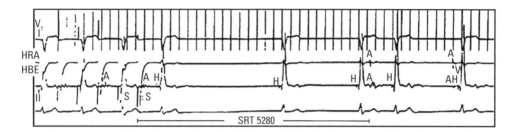

Figure 25.13 A very long sinus recovery period (SRP). Before the first sinus P wave occurs (A in EHH), two hisian deflections (H) have been recorded (Bayés de Luna and Baranchuk 2017).

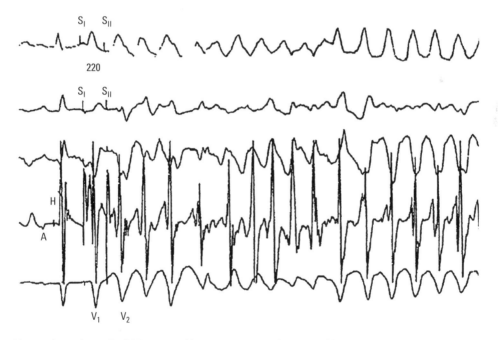

Figure 25.14 Ventricular tachycardia (VT) triggered by two extra stimuli separated by 220 ms (Bayés de Luna and Baranchuk 2017).

Body surface potential mapping

Body surface potential mapping has been used for decades for investigational purposes. Currently, portable and fast electrode placement devices allowing for good-quality ECG tracings are available.

These methods generate QRST mappings that allow us to investigate the likelihood of developing arrhythmias and allow for risk stratification, although their use in daily clinical practice is very limited (De Ambroggi *et al.* 1991; Hubley-Kozey *et al.* 1995; Korhonen *et al.* 2009). This technique has been used to demonstrate the importance of late depolarization theory to explain how the typical pattern of coved ST segment in the Brugada syndrome is produced (Postema *et al.* 2010).

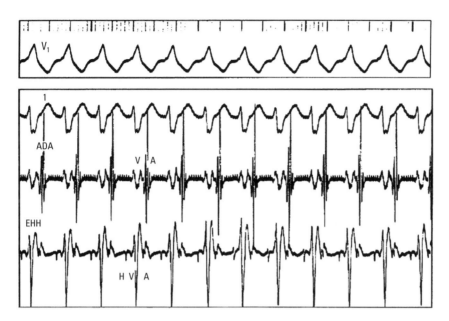

Figure 25.15 Wide QRS tachycardia (see V1). The electrophysiologic study showed that the tachycardia was supraventricular in origin, with anterograde activation by the specific conduction system (SCS) (H before V) and retrograde activation through an accessory pathway (A after V). The QRS complex was wide because of an associated right bundle branch block (RBBB) (aberrancy) (Bayés de Luna and Baranchuk 2017).

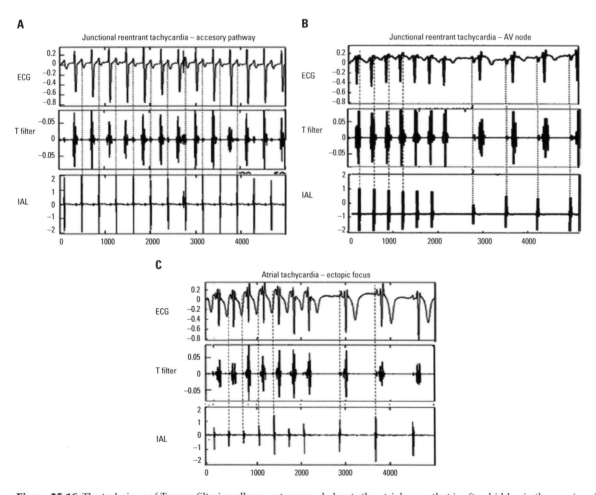

Figure 25.16 The technique of T wave filtering allows us to properly locate the atrial wave that is often hidden in the previous T wave. The figure shows three examples with a comparison of surface ECG, filtering technique (FT), and intraatrial lead (IAL) to correlate the value of the filtering technique. We can check that the FT allows us to identify the appropriate atrial wave in three types of different supraventricular tachyarrhythmias: (A) AVRT, (B) AVNRT, and (C) AT-EF (Bayés de Luna and Baranchuk 2017).

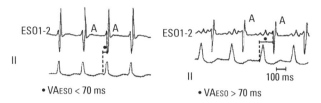

Figure 25.17 Surface lead II and bipolar esophageal ECG recordings (ESO 1–2). The distance ventricle–atria ESO (VAESO) is less than 70 ms during AV nodal reentry tachycardia (left). During orthodromic tachycardia the VAESO distance exceeds 70 ms (right). A: atrial electrogram (Based on Gallagher *et al.* 1982).

This technique has also been used to diagnose cases of myocardial infarction in the inferolateral zone, which is not easily detected by surface ECG (McClelland *et al.* 2003) (Figure 25.18). However, its use in clinical practice is very limited. Our experience shows that it is not easy to perform, and although in many cases its diagnostic capacity is better than that of automatic ECG interpretation, an expert ECG interpreter with good knowledge of the clinical history of the patient will probably make the same accurate diagnosis.

Analysis of late potentials using signal averaging electrocardiogram (SAEGG)

Late potentials are low-amplitude potentials that are detectable at the end or immediately after the QRS complex (Figure 25.19). They are caused by a late activation of myocardial zones where viable muscle tissue alternates with necrotic and/or fibrotic zones. They have been shown to be independent markers of sustained VT (Breithardt *et al.* 1983).

This technique has been used in patients with coronary artery disease to detect those at higher risk of developing VT/VF by identifying those areas with slow conduction due to the presence of a post-infarction scar. When positive, it is also useful for the diagnosis/prognosis of arrhythmogenic right ventricular cardiomyopathy and Brugada syndrome. In general, the sensitivity and specificity are quite high, but in epidemiologic reality, the PPV is usually low, whereas the NPV is high (see Chapter 8). For example, in post-infarction patients, determining the risk of VT/VF is paramount. In these cases, the PPV of late potentials is low (≈20%), so that in theory only a small percentage of post-infarction patients with positive late potentials will have malignant ventricular arrhythmias (MVAs) in the future. However, the clinical practice value

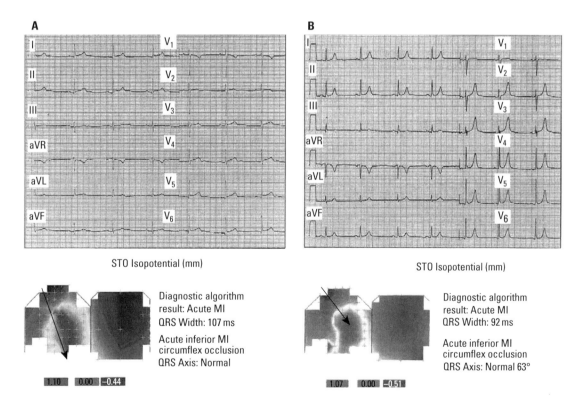

Figure 25.18 Examples of body surface mapping (BSM) and 12-lead ECGs from patients with acute myocardial infarction (AMI) confirmed by elevated troponin I or creatine kinase-MB. (A) Patient with inferior AMI diagnosed by BSM algorithm and physician but missed by the 12-lead ECG algorithm (maxima = 1.10 mm, in inferolateral area). (B) Patient with inferior AMI diagnosed by BSM algorithm but missed by physician and 12-lead ECG algorithm (maxima = 1.07 mm, in inferolateral area) (Reproduced with permission from McClelland *et al.* 2003).

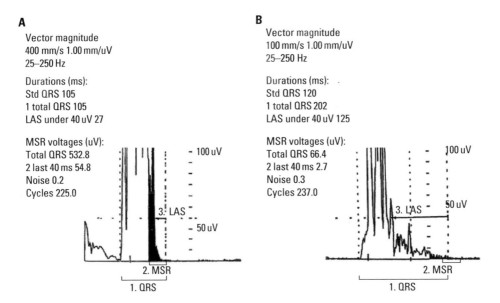

Figure 25.19 Late potential normal recording in a patient without heart disease (A) and in a patient with right ventricle (RV) arrhythmogenic dysplasia (B). In the first case, none of the three diagnostic criteria are met: (i) QRS = 105 ms; (ii) MSR (mean square root) voltage of the last 40 ms = 54.8; and (iii) low amplitude signal (LAS) under 40 μV = 27. In the second case, the three criteria are met: (i) QRS = 202 ms; (ii) MSR (last 40 ms) = 2.7; and (iii) LAS (<40 μV) = 125.

relies in the fact that the NPV is very high (99%). This means that when late potentials are negative, the risk of developing MVA is very low. In the twenty-first century, SAECG did not improve the ability to predict sudden death in patients with coronary artery disease as studies did not show additional value to the left ventricular ejection fraction.

Therefore, it is necessary to combine new parameters to increase the PPV. In this sense, the papers published by Gomes *et al.* (1987) and Kuchar *et al.* (1987) are relevant. The former demonstrated that in patients with positive late potentials and ejection fraction <40%, the number of Holter monitoring ventricular PVCs was significant and the prognosis (occurrence of malignant arrhythmias) was higher. Meanwhile, Kuchar *et al.* (1987) showed that patients with positive late potentials, Lown grade III–IV (Holter), and ejection fraction <40% had a 30% possibility of suffering from a severe arrhythmic event during a one-year follow-up. In contrast, patients with only one factor had a much lower chance of suffering from severe arrhythmia (<5%).

Tilt table test

The tilt table test technique is used to unmask the susceptibility to neurally mediated (vasovagal) syncope in patients with unexplained syncope. **It is very useful to confirm the diagnosis of neuromediated syncope, but not for evaluating the efficacy of treatments.** The tilt table test involves placing the patient on a table with a foot support, then tilting the table upward into a completely vertical position. The patient is instructed to remain resting, with the aim of assessing whether syncope occurs spontaneously or after the administration of drugs (i.e. nitroglycerin), at which point the table is returned to a flat (horizontal) position and the syncope disappears (Sutton and Bloomfield 1999).

Recently, it has been reported that during tilt table testing, the presence of oscillating systolic blood pressure, varying at ≥30 mm in patients who are nonresponders to the passive head-up tilt and glyceryl trinitrate provocation, may be considered the equivalent to vasovagal syncope, possibly obviating the need for other tests, such as the isoprenaline test (Hausenloy *et al.* 2009).

Neuromediated syncope may be of a vasodepressor, cardioinhibitory, or mixed type. Cardioinhibitory response may occur in the form of sinus bradycardia, leading to sinus arrest (20% of the cases in a tilt test) or AV block (4% of the cases) (Figure 25.20) (Brignole 2009). When it is established that the patient shows the same symptoms as the ones clinically experienced, the diagnosis is confirmed. A significant cardioinhibitory response, especially if occurring previously to the vasodepressor response, may call for pacemaker implantation, which would become activated when heart rate decreases. However, as syncope usually has a vasodepressor component, a pacemaker implantation does not provide a guaranteed lack of recurrence. The major limitation of the tilt table test is the lack of reproducibility, which led to less groups around the world using it for clinical decision-making. We consider that it still has a role as an integral part of the evaluation of the autonomic nervous system.

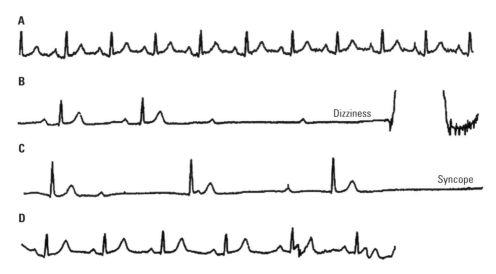

Figure 25.20 (A) A young man with syncopal attacks, probably neuromediated (vagal), and a normal ECG. Tilt testing was positive, presenting with dizziness and cardioinhibitory response with advanced atrioventricular (AV) block (B and C). After recovery in the normal position, the AV block completely disappeared (D) (Based on Brignole 2009).

Imaging techniques

Imaging techniques, especially **echocardiography,** may be useful to determine left ventricular function and to study right ventricular or aortic pathology. Echocardiography is the first-choice imaging technique for the diagnosis of structural heart disease and the study of dyssynchrony between both ventricles and is useful when deciding whether cardiac resynchronization therapy (CRT) is needed (see below). It has been demonstrated (Bouzas-Mosquera *et al.* 2009) that exercise echocardiography provides significant prognostic information for predicting mortality and MACE in patients with LBBB and no changes in the exercise ECG.

Cardiovascular magnetic resonance is a key technique to rule out or confirm the diagnosis in some diseases such as arrhythmogenic RVC/D, anomalous origin of coronary arteries, or to better study other diseases such as cardiomyopathies. It is also very useful for detecting atrial fibrosis to assess the feasibility of cardioversion or AF ablation (Oakes *et al.* 2009).

Non-invasive (multislice scanner) and invasive coronary angiography may also be necessary to assess the anatomic and functional state of the coronary circulation. The multislice scanner may be used to investigate the anatomy of pulmonary and coronary veins (AF ablation and CRT).

Genetic techniques

Genetic testing has become a necessary tool to help with the diagnosis of inherited heart diseases. Currently, it is considered to be a first-line procedure only when a genetic disease appears to be responsible for cardiac arrest in clinical test results and appropriate family history. Also, it may be useful for the study of the relatives of index cases and to plan parenting in a responsible manner.

All these techniques are used with increasing frequency, especially in young patients and athletes with exercise-related syncope or significant arrhythmias, to confirm that no structural heart disease is present (i.e. hypertrophic cardiomyopathy, coronary artery anomalies, arrhythmogenic right ventricular cardiomyopathy, etc.).

References

Alexander B, Baranchuk A. Remote device reprogramming: has its time come? *Circ Arrhythm Electrophysiol* 2020;13(10):e008949.

Bakker AL, Nijkerk G, Groenemeijer BE, *et al.* The Lewis lead: making recognition of P waves easy during wide QRS complex tachycardia. *Circulation* 2009;119:3592.

Bayés de Luna A. Baranchuk A. *Clinical Arrhythmology.* 2nd edn. Wiley-Blackwell, 2017.

Bayés de Luna A, Serra Grima JR, Oca Navarro E. *Electrocardiografía de Holter.* Enfoque práctico. Editorial Científco Médica, 1983.

Bayés de Luna A, Fort de Ribot R, Trilla E, *et al.* Electrocardiograhic and vectorcardiograhpic study of interatrial conduction disturbances with left atrial retrograde activation. *J Electrocardiol* 1985;18:1.

Bayés de Luna A, Coumel P, Leclercq JF. Ambulatory sudden cardiac death: mechanisms of production of fatal arrhythmia on the basis of data from 157 cases. *Am Heart J* 1989;117:151.

Bayés de Luna A, Martínez-Sellés M, Bayés-Genís A, *et al.* Síndrome de Bayés. Lo que todo clínico debe conocer. What every clinician should know about Bayés Syndrome. *Rev Esp Cardiol (Engl Ed)* 2020a;73:758.

Bayés de Luna A, Martínez-Sellés M, Elosua R, *et al.* Relation of advanced interatrial block to risk of atrial fibrillation and stroke. *Am J Cardiol* 2020b;125:1745.

Benchimol A, Desser KB, Schumacher J. Value of the vectorcardiogram for distinguishing left anterior hemiblock from inferior infarction with left axis deviation. *Chest* 1972;61:74.

Bigger JT, Fleiss JL, Kleiger R, *et al*. The relationships among ventricular arrhythmias, left ventricular dysfunction and mortality in the 2 years after myocardial infarction. *Circulation* 1984;69:250.

Bouzas-Mosquera A, Peteiro J, Alvarez-Garcia N, *et al*. Prognostic value of exercise echocardiography in patients with left bundle branch block. *JACC Cardiovasc Imaging* 2009;2:251.

Breithardt G, Borgreffe M, Seipel L, *et al*. Prognostic significance of late ventricular potentials after myocardial infarction. *Eur Heart J* 1983;4:487.

Brignole M. Different electrocardiographic manifestations of the cardioinhibitory vasovagal reflex. *Europace* 2009;11:144.

Cygankiewicz I, Zareba W, Vazquez R, *et al*. Relation of heart rate turbulence to severity of heart failure. *Am J Cardiol* 2006;98:1635.

Cygankiewicz I, Zareba W, Vazquez R, *et al*. Prognostic value of QT/RR slope in predicting mortality in patients with congestive heart failure. *J Cardiovasc Electrophysiol* 2008;19:1066.

De Ambroggi L, Negroni MS, Monza E, *et al*. Dispersion of ventricular repolarizaiton in the long QT syndrome. *Am J Cardiol* 1991;68:614.

Gallagher JJ, Smith W, Kerr CR, *et al*. Esophageal pacing: a diagnostic and therapeutical tool. *Circulation* 1982;65:336.

Goldwasser D, Bayés de Luna A, Serra G, Viñolas X, *et al*. New computer algorhythm to improve P wave detection during supraventricular tachycardia. *Europace* 2011;12:1028.

Gomes JA, Winters SL, Steward D, Horowitz S, *et al*. A new noninvasive index to predict sustained ventricular tachycardia and sudden death in the first year after myocardial infarction. *J Am Coll Cardiol* 1987;10:349.

Hausenloy DJ, Arhl C, Chandra N, *et al*. Blood pressure oscillations during tilt testing as a predictive marker of vasovagal syncope. *Europace* 2009;11:1696.

Hubley-Kozey CL, Mitchell LB, Gardner MJ, *et al*. Spatial features in body-surface potential maps can identify patients with a history of sustained ventricular tachycardia. *Circulation* 1995;92:1825.

Josephson ME. *Clinical cardiac electrophysiology*, 4th edn. Wolters-Kluwer, 2008.

Kadish A, Feiffel J, Clauses J, *et al*. Frequency of serious arrhythmias detected with ambulatory cardiac telemetry. *Am J Cardiol* 2010;105:1313.

Korhonen P, Husa T, Kontilla T, *et al*. Complex T-wave morphology in body surface potential mapping in prediction of arrhythmic events in patients with acute myocardial infarction and cardiac dysfunction. *Europace* 2009;11:514.

Krahn AD, Klein GJ, Yee R, *et al*. Randomized assessment of syncope trial. Conventional diagnostic testing versus a prolonged monitoring strategy. *Circulation* 2001;104:46.

Krahn AD, Klein GJ, Yee R, *et al*. The use of monitoring strategies in patients with unexplained syncoperol of the external and implantable loop recorder. *Clin Auton Res* 2004;14(suppl 1):55.

Kuchar DL, Thorburn CW, Sammel NL. Prediction of serious arrhythmic events after myocardial infarction: signal-averaged electrocardiogram. Holter monitoring and radionuclide ventriculography. *J Am Coll Cardiol* 1987;9:531.

Macfarlane PW, van Oosterom A, Pahlm O, Kligfield P, Janse M, Camm J. *Comprehensive Electrocardiology*. 2th edn. Springer-Verlag London 2010.

McClelland A, Owens C, Menown I, *et al*. Comparison of the 80-lead b ody surface map to physician and to 12-lead electrocardiogram in detection of acute myocardial infarction. *Am J Cardiol* 2003;92:252.

Nunes de Alencar Neto J, Baranchuk A, Bayés-Genís A, *et al*. Arrhythmogenic right ventricular dysplasia/cardiomyopathy: an electrocardiogram-based review. *Europace* 2018;20:f3–f12.

Oakes RS, Badger TJ, Kholmovski G, *et al*. Detection and quantification of left atrial structural remodeling with delayed-enhancement magnetic resonance imaging in patients with atrial fibrillation. *Circulation* 2009;119:1758.

Patterson RE, Eng C, Horowitz SF. Practical diagnosis of coronary artery disease: a Bayés' theorem nomogram to correlate clilnical data with noninvasive exercise tests. *Am J Cardiol* 1984;53:252.

Pehrson S. *The Oesophageal Route in Clinical Electrocardiology*. Pasquale del Bene Edit, 2004.

Postema PG, van Dessel PF, Kors JA, *et al*. Local depolarization abnormalities are the dominant pathophysiologic mechanism for type 1 electrocardiogram in Brugada syndrome. A study of electrocardiograms, vectorcardiograms, and body surface potential maps during ajmaline provocation. *J Am Coll Cardiol* 2010;55:789.

Ricci RP, Morichelli L, Santini M. Home monitoring remote control of pacemaker and implantable cardioverter defibrillator patients in clinical practice: impact on medical management and healthcare resource utilization. *Europace* 2008;10:164.

Sutton R, Bloomfield DM. Indications, methodology, and classification of results of tilt-table testing. *Am J Cardiol* 1999;84:10Q.

Zipes D, Jalife J. *Cardiac Electrophysiology: From cell to bedside*, 4th edn. WB Saunders, 2004.

Chapter 26
The Electrocardiology of the Twenty-First Century

After more than 100 years of its invention, the surface electrocardiogram (ECG) remains the most frequently used diagnostic method in cardiovascular medicine, and one of the most used in the emergency departments (Pérez-Riera *et al.* 2014; Baranchuk *et al.* 2014 and Baranchuk and Pérez-Riera 2017). A rapid question that comes to mind is, why this simple tool was not replaced by new technologies that could help in the interpretation of the heart electricity; and only few variations have been incorporated since its inception? (Nadeau-Routhier and Baranchuk 2016; Bayes de Luna and Baranchuk 2017).

The ECG has remained the flagship technique for recording electrical activity of the heart. In the field of imaging techniques, radiology, which is even older than ECG, has been widely surpassed first by echocardiography and later by magnetic resonance imaging. However, ECG has successfully outstripped the stakes of VCG, which from our point of view is still useful to understand how ECG images originate from the sequence: dipole–vector–loop–hemifield, but it is not necessary for carrying out the diagnosis, since, with few exceptions, the VCG criteria have not surpassed the ECG ones.

The answer is not easy and it could be multifactorial (Baranchuk, 2011): (i) Single method for the diagnosis of a myriad of a huge variety of conditions; from cardiomyopathies to acute myocardial infarction, from channelopathies to pulmonary embolism, etc. (ii) High reproducibility: the same type of ECG can be rapidly obtained in any corner of the world with quite similar technique and with very reasonable quality. In addition, ECGs could be obtained in the site of contact with the patient (i.e. paramedics at the site of acute cardiac arrest) helping in rapid decision-making and orientating the initial response which could save a life. (iii) Easy transferability: with the rapid evolution of communications, a single snapshot with a cell phone can be emailed to an operating center to determine the course of action to take. (iv) Diagnostic method not only useful to establish a differential diagnosis, but also to determine prognosis and evolution,

response to therapy (either drugs or cardiac devices), and identification of populations at risk (ECG & Epidemiology) (Bayes de Luna and Baranchuk 2017).

Several efforts to establish a universal ECG curriculum for pre- and postgrads have been advanced (Paul and Baranchuk 2011). More recently, two societies (International Society of Electrocardiology-ISE and the International Society of Holter and Non-invasive Electrocardiology-ISHNE) have identified gaps in the educational system and proposed a structured curriculum that defines what, when, by whom, and where to teach electrocardiology (Antiperovitch *et al.* 2018). One of the major challenges in the educational process is how to avoid erosion, and the necessary bridges between pre- and postgrad education. Another important aspect is the lack of universal tests and methodology for evaluation.

Despite these limitations, the interpretation of surface ECGs continue to attract thousands of students that renovate every year. The accessibility to rapid platforms of communication (Facebook, Twitter, Instagram) has created niches of science outside the formal academic frame, stimulating the interest of larger audiences. The disadvantage of spreading wrong concepts or ideas, we think, is overcompensated by the opportunity to teach and learn at a worldwide level, interacting with peers from all around the world and exchanging simple (not always!) but effective messages.

Do we need to teach electrocardiology nowadays?

The answer is YES. Every day, lives depend on rapid and accurate ECG interpretation. From the diagnosis of a classic ST-segment elevation myocardial infarction (pattern recognition) to the less classic ST-segment depression in precordial leads with ST-segment elevation in lead aVR (Wellens' pattern) (Zhan *et al.* 2020) indicating subocclusion of the proximal LAD. From a differential diagnosis of

Clinical Electrocardiography: A Textbook, Fifth Edition. Antoni Bayés de Luna, Miquel Fiol-Sala, Antoni Bayés-Genís, and Adrián Baranchuk.
© 2022 John Wiley & Sons Ltd. Published 2022 by John Wiley & Sons Ltd.

narrow complex tachycardia (inductive-deductive mechanisms) to the recognition of life-threatening ECG of channelopathies (pattern recognition) (Baranchuk and Bayés-Genís 2016, ECG University 2017). The huge myriad of diagnoses that an ECG reader can make are difficult to enumerate in this brief report, and we simply want to call attention on why the efforts to teach ECG should continue in the twenty-first century.

Aspects to improve about ECG teaching

Several aspects of classic ECG teaching still need to improve (Antiperovitch *et al.* 2018). Despite of decades advocating for this, the standardization of the process on ECG teaching, retention and evaluation continues to struggle. The following Table 26.1 includes some of the areas that may require specific attention in the years to come:

The challenges of the twenty-first century

The world continues to change. Some changes occur at a very slow motion, like in a movie. This is a great opportunity to adjust some "classic concepts" and give the opportunity to new strategies, fresh and young ideas; to interject in our acceptable standardized way of learning and teaching. An example of this slowly disruptive world change would be the improvement on automatic ECG diagnoses. While we remain skeptical, and test the machine toward experts (for each single ECG), we do admit that the algorithms have improved. For example, automatic measurement of corrected QT intervals (QTc), in the absence of atrial fibrillation or frequent premature ventricular

contractions; is completely reliable. Of course, other diagnoses are more difficult for the machines and further improvement is still necessary. Critical review of each ECG is still suggested (Baranchuk 2011).

On the other hand, some changes in the world occurred at high-speed, with very little time to adjust to new scenarios. This brief report is being written during the pandemic due to COVID-19 (Haseeb *et al.* 2020). All in-person teaching, educational meetings and large worldwide congresses have been discontinued. Can we stop teaching ECGs?

Of course not. But this has required (and still requires) a rapid adjustment to new educational platforms. Interactive teaching, semi-automatic use of calipers, creation of group discussions within video-conferencing teaching, and ability to communicate through a video screen are some of the current challenges to maintain ECG teaching live. We have decided not only to embrace all these new alternatives, but also to continue bidding on classic ECG teaching by promoting a new edition of this book. The new century also brings new technologies to the ECG world. Some of the most remarkable advances on ECG technology are listed in Table 26.2.

In summary, the electrocardiology of the twenty-first century is a field in expansion which will be composed by a critical review of the classic strategies of ECG teaching and learning and a dramatic change in the educational platforms. We are firmly moving into digital areas of knowledge; and the quicker we embrace this change, the more prepared we will be for the next future.

Table 26.1 Areas to be studied in the future.

Areas of deficiency	Possible actions
Accreditation of teachers	All teachers should pass a basic universal exam in order to teach ECG. Alternatively, each institution should provide accreditation.
Environment of education	Teaching could be performed in person or online. Interactive ECG teaching proved to be more efficient.
Position in the curricula	This depends on the program (medicine, nursing, technicians, etc.). The global concept is *the earlier, the better*. This provides the opportunity for escalated level of complexity as the students progress in their programs.
Topics to learn	Please refer to the ISE-ISHNE document (Antiperovitch *et al.* 2018).
Avoiding erosion	It has been well demonstrated that lack of practice evolves into knowledge erosion. New educational platforms may help in maintaining ECG interpretation skills (free access) (Nadeau-Routhier and Baranchuk 2016; ECG University).
Maintaining competence	Access to free online resources may help in maintaining certain level of comfort with basic ECG reading. Interactive tools are preferred (Nadeau-Routhier and Baranchuk 2016; ECG University).

Table 26.2 The most remarkable advances on ECG technology.

New EC technologies	Clinical and research implications
Self-detected devices	Apple Watch, Smartphones, Kardia, AliveCor. These devices change the paradigm about physicians ordering tests to patients' decision to collect information on their own; without a specific prescription. Their role in clinical practice is well-defined. There is a lack of "interface" between patient and physician (Godin *et al.* 2019).
Artificial intelligence	Possibly the biggest next challenge. Will be able to predict mortality? Will be considered within a clinical evaluation? Will transition from research into practice? As in any aspect of medicine, AI is the next revolution (Ribeiro *et al.* 2020).
Integration of ECG to imaging	Electrocardiographic imaging (ECGI) is a new imaging diagnostic test that maps (non-invasively) cardiac electrical activity on the heart epicardial surface. A very promising technique for the diagnosis of several channelopathies. (Rudy, 2017).
ECG and heart sounds	Integration of stethoscope and ECG. It may provide with a better understanding of heart sounds and cardiac cycle (EKO DUO).
ECG and heart failure	New imaging techniques can contribute to the diagnosis of HfpEF.

Furthermore, new ECG technologies are revolutionizing this area of knowledge, expanding the boundaries of anything imaginable.

We are ready for the next steps and the new challenges, following the print steps of giants such as Drs. Jospehson and Wellens and motivated by the new generation of ECG researchers (Haseeb *et al.* 2020; Çinier *et al.* 2019), the true reason to continue this journey, a journey of discoveries and joy.

References

Antiperovitch P, Zareba W, Steinberg JS, *et al.* Proposed In-Training Electrocardiogram Interpretation Competencies for Undergraduate and Postgraduate Trainees. J Hosp Med 2018;13:185–193.

Baranchuk A. How to Teach Electrocardiology? Rev Fed Arg Cardiol 2011;40(2):186.

Baranchuk A, Bayés-Genís A. Naming and classifying old and new ECG phenomena. CMAJ 2016;188:485–486.

Baranchuk A, Pérez-Riera AR. The value of learning surface ECG in the 21st century. J Thorac Dis 2017;9(10):4136.

Baranchuk A, Chiale PA, Green M, Cladwell JC. Surface electrocardiogram remains alive in the XXI century. Curr Cardiol Rev 2014;10(3):173–174.

Bayes de Luna A, Baranchuk A. *Clinical Arrhythmology.* 2nd edn. Wiley-Blackwell, 2017.

Çinier G, Haseeb S, Yeung C, *et al.* International Society of Electrocardiology Young Community. J Electrocardiol 2019;54:69–71.

ECG University. 2017 www.ecguniversity.org (Accesed October 2020).

Godin R, Yeung C, Baranchuk AM, *et al.* Screening for Atrial Fibrillation using a Mobile, Single-Lead Electrocardiogram in Canadian Primary Care Clinics. Can J Cardiol 2019;35(7):840–845.

Haseeb S, Gul EE, Çinier G, Bazoukis G, *et al.* Value of Electrocardiography in Coronavirus disease 2019 (COVID-19). J Electrocardiol 2020;62:39–45.

Nadeau-Routhier C, Baranchuk A (eds) *Electrocardiography in Practice: What to do?* iTunesUSA, 2016; https://itunes.apple.com/ca/book/electrocardiography-in-practice/id1120119530?mt=13 (Accessed October 2020).

Paul B, Baranchuk A. Electrocardiography Teaching in Canadian Family Medicine Residency Programs: A National Survey. Fam Med 2011;43(4):267–271.

Pérez-Riera A, Barbosa-Barros R, Baranchuk A. Current Value of the Electrocardiogram in the 21st century. Austin J Clin Cardiolog 2014;1(2):1–3.

Ribeiro AH, Ribeiro MH, Paixão GMM, *et al.* Automatic diagnosis of the 12-lead ECG using a deep neural network. Nat Commun 2020;11(1):1760.

Rudy Y. Noninvasive ECG Imaging (ECGI): Mapping the arrhythmic substrate of the human heart. Int J Cardiol 2017;237:13–14.

Zhan ZQ, Li Y, Han LH, Nikus KC, Birnbaum Y, Baranchuk A. The de Winter ECG pattern: Distribution and morphology of ST depression. Ann Noninvasive Electrocardiol 2020;25:e12783.

Index

Clinical Electrocardiography: A Textbook, Fifth Edition. Antoni Bayés de Luna, Miquel Fiol-Sala, Antoni Bayés-Genís, and Adrián Baranchuk.
© 2022 John Wiley & Sons Ltd. Published 2022 by John Wiley & Sons Ltd.

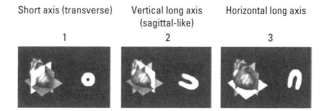

Short axis (transverse)   Vertical long axis   Horizontal long axis
                             (sagittal-like)
         1   2   3

Plate 1 The three heart planes used by nuclear medicine experts (and other imaging techniques) to transect the heart: (1) the short-axis (transverse) view, (2), the vertical long-axis view (VLA) (oblique sagittal-like)and (3) the horizontal long-axis (HLA) view.

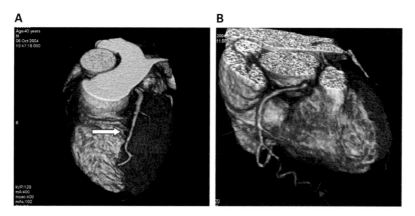

Plate 2 (A) Normal scanner multislice showing normal LAD and LCX arteries. The latter is partially covered by the left appendix. The arrow points to the LAD. (B) Normal case: showing a normal dominant RCA.

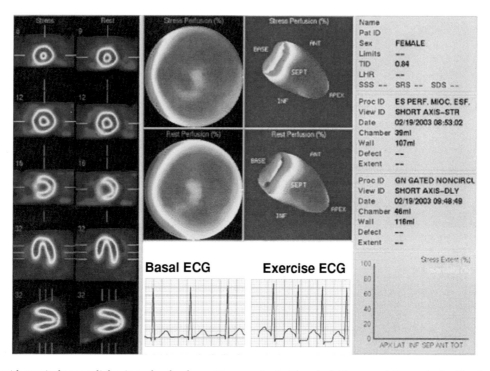

Plate 3 Patient with atypical precordial pain and a clearly positive exercise test (marked ST-segment depression) without pain during the test. The SPECT test was normal (see homogeneous uptake in red), as well as coronary angiography. It is a clear example of a false-positive exercise test.

Clinical Electrocardiography: A Textbook, Fifth Edition. Antoni Bayés de Luna, Miquel Fiol-Sala, Antoni Bayés-Genís, and Adrián Baranchuk.
© 2022 John Wiley & Sons Ltd. Published 2022 by John Wiley & Sons Ltd.

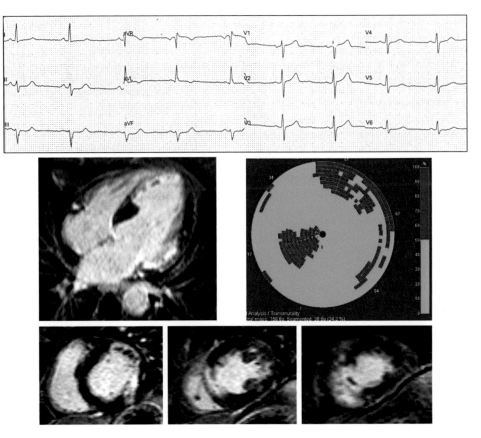

Plate 4 ECG with superoanterior hemiblock (SAH) and mild ST/T abnormalities. The patient presented with various myocardial infarctions–septal, anterior, and lateral–detected by contrast-enhanced cardiovascular magnetic resonance (CE-CMR) that masked each other.

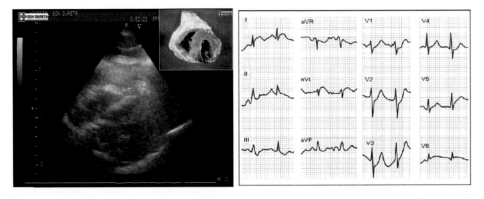

Plate 5 Rupture of inferior wall in a patient after 7 days of inferior myocardial infarction (MI) due to LCX occlusion. See the echocardiography showing large hematic pericardial effusion and the pathological aspect of the rupture. In spite of that, the ECG shows relatively small ECG changes (mild ST segment elevation in I and VL and mirror image of ST segment depression in V1–V3 that remains after a week of MI).

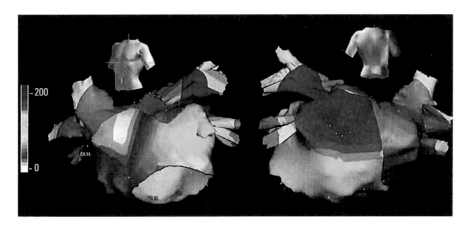

Plate 6 Virtual anatomic rendering of the LA in the other patient with typical biphasic (±) P wave in leads II, III, and aVF suggestive of Bachmann bundle block. Note that early left atrial activation (white) occurs at the high septal wall, as expected for Bachmann bundle conduction. Activation does not progress through the left atrial roof because of the presence of a large zone of low voltage (gray) that diverts activation toward the low septal (orange-yellow) then the low posterior (green) and finally the high posterior (violet) left atrial wall.

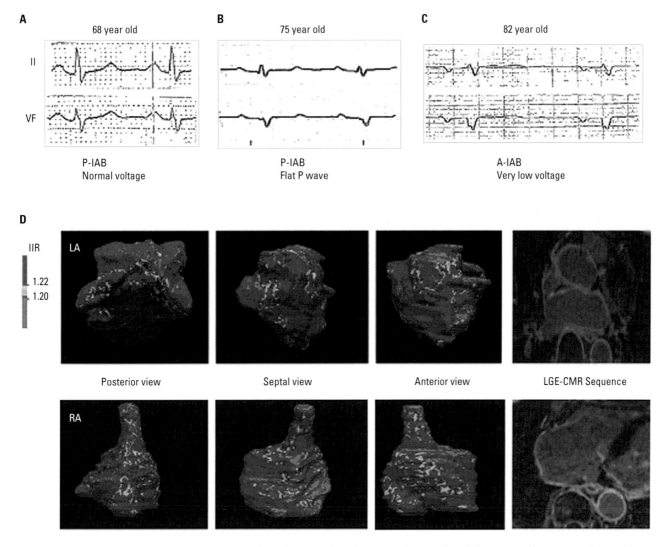

Plate 7 We present the case of an 82-year-old man. Over the years, his ECG pattern has developed from normal P wave to P-IAB and later A-IAB (Panel A) and presents short AF runs during Holter monitoring. Panel A shows that the clear A-IAB pattern with a very low voltage identifies a clear P wave with the biphasic (+) morphology. We obtained a 3D reconstruction of 3T late gadolinium enhancement cardiovascular magnetic resonance (LGE-CMR) (Panel B) showing extensive bi-atrial fibrosis with clear involvement of the upper part of the septum (Bachmann's bundle; arrows). The image intensity ratio between CMR local signal intensity of LGE and mean signal intensity of blood pool depicts the degree of fibrosis in a color scale (dense fibrosis in red).